ESSENTIALS OF FAMILY MEDICINE
SECOND EDITION

ESSENTIALS OF
FAMILY MEDICINE
SECOND EDITION

Editors

PHILIP D. SLOANE, M.D., M.P.H.
Professor
Department of Family Medicine
The University of North Carolina at Chapel Hill
Chapel Hill, North Carolina

LISA M. SLATT, M.Ed.
Lecturer
Department of Family Medicine
The University of North Carolina at Chapel Hill
Chapel Hill, North Carolina

PETER CURTIS, M.D.
Professor
Department of Family Medicine
The University of North Carolina at Chapel Hill
Chapel Hill, North Carolina

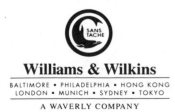

Williams & Wilkins

BALTIMORE • PHILADELPHIA • HONG KONG
LONDON • MUNICH • SYDNEY • TOKYO

A WAVERLY COMPANY

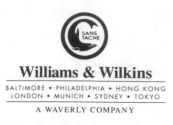

Williams & Wilkins

BALTIMORE • PHILADELPHIA • HONG KONG
LONDON • MUNICH • SYDNEY • TOKYO

A WAVERLY COMPANY

Editor: Timothy S. Satterfield
Managing Editor: Linda S. Napora
Copy Editor: Anne Schwartz
Designer: Wilma Rosenberger
Illustration Planner: Lorraine Wrzosek
Production Coordinator: Anne Stewart Seitz

Copyright © 1993
Williams & Wilkins
428 East Preston Street
Baltimore, Maryland 21202, USA

All rights reserved. This book is protected by copyright. No part of this book may be re-produced in any form or by any means, including photocopying, or utilized by any information storage and retrieval system without written permission from the copyright owner.

Accurate indications, adverse reactions, and dosage schedules for drugs are provided in this book, but it is possible that they may change. The reader is urged to review the package information data of the manufacturers of the medications mentioned.

Printed in the United States of America

First Edition 1988

Library of Congress Cataloging-in-Publication Data

Essentials of family medicine / [edited by] Philip D. Sloane, Lisa M.
   Slatt, Peter Curtis. — 2nd ed.
      p. cm.
   Includes bibliographical reference and index.
   ISBN 0-683-07759-7
      1. Family medicine.   I. Sloane, Philip D.   II. Slatt, Lisa M.
   III. Curtis, Peter, 1937–   .
   [DNLM: 1. Family Practice.   WB 110 E78]
RC46.E88 1993
616—dc20
DNLM/DLC
for Library of Congress   92-48801
                                                                       CIP

93 94 95 96 97
2 3 4 5 6 7 8 9 10

To the many practicing family physicians who generously give of their time and expertise to teach our medical students about the pleasures and challenges of caring for people and their families.

FOREWORD TO THE SECOND EDITION

Teaching medical students about family medicine will increase in importance in the 1990s. Family medicine has matured to become a core discipline in medical education. There is a renewed respect for the role of the generalist physician in health care. By assuming responsibility for the health care of a person, a family, and even a community, the generalist physician is earning increasing appreciation. As society struggles to balance the seemingly incompatible goals of universal access to health care and cost containment in public spending, family medicine is seen as a key to the health care system of the future.

As a textbook, *Essentials of Family Medicine* strikes the perfect balance for medical students on a family medicine clerkship. The size makes it readable in 4 to 6 weeks, the cost is affordable, and the content is just right to give an overview of the field. The second edition is improved by the addition of nine chapters and extensive rewriting or revising of the others. The first section, "Principles of Patient Care in Family Practice," is "must reading" for students who wish to understand the nature and scope of family medicine. Preventive care, the fastest growing area in primary care, is given a much-deserved special recognition in Section II. The bulk of the text is then devoted to a concise but adequate presentation of common health problems. Family medicine is the discipline in which common health problems, whether acute or chronic, are the focus of expertise. Medical students continue to know more than enough about pheochromocytoma, yet wonder if they have adequate information about diagnosing and treating common respiratory infections. This book is a jewel for covering common health problems; this emphasis will be appreciated by students.

Many more medical students need to choose a career in family practice or another primary care field in order to bring about a balanced physician population in America. Students often move away from a career in a generalist discipline because they feel overwhelmed by the breadth of knowledge required. *Essentials of Family Medicine* is reassuring in showing that the scope of family medicine is manageable; the book focuses on the whole person and common health problems. With a textbook that can be read in its entirety during a clerkship, students will gain substantial knowledge of the field. Teachers of family medicine will want to have this book as a ready reference to give to students they may be advising about the field. Even students who will be choosing another specialty will find this book a valuable overview of the general principles and practice of family medicine, a discipline with relevance for all physicians.

J. E. SCHERGER, M.D., M.P.H.
SAN DIEGO, CALIFORNIA

FOREWORD TO THE FIRST EDITION

Family medicine is a young academic discipline, with an evolving literature base. The changing nature of the field, coupled with its inherent breadth, challenges students and residents who seek to learn about patient care in a family practice setting. Although students with previous clinical experiences may have learned some basic aspects of family medicine in other settings, they find many of its principles and practices unique and new when applying them to unselected patients with undifferentiated problems in an ambulatory environment. They thus need a guide that orients and provides an appropriate depth of knowledge for working with patients. This book serves as such a guide.

The book began as a syllabus developed for the Family Medicine Clerkship of the Department of Family Medicine at the University of North Carolina. It provides students assigned to scattered, statewide clinical sites with access to the faculty's collective clinical wisdom. Since every student is expected to read the entire syllabus, it also provides the faculty with a practical core content for the clerkship.

Having been developed for medical students taking clinical clerkships in either family medicine or primary care, this book is particularly well-suited to that purpose. It is most useful when read cover-to-cover as a complement to standard reference textbooks. Medical educators will also find it valuable in teaching other students of primary care, such as students in physician assistant and family nurse practitioner programs. Family practice residents and practicing primary care physicians will also find the book useful, as a practical up-to-date review. Medical educators will find it exemplifies a core clinical curriculum in family medicine.

This book presents a practical, readable approach to patient care in family practice. Patient-centered, it focuses primarily on commonly encountered clinical problems in the office. Key concepts such as family, community, and health economics are discussed in informal, readable language. The reader is also provided with an up-to-date approach to the challenge of organizing and delivering cost-effective preventive services. Process and content approaches to learning are blended, with a consistent emphasis on usable information.

All of the contributors are faculty, research associates, or residents of the Department of Family Medicine of the University of North Carolina. All are clinicians actively involved in both teaching and practice. For our department, it represents a unique synthesis of knowledge and experience. For readers, this book provides a portable composite of the best teaching from a superb faculty.

KENNETH REEB, M.D.
PROFESSOR AND CHAIRMAN

PREFACE

Welcome to Family Medicine. The best way for students to learn about our specialty is in the patient care setting, usually in office practice. This is where *Essentials of Family Medicine* can be most helpful to you. You will quickly discover that primary care is diverse, challenging, and exciting. Time is limited; your preceptor, the office nurses, the technicians and laboratory staff work quickly and efficiently in managing a variety of acute and chronic problems. Everyone has a job and knows what to do. As a member of this health care team, you, too, have a special role to play. Usually this will involve taking a history and performing a focused physical examination, then presenting these data to your preceptor. You might also be asked to develop a differential diagnosis and to suggest a treatment plan. Regardless of your role, you need to approach each patient with an open mind, yet still have a game plan. This book was written to help you develop your game plans for the common medical conditions that patients bring to their family practitioner, and equally important, to help you care for each patient as a whole person.

There are three ways this book can help you during your family medicine rotation. First, it provides an overview of the discipline of outpatient family practice. This includes its distinctive features, such as working with families, integrating psychosocial with biomedical approaches, and combining long-term preventive care with treatment of acute illnesses. But it also includes the clinical "substrate" of the specialty: the spectrum of diseases commonly seen in the family practitioner's office. By reading through the entire book—which can be done with the investment of an hour or two every day—you will, over a 4- to 6-week rotation, acquire a comprehensive introduction to family medicine.

Second, *Essentials of Family Medicine* can serve as a guide for approaching individual patients. Before seeing a new patient, find out the presenting problem from the office nurse or medical assistant. Then, quickly review the appropriate chapter for clues regarding major issues and concerns you should have in mind when you see the patient. The chapters are easily skimmed, and the information presented is concise and practical.

Third, this book can help you put it all together after you have seen the patient, as you prepare to present your findings to your preceptor. Of course, this book should at times be supplemented by more in-depth textbooks and journal articles. Learn to consult those sources, as well, both in the office and when at home.

Family Medicine is a challenging specialty, and an increasingly important one. No other discipline offers such breadth. Few others offer the intimacy that comes from knowing members of an entire family and from serving a community. Practicing medicine is a special privilege; we feel that being a family practitioner is the highest privilege. We hope you can catch a glimpse of these special relationships throughout your rotation. Enjoy!

Our work in developing this book was shared among many individuals. We wish to thank our colleagues from the generalist disciplines who served as content reviewers: Ann Eyler, M.D., Bob Gillette, M.D., Bud Harper, M.D., Don Kollisch, M.D., Jake Lohr, M.D., Alan Spanos, M.D., Dick Walton, M.D., and Sam Weir, M.D. Nina Frankel, our media specialist, provided valuable computer expertise in laying out many of the figures for the new chapters.

Our textbook team at Williams & Wilkins deserves recognition for their amazingly expeditious handling of our manuscript. We wish to acknowledge Timothy Satterfield, our editor; Linda Napora, our managing editor; and Anne Stewart Seitz, our production coordinator.

Pam Carrington, our staff assistant, deserves heaps of praise for her superb organization of countless drafts of 45 chapters, for the speed of her fingers, and for her constant diplomatic encouragement to our authors.

Finally, we wish to thank our colleague, Dick Baker, M.D., for the inspiration and guidance he provided to the first edition of this book. Although his career has taken him to the West Coast, he remains fondly in our thoughts.

P.D.S.
L.M.S.
P.C.

CONTRIBUTORS

MATTHEW ALEXANDER, Ph.D.
Clinical Associate Professor
Department of Family Medicine
Carolinas Medical Center
Charlotte, North Carolina

JOHN J. ALUISE, PH.D.
Clinical Associate Professor
Department of Family Medicine
The University of North Carolina at Chapel Hill
Chapel Hill, North Carolina

GERALDINE D. ANASTASIO, Pharm.D.
Adjunct Associate Professor
Department of Family Medicine
Carolinas Medical Center
Charlotte, North Carolina

VICKIE ATKINSON, M.S.W.
Clinical Instructor
Department of Family Medicine
The University of North Carolina
School of Medicine
Chapel Hill, North Carolina

LEE A. BEATTY, M.D.
Clinical Assistant Professor
Department of Family Medicine
Carolinas Medical Center
Charlotte, North Carolina

SALLI BENEDICT, M.P.H., C.H.E.S.
Social Research Associate
Center for Health Promotion and Disease Prevention
The University of North Carolina at Chapel Hill
Chapel Hill, North Carolina

NATHAN BEROLZHEIMER, M.S.W.
Clinical Associate Professor
Department of Family Medicine
The University of North Carolina at Chapel Hill
Chapel Hill, North Carolina

THOMAS A. CABLE, M.D.
Associate Professor
Moses H. Cone Memorial Hospital
Family Practice Residency
Greensboro, North Carolina

PETER CURTIS, M.D.
Professor
Department of Family Medicine
The University of North Carolina at Chapel Hill
Chapel Hill, North Carolina

JOHN DALLARA, M.D.
Senior Staff Attending
Emergency Department
Duke University Medical Center
Durham, North Carolina

PAUL F. DUNN, M.S.N., F.N.P.
Clinical Assistant Professor
Department of Family Medicine
The University of North Carolina at Chapel Hill
Chapel Hill, North Carolina

K. BERT FIELDS, M.D.
Associate Professor
Moses H. Cone Memorial Hospital
Family Practice Residency
Greensboro, North Carolina

JEFFREY W. FURMAN, M.D.
Clinical Assistant Professor
Department of Family Medicine
The University of North Carolina at Chapel Hill
Chapel Hill, North Carolina

MARTHA GERRITY, M.D., M.P.H.
Clinical Instructor
Department of Internal Medicine
The University of North Carolina at Chapel Hill
Chapel Hill, North Carolina

ADAM O. GOLDSTEIN, M.D.
Clinical Instructor
Department of Family Medicine
The University of North Carolina
Chapel Hill, North Carolina

ROBERT E. GWYTHER, M.D.
Associate Professor
Department of Family Medicine
The University of North Carolina at Chapel Hill
Chapel Hill, North Carolina

WAYNE A. HALE, M.D.
Assistant Professor
Moses H. Cone Memorial Hospital
Family Practice Residency
Greensboro, North Carolina

MARY N. HALL, M.D.
Clinical Assistant Professor
Department of Family Medicine
Carolinas Medical Center
Charlotte, North Carolina

MARGARET R. HELTON, M.D.
Clinical Assistant Professor
Department of Family Medicine
The University of North Carolina at Chapel Hill
Chapel Hill, North Carolina

WILLIAM A. HENSEL, M.D.
Clinical Associate Professor
Moses H. Cone Memorial Hospital
Family Practice Residency
Greensboro, North Carolina

MELISSA M. HICKS, M.D.
Adjunct Instructor
MAHEC Family Practice Residency Program
Asheville, North Carolina

TIMOTHY J. IVES, Pharm.D., M.P.H.
Clinical Associate Professor
Department of Family Medicine
The University of North Carolina at Chapel Hill
Chapel Hill, North Carolina

ALBERTA KOCH-HATTEM, Ph.D.
Private Practice
Chapel Hill, North Carolina

DONALD O. KOLLISCH, M.D.
Assistant Professor
Department of Family Medicine
University of North Carolina at Chapel Hill
Chapel Hill, North Carolina

JOHN P. LANGLOIS, M.D.
Clinical Assistant Professor
MAHEC Family Practice Residency Program
Asheville, North Carolina

BEATRICE B. LEITCH, C.G.N.P.
Certified Gerontological Nurse Practitioner
Department of Family Medicine
Carolinas Medical Center
Charlotte, North Carolina

JOHN M. LITTLE, JR., M.D.
Clinical Associate Professor
Department of Family Medicine
Carolinas Medical Center
Charlotte, North Carolina

KAY LOVELACE, M.P.H.
Doctoral Candidate, Organizational Behavior
Kenan-Flagler Business School
The University of North Carolina at Chapel Hill
Chapel Hill, North Carolina

MARK MARQUARDT, M.D.
Private Practice
Chapel Hill, North Carolina

WILLIAM R. MARSHALL, Ph.D.
Clinical Associate Professor
Moses H. Cone Memorial Hospital
Family Practice Residency
Greensboro, North Carolina

DARLYNE MENSCER, M.D.
Clinical Assistant Professor
Department of Family Medicine
Carolinas Medical Center
Charlotte, North Carolina

MELANIE MINTZER, M.D.
Clinical Assistant Professor
Department of Family Medicine
The University of North Carolina at Chapel Hill
Chapel Hill, North Carolina

WARREN P. NEWTON, M.D.
Assistant Professor
Department of Family Medicine
The University of North Carolina at Chapel Hill
Chapel Hill, North Carolina

PETER J. RIZZOLO, M.D.
Professor
Department of Family Medicine
The University of North Carolina at Chapel Hill
Chapel Hill, North Carolina

JOSEPH R. SHACKELFORD, M.D.
Emeritus Clinical Assistant Professor
Department of Family Practice
The University of North Carolina at Chapel Hill
Chapel Hill, North Carolina

EDWARD J. SHAHADY, M.D.
Professor
Department of Family Medicine
The University of North Carolina at Chapel Hill
Chapel Hill, North Carolina

J. LEWIS SIGMON, JR., M.D.
Clinical Professor
Department of Family Medicine
Carolinas Medical Center
Charlotte, North Carolina

LISA M. SLATT, M.Ed.
Lecturer
Department of Family Medicine
The University of North Carolina at Chapel Hill
Chapel Hill, North Carolina

PHILIP D. SLOANE, M.D.
Professor
Department of Family Medicine
The University of North Carolina at Chapel Hill
Chapel Hill, North Carolina

SIMONE S. SOMMER, M.D.
Clinical Assistant Professor
Moses H. Cone Memorial Hospital
Family Practice Residency
Greensboro, North Carolina

ALAN SPANOS, M.D., M.A.
Adjunct Instructor
Blue Ridge Clinical Associates
Raleigh, North Carolina

CORA D. SPAULDING, M.D.
Clinical Instructor
Department of Family Medicine
University of North Carolina at Chapel Hill
Chapel Hill, North Carolina

GREGORY STRAYHORN, M.D., Ph.D.
Associate Professor
Department of Family Medicine
University of North Carolina at Chapel Hill
Chapel Hill, North Carolina

SUSAN M. THROWER, M.S.W., A.C.S.W.
Clinical Associate Professor
Director of Behavioral Medicine
MAHEC Family Practice Residency Program
Asheville, North Carolina

MICHELE MARSHALL TUTTLE, M.P.H., R.D.
Senior Health Educator
Kaiser Permanente
Mid-Atlantic States Region
Rockville, Maryland

MICHAEL J. TYLER, M.D.
Adjunct Instructor
Chatham Family Physicians
Pittsboro, North Carolina

SAMUEL G. WEIR, M.D.
Instructor
Department of Family Medicine
University of North Carolina at Chapel Hill
Chapel Hill, North Carolina

CONTENTS

Section I

Principles of Patient Care in Family Practice

chapter 1

PRINCIPLES OF FAMILY MEDICINE: AN OVERVIEW

Edward J. Shahady

Most specialties define themselves by exclusion or limitations, such as age, sex, or body organ or system. Family medicine does not limit; it is a specialty of inclusion. The focus in family medicine is on the patient and not on the disease.

When I first heard the above statement, I thought it was somewhat superficial and had little relation to what I did as a physician. As I have practiced family medicine over the past 20 years, I have begun to understand and appreciate the crucial difference between caring for the patient and caring for the disease. If one practices family medicine, then primacy is on the patient and not the disease. Patients can present to the doctor just because they are people. They don't have to have any particular or special type of problem. Family medicine is identified not by one of its principles, but by all of its principles. All of its principles put together make a very powerful and convincing therapeutic agent that can be used to help the patient no matter what the disease, sex, or age.

The six principles of family medicine are continuity, comprehensiveness, coordination, community, prevention, and family (1). Let us now look at each one of the principles and discuss the way we use them. To make this a more realistic and helpful discussion, I will use a case scenario to illustrate these principles.

This patient was presented to me while I was a visiting professor at a hospital in a Latin American country. I had just given a lecture on the principles of family medicine, and there were many doubters in the audience. They did not think these principles could be applied to patient care in a practical fashion. In response, I suggested that we review and discuss a patient currently in the hospi-tal, and I would attempt to apply the principles to this patient.

Case Example

The patient was a 36-year-old woman named Maria who, over the last 3 years, had been hospitalized six times with severe asthma. On the last three admissions, the asthma required intensive care, and she was near death on one occasion. One of the major frustrations of the house officers and attending physician was her lack of compliance with her different medication regimes. She was instructed in the use of appropriate inhalers, theophylline, and oral steroids. When she would return to the hospital, severely ill, it was discovered that she was not taking many of her medications.

I will now go through each of the principles of family medicine, first theoretically and then sharing with you how I applied it to this patient.

SIX PRINCIPLES OF FAMILY MEDICINE

Continuity of Care

Continuity of care involves one physician seeing the patient (and, ideally, the family) over many episodes of illness and during well-person visits. With continuity of care, a trusting, long-term relationship develops between the physician and the patient. If the patient does not trust the physician, the chances for effective care are minimized. Continuity is probably the most important principle of family medicine.

One has to be careful not to confuse continuity of care for a disease with continuity of care for the patient. In family medicine the continuum of care is the patient, the episode is the disease. For other

3

specialties, the continuum is the disease and the episode is the patient. Family physicians are committed to providing care to patients and their families over time. Family physicians use time as a diagnostic and therapeutic tool and are committed to contracting with patients for long-term care. The physician who practices continuity recognizes and accepts a commitment to the patient's future.

Continuity also allows the physician to use his or her personality as a therapeutic tool. The basic idea of using your personality as a therapeutic tool is one espoused by Michael Balint (2), based on his study of English general practitioners. Dr. Balint discovered that the therapeutic agent used most frequently to help patients in general practice in England was the physician's own personality.

Behaviors to Look for and Questions to Ask to Determine Whether Continuity of Care is Being Practiced. Does the physician make use of the patient's past history before making a decision? Does the physician explain the importance of follow-up to the patient? Does the physician negotiate long-term health goals with patients as well as caring for the acute problem? Does there seem to be trust between the doctor and the patient? If we looked at the medical record, would the patient be seen by that physician for the great majority of that care? This is especially important for chronic problems.

Case Discussion

Let's go back to Maria and ask some of these questions to see if continuity has been practiced in her case. Since Maria lives 30 miles from the hospital, her care has been disjointed. Nowhere in her chart could the name of her primary care physician be found. Each time she was transferred from the intensive care unit back to the regular floor her physician changed. The different specialists varied from time to time in caring for her. Also, when I asked if there was any documentation in the chart about long-term health goals being negotiated with the patient, the answer was that no documentation could be found.

Comprehensiveness

Comprehensiveness implies that the patient is viewed not only from a biological perspective but also from a social and psychological one. Thus, the family physician views total individuals in the context of their total needs. The family physician considers all these factors when designing a diagnostic or therapeutic plan. Other health care providers will also be involved in caring for the

patient, but the family physician provides access to this care.

This does not mean to say that the family physician is all things to all people. The family physician can care for 90 to 95% of the problems that are brought to the physician. Kerr White, in a review of patient care in the U.S. and Great Britain, found that in a given month, of 1000 adults living in a community, 750 reported an illness or injury, 500 of which would care for themselves without seeing a physician. Of the 250 that visited a physician, 235 received all their care in the primary care physician's office, 9 were admitted to the hospital, 5 required a consultant, and one was referred to a university medical center (3). Thus, the primary care physician—often the family physician—provides most of the care and serves as the entry into the health care system.

Evaluating for Comprehensiveness of Care. If we wish to see whether comprehensiveness is being practiced, we can look at the chart and see if the problem list and the medication list are current. Is the medical record information accessible so it can be used? Is there evidence that the physician understood what a given complaint meant to the patient? McWhinney has eloquently differentiated this type of patient care and refers to it as "patient-centered care" (4). If patient-centered care is being practiced, there is recognition that the physician and the patient may have separate agendas. For example, patients frequently come in with myths that must be dispelled before adequate care can be rendered. Many times, it is difficult to know what the patient's agenda is unless the doctor has made an effort to discover it.

In addition to considering all the biological issues, the psychosocial and fiscal issues must also be considered. Does the doctor understand the patient's ability to pay for recommended medications or diagnostic tests? Does the physician demonstrate an understanding of the psychosocial issues that are involved with the care of this patient? It is a well-known fact that 50 to 60% of patients on the general medical ward are depressed. How many times do we ask about depression? Are we aware of symptoms of depression in our patients with known medical problems? Even more important, how often do we recognize psychosomatic complaints? For example, we know that chest pain in the primary care setting is more than likely not due to heart disease (in contrast to the cardiologist's office). In fact, if a patient comes to the family physician's office with acute chest pain, the diagnosis is more likely to be panic disorder than coronary artery disease.

Case Discussion

Let's go back and look at our patient to see if comprehensiveness has been practiced. The patient had excellent care for her biological problems. There were pulmonary function tests, blood chemistries, theophylline blood levels, and so on. Nothing was listed in the chart about depressive or anxiety symptomatology. In fact, one physician said, "We first have to rule out organic before we think of psychosocial."

I challenge all physicians to not be afraid to make the double diagnosis. A patient can be depressed and have a cancer. It is important that you recognize and treat both of those. *Physicians have such a tremendous fear of missing the rare and exotic that they, unfortunately, miss the common and especially the psychosocial.*

Coordination of Care

The family physician is the orchestrator of care for the individual patient. The family physician identifies other health care providers and health care resources that are needed to assist in the patient's overall care. These include outside specialists as well as other health care professionals within the family physician's office. It is the family physician's responsibility to guide the patient through the health care system. Family physicians act as patient advocates. I often tell my patients, "It is much better to go through me to your consultant. Then the consultant must not only satisfy you but also satisfy me."

Behaviors to Look for and Questions to Ask to Determine Whether Coordination Is Being Practiced. Does the physician discuss patient care with consultants, either on the telephone or in person? Does the physician occasionally accompany patients to consultant visits? Does the physician arrange for the care of patients during her/his absence? Does the physician teach office staff how to help coordinate care? When there are multiple members of the health team involved, who tells the patient what the diagnosis is?

Case Discussion

Let's see if coordination occurred. A review of both outpatient and inpatient records revealed little communication between the respective physicians. The outpatient physicians were not aware of the number of times Maria was hospitalized or the details of hospitalization. Many of the details of her outpatient care were not known to the inpatient physicians. It was interesting to note that many of the tests ordered in one setting were repeated in another setting, thus increasing the cost of care. This lack of communication and lack of coordination places a tremendous burden on the health care system as well as burden on the patient and her family.

Community

Occupation, culture, and environment are aspects of the community that affect patient care. Knowing which diseases or health problems have the highest incidence in the community influences the diagnoses made by family physicians and helps them make decisions about community education and service. In addition to its role as a diagnostic tool, the community also serves as a therapeutic agent. There are many community resources that the family physician can use to provide optimum patient care.

Behaviors to Look for and Questions to Ask to Determine Whether a Community Orientation Is Present. Does the physician not only know what type of work the patient does but also have knowledge about the workplace that could be important in therapy of the patient and the etiology of his problem? Does the physician use community resources such as Alcoholics Anonymous and the American Heart Association? Does the physician use the knowledge of the frequency of illness in the community when assessing a diagnosis? Is the physician an active participant in the community where she/he practices? Are diagnoses made and treatments given (e.g., adjustment of insulin dosage) based on the patient's lifestyle outside the office or the hospital rather than on behavior inside the hospital?

Case Discussion

Let's now return to Maria and ask whether the principle of community was being practiced in her case. Obviously, in someone with a breathing disorder, the home and work environments may influence the disease. In Maria's case, however, the hospital chart did not discuss her occupation or the condition of her home. Physicians assumed that dust was present in the environment. Visiting nurse and social services had been asked to assess her community and home, but no report was available in the hospital chart.

Prevention

Preventing illness has many aspects. These include recognizing the risk factors of disease, delaying the consequences of chronic disease, and promoting healthy lifestyles. Prevention also means anticipating problems that will affect the emotional health of your patient and the family. An example is the "anniversary reaction," when a person develops symptoms on the anniversary of the death or the loss of a loved one. Family physicians often anticipate and counsel individuals and families about such events.

Prevention is much more than telling people not to smoke, to exercise, and to eat properly. It's also recognizing risk factors for disease, such as family history, and using screening tools to pick up disease in its early phases. Remember that you can prevent further development of a disease like chronic obstructive lung disease or heart disease by reduction of risk factors.

Behaviors to Look for and Questions to Ask to Determine Whether Prevention Is Being Practiced. Are risk factors for the patient identified and displayed in the medical record? Some clinicians believe that preventive information is so important that it should be placed on the problem list. Is there documentation that risk factors have been discussed with the patient? Is there documentation of negotiation with the patient regarding behavioral changes that may be necessary for the patient to practice prevention? Most importantly, is there evidence that the physician is anticipating normative crises that will occur in the family life cycle? For example, certain problems will occur during the first few years of marriage. It is a well-known fact that people tend to exercise less and eat differently after marriage. It's also important to recognize the normative crises that occur with the addition or departure of a child and "the empty nest syndrome." Physicians who are attentive to normative crises along with the other health care risks are practicing the principle of prevention.

Case Discussion

Let's see whether prevention was practiced. Other than discussions regarding the prevention of asthma, no other preventive measures were documented. Pap smears had not been performed for 5 years. Breast self examination had not been taught. No discussion of osteoporosis or the role of diet and exercise in the prevention of heart disease and cancer were documented in the chart. In summary, her care provided a good example of care of the disease rather than care of the patient.

Family

Family physicians regard patients as members of family systems and recognize the influence of illness on families as well as the influence of families on illness. We are trained to work with families as they adjust to predictable life transitions and unexpected illnesses. Family physicians understand the difference between functional and dysfunctional families and use this knowledge both in diagnosing and treating patients.

In defining family, we are really talking about the patient's support system. The patient need not be part of a traditional family, but usually, whether a marriage exists or not, there is some type of support system. A family is defined broadly as those individuals the patient expects to provide support, recognizing that support has a past and a future.

Behaviors to Look for and Questions to Ask to Determine Whether Family-oriented Care Is Being Practiced. Does the medical record contain a genogram, a family circle, a family Apgar and mention of the current family life-cycle stage? The family circle and family Apgar are used in special circumstances, but a genogram and family life cycle stage are necessary in all patient charts. Is the support system of the patient noted? Is there evidence that the physician is evaluating the impact of the illness on the family members and also the influence of the family on the illness?

The genogram is a biological description of the family, and the family circle is an emotional description of the family. (These will be presented in greater detail in Chapter 3.) The Apgar provides a numerical score that assesses degree of family dysfunction, and the life cycle helps the physician understand predictable normative crises that occur in a family. If the physician employs the above instruments and documents their use, the physician is probably using this information to care for the patient.

Case Discussion

Let's now return to our patient Maria. There was no documentation of the use of any of the above instruments. Her family history was stated as "noncontributory." (How many times have you put that in a chart?)

At this point I did a genogram (Fig. 1.1), which shows that Maria and her husband, Jose, have 3 children. Both of Maria's parents are deceased, and her father was an alcoholic. Jose's parents are both living. His mother is demented; his father is an alcoholic. Of the 3 children, two girls and a boy, the boy has asthma and the two girls are healthy. Jose's parents moved in with the family in their two-bedroom home 3 years ago. (When did the asthma increase in severity?)

The genogram has provided a biological description of the family. Although I have discovered a lot about family history and especially the alcoholism, I do not have an emotional description of the family. I now asked Maria to do a family circle. I first showed her a sample family circle of a husband and wife with three children. One of the children was more distant from the family because of emotional difficulties. I asked Maria to draw her circle. Maria quickly got up and went to the blackboard and drew her family circle (see Fig. 1.2). Remember, this is in another language, and I was speaking through an interpreter. As you can see, in one side is Jose (J). Behind Jose are his mother and father. In the other side is Maria (M). Behind her are the three children.

I asked Maria for an interpretation. Maria then told her story. Jose and his father would begin drinking and start to beat the son with asthma. How do you think Maria stops them from beating her son? Of course, Maria begins to wheeze. As we uncovered more of the story, it became evident that every one of Maria's acute attacks had been triggered by drinking in the family. Once Maria began to wheeze and become severely ill, her illness protected her children. It only protected them acutely, however, and she expressed deep worry about what was happening to the children now that she was not there to protect them.

CONCLUSIONS

There are numerous cases of fragmented care, just like Maria's, in the United States. For decades, our medical schools taught almost exclusively the virtues of high-tech, specialized care, and this approach remains overemphasized. Over the past few decades, the principles of family medicine have begun to be recognized, valued, taught, and learned. But there is still work to be done. Our primary health care system needs strengthening, and the principles of family medicine need to be more broadly applied. Just as principles of cardiology, endocrinology, or surgery can be used in other disciplines, the principles of family medicine can be used by other disciplines. As in other specialties, the research, cutting-edge development, teaching, and modeling of the practice of these principles of family medicine are done within the discipline of family medicine.

These principles—continuity of care, comprehensiveness, coordination of care, community, prevention, and family—help me understand and practice my specialty. They form the foundation I use when solving clinical problems. I do not use these principles on every patient at every visit, but over time I use them collectively. The hospitalized, seriously ill patient or the patient with chronic disease usually requires a more extensive use of the principles.

We now have both a theoretical and a pragmatic description of the principles of family medicine. To me these principles are vital to the fiber of family medicine. To some these principles may seem like common sense, but to practice them well is both challenging and satisfying.

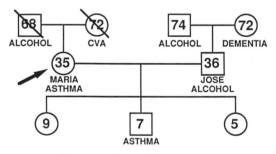

Figure 1.1. Maria's genogram.

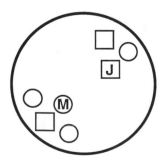

Figure 1.2. Maria's family circle.

REFERENCES
1. Shahady EJ: Teaching the principles of family medicine. *NZ Fam Physician* 10:24–26, 1982.
2. Balint M: *The Doctor, His Patient and the Illness*, rev. ed. New York, International Universities Press, 1964.

3. White KL, Williams F, Greenberg B: Ecology of medical care. *N Engl J Med* 265:885–892, 1961.
4. Levenstein JH, McCracken EC, McWhinney IR, Stewart MA, Brown JB: A model for the doctor-patient interaction in familymedicine. *Fam Pract* 3(1):24–30, 1986.

chapter 2

HUMAN LIFE CYCLE: HEALTH CARE IMPLICATIONS

Philip D. Sloane and Peter Curtis

All family physicians and other generalists should be students of human development. Understanding the challenges of each of life's stages and the impact of life events on physical and psychological health, enhances the physician's ability to help patients. Our understanding of the human life cycle tends to grow with experience, because life itself is the greatest teacher. The sensitive and interested learner can, however, gain insight beyond his or her own life experiences, through relationships with one's own family, by getting to know about the lives and families of colleagues, patients, students, and peers, and through the arts (reading, movies, and television).

The field of human development is large. A variety of scientific disciplines have contributed to our understanding of these areas, with the greatest contributions probably coming from psychology, child development, and gerontology, as well as medicine. Just as there has been a revolution in science and technology, so has our understanding and perspective of human communication, behavior, life-cycle patterns, and relationships changed dramatically since the pioneering work of Freud and his contemporaries. This chapter provides only a brief introduction to some of the issues that are important in family medicine. Chapters 3, 9, 10, 14, 15, 16, and 18 provide additional details.

Case Example

Mrs. A.G. is a 29-year-old who presents with a "cold." She states that she has had four upper respiratory infections in the past 6 months. Mrs. A.G. has been married for 6 years and has two children, aged 2 and 4. A former office assistant, she currently stays home with her children and, to augment the family income, provides day care for three additional children.

Study Question

What life-cycle-related stresses may underlie Mrs. A.G.'s decision to see a physician for a "cold?"

Case Discussion

In primary care encounters, the patient's chief complaint often does not reflect his or her most serious concerns. These underlying issues, the "actual reason for coming" (ARC), often involve problems of development of the individual patient or of relationships between the social and family systems within which the patient lives.

Parents of young children often find that the whole family gets frequent respiratory infections once the children enter day care, preschool, or elementary school. Thus, Mrs. A.G.'s frequent colds may result from her providing day care for other children. The underlying issues would be epidemiological, and the physician can reassure the patient by pointing out that being around more children increases the likelihood of catching a respiratory illness.

On the other hand, it is quite possible that other life stresses underlie Mrs. A.G.'s complaint. A couple that marries and has children in their early twenties is stressed by the simultaneous tasks of establishing themselves economically, developing their relationship as a couple, and parenting young children. In addition, the period between ages 28 and 32 corresponds to the age 30 transition, during which young adults tend to reevaluate and question their lives. These stresses can lead to marital difficulties, explaining why ages 28 to 30 are a time when marital separation and divorce frequently occur. Such life stresses may increase susceptibility to infection by suppressing T cell function; but they can also lead to office visits for minor complaints because the patient needs to talk to someone about her or his life situation. Thus, the family physician who sees Mrs. A.G. for her respiratory complaints should inquire about other concerns and stresses in her life, focusing particularly on marriage and life satisfaction.

HUMAN LIFE CYCLE

In spite of the diversity of individual, ethnic, and cultural factors that our patients bring with them to an office encounter, certain patterns and experiences occur in most normal individuals at specified times during life. On many occasions throughout the life cycle, patients in family practice see their physician for life cycle–related issues (Table 2.1). Family physicians use knowledge of normal development to guide preventive care and health education strategies. They also use this knowledge to

Table 2.1. Common Life-Cycle–related Physician Visits

Life events that generally involve a physician
  Birth
  School and college entrance (preentry examination)
  Marriage (premarital examination)
  International travel (visits for immunizations and prescriptions)
  Acute and chronic illness
  Hospitalization
  Death

Examples of life-cycle-related critical incidents often addressed by the family physician
  Failure to thrive
  Bed-wetting
  School and behavior problems in children
  Puberty/menstruation
  Sexually transmitted disease
  Contraception
  Pregnancy
  Motor vehicle accident
  Divorce
  Unemployment
  Spouse abuse
  Retirement
  Depression
  Death of a spouse
  Adjustment to disability

Life-cycle-related health maintenance visits
  Prenatal care
  Well child visits
  Preschool examinations
  Athletic preparticipation examinations
  Premarital examinations
  Preemployment physicals
  Examinations for life or health insurance
  "Annual" physical examinations
  Visits prior to international travel

anticipate, identify, and treat psychosocial issues and concerns that often underlie patient visits. Finally, family physicians provide counseling on normality during such visits as premarital examinations, physical examinations during puberty, and visits from older patients. Frequently, critical incidents, such as a missed menstrual period, provide an opportunity for counseling about normal behavior and development.

The family physician's view of human development should take into account both physiological and psychosocial factors. Often body changes and psychosocial alterations occur together. For example, adolescent sexual development and the accompanying hormonal alterations are interrelated with major behavioral changes. All these factors affect the individual, the family, and the office visit.

Stress and change are normal. Often, stressful "crises" mark necessary transitions from one stage of life to another. Since patients do not always appreciate connections between life stresses and health problems, the family physician often needs to uncover issues that underlie patient complaints. Knowing the common tasks people face throughout life helps the physician identify questions to ask and issues to explore during an office visit.

Development during Pregnancy

The prenatal period is the most dramatic and rapid period of physiological development. Beginning as a single cell (the fertilized ovum), the fetus grows and differentiates in 40 weeks to a newborn baby. At the same time, the mother experiences a variety of symptoms and body changes. Many of these changes are predictable and normal, yet they can lead to anxiety if not adequately explained to the patient. Furthermore, deviations from normal are sought by the physician, as they can provide clues to problems with the pregnancy. Table 2.2 presents a few developmental milestones that occur during the prenatal period and discusses their medical significance.

Psychosocial changes in the parents accompany development of the growing fetus. Awareness of this developing person proceeds from a vague appreciation to concrete knowledge about moods, activities, and dislikes. The mother, by virtue of being increasingly aware of the fetus' responses and cycles of movement and quiescence, generally bonds more strongly and earlier than the father, who often does not fully conceptualize the baby as a person until birth. In addition, changes generally

Table 2.2. Selected Milestones of Growth and Development during the Prenatal Period and the First Year of Life [a]

Prenatal Period		
Age from Last Menstrual Period	Milestone	Medical Care Implications
3–4 weeks	Implantation occurs	Mild vaginal bleeding can accompany implantation
3–5 weeks	Levels of human chorionic gonadotropin begin to rise	Pregnancy tests become positive; symptoms such as nausea and tiredness are noted
4–12 weeks	Major organs form	Drug and toxin effects on fetus are greatest
15–20 weeks	The fetus grows from about 4.5 inches to 9 inches in length and from about 2.5 ounces to 8 ounces	First detection of fetal movement by the mother (about 15 weeks in multigravidas and 18 weeks in primagravidas) is used to date pregnancy
22 weeks	Due to circulatory changes of pregnancy, maternal blood pressure reaches its lowest point	Failure of blood pressure to go down in midpregnancy suggests later development of preeclampsia
28 weeks	The fetus is about 14 inches long and weighs 2–2.5 pounds	Fathers can usually feel movement by placing a hand on the mother's abdomen; most fetuses born beyond 28 weeks will survive with intensive care
28–40 weeks	Rapid growth of fetus and uterus	Increasing maternal discomfort and fatigue; strong desire to prepare home for new baby ("nesting")

First Year of Life		
Age since Birth	Milestone	Medical Care Implications
0–7 days	Maternal-infant bonding takes place	The hospital and home environment can affect bonding
2–4 weeks	Can follow movement with eyes through 10–20°	Early vision screening can take place
2–3 months	Smiles in response to social stimulation	Parent-infant interaction can be observed
4 months	Turns head toward sounds	Physician can screen for hearing problems
5–8 months	Sits unsupported	Sitting comprises one common measure of gross motor development
12 months	Can recognize own name; says a few words (e.g., "mama")	Development of language skills suggests effective hearing, socialization, and brain development
9–14 months	Learns to walk on own	A period of fussiness often precedes walking; walking itself increases risk of accidental injury or ingestions

[a]Adapted from Sloane PD, Benedict S, Mintzer M: *The Complete Pregnancy Workbook*. Chapel Hill, Algonquin Books, 1986.

occur in a couple's sexual relationship and in their roles during pregnancy and after childbirth. Prenatal visits to the physician's office can help the couple adjust successfully to the pregnancy and prepare for nurturing the new baby.

During prenatal visits, the family physician carries out a variety of activities related to fetal development. Dating of the pregnancy is performed and confirmed based on developmental milestones: uterine size, the date when fetal heart tones are first audible, and the date when fetal movement is first perceived by the mother. Monitoring fetal health involves, in large measure, comparing the rate of uterine growth with that of normal pregnancies. Chapter 14 discusses the conduct of prenatal care in greater detail.

Childhood and Adolescence

As in prenatal care, developmental assessment occupies an important role in the care of children and adolescents. Developmental concerns are frequently brought up by parents; in school-age children they often manifest themselves as problems in the classroom. Thus, awareness of normal behavior at various ages is extremely important for physicians who care for children and adolescents.

Norms have been determined for a variety of developmental parameters. For example, percentiles of height and weight for various ages are represented on a "growth chart." In the physician's office, a child's height and weight (and in infants, head circumference) are plotted at each visit, comparing the individual with other American children. Next, the physician should informally screen for developmental problems by observing the child's interactions and by speaking to the parents. Often, a flow sheet is used to remind the physician of issues that should be addressed at specific ages (see Fig. 2.1 for an example of such a flow sheet). Among the areas that can be assessed are gross motor development, fine motor development, language, socialization, ability to concentrate at a task, skills, interests, and problem behaviors (Table 2.3).

Developmental milestones are commonly recorded in office practice by either nurses or physicians, using the Denver Developmental Test or adaptations of it. Figure 2.1 provides an example of a flow chart for early childhood that includes developmental assessment. Apart from physical growth, the commonest developmental issues in the first year of life involve family bonding, communication, and psychomotor skills. Parents can be helped to understand the development of their child with guidance and information about

• Sleeping patterns;
• Crying and its meaning;
• Feeding practices;
• Physical closeness;
• Talking to the baby;
• Sibling involvement;
• Separation anxiety;
• Involvement of the grandparents.

The toddler stage (12 to 36 months) is a time of great mobility and exploration. Improved coordination also means potential dangers in the house and yard. This, with increasingly skilled communication and development of personality, brings up issues of discipline and reward. Parents have to work hard at this time to agree on disciplinary and control measures as well as to spend "quality time" with their child. Areas of guidance and concern include

• Playing (alone and with others);
• Establishing routines;
• Toilet training;
• Communication;
• Modeling sibling/parent behavior;
• Daycare and baby sitters;
• Eating problems.

Development during preschool and elementary school (ages 4 to 12) involves honing of the skills of reading, communication, socialization, and the enjoyment of learning. Although school teaches these skills in mainly technical terms, parents should be encouraged to model them at home and to participate in the educational process. Many people believe that the current problems with our educational system partly result from the abdication of parents from this role. Areas of guidance and concern for the physician are

• Gender identity;
• Knowing right from wrong;
• Aggressive behavior;
• Participation in family activities;
• Learning disabilities;
• Growth of personality.

Puberty results in a variety of physical changes (e.g., breast development, menses, body hair, lower voice). *Adolescents* are generally self-conscious about such changes yet often have many questions about them. With these physical changes comes the task of developing an independent adult identity with vocational goals; moral, religious, and sexual values; and the ability to set limits based on these goals and values. This task of independence leads to questioning of parental values and advice. Conflicts with parents often arise, yet this is a normal step that is generally resolved with reacceptance of many parental values. Peer relationships are crucial to the adolescent, and conformity with peer values is often accompanied by experimentation with drugs, sexual activity, and alcohol. For greater detail on the physician's approach to adolescent patients, see Chapter 9.

Case Example

Mrs. M., the wife of a young physician newly out of residency and now practicing in a small town, is pregnant. Her son is delivered by her family physician. She is an excellent mother and bonds well with the baby, who is called Richard. Over the next 18 months, however, Richard shows delayed growth (dropping from the 65th to the 20th percentile) as well as slow mental development and sleep problems. Simple nutritional analysis, a urinalysis, and a blood count reveal no abnormality. Apart from the stresses of starting a practice and settling into a new town, Mrs. M. says that everything within the family is fine. The family physician is concerned enough to consider hospitalization for Richard to perform further

Pediatric Flow Sheet   12/91 p.2

Age 6 Months

Date: _____
Exact Age: _____

See growth chart

Tests □
(DPT, Hib) □

Exam
Review intercurrent illnesses □
Complete physical exam

Development
Use the Denver PDQ

pulls up to sitting, no headlag □
passes cube hand to hand? □
sits and takes two cubes? □

Parent-Infant Interaction:

Parent shows deep emotion
through smiles, talking
and touching
Stress level of parent (s)
Childcare responsibilities
Mom vs. Dad's role
Stranger anxiety (babysitter)

Anticipatory
Guidance □

• Compliment parents
• Comment on baby's
development

• Nutrition:

solid foods now

dental care

excessive weight gain?

iron fortification

• Safety:

Crib safety issues
car seats
baby-proofing house
small foods in airway
gate in front of stairs
stoves / heaters
sharp objects in mouth
hot water / no fear

• Sleep:
Patterns

MD _____

Age 9 months

Date: _____
Exact Age: _____

See growth chart □

Tests
check previous visits to assure
TB test □

Exam □
Complete exam/ child undressed
*exam then based on history
Dental exam/ bottle caries
obesity?

Development
Use the Denver PDQ

sits without support □
feeds self crackers □
turns to voice (see PDQ) □
works for toy out of reach □
peek-a-boo □
potty training realities □

Anticipatory
Guidance

• Compliment parents and
address parents needs

• Nutrition:
formula/breastfeeding
4 food groups
iron supplementation
food preferences
flouride

• Safety:
need for car seats
crib safety
ipecac availability
babysitting rules
electrical outlets
caustic chemical access

• Sleep:
Review child and parent
rest patterns

• Family issues:

another baby wanted?

talk about finances

MD _____

Age 1 Year

Date: _____
Exact Age: _____

See growth chart □

Tests
(no immunizations)
Hct
Hearing
Vision (acuity)
Exam
full PE □

Development
Use the Denver PDQ

imitates speech sounds □
bangs two objects together □
walks holding furniture □
stands momentarily? □
address potty training myths □

Parent-Infant Interaction:
"acceptable" child behaviors
mobility, curiosity
separation anxiety

Anticipatory
Guidance

• Compliment parents
• Nutrition: □
4 food groups
still drinking bottle?
non-nutritious foods
iron supplementation
need for whole milk

• Safety:
need for car seats
crib safety
ipecac availability
babysitting rules
electrical outlets
caustic chemical access

• Sleep:
Normal Variability
• Parent skills:
taking a temperature
signs of infection
head injuries
Heimleich maneuver tng.

MD _____

Age 18 Months

Date: _____
Exact Age: _____

Measure
See growth chart □

Tests
(15 mo. get MMR, Hib#4) □
(18 mo. DPT, OPV) □

Exam
Based on history □

Development
Use the Denver PDQ

Walking with ease □
Indicates wants without cry □
Can throw a ball you roll to him/her □
Drinks from cup □
Imitates housework? □
Stacks objects? □

Parent-Infant Interaction:

Parent expectations of behavior
Discipline types
Management of separation
Toilet training?
Sleep issues
Need for positive self-image
development

Anticipatory
Guidance

• Compliment parents
• Comment on baby's
development

• Nutrition:
Fluoride supplementation
sugar containing snacks
patterns/ habits
food likes and dislikes

• Safety:
car seats
Do not leave child
unattended
Cigarettes/hot liquids
Unbreakable/ swallow-
proof toys
Babysitter rules

• Sleep:
Patterns
nightmares? / soothing

MD _____

Figure 2.1. Sample page from a pediatric flow sheet, illustrating the incorporation of developmental screening and education about developmental issues into routine office procedure.

Table 2.3. Developmental Areas to Assess during Pediatric Examinations

Domains	Examples (Appropriateness Varies Depending on Age)
Gross motor skills	Rolling over, walking, running, playing sports
Fine motor skills	Stacking blocks, writing
Language	Receptive, spoken, written
Socialization	To family, to peers, to children and adults of varying ages
Ability to concentrate at a task	Length of time the child is able to stick with a specific task, such as reading a book or practicing tennis
Habits	Toilet training, eating patterns
Interests	Dolls, sports, favorite television programs, peers of the opposite sex
Problem behaviors	Fighting with siblings, withdrawal, refusal to go to school, truancy, drug or alcohol use

studies in a controlled environment, but before this occurs, Dr. M. is arrested for driving while intoxicated and damaging property. When asked about this incident, Mrs. M. breaks down and sadly admits that her husband has been a heavy drinker for several years and sometimes physically abuses her when drunk. Dr. M. eventually enters and successfully completes a residential treatment program, and at the same time Richard begins to regain weight and developmental milestones.

Case Discussion

Most problems of growth and development in the United States are not due to disease but to psychosocial problems such as stress, abuse, and lack of affection, which then lead to malnutrition. Whether primary (as in many third world countries) or secondary (as generally occurs in this country), malnutrition causes serious and often irreversible effects on motor and intellectual skills. No social class or occupation is immune from family, social, or substance-abuse problems, which have profound effects on growth and behavior. The physician's understanding of all stages of the life cycle, both norms and problems, is vital in helping patients and their families.

Early and Middle Adulthood

Early studies of human development concentrated on childhood. It has become increasingly evident, however, that change and evolution continue throughout adulthood and tend to occur in predictable stages (see Table 2.4). Among the most influential studies of adult development have been those of Levinson, which were popularized by Sheehy. Levinson views adulthood as a series of stable periods separated by developmental transitions ("crises"), during which the adult more actively reevaluates his or her life, and during which both conflict and change are more likely to occur. According to Levinson, these developmental transitions occur because no life course can fulfill all aspects of one's self (dreams, goals, aspirations).

Choosing a path in life involves rejecting other possibilities. Transitions occur when one reexamines one's life, considering alternatives again.

Adolescence ends with the *early adult transition* (ages 17 to 22). During this period the individual must modify or terminate relationships with parents and institutions (such as a religious denomination) and begin exploring the adult world. As part of the same process, the individual makes choices regarding occupation, love relationships, peer relationships, values, and lifestyle. This transition is followed by *early adulthood* (ages 22 to 28), during which the individual builds upon these initial choices.

The next life transition, the *age 30 transition*, occurs between ages 28 and 33. During this period, the individual actively reexamines his or her life. The result is either change (e.g., a new career direction, marriage, or divorce) or a smoother transition, where the individual continues to build on the foundation of the 20s. This transition is followed by the period of *settling down*, where one focuses on establishing a place in society. Often, the individual concentrates on "making it" in his or her chosen career, and the couple focuses on child rearing. Individuals who do not have children develop expanded committments to work, friendships, community, and/or leisure—whatever is most central to their values.

Between ages 33 and 45 for women, and between 37 and 45 for men, the next life transition occurs. This *midlife crisis* involves a confrontation with the limitations of one's life, in terms of both physiological aging and the likelihood that one will not achieve all of one's life goals. For both men and women, this crisis is usually brought on by an accumulation of signs of aging—everything from being passed over for a promotion at work in favor of a younger person, to developing an injury that prevents participation in a favorite sport, to

Table 2.4. Life Stages and Transitions of Adulthood

Age	Life stage	Transition	Tasks/Goals/Issues
17–22		Early adult transition	Establishment of independence from family of origin; definition of personal goals and values; career choice; initial attempts at partnering
22–29	Early adulthood		Career launched; early parenting or deferral of reproduction; balancing individual/partnership roles; mentorship relationships can be helpful
28–33		Age-30 transition	Reevaluation of initial choices results in either change or recommitment; lack of perceived choice can lead to depression, alcoholism, marital conflict/abuse
30–39	Settling down		Establishing a place in society through career success, child rearing, or community involvement; nurturance and accommodation to partner and children
33–45		Midlife crisis	Major reassessment of life goals and activities; initial adjustment to early signs of aging; career changes and marital crises are common; completion of childbearing
45–60	Middle adulthood		Movement from career establishment to mentoring others; facilitation of children in obtaining independence; reestablishment of marriage as a dyad after children leave home; interest in individual expression and growth is common among women who have been full-time mothers
47–55		Age-50 transition	Reevaluation of lives; may be particularly traumatic in individuals who changed little during their 30s and 40s; menopause triggers physiological and psychological responses in women
58–68		Transition of the early 60s	Anticipation of retirement; greater identification with family and culture; acceptance of one's life
65–79	Young old ("golden years")		High levels of life satisfaction; maintaining connections with family; grandparenting; ability to pursue deferred leisure and community interests; concern about maintaining health and independence
70–84		Transition to physical dependency	Chronic illness and disability reduce independence; help needed with activities of daily living; dependency increases reliance on family
75+	Older-old ("frail elderly")		Deaths of partner(s), friends, and siblings; acceptance of physical changes; physical discomfort; considerable social contact with and support from health care providers; desire to share life experiences with others, especially younger persons; readiness for death

the death of a parent. Whatever the precipitating factors, men and women at this stage of life reassess their lives, often feeling that they have very little time in which to achieve their goals. An intense questioning of commitments, goals, and activities results, often leading to disruptions in career and in personal relationships. This is a time during which career changes often occur, marriages may end, and depression is frequent. For women without children, a major component of the midlife crisis is a sense of urgency about becoming a parent, since the incidence of Down's syndrome, infertility, and pregnancy risk rises more steeply after age 35.

After committing themselves to (new or old) choices, individuals in their mid-40s enter *middle adulthood*. For some, this period is a time of great satisfaction. For others, who have not been able to satisfactorily resolve their conflicts, this is a time of resignation and/or depression. Moving into their late 40s and their 50s, adults who have heretofore climbed a career ladder move more into mentoring others' careers, often through rising in managerial positions. Among couples who have had children, men tend to exhibit greater interest in family and personal relationships, women in individual expression and growth.

Middle adulthood continues until around age 60. During this period, however, a milder transition occurs, the *age 50 transition*, during which adults again reevaluate their lives. For individuals who changed little during their 40s, this period may be a time of intense crisis and change. For women, this transition is heralded by a major physiological event, *menopause*. The hormonal and body changes of menopause occur over several years, with the average age of cessation of menses being 48. Many women who are heading into menopause view it as the end of their attractiveness, usefulness, and sexuality. Most women successfully overcome these concerns, however, and after menopause find themselves feeling freer to do things for themselves and satisfied with their lives.

Another transition tends to occur in the early 60s, as the adult anticipates retirement and old age. The task of this stage of development is for the individual to accept the course of his or her life and to give up striving for personal accomplishment in favor of feeling a part of the larger flow of family, cultural, and historical events. This acceptance of one's life also leads to acceptance of the inevitability of death. The result of successfully completing this transition is that the "proximity of death" adds "value to living" (1).

Older Adulthood

Successful aging involves a combination of good health and adjustment to losses. Goals and interests continue to be important to good health throughout older age. Studies of "successful" adults in their 70s and 80s indicate that they tend to have routines that involve regular exercise and social contacts, productive activity through a profession or community service, and good nutrition. Examples of physical losses to which older adults must often accommodate are reduced hearing, diminished stamina, and disability due to disease. Social losses vary from retirement (loss of the role of worker and its consequent sense of productivity to society), to relocation (e.g., movement from a house to an apartment), to the loss of friends and siblings through death.

For family physicians, it is useful to differentiate between the younger-old, who are similar to adults of late middle age, and the older-old, who tend to have significant physical impairment. For many, the *young-old* period truly represents the "golden years." Studies indicate that adults aged 65 to 74 express greater life satisfaction than adults at any other age. This occurs because, in spite of physical limitations, the young-old possess the ability to do many things they enjoy, are freed of many financial and time pressures, and recognize

(at last) that they must live each day for its own sake rather than looking to the future. Health concerns are common in this age group, and the young-old tend to be highly responsive to health education and physician recommendations.

The *transition to physical dependency* characterizes entry into the *older-old*. There is considerable age variation, but by 80 most individuals have begun this transition. Couples frequently approach age 75 in good health, but few reach age 80 without at least one member suffering death or major disability. For the older-old, important issues are maintaining independence and mending relationships with family members. Disability, being a burden to family, and dying (rather than death) are major concerns; being with family and sharing life experiences with others are particularly valued. Physicians and other health care workers occupy a prominent role in the lives of the older-old, since health issues are a central focus of this stage of life. Physician openness about disability, death, and dying is generally welcomed.

LIFE STAGES AND THE IMPACT OF CHRONIC ILLNESS

Chronic and disabling illness generally has a major influence on the individual at any stage of life. Successful accomplishment of developmental tasks is often hampered, making it difficult for the individual to progress to the next life stage. The result can include depression, anxiety, overdependency, and significant family stress.

Illness in children has profound effects on both the individual and the family. The child often regresses to earlier patterns of dependency, and the parents go through a difficult and often prolonged period of adjustment. Changes in life goals and roles of many family members are often necessary to accommodate a chronic disease such as sickle cell anemia, cystic fibrosis, or autism. Depression, marital breakup, alcoholism, and illness among other family members can result.

At later stages of life, illness is particularly difficult to cope with if it occurs during a period of transition. For example, acute myocardial infarctions in men occur, not uncommonly, during a midlife crisis or an intense age-50 transition. The illness itself, with its temporary dependency on others and its threat of death or permanent disability, precipitates further self-doubt. Patient reactions vary. One may deny the seriousness of the problem, becoming noncompliant with medications, insisting on early resumption of vigorous physical exercise, and making sexual advances on nursing staff. Another may enter a severe depression, paralyzed by fear that resumption of activity will precipitate another heart attack.

In caring for all patients, the family physician should be sensitive to life stages and the potential problems that can result from them. When caring for a patient with a serious illness, the physician should evaluate the impact of the illness on the individual and the family. Part of that process involves understanding the needs and developmental tasks of the patient and of each family member who is affected by that illness. Often, counseling around these issues can help the patient and family adjust more successfully to the illness.

OPPORTUNITY IN EACH PATIENT ENCOUNTER

The developmental stages of life are often accompanied by visits to the family physician's office. Frequently, the patient's stated reason for the visit is to complete a required examination form, such as a premarital certificate or a vaccination certificate. At other times the patient will have a physical problem but also have concerns related to life transitions. Knowing, identifying, and managing developmentally linked health and psychosocial issues is one of the key aspects of health maintenance. These issues are expanded upon in the second section of this text. Whatever the focus of the patient encounter, the family physician can provide more sensitive and appropriate care if he or she approaches the patient within a perspective of human development.

REFERENCES

1. Comfort A: *A Good Age*. New York, Crown Publishers, 1976.

SUGGESTED READINGS

Erikson, EH: The eight stages of man. In Erikson EH: *Childhood and Society*. New York, WW Norton, 1963.

A classic paper. Enumerates and describes 8 stages of personal development. Ericsonian theory provides the basis for much of child and adult development theory.

Fraiberg SH: *The Magic Years*. New York, Charles Scribner's Sons, 1959.

A delightful, readable book about the growth and development of preschool children. Emphasizes Freudian principles.

Levinson DJ, Darrow CN, Edward B. Klein, Levinson MH, McKee B: *The Seasons of a Man's Life*. New York, Ballantine Books, 1978.

One of the first scholarly studies of adult development, this book traces the lives of primarily professional men between ages 20 and 60.

Sheehy G: *Passages*. New York, EP Dutton, 1976.

A popular book on adult development, which builds upon the work of Levinson.

chapter 3

WORKING WITH FAMILIES

Nathan Berolzheimer, Susan M. Thrower, and Alberta Koch-Hattem

The family physician has a unique role in combining psychosocial with biomedical expertise in clinical practice. Because family practice is not limited by age, gender, or type of problem, the family physician can provide lifelong care to the entire family. Understanding individual and family development enables the physician to help with psychological as well as medical problems. This chapter introduces family systems theory and some of its key applications to patient care in family practice.

BIOPSYCHOSOCIAL MODEL

The biopsychosocial model of health care, proposed by Dr. George Engel in 1977, extended the traditional biomedical model to include the personal and social context in which health and illness occur. Psychosocial influences on illness include the patient's intellectual, physical, and emotional capacities; life experiences; and role as a member of a nuclear and extended family, a school or occupational group, and a community.

Psychosocial factors both affect, and are affected by, disease processes. To successfully treat their patients, physicians must pay attention to these issues.

Psychosocial factors in the patient's life often play a key role in treatment compliance. For example, effective treatment for the diabetic patient involves changing family habits and altering patient attitudes as well as attending to traditional medical interventions.

DEFINING THE FAMILY

The family is a basic building block in most cultures. It provides support and nurturance, guidance and socialization of children, affiliation and identity, legitimization of sexual relationships and

procreation, and social and economic organization. Urbanization and two world wars have brought changes in family structure and function in the United States. The traditional family structure, or nuclear family (husband, wife, and offspring living in the same household) with strong ties to extended kin (those beyond the nuclear family, related by blood or marriage), is no longer the dominant family form in our society. In fact, only 26% of all households in the United States in 1991 consisted of a married couple with children living together.

Detailed information about the number of people who are geographically distant from the social support of their extended families is not as available. The 1990 census provides examples of increasingly common family forms (1):

- Adults living alone—25% of all households (a 75% increase in numbers from 1970);
- Unmarried cohabiting couples—3 million households had cohabiting couples (this represents an increase of 2.5 million since 1970);
- Children living with one parent—25% of all children under 18 (16.6 million children, which is a 5% increase from 1980).

Due to economic changes in the 1980s, experts anticipate a decline in the more expensive lifestyle, namely the number of adults living alone. Divorce rates are projected to decline, in part because of the cost of maintaining two separate households. Other predictions for the 1990s include increases in the following: (*a*) the number of women in the work force, particularly mothers of preschool children; (*b*) the number of children living in single-parent families, most of whom live with women at or below the poverty level; (*c*) the

19

diversity of living arrangements, including adult children returning home and aging parents living with children; (*d*) home-based jobs; and (*e*) the geriatric population. These changes will affect primary health care. Stress-related problems, such as depression, psychosomatic illnesses, chemical dependence, and physical violence may increase in frequency. As a result, family physicians will require greater diagnostic and treatment skills for successful management of such family-related problems.

Treating patients whose lifestyle differs from yours requires personal assessment of your own values and expectations about families. For example, an upper-middle-class background may make it difficult for you to view poverty-related health problems as beyond the control of a patient. Similarly, you may experience value conflicts when asked to provide obstetric care to an adolescent who wants to raise her child.

The diversity of families precludes agreement about a definition. The following, however, is general enough to apply to most families: A family is a group of individuals sharing emotional bonds, a history, and a future. This group accomplishes special functions or tasks, including provision for security and survival, socialization of children, and support for individual growth.

The family physician's knowledge of the patient's family benefits the routine care of individuals. Knowledge of parents' separation is important when treating functional abdominal pain in a child. Knowledge of family functioning also helps the physician anticipate future problems for the patient. For example, a physician, aware of marital distress accompanied by a financial inability to dissolve the marriage, should be alerted to symptoms of distress like alcohol abuse, depression, child behavior problems, and family violence.

FAMILY LIFE CYCLE

Just as knowledge of normal development (see Chapter 2) is important for individual care, you need to understand how a family develops: how it begins; the stages through which it passes; and how it ends. The sequential stages of a family occur concomitantly with the developmental stages of the individual members. Developmental stages involve both normal and expected transitions, such as developing a commitment to a new family at the time of marriage, adjusting to living with three at the birth of the first child, and adapting to aging parents. Families also experience unanticipated crises, such as early death, divorce, birth defects, onset of a chronic illness, or unemployment. Table 3.1 describes individual and family life cycle stages, with corresponding health issues.

Understanding the family life cycle helps family physicians distinguish between normal and abnormal development, anticipating potential problems in order to provide education and counseling. For example, a physician might make a house call to a young couple immediately following the birth of their first child, anticipating the anxiety of caring for a newborn. This physician might also see the new family in the office a month after the birth, to assess the couple's ability to maintain their relationship while also adjusting to being parents.

HOW FAMILIES WORK: FAMILY SYSTEMS THEORY

Conceptualizing the family as a system helps in patient care. Viewing individuals as acting and reacting members of a social group resembles the interactions that occur within organ systems. Three concepts help explain how family members work together: (*a*) the interdependence of members within the family system, (*b*) system boundaries, and (*c*) triangulation.

Table 3.1. Traditional Family Life-Cycle Stages and Their Relationship to the Individual Life Cycle

Age	Family Life Cycle	Individual Life Cycle
18–21	Between families: the unattached young adult	Late adolescence, early adulthood, age-30 transition
22–27	New couple: the joining of families through marriage	Early adulthood, age-30 transition, settling down
28–39	The family with young children	Early adulthood, age-30 transition, settling down
35–49	The family with adolescents	Settling down, midlife crisis, middle adulthood
40–59	Launching children and moving on	Middle adulthood, age-50 transition
45–60	Empty nest	Middle adulthood, age-50 transition
60+	The family in later life	Transition to the early 60s, young-old, transition to physical dependency, older-old

Interdependence

The characteristics of a family are related to, but distinct from, the characteristics of individual members. The old adage "the whole is greater that the sum of its parts" applies to families. The interaction between individual members is what distinguishes the family group from its members.

Family interactions tend to be repetitive, thus forming patterns. Families develop rules that support these patterns. These generally unstated rules may prohibit members from questioning the status quo, thereby sustaining interaction patterns. For example, in families where females cannot express anger openly, a family rule often prohibits them from questioning or even commenting on the rule. Psychophysiological changes, such as hyperacidity or tension headaches, or behavioral changes, such as increased drinking or lowered libido, may result. When patterns and rules resist change, the situation is called *entrenched*. Even when circumstances require new patterns of interaction, change is extremely difficult.

Interaction patterns and their accompanying rules are more clearly observed by someone outside the family than by family members themselves. Thus, the family physician or family therapist can promote change by identifying a family's malfunctioning patterns and changing the rules that support those patterns. By viewing the family and change this way, the blame for family problems is ascribed to family interactions, rather than the behavior of any given family member. It is not the parents' fault that the children do not obey them; rather, interactions within the family allow for the disobedience. Successful attempts at changing families are directed toward these interactions and the rules that sustain them, rather than toward individual family members.

Boundaries

Boundaries define what is considered acceptable and unacceptable behavior for family members. Boundaries, like fences, demarcate the family as a whole from outsiders, or demarcate subgroups within the family such as adults and children. Boundaries define acceptable interactions from both within and without. Like all interactions, those defined by boundaries become patterned, are governed by rules, and are often difficult to change. For example, many families have a rule that only married couples can sleep in the same room while visiting. In that case, marriage defines the boundary between certain acceptable and unacceptable behaviors.

Boundaries differ in their permeability; in other words, how easily the fence can be crossed. When boundaries are excessively permeable, the distinctions among individual members may become blurred, and the family becomes *enmeshed*. These families are characterized by intense relationships in which conflict is not expressed or resolved, and relationships outside the family are viewed as threatening. Members of enmeshed families often have difficulty developing independent identities, engaging in activities outside the family, and leaving the family. Family members tend to speak for one another when the family meets with health professionals, and they present a happy facade no matter how bad the situation. In working with these families, the physician may find herself inadvertently speaking for others and accepting the facade. Feelings often reverberate through these families; if father had a rough day at work, everyone in the family is upset.

When boundaries around individuals are extremely impermeable, the family and its members are isolated from one another and from the world. Members of such *disengaged* families cannot present a consensual picture of the entire family, nor can they accurately relay information from the physician back to the family. Disengaged families are recognizable if after a family conference, there are many unanswered questions and unaddressed issues or if there is strong family unwillingness to accept outside help. In working with disengaged families, the family physician may feel rejected and angry, as if members just do not care. In this case, family rules prevent outsiders from crossing the boundaries into the family; it is not a personal rejection.

Healthy families balance closeness and distance. Members are caring, yet they recognize, accept, and foster each others' individuality. Boundaries are sufficiently permeable to allow for development. Boundaries also need to be well defined to allow for the support, nurturance and protection of family members.

Triangulation

Triangulation is of particular importance to family physicians because of the potential role they are recruited to play. Most interactions within a family involve two persons. When stress occurs within this dyad, there is a natural tendency to involve a third person. The role for this triangulated person is to "rescue" the pair. Stress is thus reduced, and the focus of the problem is shifted from the dyad to the rescuer.

Since triangulation appears to reduce stress, family members repeat it, hoping to maintain control and to keep the family together. Triangles are ineffective coping mechanisms, because the stress is not permanently reduced, and they usually have detrimental consequences.

School phobia in a child whose parents are having marital problems is a common example. In that case, the child "comes to the rescue" of a distressed parental relationship by refusing to go to school. This shifts attention from the parents' own distress to their child's fear of leaving home. Another example occurs in the alcoholic family, when the child develops a depression or psychosomatic problems. To make an accurate diagnosis in these cases, the physician must identify the triangles in the family. By focusing on the source of stress, the dyad, and blocking the triangulation of the third person, the family physician can help the family cope more effectively with the true problem and thus prevent recurring symptoms.

The family physician can be enrolled as the object of triangulation. This happens whenever a patient colludes with the physician to treat a single family member for a family problem. The physician who treats school phobia or depression without attending to the underlying problems is, in fact, colluding with one patient and is thus being triangulated into the distressed patient-family dyad.

FAMILY PHYSICIAN'S INVOLVEMENT WITH THE FAMILY

While thorough patient care involves attention to the individual's social context, physicians vary in their involvement with families. The physician, concerned about the family's role in the patient's illness and treatment, may occasionally include the family in the patient's care. Meeting with a patient's entire family on a regular or even intermittent basis is time-consuming and logistically difficult, however. Not meeting with the entire family entails few consequences if the patient's problem is minor. At other times, as when a diabetic patient fails to mention dietary prescriptions to his wife, the consequences may be more serious.

Each family physician must decide how involved to be with families. The five types of involvement, ranging from minimal to maximum, are illustrated in Table 3.2. New family medicine interns usually operate at level 1 or 2, while more seasoned family physicians operate at level 3 or 4. Level 5 requires specialized training in family therapy, and only a handful of family physicians practice at this level. Involvement with families at level 4 is called primary care counseling. After completing a family medicine residency, graduates should be functioning at this level.

Table 3.2. Five Levels of Physician Involvement with Families[a]

Level	Physician Perspective	Physician Behavior
1. Minimal emphasis on family	Communicating with families is useful for practical and medical/legal reasons	Meet with families to discuss only biomedical issues
2. Medical information and advice	Family useful in diagnosis and treatment decisions, a general openness to engage families	Meet with families to facilitate diagnosis and treatment decisions, identify gross family dysfunction, and refer
3. Feelings and support	Feelings and mutual impact of patient, family, and physician important to diagnosis and treatment	Meet with families to emphatically discuss stresses and members' emotional reactions to illness and treatment
4. Assessment and intervention	Family systems, dynamics, and family development important to diagnosis and treatment	Meet with families and help them alter roles and interactions to more effectively cope with stress, illness, and treatment
5. Family therapy	Family dynamics and patient health sustain one another; the patterns that allow this can be changed	Meet regularly with families to change underlying dynamics and rules that are associated with the development and maintenance of physical and mental illness

[a]Adapted from Doherty WJ, Baird MA: Developmental levels in family-centered medical care. *Fam Med* 18:153–156, 1986.

Primary Care Family Counseling

Primary care family counseling is illustrated in the case of a patient who has recently suffered a myocardial infarction. Several months after discharge, the physician meets with the whole family to assess how they have coped. If the family is overstressed, members other than the patient may exhibit emotional or physical problems. For example, a previously healthy young child may have more frequent colds, stomach problems, or croup. An older child may become withdrawn, or school performance and peer relationships may decline. Adolescents may act out with antisocial behavior, such as truancy, reckless driving, or shoplifting. The spouse may become depressed, lose interest in sex, or become preoccupied with multiple new activities outside the family. Most likely, a family will display only one or two of these symptoms. Without a family conference, the family physician will not know of the problem until it is mentioned during an office visit or someone contacts the physician by telephone to express concern.

Primary care family counseling requires assessing the developmental level of each family member, the roles each plays in the family, and the patterns of interactions. When using primary care counseling, the physician's goal is to help families alter their roles and interactions to cope more effectively with stress, including illness-related stress. The physician must be competent in diagnosing psychopathology in an individual or dysfunction within the family that requires treatment by a mental health professional. While providing primary care family counseling, the physician maintains interest in the treatment of the patient's biomedical disorder.

When to Meet Families

A family conference is useful when a serious and/or chronic illness is diagnosed or when a patient has been hospitalized. Family conferences are also useful when a patient has a recurring problem, whatever its severity. Examples include recurrent back, chest, or abdominal pain; depression; gastrointestinal complaints; and coughs, colds, and flu. Here family conferences are used to educate the members about diagnoses and treatment plans, to obtain information, to facilitate diagnosis and adherence to treatment, and to assess family functioning.

Unexplained, recurrent symptoms may indicate previously unobserved problems, such as alcohol abuse, for which early detection and treatment can prevent morbidity and mortality. Additional indicators for a family conference include these six clinical "red flags" of family dysfunction: recurrent atypical migraine headaches that have responded poorly to treatment; long-term depression; chronic anxiety accompanied by vague symptoms with no biomedical diagnosis; chronic fatigue; pediatric problems that have not subsided with parental education; and chronic insomnia, which may be indicative of underlying depression or chemical dependency (2). While these conditions require medical intervention, family conferences can identify family problems that contribute to the illness. Relieving these problems, either through primary care counseling or referral to a family therapist, may then result in decreased symptomatology.

The Family and Chronic Illness

Chronic illness, unlike acute conditions, increasingly permeates all aspects of the patient's and family's life. Because of this, the physician's involvement with the patient and the family broadens. Frequently, the relationship of the physician to the patient and the family becomes more important. In coping with chronic illness, the patient and family must adapt to the medical team, the treatment, the uncertainties of crises and death, changes in the patient's appearance and behavior, and the patient's dependence on the family for care. The family's adaptation is influenced by, and influences, the patient and the illness.

When family resources are sufficient to overcome family stresses, successful adaptation occurs. Resources include finances to cover the costs incurred during illness, the psychological strengths of family members, the social supports available to family members, and positive family dynamics. If the family has insufficient resources to manage the stresses or if resources become depleted during the course of the illness, other symptoms of distress may appear in either the patient or other family members. Issues of family stress theory and family adaptation to a chronic illness may be summarized as follows:

Family stresses
Patient's chronic illness
Work
School
Legal issues
Illnesses

Mental disorders
Substance abuse
Births
Marriages
Deaths
Life cycle changes
Marital and family distress

Resources for coping with stress
Finances to cover costs incurred
   (savings, insurance)
Maturity and emotional stability
Support from Friends
Extended family members
Community
Medical team
Flexible family organization
Family closeness
Family members sense of identity
Communication skills
Problem-solving skills
Belief that family can cope with the chronic
   illness

Outcomes
When stress is greater than resources
Family distress
Biomedical and psychosocial symptoms appar-
   ently unrelated to the chronic illness
New stresses that appear unrelated to the
   chronic illness

When resources are greater than stress
Nondistressed family
All biomedical and psychosocial symptoms
   predictable given the nature of the chronic
   illness
All new stresses are predictable given family
   life-cycle changes.

Family in Crisis

When the magnitude of a stress far outweighs a family's resources, problem solving will fail. The family in crisis is characterized by:

• Chaotic or disorganized behavior and thinking;
• Impeded day-to-day functioning;
• Loss of confidence;
• A sense of reduced options and less autonomy.

Family crises include prolonged unemployment, death, divorce, unwanted pregnancy, and battering of women.

Violence against women (battering and sexual assault) is an example of a family crisis in which the family physician can intervene. The incidence of husband-to-wife violence ranges from 11 to 21% of couples. Estimates of lifetime prevalence for sexual violence against women are as high as 30% (3). These women seek health care frequently, usually through emergency room visits for acute injuries and office visits for abdominal pain, headaches, irritable bowel syndrome, depression, and anxiety. The incidence of physical assault of women by their partners within the past year was 22% in one family practice setting (4).

A victim of violence should be treated with sensitivity, support, and directness. These women are usually ashamed and are, therefore, unlikely to volunteer information. The family physician must sensitively inquire about and assess the extent of the problem, the degree of psychological and physical injury, and the degree of present danger. Intervention should include treating the acute problems, expressing support, and outlining concrete suggestions aimed at helping the woman (and children) gain structure and stability. Referrals to social service agencies, women's centers, rape crisis and domestic violence centers, and the legal system are all possibilities, depending on the severity of the problem and the personal and family resources available (3).

ASSESSMENT OF FAMILIES

The family circle and the family genogram are two family assessment tools. The *family circle* provides information about current relationships and may require updating from time to time, particularly during life transitions or when serious illness occurs. The *genogram* provides a diagram of the family structure, medical history, family relationships, and critical events, enabling the clinician to grasp a large amount of information quickly. Genograms change less frequently than relationships depicted in the family circle.

The family circle illustrates the patient's perspective of the family and his or her social network. The patient is asked to draw a large circle and then add smaller circles or other symbols to represent himself or herself and personally important people. Each symbol represents a specific person and should be identified. The location of the symbols within the circle represents the patient's perception of that relationship. For example, symbols that touch show the closeness of the patient to that person. Reassure the patient that there are no right or wrong family circles. The physician can leave the room while the patient draws the circle. The patient then explains the family circle to the family physician, who asks clarifying questions. These may cover relationships, such as who has the decision-making power (hierarchy), roles and communication patterns, personal boundaries, life cycle changes, alliances, and openness. Table 3.3 illustrates such questions. When time permits, the physician can also ask questions, such as, How would you like to change your circle? What are some ideas of how you would accomplish this? If one person in the circle changes, what effects will this have on others?

The family circle can be used to review family information during the course of routine care or it can be a springboard for goal setting in dysfunctional families, with follow-up appointments for primary care counseling. For example, conducting a family circle is helpful in counseling couples during routine prenatal care. To do so, arrange a 45-minute visit with the couple. Explain the family circle and ask each parent-to-be to complete a personal family circle without consulting the other. Then use each person's family circle to open up a discussion of expectations of parenting, to explore the dynamics of their relationship, and to talk about the anticipated role of the new grandparents. Often, in this setting, you will uncover important clinical information, such as a previous marriage or a lack of communication about differing expectations of parenthood.

The family genogram is a three-generational family tree. The family physician or other health professional usually draws the genogram, asking the patient very specific questions to obtain the required information. You can start with the youngest generation and diagram upward, or start with the middle generation and move downward and upward. Sibling order is significant, and is drawn with the oldest on the left and the youngest on the right. Include both spouses' families. Record ages or birth dates of family members and significant family events (including dates), such as marriages, deaths, divorces, and retirement. Noting anniversaries is important because they often contribute to stress. Genogram symbols are shown in Figure 3.1.

The family circle can be administered to patients in 15 to 30 minutes, while the genogram can be completed in 5 to 15 minutes; the differences in length depend on the physician's time and interest and the depth to which questions are asked and answered. In addition, the genogram can become a working document in the medical record, added to as the physician gathers more information over time.

The family circle and the family genogram, used together or separately, help define the patient-family relationship for both the family physician and the patient, and expands the data base for that patient. The family circle provides one member's perception of relationships within the family. Discussion of it can be emotional for the patient and thus can help draw out feelings. The genogram, a more cognitive tool, provides a historical, factual, and structural family diagram. It is a convenient and comprehensive "ready-reference" for the physician/health care team. Both the family circle and the family genogram are adaptable to the needs and constraints of office practice. Each yields single-page, graphic results that can fit easily into the medical record.

Case Example

J.B. is a 29-year-old man who was hospitalized with thrombophlebitis complicated by his obesity and de-

Table 3.3. Questions to Ask as Part of a Family Circle Assessment

Relationship Issue	Questions
Life cycle	Does this configuration represent any changes?
Support	Who do you go to for support?
Support, boundaries	Size of family; how many are included, excluded? sheer quantity
Boundaries	What does the distance between people mean? What does being inside or outside the circle mean?
Openness	Who is missing? Any family ghosts? Losses (death, separation, divorce, etc.)
Hierarchy	Who are in power positions and control positions? Which are central or peripheral positions? What are the sizes of symbols?
Triangles, alliances	What do the groupings mean?
Interdependence, communication	Who is connected to whom?

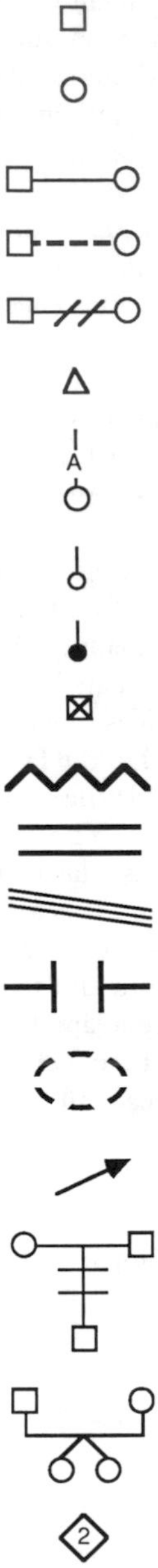

Common Symbols

□	Male
○	Female
□——○	Marriage
□----○	Unmarried Relationship
□—//—○	Divorce
△	Pregnancy
⊙ (A)	Adopted
○ (induced)	Induced Abortion
●	Spontaneous Abortion
⊠	Death
∿∿∿	Conflictual Relationship
═══	Supportive Relationship
≋	Overclose Relationship
⊣├	Relationship Cut off
(⸰ ⸰)	Members of one household
↗	Identified patient
○═╤═□	In household- living away (school, jail, etc.)
□ ○ ⋀	Twins
◇②	2 offspring, gender unknown

Common Abbreviations

ALC	Alcohol
ANX	Anxiety
ARTH	Arthritis
B DEFECT	Birth defects
BLOOD D	Blood disorder
CA	Cancer
↓HEAR	Deafness
DEP	Depression
DM	Diabetes mellitus
GI, GB, HEP	GI tract, gall bladder and liver disease
GLAUC	Glaucoma
HRT DIS	Heart disease
↑CHOL	Hypercholesterolemia
↑BP	Hypertension
REN DIS	Kidney disease
M RETARD	Mental retardation
MI	Myocardial infarction
RF	Rheumatic fever
CONVUL	Seizures
CVA	Stroke
LUES	Syphilis
↑THY↓	Thyroid, hyper or hypo activity

Figure 3.1. Symbols and abbreviations commonly used in genograms.

pression. His family circle and family genogram appear in Figures 3.2 and 3.3.

In his family circle (Fig. 3.2), J.B. placed himself in the center of an older persons' network, close to and between both parents. The family system and neighborhood group appear to have J.B. surrounded. In fact, J.B. described his family as supportive, but also talked of feeling "trapped." The picture exemplifies family enmeshment, as well as J.B.'s triangulation into his parents' marriage.

J.B.'s age is important in his family's life cycle. If J.B. were an infant or a young school-age child, his current position in the family circle would be of much less concern. But J.B. and his parents appear to be stuck in the task of launching a young adult, which usually occurs in late teens. Concurrently, J.B. is unable to progress toward intimacy with peers, which is characteristic of young adulthood. Eating disorders, including anorexia nervosa, bulimia, and obesity, often appear when an enmeshed family faces the task of launching children. Eating disorders appear to solve the family conflicts around launching, as the patient effectively regresses to the status of a young child who requires eating to be monitored by parents and therefore cannot leave the family. The parents' marriage, which by now has become dependent on

the triangulation, therefore remains unthreatened by the adult child leaving home or developing an intimate peer relationship that might supercede family loyalty.

The genogram drawn by J.B.'s physician during a hospital interview (Fig. 3.3) also emphasizes J.B.'s triangulation into his parents' marriage and the family's enmeshment. These family dynamics have developed over a long period of time, with numerous contributing events. Such events might include the parents' families of origin, the father's long-term blindness and recent myocardial infarction, and J.B.'s only child status. Effective treatment of J.B's obesity and depression must account for his current family dynamics and some aspects of the family history.

CONCLUSIONS

By using the knowledge of individual and family development and the skills of interviewing, assessment, and brief counseling, the family physician can have a tremendous postive influence on the health of patients. Understanding the patient's life, through the family history (genogram) and support networks (family circle), greatly increases the physician's healing potential.

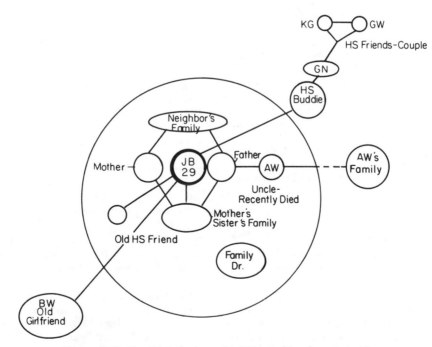

Figure 3.2. Family circle drawn by 29-year-old male patient, J.B.

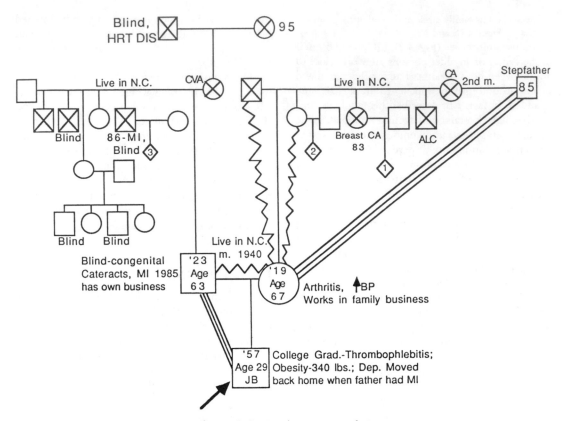

Figure 3.3. Family genogram of J.B.

REFERENCES

1. Ahlburg DA, DeVita CJ: New realities of the American Family, *Popul Bull* 47(2), 1992.
2. Doherty WJ, Baird MA: *Family Therapy and Family Medicine: Toward the Primary Care of Families.* New York, Guilford Press, 1983, pp 46–49.
3. Burge SK: Violence Against Women As A Health Care Issue. *Fam Med*, 21(5):368–373, 1989.
4. Hamberge LK, Saundes DG, Harvey M: Prevalance of domestic violence in community practice and rate of physician inquiry. *Fam Med* 24(4):256–260, 1992.

SUGGESTED READINGS

Carter EA, McGoldrick M: *The Family Life Cycle: A Framework for Family Therapy*. New York, Gardner Press, 1980.

This book examines normative family development and the ways in which American families currently deviate from this model. The writers then use developmental theory to predict problems that families encounter as they move through their life cycles and ways professional intervention might help them.

Doherty WJ, Baird MA: Developmental levels in family-centered medical care. *Fam Med* 18:153–156, 1986.

This article presents a model of the stages physicians commonly go through to develop comfort and skill working with families. It is simple to use their model to set goals for oneself and to monitor one's progress in achieving the long-range goal of working effectively with families each step along the way.

Doherty WJ, Baird MA: *Family Therapy and Family Medicine: Toward the Primary Care of Families*. New York, Guilford Press, 1983, pp 46–49.

This book looks at ways in which physicians and therapists can collaborate to treat the patient and the family. Family problems that are commonly seen by family physicians, clues that these problems exist, and methods of helping families are described.

Minuchin S, Rosman BL, Baker L: *Psychosomatic Families: Anorexia Nervosa in Context*. Cambridge, Harvard University Press, 1978.

This book discusses the development of psychosomatic problems in families, specifically the problem of anorexia nervosa. A clinical model is stated, research findings are cited, and case examples are generously utilized.

Schleifer SJ, Keller SE, Camerino M, Thornton JC, Stein M: Suppression of lymphocyte stimulation following bereavement. *JAMA* 250:374–377, 1983.

This is an example of a well-designed research study. Additionally, it tests the biopsychosocial model and presents very convincing results from a biomedical perspective.

chapter 4

ROLE OF THE COMMUNITY
Salli Benedict

Most American medical students have little opportunity to focus on the community. This is inevitable, since most student training takes place in tertiary care centers. Yet family physicians do not share this isolation from the patient's community. On the contrary, one key to the family physician's effectiveness is understanding the interaction between a patient's complaints and his or her community environment. Drawing from their knowledge of the community, effective family physicians use community resources to help care for their patients. Thus, a thorough understanding of the community's role in health and medicine is critical to primary medical care.

DEFINING A COMMUNITY

A community is a group of people who have some things in common and who recognize and are aware of that commonality. Using this very broad definition, a community can take different forms. Geographic communities can consist of a neighborhood, a town, or a group of farms spread over many miles. A community of identity is a group of people who have common interests based on similar professions, cultures, background, religion, or recreational activities.

As traditional neighborhoods and extended families have become less of a focal point in people's lives, these communities of identity have assumed greater importance. Individuals may belong to several communities at one time, and membership tends to be fluid. A community-oriented family physician must be aware of the multiple sources of support that are available to patients and be prepared to use them to provide optimal care.

ROLE OF SOCIAL SUPPORT IN HEALTH

The family, friends, co-workers, and neighbors that make up an individual's social support network contribute to his or her life satisfaction and medical health. A strong relationship between social support and individual health was demonstrated by Berkman and Syme (1), who followed 4725 subjects for 9 years. Berkman and Syme found that people with a supportive social environment tended to be healthier and to deal better with stress than those who lacked a supportive environment.

There are practical implications from this and similar studies for family physicians. For example, the family physician can use knowledge of the patient's current support networks to mobilize home care for a patient who has recently been released from the hospital. Where such support is lacking, the physician can help individuals and families establish support networks and can refer to appropriate community resources when needed.

One method of assessing the strength of an individual's support network is the Social Network Inventory (Fig. 4.1). Ideally, this inventory will be completed at an initial patient visit, updated periodically, and placed in the medical record, thus providing a ready source of valuable information for the physician.

Another way to conceptualize how a person's social support affects health is illustrated in Figure 4.2. People respond to similar stressful events, such as the death of a loved one, accidents, or illness, in different ways. In addition, many societal stresses, such as racism, sexism, and poverty, simply cannot be eliminated or reduced by individuals. It is important, therefore, to recognize individual variations in reacting to stress, and to strengthen individuals' social supports, coping skills, and competence when appropriate. When lack of social support is a problem for a patient, the family physician is in a position to teach the patient about the health benefits of social support and to prescribe activities that strengthen

Please indicate below:

Person	Does this person exist in your life? Check One		IF YES: Is this person living now? Check one		How supportive is this person for you in general? Not at all supportive / Extremely supportive 1 2 3 4 5 6 7 8 9 10
	Yes	No	Yes	No	
Mother					
Father					
Spouse					
Live-in Partner					
Children					
Sister					
Brother					
Grandmother					
Grandfather					
Other Family					
Supervisor (Job)					
Fellow Workers					
Neighbors					
Female Friends					
Male Friends					
Minister/priest					
Religious Faith					
Doctor					
Agency Helper					
Clubs or Orgs.					
Community you live in					
Pet:					
Other:					

Figure 4.1. Social Network Inventory.

social and community ties. For example, a patient who tends to be isolated (such as many elderly, handicapped, recently widowed, or divorced individuals) can be referred to programs or community agencies that will increase social contacts. In doing so, you should help the individual identify an activity that pursues an interest or goal and that enhances the development of meaningful social relationships. Recreation programs, classes, self-help groups, and hot lunch programs in community centers are examples. Encouraging retired persons to volunteer has the extra benefit of adding time and energy to the community's volunteer pool.

Other health professionals in the practice can help people who share a common problem contact each other, and can provide the impetus for starting support groups around these problems. For example, if the practice has a number of families with young children who have recently moved to the practice community, the nurse might suggest that they contact each other to form a cooperative babysitting or play group. This not only provides a service (child care) for the parents, but also puts them in contact with others with similar interests. Many long-term friendships among parents and children are formed this way. The only time commitments on the nurse's part involve putting up a notice in the waiting room asking for interested families to sign up with their phone number, and recruiting one family as coordinators of the first meeting.

COMMUNITY RESOURCES

Community resources cover a wide range of services, agencies, and support groups that provide help to members of the community. Table 4.1 lists categories of community resources.

Appropriate use of the many available community resources is an important skill in family practice. Using these resources requires the physician to be aware of what is available in the community. While it is unrealistic to expect a family physician to learn everything about all of the resources in the community, it is the physician's responsibility to know those resources that are commonly used and to know how to find new resources when they are needed. Unfortunately, many patients who would benefit from services offered by local agencies never receive these services because physicians either are not aware that they exist or fail to make a referral.

Lists and descriptions of community resources can be found in several ways. Many communities publish resource guides compiled by local agencies or the Chamber of Commerce. If a guide does not exist for a community, consult your local telephone directory, since many have special sections listing resources. The Department of Social Services, nurses, social workers, home health agency

$$\text{An Individual's Illness} = \frac{\text{Stresses} + \text{Physical Vulnerability}}{\text{Social Support Systems} + \text{Coping Skills}}$$

Figure 4.2. The importance of social support in preventing illness.

Table 4.1. Some Categories of Community Resources

Type	Examples
Health agencies	Health departments, hospitals, clinics, home health
Emergency services	Fire, rescue, police
Women's services	Women's resource centers, rape crisis centers, services for abused women and children
Municipal and government services	Recreation, transportation, library
Recreation and exercise program and facilities	Schools, YMCA, YWCA, public pools and parks
Services for special population groups	Handicapped, elderly, teens, and children
Alcohol and drug-related services	Help lines, Alcoholics Anonymous
Mental health and counseling services	Stress management, mental health centers, therapists
Dispute settlement center, legal aid services	
Hotlines/clearinghouses for information	
Self-help and support groups	Alzheimer's support group, Parents Without Partners
Family planning, pregnancy, abortion-related services	Planned Parenthood, abortion clinics
Employment counseling, job referrals, vocational rehabilitation	
Hospice	
Churches, clubs, civic organizations	
Social services	Aid to dependent children, nutrition services, emergency aid
Weight management resources	Weight Watchers, Overeaters Anonymous

workers, and other physicians are also valuable sources of information. As you identify agencies and resources, you should create a card catalogue or file of the ones you use most often. Categories to be aware of are listed in Table 4.1.

Frequently used community agencies are home health agencies, departments on aging, Meals on Wheels, Department of Social Services, and Hospice. Often, these agencies work together to coordinate services for homebound patients. With the advent of diagnostic-related groups (DRGs), home health agencies are caring for sicker patients than they have in the past. It therefore is more crucial to coordinate services. Intravenous therapy, dressing changes, and physical therapy are now routinely performed by home health professionals. Typically, patients served by these agencies do not have sufficient friends, neighbors, and family available to meet all their needs.

Advantages of the appropriate use of community resources include:

• Support for home care, which can shorten hospitalization or prevent institutionalization. For example, an elderly invalid may be able to live at home with the help of home health nurses, homemaker aides, and a Meals on Wheels program. Hospice and the home-birth movement are examples of grassroots movements that provide alternatives to hospitalization.
• Avoidance of unnecessary technological intervention, a result of keeping people out of hospitals.
• Cost containment, since community resources often employ nonphysician health professionals or volunteers, and have sliding fees or government grants that help them provide lower cost services.
• Strengthening of community and social networks.
• Provision of services, such as education and counseling, which are too time-consuming for physicians to provide. Preventive and promotive services offered by health departments are examples.

Working together, agencies in a community can enhance the level of well-being of the entire community. The following is an example of how an agency's referrals can have a significant influence on the health and well-being of an individual and her family.

Case Example: Cook with Osteoarthritis

Judy Leigh is a 35-year-old woman with two children who has been Dr. Jones' patient for 3 years. She makes her living as a cook, spending 8 hours a day on her feet, often lifting heavy pots and pans. Fifteen years ago she suffered a broken hip in a car accident and spent several weeks in traction. She was told by her surgeon at that time that she would probably develop osteoarthritis of the hip. Since the accident she has remained very active: biking, camping, and backpacking are family pursuits. For the past few years she has complained increasingly of hip and leg discomfort, and Dr. Jones has recommended physical therapy and exercises. X-ray films over the years have shown gradual deterioration of her hip, and when she presents to Dr. Jones with severe pain after a weekend backpacking trip, x-ray films are ordered again. A consulting orthopaedic specialist recommends surgical hip replacement. Dr. Jones suggests that Judy stop working on her feet and tells her to plan for surgery as soon as possible.

Neither Judy nor her husband, who is also a cook, has health insurance. Their combined income is approximately $18,000 a year, and although this income is below the poverty level for a family of four, they are ineligible for any substantial help from Medicaid. The family depends on Judy's income, but she has no training that will allow her to find a desk job.

Since the family has determined that Medicaid is not an option, other resources for both financial and medical help must be explored. Dr. Jones begins by calling the Department of Social Services to discuss options for direct financial aid but discovers that the family's income is too high for welfare. Next, she looks into the policies of the state hospital for providing services for indigent persons. Dr. Jones is referred to the hospital's social worker who, when she has heard about Judy's case, refers her to the State Division of Vocational Rehabilitation. With the aid of a rehabilitation counselor, Judy enrolls in a 2-year computer programming program at a local technical school, starting classes after the hip replacement surgery. Income supplementation while she is recuperating from the surgery will be made available to the family.

Case Discussion

Each state has a Division of Vocational Rehabilitation. The services offered differ from state to state, but the intent is federally mandated: to provide counseling, guidance, and appropriate services for vocational rehabilitation and to obtain and maintain employment restoration. In Judy Leigh's case, these services will include financing her surgery and paying for her reeducation. A vocational rehabilitation counselor will counsel, evaluate, and prescribe appropriate services for each individual.

Solutions to complicated cases are not always this simple, but it is important to realize that sources for substantial help exist in the community. Although in this case one agency handled all aspects of the family's problems, often more than one agency must be called upon, and the services coordinated. Families who are not sophisticated in the use of the health care system need help; when their medical providers are unaware of referral sources the consequences can be severe. Thus, a physician should always consider how the patient and family will cope with the consequences of their medical problems after they leave the office.

Self-Help Groups

An important category of resources, but one that is often overlooked by medical professionals for referrals, is self-help groups. Self-help groups are organized around an issue or problem such as single parenting, arthritis, or alcohol abuse. They seek to help members through information sharing, discussion of coping strategies, and mutual support. They usually do not involve health professionals except as resources or occasionally as initiators of the group. Leadership comes from the group, and the knowledge base tends to be experiential. The self-help movement is a strong and growing social movement. It fosters self-responsibility and returns a sense of control and power to people, seeking to convert people with problems into resources for solving those problems.

These groups are powerful tools for helping individuals cope with problems, and they are much less expensive than professional services. They can be alternatives to traditional medical care, but they can also be effective additions to medical management, which family physicians should encourage their patients to utilize. Family physicians can help patients with similar problems contact each other to start groups or can refer patients to groups already in progress. Physicians can act as resources for groups or actually start groups by putting announcements in their offices or the local media. Not only do these self-help groups benefit patients by giving them coping skills and knowledge about problems, they also act as support groups.

COMMUNITY-ORIENTED PRIMARY CARE: THE PHYSICIAN AS ACTIVIST FOR COMMUNITY HEALTH

The philosophy of family medicine recognizes three levels of care: the individual, the family, and the community (see Fig. 4.3). Caring for the community uses the public health skills of community diagnosis, epidemiology, biostatistics, and health education. Community-related influences (environmental, socioeconomic, educational, and cultural) exert a far greater influence on health and disease than specific medical interventions, so primary health care providers must take these community aspects into account to be effective.

Historically, physicians have been seen as community leaders, and they are often held in high regard as public figures. Many would also argue that the physician, as a health professional, has a responsibility to assume a public role in health issues. There are many ways physicians can participate in the health of their communities:

- Serving as advisors or board members for community agencies and schools.
- Taking an active role in community politics, which may include speaking at town council meetings on health issues and writing letters to newspapers as advocates for political candidates or issues that support community health.
- Monitoring and reporting changes in community health, including reporting communicable diseases (see Fig. 4.4) and raising public awareness about health hazards.
- Working as change agents with grass roots organizations which work for better health conditions.

Traditionally, public health has focused on groups of people and the communities in which they live, while medicine has concerned itself with the care of individuals. Family practice has extended medicine's traditional focus to the care of families.

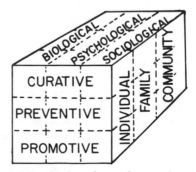

Figure 4.3. The three faces of comprehensive care. (Adapted from: Medalie, JH(ed): *Family Medicine Principles and Applications*, Baltimore, Williams & Wilkins, 1978, p 18.)

☐ Surveillance Form Required   **PLEASE ENTER CODE NUMBER IN BLOCK ON FRONT OF CARD**   *Add'l Information Required on Other Side of Card

GENERAL

REPORT WITHIN 24 HOURS		REPORT WITHIN 7 DAYS			
ANTHRAX	3	ACQUIRED IMMUNO-DEFICIENCY SYN. (AIDS)	1	MALARIA	21
BOTULISM	10			MENINGITIS, PNEUMOCOCCAL	*25
CAMPYLOBACTER INFEC.	50	AMEBIASIS	2	MENINGITIS, VIRAL	*26
CHOLERA	6	BLASTOMYCOSIS	4	MUMPS	28
DIPHTHERIA	8	BRUCELLOSIS	5	PSITTACOSIS	31
FOOD BORNE DISEASE:		DENGUE	7	Q FEVER	32
C. perfringens	11	ENCEPHALITIS	*9	REYE'S SYNDROME	34
STAPHYLOCOCCAL	12	HEPATITIS B CARRIER	115	ROCKY MOUNTAIN SPOTTED FEVER	35
OTHER or UNKNOWN	*13	HEPATITIS, NON-A, NON-B	16	RUBELLA CONGENITAL SYNDROME	37
HEMOPHILUS INFLUENZAE, INVASIVE DISEASE	*23	HIV INFECTION 101 (1. Repeatedly reactive EIA and positive confirmatory test; or 2. Positive virus culture)			
HEPATITIS A	14			TETANUS	40
HEPATITIS B, ACUTE	15			TOXIC SHOCK SYNDROME	41
MEASLES (rubeola)	22			TRICHINOSIS	42
MENINGOCOCCAL DISEASE	*27	KAWASAKI SYNDROME	52	TYPHOID CARRIER	144
PLAGUE	29	LEGIONELLOSIS	18	TYPHUS, EPIDEMIC (louse-borne)	46
POLIO, PARALYTIC	30	LEPROSY	19		
RABIES, HUMAN	33	LEPTOSPIROSIS	20	YELLOW FEVER	48
RUBELLA	36	LYME DISEASE	51		
SALMONELLOSIS	*38				
SHIGELLOSIS	39				
TULAREMIA	43				
TYPHOID, ACUTE	44				
WHOOPING COUGH	47				

TUBERCULOSIS — REPORT WITHIN 24 HOURS

Bacteriologic Status

	POS. SMEAR	POS. CULTURE	NEGATIVE	NOT DONE OR UNKNOWN
PULMONARY	601	701	801	901
PLEURAL	602	702	802	902
LYMPHATIC	603	703	803	903
BONE-JOINT	604	704	804	904
G.U.	605	705	805	905
MILIARY	606	706	806	906
MENINGEAL	607	707	807	907
PERITONEAL	608	708	808	908
OTHER*	609	709	809	909

SEXUALLY TRANS. DISEASES — REPORT WITHIN 24 HOURS

SYPHILIS

PRIMARY (lesion present)	211
SECONDARY (skin or mucosal lesions)	221
EARLY LATENT (<1 yr)	232
LATE LATENT (>1 yr)	243
LATE	*277
CONGENITAL	284
EPIDEMIOLOGIC Rx	200

GONORRHEA

GENITO-URINARY (non-PID)	*315
GONOCOCCAL PID	*385
OPHTHALMIA NEONATORUM	345
OTHER	*395
EPIDEMIOLOGIC Rx	300
CHANCROID	466
GRANULOMA INGUINALE	576

OTHER STD — REPORT WITHIN 7 DAYS

CHLAMYDIA Lab confirmed EPIDEMIOLOGIC RX	*500 515	Other than lab-confirmed CHLAMYDIA: NONGONOCOCCAL URETHRITIS (NGU) EPIDEMIOLOGIC RX	365 400
LYMPHOGRANULOMA VENEREUM	686		

Figure 4.4. Communicable disease reporting: a vital community service. Physicians are required to report communicable diseases to local health departments, which then forward the information to the federal Centers for Disease Control in Atlanta. Each state provides reporting cards for physicians to use.

A growing body of theory, practice, and research, based on the writings of Sydney Kark (2), Fitzhugh Mullen (3), Paul Nutting (4), and others, seeks to incorporate public health principles into primary care theory and practice. Community-oriented primary care (COPC), as this combination is called, emphasizes applying community survey, community diagnosis, and community-wide treatment efforts to the physician's community of practice.

Unfortunately, it has proven difficult for most family practices to move from acceptance of the abstract theory of COPC to actually practicing it. One successful example is the primary care clinic and training program for residents at Montefiore Medical Center, the Bronx, NY. The curriculum of the Montefiore Medical Center Residency Program includes a major focus on COPC. Residents are exposed to people working in the community during their orientation, analyze their practice profile in light of the community profile, and work on their own social medicine projects. One successful project involved an apartment building directly across from the Montefiore Family Health Center. A successful rent strike and housing court suit, visible improvements in the landlord's upkeep of the building, and improved communication between the buildings' Hispanic and Cambodian tenants were results. Other projects initiated by the family practice residents at Montefiore are a lead poisoning prevention program, a middle-aged Hispanic women's self-help and mutual aid network, and an outreach team for health care for the homeless in the Bronx. Three special circumstances have made Montefiore a natural place for training in COPC: the practice clinic is a federally funded community health center serving a defined inner-city area; the residency program has always focused on serving that community; and the faculty are committed to the concept.

In office practice, COPC involves taking advantage of available opportunities for influencing community health. In your practice community, census and other data are readily available to learn what the major community health problems are and where they occur. If, for example, hypertension and alcoholism are especially prevalent, then your practice should set goals to bring about community change, working through schools, churches, and public officials. In this way the practice seeks to actively monitor and shape community health.

Case Example: A Community-Oriented Family Physician

To see how a family physician lives and works in a community, we will follow Dr. Ann Paxton during a typical day. Dr. Paxton is a young family physician in a small town in North Carolina. Many people in town work at one of the two factories, a textile mill and a small furniture factory. She moved to town when she joined the growing family practice center in town 4 years ago, upon completing her residency in family medicine.

Dr. Paxton leaves for work 30 minutes early to make a house call. The patient, Mary Kraft, is a 70-year-old alcoholic who lives alone and whose many visits to Dr. Paxton over the past 4 years have been alcohol-related. Recently, however, she was admitted to the local hospital for tests, and was found to have colon cancer. When she returned home, she began drinking again and was not eating well or taking her medications. Dr. Paxton made arrangements for Meals on Wheels to deliver hot lunches and arranged for a home health nurse to visit three times a week to monitor her chemotherapy. Using these community resources has allowed Mary to stay at home and has ensured that she receives the care she needs. Dr. Paxton's visit is brief, but Mary is doing well and responds positively to a suggestion that she attend an Alcoholics Anonymous meeting.

During the day of seeing patients, Dr. Paxton has several other opportunities to call upon community resources. On hospital rounds, she arranges home phototherapy on a newborn with jaundice due to ABO incompatibility. In the office, she refers one patient to the mental health center, advises a mother about a child care information service, and encourages the spouse of an elderly patient to attend a support group for families of patients with Alzheimer's disease.

Dr. Paxton serves on the board of directors of the local mental health center and is active in an environmental group. Dr. Paxton feels that it has been crucial for her to live in the town where she practices, so she can be familiar with the places her patients work, the neighborhoods in which they live, and the schools the children attend. She feels that it makes a big difference to her patients to see her in the supermarket or library or working in her garden. This knowledge and trust between patient and physician is not only crucial to Dr. Paxton's patients but also adds to the satisfaction she receives by caring for her patients in their community.

MEDICAL STUDENT'S GUIDE FOR VISITING AND ANALYZING A COMMUNITY AGENCY

During the course of your medical education you will probably be asked to visit a community agency. This can be an exciting opportunity for you to get out of the hospital and classroom and into the community, especially if you choose an agency that, because of its services, interests you. For example, if you are interested in emergency medicine, you could contact a rescue service squad and make arrangements to spend a night with the crew. If alcoholism interests you, attend the local Alcoholics Anonymous, Al-Anon, and Al-Ateen meetings. There is a community resource pertinent to almost any health-related interest you have.

Telephone directories often have lists of community resources, and many communities publish directories of resources. Other resources are social workers, nurses, and primary care physicians who have been in the community long enough to be familiar with its resources. When you have decided on an agency, call and ask to set up an appointment with the director or someone whom you can interview about the agency. Also let them know your need to arrange for a client interview. Be sure to tell them you are a medical student and the reason (course requirement, personal interest, etc.) you want to learn about their program.

During the visit, the following outline can be used as a guide for your interview. Be flexible enough, however, to add or delete questions as is appropriate to your agency.

Outline for Conducting a Community Agency Visit
Briefly cover the relevant items:
I. Background, purpose, and target population
   A. When it came into existence
   B. Whose instigation
   C. Demographic, socioeconomic, and cultural description of clients to be served
   D. Services offered
   E. Changes in clientele or services over time
II. Organizational structure
   A. Administrative body
   B. Advisory group
      1. Professional representation
      2. Community representation
      3. Client representation
   C. Staffing patterns
      1. Kinds of health professionals used
         a. Number
         b. Training received
      2. Utilization of health professionals
         a. Services rendered
         b. Support staff and their role
III. Sources of agency income
   A. Funding agencies (private and government)
   B. Clients

    C. Third-party
    D. Other
IV. Problems defined by agency personnel
    A. External
    B. Internal
V. Client interview
    In order to obtain a consumer's perspective on the resources, spend some time talking with at least one client. Be able to describe the client (age, occupation, socioeconomic description). What are the most obvious problems? How is the agency serving the client? What is the client's response? If a client interview is not possible because of confidentiality or other problems, identify a patient of your preceptor's who has used that community resource and request an interview by phone.

REFERENCES

1. Berkman LF, Syme SL: Social networks, host resistance, and mortality: a nine-year follow-up of Alameda County residents. *Am J Epidemiol* 109:186–204, 1979.
2. Kark SL: *The Practice of Community-Oriented Primary Care*. East Norwalk, CT, Appleton-Century-Crofts, 1981.
3. Mullan F: Community-oriented primary care: an agenda for the 80s. *N Engl J Med* 307:1076–1078, 1982.
4. Nutting PA, Wood M, Connor EM: Community-oriented primary care in the United States: a status report. *JAMA* 253:1763–1766, 1985.

SUGGESTED READINGS

Connor E, Mullan F (eds): *Community-Oriented Primary Care: New Directions for Health Services Delivery*. Conference Proceedings of the Division of Health Care Services, Institute of Medicine. Washington DC, National Academy Press, 1983.

This book, recommended for anyone who is interested in the theory or practice of community-oriented primary care, includes chapters by many of the best known theorists and practitioners of COPC. Discussions on topics that range from medical education for COPC in the American context make this a very useful book.

Gumas P: A physician's responsibility in a community health problem. In Houts PS, Leaman TL (eds): *Case Studies in Primary Medical Care: Social, Psychological and Ethical Issues in Family Practice*. University Park, The Pennsylvania State University Press, 1983.

Presented as a case study, this chapter addresses the issues facing a family physician when he becomes involved in a public health issue (a dangerous highway). The chapter includes two selected readings that deal with the conflicts that face physicians when they become activists.

Maxcy KF (ed): *Maxcy-Rosenau Public Health and Preventive Medicine*, ed 11. New York: Appleton-Century-Crofts, 1980.

This is the encyclopedia of public health and is a must for primary care practitioners. It includes chapters on public health methods, communicable diseases, environmental health, behavioral factors affecting health and health care planning, organization, and evaluation.

Prime B: Patient education and community resources. In Shires DB, Hennen BK (eds): *Family Medicine: A Guidebook for Practitioners of the Art*. New York, McGraw-Hill, 1980, pp 442–459.

This chapter addresses the topic of patient education in general but also includes good discussions of the use of formal and informal community resources, voluntary agencies, and self-help groups. Guidelines for obtaining and discussion of developing educational resources and the referral process make this a very useful chapter.

chapter 5

ENVIRONMENTAL AND OCCUPATIONAL HEALTH

Mark Marquardt and Kay Lovelace

We are in an era of increased public attention and knowledge about the interaction of the environment and health. The public, the medical profession, and the government have become increasingly aware of health hazards both in the workplace and in the general environment. Concern about regulating worker safety resulted in the Occupational Safety and Health Act in 1970, which created the Occupational Safety and Health Administration (OSHA) and the National Institute for Occupational Safety and Health (NIOSH).

SCOPE OF OCCUPATIONAL/ ENVIRONMENTAL MEDICINE

The American College of Physicians has defined environmental and occupational medicine as a field "concerned with the diagnosis, treatment and prevention of disease caused by agents in the environment. Its preventive approach stresses the physical, chemical and biologic properties of the external environment that affect human health" (1). The family physician's definition should be expanded to include (*a*) the emotional and psychological components of work, (*b*) the interaction of work with family and community, and (*c*) the workplace's impact on health through its impact on the environment. A job may have a negative or a positive effect upon a worker's self-image, financial status, family, community, and personal health. Patients, families, and communities may be exposed to chemical, physical, psychological, or infectious hazards that cause or exacerbate acute or chronic health problems and produce anxiety or depression.

Depending on the source of the estimate, from 85 million (2) to 104 million (3) Americans are employed, working in about 5 million businesses.

Nearly 90% of the businesses employ fewer than 100 workers (2). It is estimated that 85% of American workers do not have access to physician services through their workplace, and only 2% have access to an industrial hygienist and workplace-monitoring programs (4). When there is a concern about ill health as a result of an exposure or injury at work or from the environment, primary care physicians are often the first contact with the medical profession.

A study for the National Institute for Occupational Safety and Health (NIOSH) found that 31% of the conditions seen in a primary care population are related to work (5). The overall incidence of work-related injuries in 1983–1985 was 10.2 per 100 workers per year, with a low of 3.6 for workers in personal services to a high of 26.9 for workers in construction. Ninety percent of the work-related injuries received medical attention (6). Nine percent of all persons in the labor force have limitation of activity due to a chronic medical condition(s) (7). Exposure to toxic substances has become an increasingly important problem. There are over 60,000 chemicals used in industry, and only 10,000 have been tested for toxicity in animals (2).

Occupational health is a subset of environmental health. In fact, the substances present in the workplace may be emitted into the community, often with profound effects on community health. Environmental factors outside the workplace also affect health. As the Surgeon General's report *Healthy People* states, "There is virtually no major chronic disease to which environmental factors do not contribute, either directly or indirectly" (8). Factors such as ethanol use and abuse, tobacco abuse, and diet are not specifically addressed in this chapter, even though they may have significant interactions with occupational and environmental exposures.

Family physicians must be knowledgeable about occupational and environmental health because family physicians will see occupationally- and environmentally-related disease in their practices. In addition, many family physicians will be asked to provide preventative services for employees. Finally, they will often be looked upon as advocates for community health issues, some of which will be environmental.

TAKING AN OCCUPATIONAL/ ENVIRONMENTAL EXPOSURE HISTORY

The most basic skill needed by physicians is that of taking an occupational/environmental-exposure history to uncover links between work, the environment, and health. Physicians can use three questions, along with a self-report occupational exposure form, to screen patients with medical complaints for occupational disease (9).

1. Do any other persons where you work have similar symptoms?
2. Do these get better or worse on any day of the week, or go away on weekends or vacations?
3. Do you think that these problems are related to your job?

- Question 1 screens for work relatedness, because occupational exposures frequently affect more than one worker at a time.
- Question 2 deals with the temporal relationship of symptoms to work. For example, workers in cotton textile mills often have more difficulty breathing when they have been at work several hours Monday morning after being off for the weekend. It is important to realize, however, that many persons have work schedules that vary in a way that will not enable them or you to make this link easily. Also, long-term, cumulative exposures may cause health problems that will not vary with days off work.
- Question 3 is a way of obtaining patients' perceptions about what is going on in the workplace. It is important to recall that many epidemics of workplace disease have been first noted by the workers themselves.

Taking a thorough occupational history requires a structured approach. In family practice

settings, this is sometimes not practical unless exposures and symptoms suggest the need for an in-depth history. Family practitioners are encouraged to use a self-reporting occupational/environmental history form with their patients. An example is shown in Figure 5.1. This record can be kept in the patient's chart and be periodically updated. After gathering and reviewing information on occupational and environmental exposures, you may think that the patient's condition is work-related or decide that you need more information. Evidence that can support a work-related diagnosis includes the following (10):

1. Symptoms compatible with the suspected exposure.
2. Previous work-related exposure that resulted in illness.
3. Symptoms in other workers with similar exposures.
4. Suggestive or diagnostic physical signs.
5. Known exposure to a sufficient amount of a suspected causative agent, with the proper temporal relationship between exposure and symptoms.
6. Confirmatory industrial hygiene data. Environmental sampling data may be available through NIOSH Health Hazard Evaluations, OSHA inspections, or company records.
7. Scientific plausibility. (Are the exposures known to cause the symptoms? Are routes of entry likely considering the control measures?)
8. Biological (tissue or fluid) confirmation in the patient. By taking laboratory tests for specific agents (e.g., blood lead), it may be possible to measure exposure.
9. Lack of a nonoccupational cause.

Any of the above conditions should raise suspicion that a work-related problem is present, but none alone is enough to establish a diagnosis. Often, following up a suspicion takes considerable time. Uncovering and helping to manage occupational health problems is, however, one of the ways physicians can make a unique contribution to both patient and community health.

WHEN A PATIENT HAS A WORK-RELATED CONDITION

Once you have determined or strongly suspect that a patient's condition is work or environmentally related, you have several options:

Part I: Work and Exposure History

The following questions refer to your current or most recent job:

1. Job title _____
2. Type of industry _____
3. Name of employer _____
4. Year job began _____
   Are you still working in this job? Yes _____ No _____
   If *no*, what year did the job end? _____
5. Describe this job, especially any part of it that you feel may be hazardous to your health.
   _____
   _____
6. Do you wear protective equipment on this job?
   _____ Yes _____No If yes, mark any of the following that are used:
   _____ Gloves _____Coveralls/apron _____ Safety glasses
   _____ Hearing protection _____ Paper mask _____ Respirator
7. In this job, are you exposed to any of the following?
   _____ Fumes and dusts _____ Metals _____ Solvents
   _____ Other chemicals _____ Heat or cole _____ Noise
   _____ Emotional stress _____ Heavy lifting, physical strain
   _____ Radiation _____ Other
8. Is there any particular hazard or part of your job that you think is related to your health problems?
   _____ Yes _____ No
9. Are there any other employees at your place of work who have problems or complaints similar to yours?
   _____ Yes _____ No

Part II: Employment History

It is important that we know as best as you can remember all the jobs you have had. Job #1 is the one you mentioned in the beginning of this questionnaire–your current or most recent job. Beginning with the job before thi sone–call it Job #2–please fill in the information asked below, working back in time. Include any military service you have had.

	Years from-to	*Description of work*	*Exposures*
Job #2			
Job #3			
Job #4			
Job #5			
Job #6			
Job #7			
Job #8			

Part III: Other Exposures

1. Does anyone in your household work at a job that you think may involve exposures which may be brought home from work (for example, asbestos fibers on clothes)? _____ Yes _____ No
2. Do you have any hobbies that expose you to chemicals, metals or other substances?
   _____ Yes _____ No
3. Are there any industries in the area where you live that may pollute your environment?
   _____ Yes _____ No

(Adapted from Rosenstock L. The Role of the physician in the recognition and management of occupational disease. Univ WA Med 1982; 9:18–24.)

Figure 5.1. Suggested format for obtaining an occupational history.

1. Treat the patient and inform him or her of the consequences of the exposure.
2. Report the incident or encourage the patient to report the incident to the appropriate authorities and peers, including the patient's labor union.
3. If the patient is impaired because of his or her condition, refer the patient for competent legal advice in the case that the patient may be eligible for workers' compensation benefits.
4. Notify the company.

The way in which you carry out the above actions may have serious ramifications for the patient. All options should be considered carefully. For example, you may treat the patient, but if he or she returns to the same workplace, the same exposures may be there and the risk of recurrent illness remains. It is also important to follow up the patient who has chronic exposures that may cause problems in the future (e.g., low-level metal and carcinogen exposures).

In reporting an incident of suspected hazards to agencies responsible for worker health (e.g., Occupational Safety and Health Administration (OSHA), the National Institute of Occupational Safety and Health (NIOSH), or the state Department of Health), it is imperative to remove any information that may identify the patient unless you have the patient's permission. Section 11(c) of the Occupational Safety and Health Act (OSH Act) theoretically protects workers against discrimination when they report health and safety violations, but there are few instances of Section 11(c) being enforced. Far more commonly workers have faced discrimination or have been fired because of health problems, even when the problems were caused by the workplace.

ETHICS IN OCCUPATIONAL MEDICINE

Family physicians sometimes provide occupational health services under contract from one or more companies. In such situations, this question might arise: Whose agent is the occupational physician? The answer, as stated by Tabershaw, is that "the physician works for no other purpose than the benefit of his patients. In occupational medicine, this is the worker. As with other third-party payers, the patient is still primary. The physician is not an agent of industry" (11). A similar response by the American Occupational Medical Association Code

of Ethics stresses that "(1) the highest priority is to be given to the health and safety of the individual (patient), (2) the physician must practice on a scientific basis, with objectivity and integrity, and (3) the physician must give an honest opinion and avoid having his or her medical judgment influenced by any conflict of interest" (12).

Confidentiality applies in occupational health cases, as it does in all doctor-patient relationships. Therefore, any identification of the patient to the employer or to agencies should be done only with the patient's permission, with two exceptions: (*a*) imminent danger of death or injury to the patient or other workers and (*b*) overriding public health concern.

Preplacement physical examinations are an exception, however. OSHA has ruled that the patient has waived rights to confidentiality with a preplacement physical examination, and that the information is the property of the employer. Another exception is workers' compensation cases, in which the employer, the workers' compensation agent, and the workers' compensation courts are entitled to access to all records pertinent to the particular incident. In both situations, however, the patient has the right to know of your intent to notify the company or relevant agencies. A more comprehensive discussion of ethical issues involved in providing occupational health services can be found in *Ethical Dilemmas Facing Clinicians Who Provide Health Services to Workers* (13).

WHEN YOUR PATIENT CANNOT WORK

Inevitably, you will find patients who cannot work because they are impaired or disabled. *Impairment* is defined as any anatomical or functional abnormality or loss. *Permanent impairment* is impairment that has become static or well established with or without medical treatment, or that is not likely to remit despite medical treatment of the impairing condition. *Disability* is not a purely medical condition. Disability is the limiting loss or absence of the capacity of an individual to meet personal, social, or occupational demands, or to meet statutory or regulatory requirements (14).

The role of the physician is to determine impairment. The determination of disability is a complex process including assessment of nonmedical factors such as age, sex, education, and economic and social environment, in addition to medical impairment. Disability determination is done by either the state workers' compensation board or industrial commission (in the case of disability caused or aggravated by work) or the Social Security Administration (for nonoccupational disability).

Workers' Compensation Law

Workers' compensation is the major resource available to patients who cannot work because they are impaired (15). A legal mechanism to compensate work-related injury and illness in the United States, workers' compensation is based on a no-fault principle; proof of negligence on the part of the employer is not required. Types of benefits include medical payments, income replacement, and death benefits. This law is a compromise between workers and employers. It provides payment of medical expenses and partial payment of lost income, but prohibits the worker from winning large jury verdicts (2). The law compels every employer to compensate workers who are judged to be entitled to compensation. Workers are responsible for reporting the injury to their employer. In some states, workers' compensation benefits pay for vocational rehabilitation. Each state is responsible for its own workers' compensation system; therefore, the type and extent of coverage varies by state. Statutes of limitation for filing also vary from state to state.

Physicians are not expected to be experts on workers' compensation law. Your responsibility as a physician includes notifying a patient if you think a condition might be work-related, explaining about the statutes of limitations in your state, referring the patient to competent legal counsel and filing a doctor's report of the work injury with the employer (or the employer's insurance company). Once an occupational injury is reported to an employer, an adjustor will be in communication with the physician about the worker's claim. Physicians who expect to care for workers with occupational injuries/illness must keep on hand a supply of forms required by the state Workers' Compensation Act. The physician needs to understand the terminology and mechanics involved in workers' compensation.

Social Security Disability Insurance

For patients with a long-standing disability, Social Security Disability Insurance (SSDI), an income replacement program covered under the Social Security Act (SSA-20), provides income. It serves disabled workers under age 65 and their families, people who became disabled before age 22 (if a parent covered under Social Security retires, becomes disabled, or dies), and disabled or dependent widows and widowers age 50 or over, if the deceased spouse had worked long enough under Social Security. Medical expenses are not covered. The etiology of the patient's impairment does not have to be related to work. The formula for determining eligibility and benefits is complex, and nonmedical considerations often override (15).

When a patient applies for SSDI, your responsibility as a physician is to provide evidence to allow the Social Security Administration reviewing team to make a determination. The book *Disability Evaluation Under Social Security, A Handbook for Physicians*, which is available through the Social Security Administration, will be helpful in determining how to assist your patients.

MAKING A WORK SITE VISIT AND DEVELOPING A COMMUNITY PROFILE

One method of obtaining valuable information about a patient's job is to supplement the occupational/environmental exposure history with a work site visit. Not only does this visit provide information that the history does not, such as a visual picture of a repetitive, complex, or technical task for which the patient's description may be inaccurate, it helps the physician develop a richer and more thorough understanding of the community (16). When making a work site visit, it is useful to collect the information listed in Table 5.1.

While at the workplace, it is important to observe your patient's job in detail, noting the chemical, physical, biological, and psychological hazards to which the patient is exposed. The following format is a useful way to organize the specific information on your patient's job:

1. Potential hazards;
2. Control measures;
3. Potential effects;
4. Medical surveillance;
5. Prevention.

For physicians whose time and expertise in this area are limited, resources are available to help gather information on the workplace. The

Table 5.1. Information to be Collected during a Work Site Visit[a]

1. Specifics: (can be completed prior to visit via letter or telephone).
   Plant name, location, directions
   Contact person, health professional
   Major or minor products or processes
   Demographics:
      Number of employees: blue collar, white collar
      Hours worked each week
      Union or nonunion
      Health services available
2. Kinds of jobs: (to be completed on site)
   Waste disposal: liquid, solid, gas
   Safety measures and equipment: required or provided, protective equipment
   Kinds of jobs: terminology, descriptions, psychological and physical hazards
3. Observer impressions (to be completed after the visit):
   Profile
   Selected hazards
   Specific health maintenance and monitoring by laboratory tests needed by patients
   References for specific chemical processes

[a]Adapted from Larsen ME, Schuman SH, Hainer BL: Workplace observation: key to a meaningful office history. *J Fam Pract* 16:1179, 1983.

occupational health division of each state's health department may send out an industrial hygienist to work sites at a physician's request. Also, occupational physicians and schools of public health can provide expertise when needed to assist the family physician in gathering occupational and work site data. One of the most effective ways to increase your understanding of the types of work and environmental hazards to which your patients are exposed is to talk with your patients about their work in detail. Visiting the workplace also provides a powerful understanding of the conditions and hazards to which your patient is exposed. As your knowledge about individual patients and their work sites increases, you will begin to develop a picture of the community's work life. To enhance this community profile, you can obtain a list of the major industries and types of work in your state or community, keep a file that lists hazards by industry and information gained from your patients on any particular industry, and keep information on the workplaces that you visit in a central location. You will then be able to refer to this file for information when you see other patients who work in these plants or when community environmental health problems are suspected.

Hazardous Substances

The federal Hazard Communication Standard (covering manufacturing industries in the Standard Industrial Classification Codes 20 to 39), published by the United States Occupational Safety and Health Administration, is a tool that should prove valuable to physicians and their patients. This regulation, known as a "right-to-know" standard, provides workers with a right to obtain information about hazardous chemicals at work. A number of states have enacted separate right-to-know legislation that is generally more comprehensive than the federal hazard communication standard, often providing information to the public about hazards used and stored in the community. By contacting your state Department of Labor, you can find out about the specific regulations and laws governing disclosure of information about toxic substances in your state.

In general, unless a substance is classified as a trade secret, a worker should be able to obtain information on it from the employer. This information is generally given in the form of a Material Safety Data Sheet (MSDS), a fact sheet developed by the chemical manufacturer to provide information on the product name; the chemical ingredients; instructions on handling the chemical; physical properties, including the boiling point, vapor pressure and flash point (helpful in case of fire); what protection to wear; what to do in case of a chemical spill or emergency; and the health effects of the chemical (acute effects are usually listed, chronic effects are often omitted). If a substance is classified as a trade secret and the situation is considered an emergency, the physician can require the industry to reveal the names of the chemicals they are using. The physician will, however, be asked to sign a confidentiality agreement that states that the name of the chemical will not be revealed to the worker. If the substance is classified as a trade secret and the situation is not an emergency, the physician must file a written request with the company for release of the information. If the company refuses to respond or has not responded within 30 days, the physician has the right to file a request with OSHA officials.

LEADING WORK-RELATED DISEASES AND INJURIES IN THE UNITED STATES

Reliable data on prevalence of occupational disease and fatalities are lacking. Surveillance for occupational disease began only in the late 1980s (17).

One estimate of 125,000 annual fatalities as a result of 500,000 incident cases is not based on verifiable data (18).

Better data are available for accidental injuries and fatalities. Between 1912 and 1988, accidental work deaths per 100,000 population were reduced 81%, from 21 to 4. There were 10,600 work-related deaths in 1989. Agriculture had the highest death rate (48/100,000), followed by construction (34/100,000), and mining and transportation (24/100,000). Motor vehicle deaths accounted for 35% of all work-related deaths (19).

The National Institute for Occupational Safety and Health has developed a list of the ten leading work-related diseases and injuries based upon the following criteria: the disease's or injury's frequency of occurrence, its severity in the individual case, and its amenability to prevention (20). Table 5.2 lists these leading work-related health problems. They are summarized below.

Occupational Lung Diseases

Occupational lung diseases are often difficult to recognize because the latency period may be long (e.g., up to 30 years or more for asbestos-related

disease). Six of the major types of occupational lung disease are listed in Table 5.3 (20).

Musculoskeletal Injuries

NIOSH estimates that musculoskeletal injuries account for 580,000 (18%) of the estimated 3.2 million emergency room–treated occupational injuries (21). Data from the Bureau of Labor Statistics indicate that approximately one of every five injuries in the workplace is a back injury (i.e., about 1 million workers in 1980).

Repetitive motion injuries, caused or aggravated by repeated twisting or awkward postures (especially when combined with high force), accounted for about 23,200 occupational injuries in 1980, according to the Bureau of Labor Statistics. Persons at risk include about 15 to 20% of those working in construction, food preparation, clerical work, product fabrication, and mining.

Table 5.2. Ten Leading Work-related Diseases and Injuries in the United States, 1982[a,b]

1. Occupational lung diseases: asbestosis, byssinosis, silicosis, coal workers' pneumoconiosis, lung cancer, occupational asthma
2. Musculoskeletal injuries: disorders of the back, trunk, upper extremity
3. Occupational cancers (other than lung): leukemia, mesothelioma; cancers of the bladder, nose, liver
4. Amputations, fractures, eye loss, lacerations, traumatic deaths
5. Cardiovascular diseases: hypertension, coronary artery disease, acute myocardial infarction
6. Disorders of reproduction: infertility, spontaneous abortion, teratogenesis
7. Neurotoxic disorders: peripheral neuropathy, toxic encephalitis, psychoses, extreme personality changes (exposure-related)
8. Noise-induced hearing loss
9. Dermatologic conditions, dermatoses, burns (scaldings), contusions (abrasions), chemical
10. Psychological disorders, neuroses, personality disorders, alcoholism, drug dependency

[a]The conditions listed under each category are to be viewed as selected examples, not comprehensive definitions of the category.
[b]Adapted from Centers for Disease Control: Leading work-related disease and injuries—United States. *MMWR* 32:25, 1983.

Table 5.3. Selected Occupational Lung Diseases

1. Asbestosis. Diffuse, extensive scarring of the lung. Disease progresses after exposure ends. Latency can be 10 to 20 years after exposure. Smoking increases the risk 2 to 3 times. Estimated that 10 to 18% of asbestos insulation workers and shipyard workers will die of asbestos-related diseases.
2. Byssinosis. Consists of acute (reversible) and chronic lung disease as a result of the inhalation of cotton, flax, hemp. Smoking greatly increases the risk of this disease. Symptoms are "chest tightness," cough, and obstruction of small airways. Estimated that there are 35,000 current and retired textile workers disabled from this disease.
3. Silicosis. Prevalence of disabling silicosis is still high in certain groups of workers: in mines and foundries, abrasive operations, and in stone, clay, and glass manufacturing.
4. Coal workers' pneumoconiosis. Estimated prevalence in currently employed coal miners is 4.5%. In 1974, there were an estimated 19,400 cases of coal workers' pneumoconiosis, resulting in 4,000 deaths annually.
5. Lung cancer. Although tobacco smoke is the single most important cause of lung cancer, the following occupational agents are also associated with it: arsenic, asbestos, chloroethers, chromates, ionizing radiation, nickel, and polynuclear aromatic hydrocarbon compounds. Tobacco smoke interacts synergistically with some of these agents, thus sharply increasing the risk.
6. Occupational asthma. Asthma and hypersensitivity pneumonitis may be caused by a variety of organic and inorganic substances. Prevalence varies from 10% to nearly 100% of workers in some occupations. Agents that have been shown to cause occupational asthma include grain dusts, flour, metals, inorganic chemicals, isocyanates, enzymes, and fungi.

About 7 million workers in jobs such as vehicle operation are exposed to whole body vibration, which places significant stress on the musculoskeletal system, and about 1.2 million workers are exposed to segmental or body part vibration, the sources of which are hand-held power tools. This exposure can result in the vibration syndrome, or intermittent numbness and blanching of the fingers with reduced sensitivity to cold, heat, and pain (21).

Occupational Cancers (Other Than Lung)

Estimates for the proportion of cancers related to occupation range from less than 4% to more than 20%. Evidence for extragenetic factors (behaviors such as cigarette smoking, alcohol use, and toxic environmental exposures from the workplace and the community) as a cause for cancer has been developed through epidemiologic and toxicologic studies (22). Table 5.4 shows a selected list of types of cancer and occupational risks.

Amputations, Fractures, Eye Loss, Lacerations, and Traumatic Deaths

NIOSH estimates that about 10,000,000 persons are traumatically injured on the job each year; approximately 30% are severe (3,000,000), and 10,000 are fatal. These figures include deaths from motor vehicle accidents, falls, industrial vehicle accidents, blows, and electrocutions. The following occupations are associated with the highest rates: (*a*) mining and quarrying; (*b*) agriculture (including forestry and fishing); and (*c*) construction. Approximately 21,000 workers suffered amputations in 1982; there were 400,000 fractures, 900,000 eye injuries (84% were minor), and about 2,250,000 lacerations (23).

Cardiovascular Diseases: Hypertension, Coronary Artery Disease, Acute Myocardial Infarction

Although the role of occupation as a factor in cardiovascular disease is not clear, evidence on associations with some occupational factors is accumulating. An ad hoc task force of the American Heart Association published a report in 1981, "The Impact of the Environment on Cardiovascular Disease," which identified and reviewed six environmental factors that have potential impact on cardiovascular health: water hardness, trace elements, inhalant occupational exposures, carbon monoxide, noise and radio frequency, and physical and psychosocial stress (24). These are summarized in Table 5.5.

Because heart diseases are so prevalent in the United States, even a small decrease in the relative

Table 5.4. Selected Occupational Cancers[a]

Condition	Industry/Occupation	Agent
Hemangiosarcoma of the liver	Vinyl chloride	Polymerization; monomer
Malignant neoplasm of nasal cavities	Industry vintners, woodworkers, cabinet/furniture makers, boot and shoe producers	Arsenical pesticides, hardwood dusts
Malignant neoplasm of the larynx	Asbestos industries and utilizers	Asbestos
Mesothelioma, (peritoneum), (pleural)	Asbestos industries and utilizers	Asbestos
Malignant neoplasm of bone	Radium chemists, processors, watch dial painters	Radium
Malignant neoplasm of scrotum	Automatic lathe operators, metalworkers, coke oven workers, petroleum refiners, tar distillers	Mineral/cutting oils, soots and tars, tar distillates
Malignant neoplasm of bladder	Rubber and dye workers	Benzidine, alpha and beta naphthylamine, auramine, magenta, 4-amino-biphenyl, 4-nitrophenyl
Malignant neoplasm of kidney; other and unspecified urinary organs	Coke oven workers	Coke oven emissions
Lymphoid leukemia	Rubber industry	Unknown
Acute myeloid leukemia	Radiologists; Occupations with exposure to benzene	Ionizing radiation, benzene

[a]Adapted from Centers for Disease Control: Leading work-related diseases and injuries—United States. *MMWR* 33:125, 1983, and Rutstein DD, Mullan RJ, Frazier TM, Halperin WE, Melius JM, Sestito JP: Sentinel health events (occupational): a basis for physician recognition and public health surveillance. *Am J Public Health* 73:1054–1062, 1983.

Table 5.5. Selected Occupational Contributions to Cardiovascular Disease

Agent	Health Effect
Metals, dusts, trace elements	Congestive heart failure may result from restrictive lung disease. Antimony, cobalt, and lead have also been implicated as possible causes of cardiovascular disease.
Carbon monoxide	Decreases oxygen-carrying capacity of hemoglobin and thus reduces the oxygen supply available to heart muscle and other tissues. Exposure may precipitate acute cardiovascular events. Short-term exposures at levels within the OSHA permissible exposure limit have been associated with decreased exercise tolerance and ECG evidence of myocardial ischemia.
Carbon disulfide	Increases the risk of coronary artery disease and hypertension.
Halogenated hydrocarbons	Acute exposures to solvents (e.g., chloroform, trichloroethylene) and fluorocarbon aerosol propellants have precipitated sudden death, probably due to cardiac arrhythmias.
Nitroglycerin and nitrates	Increased risk of cardiac chest pain, myocardial infarction, and sudden death, particularly after a time away from work. Mechanism thought to be "rebound vasospasm."
Noise	Single exposures can cause transient increases in blood pressure. Chronic exposure associated with sustained increases in blood pressure, particularly in workers with noise-induced hearing loss. Other effects include increases in serum cholesterol, changes in circulating hormones, and abnormalities in platelet aggregation.
Psychosocial stress-cardiovascular	Correlation with "type A personality." Association between "work-overload," role conflicts, thwarted career goals and cardiovascular disease. Association between "nonsupportive supervisor," decreased job mobility and cardiovascular disease. Association with limited autonomy and heavy workloads.

risk of heart disease would involve large numbers of persons and would have major consequences to the public's health.

Disorders of Reproduction

Occupational exposures are known to produce a wide range of adverse effects on reproduction. Parental exposures to reproductive toxins prior to conception may result in reduced fertility, unsuccessful fertilization or implantation, or an abnormal fetus. Exposure after a woman has conceived may cause death of the fetus or congenital defects if it survives to term. Spontaneous abortion (early and late), major and minor birth defects, perinatal death, low birth weight, altered sex ratio, developmental or behavioral disabilities, and transplacental carcinogenesis are also possible. About 560,000 infant deaths, spontaneous abortions, and stillbirths occur each year, and 200,000 live infants with some type of birth defect are born in the United States each year. The causes of most of these are unknown. Table 5.6 summarizes some of the known adverse reproductive effects and their causes (25).

Neurotoxic Disorders

Neurotoxic disorders are on the NIOSH list of 10 leading work-related diseases and injuries because of their potential severity and because of the large number of workers at risk (more than 7.7 million)

Table 5.6. Selected Reproductive Hazards

Exposure	Agent	Outcome
Maternal	Lead, ethylene oxide, and anesthetic gases	Spontaneous abortion
	Ionizing radiation	First trimester: microcephaly and mental retardation
		Third trimester: low birth weight, neonatal death
Paternal	Dibromochloropropane	Azoospermia
	Lead	Poor semen quality

(26). There are over 850 neurotoxic chemicals in the workplace. Clinically, either central or peripheral effects may be more dominant. When peripheral neuropathies develop, early symptoms may include numbness, tingling, or pain in the feet or hands. Clumsiness or uncoordination due to sensory and motor changes will follow as the disease progresses. Effects on the central nervous system may include mood and personality changes or cognitive dysfunction (such as reduced attention span, lack of alertness, and memory loss). Other neurological effects of toxins may include ataxia, myoclonus, paraplegia, parkinsonism, seizures, tremor, nystagmus, constricted visual field, and impaired visual acuity (26).

Noise-Induced Hearing Loss

The Occupational Safety and Health Administration indicates that about 9.4 million United States production workers now work or have worked in industrial locations where noise exposure levels are 80 decibels (dB) or higher (27). This is the level at which hearing loss begins to develop.

Unfortunately, noise-induced hearing loss is an irreversible sensorineural condition that progresses with exposure. It is caused by damage to the nerve cells of the inner ear (cochlea) and cannot be treated medically. Among those workers, the following excess hearing loss has been estimated: 17% of production workers have mild hearing loss; 11% have material hearing impairment; 5% have moderate to severe impairment. Most, if not all, of this hearing loss could be prevented with proper protection.

Dermatologic Conditions

Dermatologic conditions other than injuries accounted for 37% of the occupational illnesses recorded in 1983 Bureau of Labor Statistics Annual Survey of Occupational Injuries and Illness. The Bureau of Labor Statistics has also indicated that 20 to 25% of all occupational dermatologic conditions result in lost work time, averaging 10 to 12 lost work days. NIOSH assumes that only 2 to 10% of cases are reported and estimates the annual cost of occupational dermatologic conditions resulting from lost worker productivity, medical care, and disability payments to range between $222 million and $1 billion (9).

Approximately 23 to 35% of all reported occupational injuries are dermatologic, resulting in an estimated annual skin injury rate of 1.4 to 2.2 per 100 full-time workers. Most of these skin injuries are lacerations/punctures (82%), followed by burns (11.9%), abrasions (3.4%), and chemical burns (2.2%). Other frequently reported occupationally-related dermatologic conditions include contact dermatitis (90%), infections (5%), acne, and skin cancer (28).

Psychological Disorders

Increasing evidence suggests that an unsatisfactory work environment may contribute to psychological disorders (29). These may be classified as: (a) affective disturbances (e.g., anxiety, irritability), (b) behavioral problems (e.g., substance abuse, sleep difficulties), (c) psychiatric disorders (e.g., neuroses), and (d) somatic complaints (e.g., headache, gastrointestinal symptoms). Recent studies of stress-related immunologic suppression suggest that stressful working conditions may have a systemic influence and may affect the etiology and/or prognosis of other disease states. Data available for determining the extent of work-related psychological disorders are limited; however, there are several indicators of the financial and health costs of these disorders. One study in California showed that workers' compensation claims for "work-related" neuroses doubled between 1980 and 1982, while claims for all other disabling injuries were reduced by one-tenth during that time. Another study showed that during the same 2-year period, claims for "mental stress" that developed gradually were about 11% of all occupational disease claims (29).

Specific working conditions that cause negative psychological outcomes include repetitive tasks, role ambiguity, lack of control over the job by the worker, shift work, a responsibility for others (such as in health care), and poor physical environment.

CONCLUSIONS

As a family physician, you will need to develop a clear understanding of the community in which you work: its industries, environmental hazards, and the overall standard of living. This information will greatly enhance your ability to provide quality medical care to your patients. When you find an illness that recurs because it is caused or exacerbated by an exposure in the work environment, you will need to obtain information on protection from, or elimination of, the hazard. When you assist in preventing your patient from developing a disease related to work or the environment, you may help co-workers, community members, and families as well.

RESOURCE LIST

Institutions and Agencies That Can Help with Occupational and Environmental Health Problems

A. The National Institute for Occupational Safety and Health (NIOSH), located in Atlanta, Cincinnati, Morgantown, WV, and in ten regional offices. NIOSH researches causes of occupational disease and methods of prevention. Contact NIOSH to obtain information on hazards in specific industries, to obtain information on prevention and control strategies for specific hazards or industries, for recommendations on worker screening, and to request a study of a particular workplace (Health Hazard Evaluation) when a hazardous situation is suspected.

NIOSH
1600 Clifton Road, NE
Building 1, Room 3007
Atlanta, GA 30333
404-639-3771

NIOSH Cincinnati Installation
Robert A. Taft Laboratories
4676 Columbia Parkway
Cincinnati, OH 45226
513-533-8302

Appalachian Laboratory for Occupational Safety and Health
944 Chestnut Ridge Road
Morgantown, WV 26505
Division of Safety Research 304-2991-4595
Division of Respiratory Disease Studies 304-291-4474

B. Occupational Safety and Health Administration (OSHA):
U.S. Department of Labor
Room N3647
200 Constitution Avenue NW
Washington, DC 20010
202-523-8148

OSHA sets and enforces workplace health and safety hazards, investigates occupational health and safety complaints, and inspects work sites. The Occupational Safety and Health Act is enforced in each state by federal OSHA or by the state. The Department of Labor publishes a document entitled *All About OSHA* 1985 (Revised). *The Federal Register* publishes all federal OSHA standards as well as all amendments and corrections. *The Federal Register* is available in many libraries and from:

Superintendent of Documents
U.S. Government Printing Office
Washington, DC 20402

C. State Workers' Compensation Agencies are responsible for implementation of workers' compensation legislation

D. The Environmental Protection Agency (EPA) assesses and controls environmental problems such as air and water pollution, hazardous wastes, pesticides, radiation, noise, and toxic substances. Information can be obtained from:

Toxic Substances Control Act Assistance Office
EPA (TS-7999)
Washington, DC 20470
202-554-1404

E. Poison Control Centers provide the public and health professionals with rapid information on poisonings and can assist in the diagnosis and management of toxic exposures and the identification of nameless or brand name toxic substances.

F. Educational Resource Centers are regional centers established and funded by NIOSH to train occupational safety and health professionals and to conduct research and continuing education programs in occupational safety and health. Contact NIOSH to locate the center nearest you.

REFERENCES

1. American College of Physicians: Position Paper; Occupational and environmental medicine: the internist's role. *Ann Intern Med* 113:974–982, 1990.
2. LaDou J. The practice of occupational medicine. In LaDou J (ed): *Occupational Medicine*. Norwalk, CT, Appleton & Lange, 1990, pp 1–17.
3. *Vital Health Stat (10)* 170: 1–151, 1989.
4. Rosenstock L, Hagopian A: Ethical dilemmas in providing health care to workers. *Ann Intern Med* 107:575–580, 1987.
5. Discher DP, Kleinman GD, Foster FJ: *National Occupational Hazard Survey: Pilot Study for Development of an Occupational Disease Surveillance Method*. Cincinnati, National Institute for Occupational Safety and Health, 1975.
6. *Vital Health Stat (10)* 170: 95, 1989.
7. *Vital Health Stat (10)* 170: 13, 1989.
8. U.S. Department of Health and Human Services: *Healthy People: The Surgeon General's Report on Health Promotion and Disease Prevention*. Rockville, MD, US Government Printing Office, DHEW publication no. (PHS) 79-55071, 1979.
9. Coye MJ, Rosenstock L: The occupational health history in a family practice setting. *Am Fam Physician* 28:229–234, 1983.

10. Warren-Gray B, Gray MR: *The Occupational and Environmental History*. Project module developed by the Department of Community and Family Medicine, Arizona Center for Occupational Safety and Health, University of Arizona, 1979.

11. Tabershaw IR: Whose "agent" is the occupational physician? *Arch Environ Health* 30:412–416, 1975.

12. Welter ES: The role of the primary care physician in occupational medicine: principles, practical observations and recommendations. In Zenz C (ed): *Occupational Medicine, Principles and Practical Applications*. Chicago, Year Book Medical Publishers, 1988, pp 62–73.

13. Rosenstock L: *Ethical Dilemmas Facing Clinicians Who Provide Health Services to Workers*. Project module developed by the Department of Family and Community Medicine, and Arizona Center for Occupational Safety and Health, University of Arizona, 1983.

14. American Medical Association: *Guide to the Evaluation of Permanent Impairment*, ed 2. Chicago, American Medical Association, 1984.

15. Lea JL, Edwars WV, Cordes DH: *Physician Evaluation of Impairment/Disability*. Project module developed by the Department of Family and Community Medicine, Arizona Center for Occupational Safety and Health, University of Arizona, 1983.

16. Larsen ME, Schuman SH, Hainer BL: Workplace observation: key to meaningful office history. *J Fam Pract* 16:1179–1184, 1983.

17. Cullen MR, Cherniack MG, Rosenstock L: Occupational medicine. *N Engl J Med* 322:594–601, 1990.

18. Pollack ES, Keiming DG (eds): *Counting Injuries and Illnesses in the Workplace: Proposals for a Better System*. Washington, DC: National Academy Press, 1987.

19. National Safety Council: *Accident Facts*. Chicago, 1989.

20. Centers for Disease Control: Leading work-related diseases and injuries in the United States. *MMWR* 32:24–32, 1983.

21. Centers for Disease Control: Leading work-related diseases and injuries in the United States. *MMWR* 32:189–191, 1983.

22. Centers for Disease Control: Leading work-related diseases and injuries in the United States. *MMWR* 33:125–128, 1984.

23. Centers for Disease Control: Leading work-related diseases and injuries in the United States. *MMWR* 33:213–215, 1984.

24. Harlan WR, Sharret AR, Weill H, Turino GM, Berhani NO, Resnekov L: Impact of the environment on cardiovascular disease, report of the American Heart Association Task Force on environment and the cardiovascular system. *Circulation* 63: 243A–246A, 1981.

25. Centers for Disease Control: Leading work-related diseases and injuries in the United States. *MMWR* 34:537–540, 1985.

26. Centers for Disease Control: Leading work-related diseases and injuries in the United States. *MMWR* 35:113–123, 1986.

27. Centers for Disease Control: Leading work-related diseases and injuries in the United States. *MMWR* 35:185–188, 1986.

28. Centers for Disease Control: Leading work-related diseases and injuries in the United States. *MMWR* 35:561–563, 1986.

29. Centers for Disease Control: Leading work-related diseases and injuries in the United States. *MMWR* 35:613–621, 1986.

chapter 6

HOME CARE

Peter J. Rizzolo and Vickie Atkinson

Home care today has come to be synonymous with the services rendered by organized home health agencies (HHAs) and *not* with physician services for homebound patients. Home health care has been the fastest growing segment of the health field in recent years, with the number of HHAs growing from approximately 3000 to over 8000 nationally during the past 10 years (1). These professional in-home services include nursing care, physical therapy, occupational therapy, speech therapy, and social work. Other available services are home health aides, chore workers, Meals on Wheels, transportation, and a variety of community volunteers (e.g., those doing home repairs).

The tremendous recent growth in home care has taken place largely without physician involvement, other than the requirement for an initial referral. When a patient needs to see a physician, he or she is typically transported by ambulance to a medical center for an appointment, often with a subspecialist. That physician rarely has the time, training, or interest to adequately treat the whole person.

In fact, home visits by physicians have declined over the past decades, while other aspects of home care have been booming. Not surprisingly, family physicians and general practitioners have the highest home visit rates, although even they make infrequent visits as a rule. Recently trained physicians are less likely to make home visits than are older physicians. The high cost of running a medical practice, the inefficiency of going to the patient's home, poor reimbursement, and concern about possible compromised quality are most often cited as impediments to physicians making home visits (2).

Yet patients value home care, including home visits by physicians. Most older persons want to remain in their own homes rather than move to in-stitutional settings, even when getting around is very difficult, and home care can help facilitate this. Furthermore, younger patients often consider a home visit to be an event that bonds them to a physician, and physicians who have visited the home generally leave with a far deeper understanding of the patient. Given the rising older population, physician home care can be expected to rebound in the future. Recent increases in Medicare reimbursement for physician home services may facilitate this development.

WHO CAN BENEFIT FROM A PHYSICIAN HOME VISIT

There are three general types of home visits by physicians to patients: assessment visits, continuing-care visits, and acute problem visits. *Assessment visits* generally occur on a one-time basis and can often involve several members of the health care team. Geriatric patients are particularly suitable for home assessment visits. *Continuing-care visits* involve a physician committing to provide care for the patient by way of regular visits to the home. In general, this type of home visit contract is provided to people who are bed-bound, often in the terminal phases of a chronic disease. *Acute problem visits* occur often because it is more convenient for the physician to visit the home. A typical example is the patient with a fever who lives near the physician and who has no transportation.

Among the types of patients that you should consider as candidates for home visits are

- **Couples with a newborn child.** Generally, a couple that has had a child will be fatigued and stressed during the initial weeks after childbirth. If they are first-time parents, they often have a long list of questions for the physician. Visiting

51

the home (ideally about 2 weeks after delivery) will allow you to observe more accurately the impact of the new baby on the family. The home visit also provides a more comfortable atmosphere for talking about parenting. Thus, the first well-child visit can be conducted very successfully in the home.

- **Patients with an acute back strain.** It is extremely uncomfortable for a patient with an acute back problem to come into the physician's office. Since rest and medication often accelerate improvement, a home visit is the best way to initiate therapy in selected patients.
- **Patients with unexplained compliance or psychosocial problems.** A common truism in family medicine is that when a patient is frustrating, the physician should find out about the home situation. A home visit is often the best way to gather this information.
- **Chronically disabled individuals, especially those who are bed-bound.** Most family physicians care for persons whom they visit at home because it is so difficult to get them into the office. Patients with severe strokes, advanced multiple sclerosis, and degenerative diseases such as muscular dystrophy all tend to have long periods in which the patient is bed-bound. Family care givers, who sacrifice so much to keep their loved one at home, appreciate a physician who will come to the house.
- **New geriatric patients with multiple problems.** Home visits in the elderly add a critical dimension to assessment. Looking in the medicine cabinet and on the bedside table is generally the best way of finding out what medicines the patient is taking. Speaking to care givers and other family members can reveal unexpected problems and assets. Finally, a home visit is the only way to look for hazards that may precipitate a fall.
- **Patients with dementia.** Many patients with Alzheimer's disease and related dementias resist going to the doctor or become agitated in the unfamiliar office environment. Home visits are less disruptive, allow you to view the patient in the living environment, and provide an excellent opportunity to meet with family.
- **Suspected abuse.** Both child abuse and elder abuse are not infrequent. Most states now have legislation to encourage or mandate reporting suspicions of abuse or neglect. The physician needs to be attuned to the possibility of abuse or neglect and know the procedure for involving the agency assigned to investigate referrals.

Often a social service agency worker will visit the home as part of the abuse evaluation.

These are some of the situations in which a home visit is most productive. In order to make home care part of your practice, you will need to develop the skills to conduct efficient, productive visits.

SKILLS NEEDED FOR HOME CARE

Overcoming the Fear of Making Home Visits

Medical students often are assigned a patient or family to visit at home during the first year of medical school. These visits tend to be social and easy to make. As their training becomes more advanced, however, students and residents often are fearful of making house calls. This is understandable. The availability of nursing staff, radiology, laboratory, and faculty backup helps make the office environment more secure for physician trainees. It is easier to be in control in the office; the patient is on her or his own ground when you make a home visit.

Students and residents often worry about what equipment to take on house calls. There are published lists of the contents of home visit bags, but the amount of equipment needed really depends on the type of home visit. Assessment visits generally require nothing other than the eyes and ears of the physician and perhaps a stethoscope; therapeutic visits may require medications, blank prescriptions, or equipment (e.g., a catheter kit for a patient whose Foley catheter needs replacement).

The best way to overcome the fear of making home visits is to make them. It takes about two dozen visits to a variety of patients before you will begin to feel comfortable with this important care modality. Therefore, you are encouraged to look for and to take advantage of home visit opportunities that arise as you see patients. Also, since the subtle aspects of home visiting take years to perfect, you are encouraged to look for opportunities to make your visits accompanied by an experienced community physician, faculty member, or home health care provider.

Initiating the Home Visit

Patients rarely refuse a physician home visit. They do, however, generally appreciate knowing in advance when the physician plans to arrive. If you are running late, you should call and let the patient know of your new timetable. Scheduling home visits in advance can also allow family members to make arrangements to be present when you are there.

Any visit begins with greetings and generally with social interchange. In the home, this may take several minutes. Your host may wish to give you a tour of the house (and possibly the garden) or offer to serve you something to eat or drink. These social activities help the patient and family feel more comfortable with the physician.

The clinical portion of the visit is not infrequently mixed with socializing. For example, in visiting a 2-week-old infant, you may admire and play with the baby while beginning your physical assessment. Similarly, a tour of the home may provide the opportunity to review the contents of the bathroom medicine cabinet.

Completing a home visit takes a little longer than an office visit. Familiarity with the patient and with the home makes visits more efficient, however. Also, if you have formulated a clear idea beforehand of your goals for the visit, you will be able to conduct the visit in a purposeful manner, and you will know when you are finished.

Specific Home Visit Skills

In addition to appreciating the uses of a home visit, the physician should acquire specific knowledge and skills appropriate to caring for a person in the home. These include: (*a*) assessment of activities of daily living (ADLs) and instrumental activities of daily living (IADLs), (*b*) evaluation of the physical environment, (*c*) social assessment, (*d*) knowledge of available community home care services, (*e*) the ability to formulate a comprehensive treatment plan, and (*f*) some knowledge of Medicare benefits and what services they provide in the home.

Activities of daily living (ADLs) include feeding, dressing, toileting, ability to transfer from the bed or chair to a standing position, and the ability to walk about the house. In the home, the physician can observe one or several of these activities to assess the individual's ability to function independently. Instrumental activities of daily living (IADLs) include shopping, cooking, housecleaning, telephoning, paying one's bills, and driving a car. The physician may pick up clues about problems with IADLs by observing unopened mail, newspapers lying about the front yard, or the home looking unattended.

Environmental assessment requires an observant eye. Cleanliness and decor provide obvious clues to the mood and habits of the family. For people with small children at home, safety concerns such as outlet protectors and the placement of toxic substances on high shelves can be observed. Smoke and fire alarm devices should be looked for. A fire extinguisher should be available in or near the kitchen. For older persons, falls are a serious problem, and the home should be evaluated for risk factors. Loose or uneven carpeting, slippery floors, and scatter rugs may cause an accidental fall. Poor or uneven lighting, especially in stairways and hallways, is hazardous, since vision in low light is significantly diminished in the elderly. Night lights in hallways and along the route to the bathroom are useful. Nonskid mats are useful in the bathtub or shower. Wall-mounted "grab bars" are useful in the bathroom, in the tub/shower areas, and next to the toilet. An elevated toilet seat may be helpful for individuals who experience difficulty rising from a sitting position.

Social assessment is far better done at home than in the office. Meeting family members living in the home will greatly enhance your understanding of at least part of the patient's social supports. Often family portraits offer the physician the opportunity to inquire and learn about the extended family.

A variety of home health services are available in most communities. Physicians should build an awareness of as many as possible. An office nurse or social worker can serve as a home services resource. Many telephone companies have special community service numbers listed somewhere in the phone book. They may be listed as "Aging," "Senior Citizens," or "Elderly Services." Councils on aging, departments on aging, and senior centers usually have available directories of services available in the community.

Treatment plans vary, depending on the problem. A good home care plan addresses the medical needs within the context of the home environment and social situation. For patients who are homebound, the care giver and the patient must be cared for.

Many family physicians are part of an informal community-based multidisciplinary team, usually through affiliation with a private or public home health agency. Core team members generally include a physician, a social worker, and a home health nurse. Additional team members may include a physical therapist, occupational therapist, and other medical specialists. Often, it is up to the physician to pull together a general care plan; but when a home health agency is involved, the "case manager" formulates a plan for approval by the physician prior to implementation. Team members often communicate entirely by telephone. Increasingly, however, family practices with large home care caseloads meet weekly, often over breakfast, to review patients with home care agency staff.

Physicians will usually find social workers, case managers, and other allied health professionals knowledgeable about the patient's environment and support system. They are interested in hearing what the physician has to say, are ready to assist the patient in following medical advice, and are capable of reporting physical and psychosocial changes in the patient's life. The attitude of physicians in talking with these professionals will be a significant factor in how information is shared and used. Showing respect for the expertise of these professionals is likely to yield much useful information about the patient and provide assistance in caring out the treatment plan.

Caring for the Caregiver

For patients who are homebound because of chronic illness, the primary care giver often is the main reason the homebound patient is not in a nursing home. Any patient care plan designed to maintain the patient in the home must address the needs of the care giver as well. Empathetic listening is important, but occasionally more help is needed. Services that make life more tolerable for the overburdened care giver include day care, respite care, home health aides, senior centers, Meals on Wheels programs, peer counselors, and support groups. These services are often listed in the telephone directory, or they can be located by contacting the local department on aging or social service department.

Case Example

Mrs. E.R., a 79-year-old woman with a history of hypertension, anemia, mitral valve prolapse, and Parkinson's disease, comes to the office accompanied by her daughter. She shares a mobile home with the daughter, a granddaughter, and a grandchild. Her daughter, a full-time waitress, expresses concern about her mother's worsening condition. She has had several passing-out spells in the past 2 months, and most recently, she required several stitches when she struck her head against a countertop as she fell. The emergency room physician who repaired the laceration suggested a walker, which her daughter purchased for her. The daughter reports that Mrs. E.R.

is not using the walker and continues to fall once or twice a week.

Her former physician, in evaluating the cause of her falls, had done a complete blood count, blood sugar and electrolyte determinations, ECG, chest x-ray, and Holter monitor. A mild anemia was noted, but the remainder of the results were within normal limits.

Physical examination reveals absent facial expression, generalized muscle stiffness, lack of arm swing with walking, and a stooped posture. Her blood pressure is 160/85 sitting, but on standing it drops to 90/50. If made to stand for more than a few minutes she becomes lightheaded and has to sit down to keep from falling.

The physician's problem list is as follows: (*a*) anemia of undetermined cause, thought to be most likely due to chronic disease, (*b*) Parkinson's disease (PD), inadequately treated, (*c*) postural hypotension secondary to PD, and (*d*) gait instability secondary to PD. The initial impression is that she would benefit from more vigorous antiparkinsonian drug therapy. Her falls are attributed to postural hypotension.

The patient and her family are asked to keep a record of any falls, recording the time, location, activity, and relationship to meals and medication dosage. A second antiparkinson drug is added to her regimen; she is urged to use her walker and to keep several chairs strategically located in her home so that she can sit down if she feels faint.

One week later she falls in her bathroom, contusing her right shoulder and ear, again requiring a trip to the emergency department. As a result, a physician home visit is arranged.

At the home visit, significant findings include:

- Her granddaughter, the primary caretaker, has a 16-month-old toddler and cares for a neighbor's 1-year-old child. Thus, she has little time to supervise her grandmother.
- The trailer is small and cluttered with excess furniture from a previous larger apartment. The walkways are too narrow for the patient to turn in while using her walker.
- There are no grab bars in the bathroom or shower.
- The patient's bedside table is cluttered with prescription bottles. Many are from her former physician, including several duplicates of medicines that her current physician has prescribed.
- There is no ramp leading to the front door, and the ground outside the house is cluttered and uneven. As a result, she rarely goes outside. There are no sidewalks; so even if she were to walk outside, she would have to walk on the road.

• There is only one car in front of their trailer; it belongs to her daughter.

Case Discussion

This home visit yielded important information that had not been apparent on the patient's visits to the office. First, it became obvious that the granddaughter, not the daughter, is the primary caretaker. In addition, the granddaughter's attention was mostly directed to the care of her small child and the second toddler. Secondly, the physician's advice to use a walker was unrealistic, given the physical dimensions of the trailer and very limited floor space. It was impossible to turn around in the bathroom while using the walker, making the bathroom a particularly dangerous place for a potential fall. Finally, the patient had been advised to walk every day to strengthen her legs, but she was forced to ignore that advice because there is no place to walk safely.

As a result of the home visit, a series of new recommendations are made. A social worker is contacted, who helps arrange for a ramp to be built, for storage of excess furniture, and for additional handrails to be installed in the home. In addition, the physician has a better understanding of the patient's living situation and can, in future recommendations, better take the environment into account.

REFERENCES

1. Wieland D, Ferrell BA, Rubenstein LZ, et al.: Geriatric home health care. *Clin Geriatr Med* 7:645–664, 1991.
2. Keenan JM, Fanale JE: Home care: past and present, problems and potential. *J Am Geriatr Soc* 37: 1076–1083, 1989.
3. Keenan JM, Hepburn KW: The role of physicians in home health care. *Clin Geriatr Med* 7:665–675, 1991.

chapter 7

HEALTH ECONOMICS AND PRACTICE MANAGEMENT

John J. Aluise

Until the latter part of the twentieth century, medicine was seldom referred to as a business. Its function was simple, solo physicians and small groups of practitioners worked independently in their practices and in small- to moderate-sized community hospitals. Patients or insurance companies paid for most medical care, and the government reimbursed hospitals for costs associated with Medicare patients. Billing patients, insurance companies, and the government was a routine procedure, and third-party payers normally reimbursed physician charges and hospital costs with little or no scrutiny.

All this has changed in the past 25 years, and the pace of change continues to be rapid. Medicine has been transformed from a cottage industry to a complex regional and national health care system. Many factors, most of which are discussed in this chapter, contribute to rapid flux in the delivery and financing of medical services. Physicians must know and understand these changes or risk being frustrated by the world in which they practice.

The first part of this chapter presents a macroanalysis of the economic environment of medicine, including an overview of governmental programs and commercial insurance companies, and a discussion of the growth and impact of managed-care plans and multispecialty organizations. The second part of the chapter is a microanalysis, focusing on the managerial features and functions of the family practice office. The information presented in this chapter is by no means exhaustive. As you train for your career in medical practice, you are encouraged to expand your professionalism to include continued learning about the business of medicine.

ECONOMIC ENVIRONMENT

Government Programs

Currently, the federal government subsidizes nearly 40% of the $900 billion dollar cost of medical services nationwide. Medicare is the largest medical insurance program of the federal government. Because of the dramatic increase in Medicare expenditures (1400% increase between 1965 and 1984, compared with a 240% increase in the consumer price index for the same period), the government legislated two cost-containment initiatives. In 1983, the Tax Equity and Fiscal Responsibility Act (TEFRA) legislation created a prospective payment system (PPS) for hospitalized Medicare patients. In 1992, a resource-based relative value system (RBRVS) established a system of standard fees for physicians offering primary and specialized care to Medicare patients.

Medicare is a health insurance program for those aged 65 and older, regardless of income or wealth; it also covers disabled people under 65 who have been entitled to Social Security disability benefits. The program consists of Parts A and B. Part A is the hospital insurance portion, providing coverage for in-hospital care, skilled nursing facility care, and home health care. Part B of Medicare covers reasonable physician charges, outpatient, ambulance, and emergency room services and other services and supplies. Payment under Part B is not full payment, only 80% of what Medicare determines to be reasonable. If the physician accepts "assignment" (i.e., agrees to accept the Medicare fee), the physician bills Medicare, receives 80% of the fee, and is allowed to bill the patient for the remaining 20% of the reasonable fee. If the physician declines to accept assignment of the fee, the patient is responsible for whatever the physician feels is an appropriate fee. The amount of reimbursement from both Part A and Part B is not intended to cover the total costs, and various stipulations in each part determine how much the patient pays through deductible or copayments. Because of the increasing costs of medical care, the government encourages providers (hospitals and physicians) to accept the Medicare reimbursement as payment in full and not bill patients for the percentage of the fee that is not reimbursed by Medicare. During the 1980s, government payments for Medicare costs rose an average of 15% per year. Trustees of the Medicare Health Insurance Trust Fund have warned that at the present rate of growth, the trust fund will be unable to meet its obligations by the turn of the century. The aging population, all of whom will become Medicare beneficiaries, and the rising costs of medical care have forced the government to assume a dominant role in the financing of medical services.

Medicaid is a jointly federal/state-financed program to pay for health services for indigent persons. Each state defines income eligibility for classification of the medically needy. The Medicaid benefit structure varies from state to state; however, it must at least provide for inpatient and outpatient medical services, skilled nursing facility services, physician services, home health care, family planning services, and periodic screening, diagnosis, and treatment of children under 12. A state may elect to pay for dental services, prescribed drugs, eyeglasses, and other services. The federal government's share ranges from 50% in the wealthiest states to 77% in states with the lowest per capita personal income. In most states, the increasing costs of Medicaid are outpacing general revenues. Many states are reducing the number and scope of services being subsidized and are being more restrictive about eligibility requirements.

To combat the rising costs of hospital expenditures for Medicare beneficiaries, the government introduced a **prospective payment system (PPS)** for hospitalized Medicare patients. Hospital care represents approximately 70% of Medicare payments. To implement the PPS system, the government adopted a plan that assigns every hospital patient to one of 478 diagnosis-related groups (DRGs), such as congestive heart failure (several groups depending on severity), diabetes (again with several groups), and acute cholecystitis. Reimbursement was predetermined for each group,

based on historical data from Medicare costs for patients previously discharged in that DRG.

The PPS system assigns each disease classification a predetermined length of stay and assigned payment. Only under exceptional circumstances can a hospital receive additional payment for a patient with a specified DRG illness or disease. Under the PPS, a hospital's profitability from Medicare patients is tied to (a) strict discharge planning and shorter lengths of stay; (b) eliminating unnecessary tests and services; and (c) seeking economies of scale and productivity improvements through more selective use of staff and high-technology equipment. Potential abuses of PPS by hospitals, such as increasing nonacute admissions to collect more DRG fees, discharging patients "sicker and quicker," and manipulating loopholes in the discharge coding system to get higher-priced DRG payments are monitored by federal Professional Review Organizations (PROs). PROs employ physicians and nurses to review 25% of all Medicare patients' medical records, with the authority to deny payment and to screen quality problems. The impact of the PPS system, specifically the DRGs, has been evidenced by reducing the length of hospital stay, revamping hospitals' case mix, forcing smaller hospitals to reconsider their "full-service" abilities, strengthening utilization review procedures, and creating sophisticated information systems to report the cost-effectiveness of physicians' clinical decisions.

The **Physician Payment Review Commission** was created in 1986 to advise Congress on reform methods used to pay physicians for services to Medicare beneficiaries. In 1989, following extensive research by Professor William Hsiao and his colleagues at Harvard, the Commission proposed a Medicare Fee Schedule called the **Resource-Based Relative Value Scale (RBRVS)**. RBRV designations for physician-patient encounters are based on a complex formula that includes the amount of time required, the degree of training needed, the complexity of the problem, and the risks associated with poor care. If physicians of a similar specialty in two regions of the country provide the same service to Medicare beneficiaries, they will earn the same net income from these services, allowing for geographical variations. A conversion factor converts the relative value scale to a dollar amount. The proposed conversion factor as of 1992 is $31, which means if a particular service or procedure has a unit value of 5 then the payment from Medicare would be $151. The government will establish a list of standard unit values for several thousand physician services and procedures. Fee schedules will be phased in between 1992 and 1996. To control costs, the commission also recommended expenditure targets (specifying a desired annual rate of increase in expenditures for physician's services), strengthened quality assurance and utilization review, and increased research on the effectiveness of medical services and the development of practice guidelines.

One of the transformations occurring in the financing of health care can be seen in the shift from the retrospective, cost-based, payment mechanisms originally established in the Medicare and Medicaid programs to the prospective payment schemes the PPS-DRG and RBRVS plans. Retrospective payment merely reimbursed physicians for their charges and hospitals for their costs. Medicare and many other third-party payers were not stringent in their monitoring of services, fees, and charges, until the monies that were being spent to reimburse medical costs exceeded the budgeted reserves for medical costs. The change to prospective systems for payment of hospital care (DRGs) and standard fee schedules for physician services (RBRVS), along with a stronger emphasis upon utilization review and evaluation of physician practice patterns, marks a major change in the financing of health care. Commercial insurance companies face similar financial constraints and are implementing their own prospective payment programs.

Commercial Insurance Companies

The year 1929 marked the birth of modern health insurance: Baylor University Hospital established a hospital insurance plan for schoolteachers in Houston. This plan included 21 days of hospital care in a semiprivate room for a rate of 50 cents per month. This plan became a model for **Blue Cross** hospital coverage plans, which gained nationwide acceptance in the 1940s and 1950s, when unions and industries began offering health insurance as an employee benefit.

The first **Blue Shield** plan to cover physician's costs was started in 1939 in California. All physician's services were covered for a premium of $1.70 per month. California was also the first state to establish a relative-value scale for physician services. Blue Shield plans did not work as well as the

Blue Cross plans because the reimbursement was tied to physician charges, and in those days physicians normally charged patients on a sliding scale, overcharging the wealthy to pay for the care of the poor. Thus, patients with health insurance were often charged high rates because they had the benefit of a third-party payer. Another problem the Blue Shield plans faced was the coverage of radiology, anesthesiology, and pathology services when these specialties moved outside the hospital, where they were formally covered by Blue Cross plans. Blue Shield rates were not structured for these high-cost services, and it took a while for premiums to increase to cover the higher fees. Blue Cross and Blue Shield merged in 1978, and now these plans provide a network of regional coverage throughout the U.S.

Today nearly 50% of health care costs are paid by commercial insurance companies and Blue Cross/Blue Shield plans. Blue Cross/Blue Shield plans offer both individual and group coverage. Prudential and Equitable companies restrict their insurance to group coverage.

To combat the rising costs of health care, commercial firms have expanded their coverage to include prepaid plans, health maintenance organizations (HMOs), and preferred provider plans (PPOs). Corporations and large service organizations, such as hospitals and universities, have become self-insured, and are essentially organizing and funding their own insurance coverage. Another cost containment initiated by industry and commercial insurance firms shifts more of the burden of payment to the patient through copayments and deductibles. In addition to financial restrictions, insurers and companies have now realized the value of wellness programs and other preventive medicine programs that have long-term cost-saving implications.

Managed-Care Plans

As business, government, and commercial insurance companies explore ways to decrease medical costs, the fee-for-service system of medical care payment and reimbursement is being replaced with various prospective and prepayment plans. Prepayment plans similar to the health maintenance organization (HMO) model pioneered by Kaiser in California demonstrated positive results in modifying medical costs without jeopardizing the quality of medical care. To support the HMO movement, the government enacted a law in 1973 requiring employers to offer employees at least one HMO that met federal standards, if one was available. By the end of the century approximately 50% of the population is expected to be enrolled in some form of prepaid, or managed, health plan.

The typical managed-care plan has five basic features: (*a*) a contractual relationship among the employer (or government agency), the individual employee or beneficiary, and the managed-care plan to provide medical care; (*b*) a defined population enrolled for a period of time, usually 1 year; (*c*) voluntary participation by clients and providers; (*d*) fixed payments or predetermined fees, regardless of utilization; and (*e*) assumption of a portion of the financial risk by the physicians and other providers.

Managed-care plans have four organizational patterns: staff-model HMO, group-model HMO, Independent Practice Association (IPA), and preferred provider organization (PPO).

In the **staff-model HMO**, a company or large organization such as a union employs physicians to provide medical services to its employees and their dependents. Companies may own and operate their medical and dental facilities as a mechanism for controlling costs and budgeting services. Since physicians and other health professionals work on a salary basis, the cost of the services rendered will be relatively fixed, with the exception of medical supplies and other expenses directly associated with the number of procedures performed. Many physicians find the staff model advantageous because the workload is moderate, facilities tend to be well-equipped, and the administrative responsibilities and financial risks of private practice are absent.

The **group-model HMO** consists of physicians, usually in a multispecialty practice, serving as the providers for all or a portion of an enrolled group. This model has different variations. The group can be the exclusive provider group, such as Kaiser Permanente. Under this system, a monthly premium (capitation) for each client is paid to the group. The physicians agree to provide all their services for this prepayment. All clients must go to the designated Kaiser facility for their medical care or for referral to services that may not be provided by Kaiser physicians. Another example of a group model is Pru-Care (Prudential's HMO), which negotiates with an established group practice in a large community to be the provider for the Prudential subscribers who select their HMO plan. The group practice receives a capitated payment

or negotiates a fee schedule for the services they perform for Prudential's enrolled clients. The group is not restricted to Prudential's patients and may provide services to other HMOs and to patients on a fee-for-service basis. Large multispecialty groups are the most desirable provider group for a group model HMO because they can provide the full range of outpatient and inpatient services, including ancillary tests and diagnostic procedures.

The **Independent Practice Association (IPA)** establishes a network of community physicians, both primary care and medical and surgical specialists, and then markets this association of physicians to employers under a prepaid plan similar to the HMO systems previously discussed. Patients who enroll in the IPA can select from the list of primary care providers and specialists. The IPA plan usually pays physicians on a capitated basis, a specified amount per member per month. Most IPAs establish primary care physicians as case managers to provide the majority of primary care and preventive medicine services and to authorize referrals and consultations. IPAs also require physicians to participate in a utilization review process to monitor medical care expenditures, including surgical procedures, admissions, and laboratory and radiology usage. Physicians who join an IPA maintain their traditional fee-for-service practice and may also contract with other HMO or PPO organizations.

Another type of managed-care plan is the **preferred provider organization (PPO)**, which combines the fee-for-service approach with some of the HMO concepts. PPOs have several features: (*a*) a panel of physicians so that clients have a choice of service provider; (*b*) a negotiated fee schedule, usually 10 to 20% below the regular charges; (*c*) primary care providers providing basic services and authorizing referrals; and (*d*) a utilization review system to monitor physician practice patterns and quality-of-care standards. Discounted rates may produce cost savings initially, but clients and providers may compensate for lower rates by performing additional services or increasing the frequency of visits and services offered.

IPAs and PPOs are still in their infancy, compared with the staff- and group-model HMOs. Their capability to provide a cost-effective, high-quality health care plan is still uncertain. Several concerns have been raised concerning these plans. They contract with a large number of independent providers, who may not be fully committed to the procedures and principles of prepaid care. Physicians may have to pay a sign-up fee, yet they have little or no control over the number or type of clients who may select them as providers. Administrative responsibilities of physicians and their office staff may not be adequately compensated by the plans.

Nearly 50% of all practicing physicians participate in some form of managed-care affiliation, either HMO or PPO. In 1990, HMO enrollments in the more than 600 plans nationwide rose to 39 million people. The most recent growth in HMO enrollment is due to the addition of a new feature in HMO guidelines referred to as the "point of service" option, which gives members the choice of seeking care outside the HMO setting from any doctor they choose, although at significantly lower benefit levels. Table 7.1 is a list of some of the largest HMOs. Though the HMO movement is nationwide, the impact of managed care is mainly in the large urban areas.

Under the managed-care system, primary care physicians are exposed to several risks since they will be the personal physician for most medical services. Risks are associated with three main areas of concern:

- *Panel size.* Smaller populations contain more risks, and a major illness for a few patients may absorb most of the capitation money.
- *Adverse selection.* HMO members with unusually high risks may prefer going to a physician where they are not charged on a per visit or per procedure basis. These patients will obviously have a higher than normal utilization rate.
- *HMO solvency.* When a plan cannot meet its obligations to its members or its physicians, then the practice may lose a large portion of its client base and the revenue from these patients.

Table 7.1. Top HMOs in the United States

Rank	Plan	1990 Enrollment
1.	Kaiser Permanente, Oakland, CA	6,200,000
2.	Blue Cross/Blue Shield, Chicago, IL	4,400,000
3.	Cigna Healthplan, Bloomfield, CT	2,100,000
4.	Aetna Health Plan	1,100,000
5.	Health Ins. of New York, NY	1,100,000
6.	US Healthcare, Blue Bell, PA	1,100,000
7.	United Health Care, Minneapolis, MN	700,000
8.	Prudential Health Care, Roseland, NJ	700,000
9.	PacifiCare Health Systems, Cypress, CA	600,000
10.	Humana, Louisville, KY	500,000

Before entering into a managed-care contract, physicians should carefully review the following features of the contract: types of services required of the primary and secondary physician; the authorization process for consultations, admissions, mental health services and diagnostic and surgical procedures; the risk pools; utilization review; renewal and termination provisions; referral restrictions; confidentiality and access to records; "hold-harmless" clauses; information reporting requirements; and other features that require the physician to become an agent of the managed-care system.

Participation in a managed-care system requires physicians to educate patients about the appropriate amount and type of medical services, establish cooperative associations with medical and surgical colleagues, and organize a comprehensive system of cost-effective primary medical care for outpatient and inpatient services, including diagnostic and surgical procedures. A management information system is also necessary to monitor patient care services, determine if the prepayment is adequate for the type and volume of patients enrolled, and evaluate the practice habits of the physicians.

Multispecialty Medical Organizations

Another transformation occurring in the health care industry is the increasing size and complexity of large group practices, particularly multispecialty organizations. This is another indicator of the demolition of the cottage-industry mode of medical practice that survived well beyond other occupations. Health care organizations, medical practices, and hospitals in particular are in the transition from a system that paid for medical services on a fee-for-service, cost-based method to a system that pays for medical services in a more predictable manner, using standard fees between large purchasers and large numbers of providers. This corporate structure of health care does not mean that physicians have no role in leadership and management. On the contrary, physicians played a key leadership role in several national and regional health care organizations during this transition to larger medical systems.

Table 7.2 contains a list of some of the largest medical group practices in the country. Kaiser Permanente Medical Group stands out as the largest exclusively prepaid medical group. In several metropolitan areas, large medical groups combine their traditional fee-for-service practice with HMO and PPO affiliations. Large, multispecialty

Table 7.2. Largest Multispecialty Medical Practices in the U.S.

Medical Group	Nos. of MDs	Nos. of Specialties
Kaiser Permanente Group, Oakland, CA	3000	41
Kaiser Permanente Group, Southern California	2700	34
Mayo Clinic, Rochester, MN	1000	100
Henry Ford Medical Group, Detroit, MI	800	40
Group Health of Puget Sound, Seattle, WA	550	56
Cleveland Clinic, Cleveland, OH	550	78
NW Permanente Group, Portland, OR	500	49
Geisinger Medical Group, Danville, PA	480	65
Capital Area Permanente, Washington, DC	420	29
Marshfield Clinic, Marshfield, WI	360	100

group practices have been successful in expanding their patient care base through networking with managed-care plans and also by merging with other medical practices, particularly primary care groups.

It is not uncommon to see mergers between multispecialty practices and local family physicians, internists, and pediatricians. Physicians in large groups understand the positive economic and professional implications for large, well-managed health care organization, and they have assumed their rightful role as executives of these organizations. For example, the Mayo Clinic owes much to Henry Plummer, M.D., who designed Mayo's revolutionary patient record system and the mechanical apparatus to transport records quickly and efficiently. Plummer created the systems and process improvements that allowed Mayo Clinic to consistently meet patient expectations. Mayo Clinic did not sacrifice quality medical services and responsiveness to patients' needs as they became one of the largest medical groups, now with satellite and computer linkage between their Minneapolis home site and their "branches" in Arizona and Florida.

Large, multispecialty medical organizations are positioned to respond to the challenges set forth by the government, commercial insurance companies, and industry for a well-managed, cost-effective health care system. Because of their size, and the diversity of their physicians, and the capacity to offer full-service medical care within one organized system, large medical groups will be attractive to government-funded medical programs, large employers, and insurance companies.

MANAGING A MEDICAL PRACTICE

The mechanisms developed by industry and government to lower health care expenditures have a direct relationship on how the individual physician runs his or her practice. Regardless of whether a physician is a salaried employee of Kaiser Permanente or a solo practitioner, the physician must understand, and become comfortable with, the business aspects of the practice. This requires knowledge of how personnel, time, finance, and office-management systems work together to create an efficient and effective business.

Personnel

The office staff is a vital part of any practice. From the receptionist who answers the phone, to the nurse who takes the blood pressure, to the clerk who fills out insurance forms, the way your office staff treats your patients has a direct bearing on the success of your practice. Typically, personnel accounts for 80% of a practice budget; so recruiting, training, and supervising competent office staff should be a high priority in any practice. Gone are the days when office personnel reported directly to the physician. Today's practices usually rely on supervisory personnel who are charged with maintaining a competent and dedicated staff.

Personnel management consists of these key questions: What task has to be performed? Who is the right person? What is the right job for each person? Who will monitor the work of others? Answering these questions requires a personnel system that includes well-defined job descriptions, a thorough selection and training process, and an appropriate supervisory system.

JOB DESCRIPTIONS

Job descriptions, which define each office worker's role and responsibility, consist of six features: (*a*) title of the position; (*b*) summary of the work; (*c*) primary responsibilities; (*d*) knowledge and skill requirements; (*e*) accountability/

results; and (f) supervision. Creating a job description is the first step in recruiting for a new position, and revising an old job description is equally important before filling an existing position. After selecting a new employee, periodic review of the job description allows for modifications based upon changes in clinic needs or the unique qualities of the individual.

SELECTION AND TRAINING

The knowledge and skills needed for the job determine the qualifications of the candidate you will recruit and will serve as the basis for your advertisement. After publicizing the position and identifying several desirable candidates, a set of specific questions should be developed before interviews begin. These should include previous work experience, reasons for leaving the last position, knowledge and skills relevant to the position being offered, and other pertinent information to assess the individual's compatibility with the organization and future responsibilities. The top four or five candidates should be interviewed by two different members of the practice, so that impressions and responses to questions can be compared and individual bias eliminated.

When the top candidate has been hired, a 3-month orientation and training period allows both the practice and the individual to see if the match of person and job is satisfactory. This orientation and training process is critical when a person fills a newly created position. The training period should have a structured orientation program, including formal educational sessions with the supervisor, and several opportunities to evaluate the person's skills in the new role and working relationships with other members of the office staff. At the conclusion of the training period, the supervisor should meet with the individual to determine if the job description is accurate, to provide feedback on the initial assessment of the person's skills, and to plan the first performance appraisal session.

SUPERVISION

Each employee deserves to have a supervisor who understands his or her role and is available for support and direction. As medical practices increase in size and sophistication, supervisors are needed for the business, nursing, and ancillary functions. This middle-management tier of practice supervisors insures close monitoring of the daily operations and allows the physicians in the practice to function at the executive-management level.

One tool to help supervisors and employees monitor work performance is the performance appraisal system. In this system, the job expectations and goals are clearly outlined when the employee assumes them. At predetermined intervals, the employee and supervisor meet to discuss the employee's actual performance. During these meetings, the supervisor may introduce changes in responsibilities and areas for improvement. The employee can discuss satisfactions and dissatisfactions and explore future roles and responsibilities. The first appraisal should occur within a few months of an employee beginning a new job, to help insure that he or she understands the job and that skills match the demands of the work. Thereafter, they should occur semiannually.

The employee's self-assessment of skills is crucial to the performance appraisal system. This assessment should include some of these questions: What would increase your effectiveness on the job? What do you enjoy about your work? How can your supervisor help you in your work? Are your capabilities being used in this job? What are your long-range plans?

TIME

The most difficult resource to manage in a medical practice is time. Mismanaged time victimizes physicians, staff, and patients. As a budget item, a doctor's time is valued at $200/hr. If your time is not planned wisely, something of value is lost. Office personnel and patients are quite candid about physicians' inability, or unwillingness, to manage their time. Time wasters that cause disruptions and frustrations in medical practice include:

- Inadequate time set aside for planning or problem-solving;
- Not adhering to scheduled appointments and meetings;
- Accepting interruptions irrespective of urgency or importance;
- Failure to end patient and colleague encounters;
- Lack of preparedness for key events and meetings;
- Reluctance to delegate responsibilities;
- Overcommitment, which results in fatigue and/or ineffectiveness.

Managing your time efficiently can be a difficult task. By analyzing your use of time from different perspectives, however, you can gain an understanding of which time-management areas you need to improve. Two perspectives of time that can be useful to explore are self-management and the qualitative aspect of time.

To be a good self-manager, you should assess how your personal, family, and career needs are influencing your life. How are the inevitable conflicts between personal and professional goals being addressed? Have priorities been set for personal, family, and career needs? What obstacles lie in the way and how can they be resolved?

A self-management plan is a structured way of analyzing your personal, family, and professional goals. The plan includes developing long-term goals (1 to 5 years) and short-term goals (less than a year); outlining obtainable objectives for each goal; and identifying personal strengths, areas for improvement, and resources, including other individuals, that will help accomplish your personal and career goals.

The first attempt at creating a self-management plan may be awkward, and obtaining advice or consultation from a colleague or mentor can be useful. Once the initial effort is under way, this process will be an invaluable guide for understanding yourself and determining obstacles to your personal and professional satisfaction.

Another strategy for managing time is to analyze the events and activities within the practice. Patient visits in the office require a different time allocation than patient visits in the hospital or nursing home. Staff meetings involve several as opposed to one-to-one performance appraisal sessions. Physician group meetings with advisors necessitate considerable premeeting activity, as opposed to a morning briefing on patients seen the night before. In their article entitled "Psychological aspects of the problem of time in practice management," Bibace and associates describe six qualitative dimensions of time: duration, density, location, succession, grouping, and vividness (1). Table 7.3 describes these dimensions and provides examples.

These dimensions of time interact with one another, and a careful analysis of specific problems in the practice or of an individual physician's time management may reveal that not enough attention is being paid to one or more of these factors.

Besides looking at time from these two perspectives, there are other specific strategies which can help you manage your time. They are outlined below.

PRACTICE SITE SELECTION

One of the most important decisions you will make affecting your time is the type of practice you wish to have. Solo practice is less popular today than several years ago because of the intense time commitment required. Group practices, where several doctors in the same or different specialties practice together, allow for greater time flexibility. In addition, whether you maintain a hospital practice or choose to do obstetrics will affect your time both in and out of the office.

SCHEDULING

Managing the many different tasks a physician must perform—seeing patients during office hours, making hospital rounds, and covering the practice at nights and on weekends—is not an impossible task. Several strategies will help the individual physician manage time in the most efficient way possible. Ideally, office hours are planned 2 to 3 months ahead. Vacation and other out-of-office commitments should be decided 3 to 6 months in advance. In addition, each day's patient care and other professional activities should be organized to allow physicians and their office personnel to work efficiently.

Good time management takes into account unexpected events. For example, allowing two or three openings each day for emergency visits will keep the practice from getting behind schedule. The following rules will help: only one physician out of town at a time; staff must give 4-weeks notice for vacation times; once the practice schedule is put on the appointment books, only emergencies will precipitate changes; and coverage and office hour schedules will be sent home to spouses and family so they can plan personal activities.

DELEGATION

Physicians must be willing to delegate some of the authority to plan, make decisions, and problem-solve in their absence. To effectively delegate authority, tasks or functions must be well-defined. If the physician does not understand the work to be done, then the person assigned the responsibility may not be given adequate information about what is expected or the desired outcomes. Another obstacle to delegating is the physician's unwillingness to hire and train midlevel, supervisory

Table 7.3. Qualitative Dimensions of Time and Their Applicability to Office Practice[a]

Dimension	Definition	Example
Duration	Length of time an event requires, including preparation and after-math	Committee meetings or meetings with financial advisors require preparation and summarization time, which physicians in practice rarely allot.
Density	Actual number of tasks/activities that can be completed in an ac-ceptable manner in one period of time	Counseling sessions require one long uninterrupted period, while returning several phone messages or reviewing the previous day's laboratory reports can be done intermittently or consolidated into a relatively brief period at the conclu-sion of a day.
Location	Temporal or physical position of an event	(1) Conducting a staff meeting in the local restaurant may not be conducive to discussion of difficult issues. (2) If an em-ployee is to be reprimanded, the meeting should be at the end of the working day.
Succession	Sequence and relationship of sev-eral events	The hectic pace of a busy physician cannot be ordered in a smooth fashion each day, but some thought should be given to when events take place, such as staff meetings, family counseling and reading professional journals. Otherwise, day-to-day patient care demands will consume the entire workday. Also, the daily appointments schedule for physical examinations, routine follow-ups, new patients, and diagnos-tic and surgical procedures should be organized to maxi-mize physician and staff efficiency.
Grouping	Involves the clustering of tasks to produce most effective results	(1) Schedule patient appointments for laboratory and x-ray, and return visits for diabetic and hypertensive patients when laboratory and nursing personnel can work independently of the physicians. (2) Consider blocking out 1 day every other week for administrative meetings, instead of trying to squeeze them into a busy schedule. (3) Staff and physicians should take vacations of at least one week at a time, preferably out-of-town.
Vividness	How much one event stands out from other events	An unexpected death of a patient, firing an employee, or the joining of a new physician to the practice, are significant events that have dramatic influence upon the practice rou-tines. Similarly, computerizing a medical practice, or affiliat-ing with an HMO will alter "the way things work around here."

[a]Adapted from Bibace R, Beattie K, Catlin R: Psychological aspects of the problem of time in practice management. *Continuing Educ Fam Phys* 18(3):203–298, 1983.

people who can eventually assume increased re-sponsibilities. Rules of thumb when delegating are: choose the right person; take time to carefully instruct; monitor work when assigning new or dif-ficult tasks; and allow staff to try out new and cre-ative methods.

Finance

To understand the basics of financial revenue, the physician must monitor the practice expenses and understand third-party reimbursement systems. Government and industry make up the bulk of third-party payers and usually account for 80% of all reimbursements. Financial management is one responsibility that cannot be abdicated, and physi-cians must allocate a portion of their administra-

tive time to reviewing productivity reports, plan-ning for major investments, negotiating contracts, and meeting with financial advisors.

Financial management requires the same de-gree of planning and critical decision-making as the management of clinical problems. The eco-nomic viability of the practice will depend upon a well-designed financial system that includes bud-geting, cost control, financial analysis, and compe-tent advisors.

BUDGETING

Budgets guide management decisions and assist in evaluating how revenues and expenses are meeting previous goals. The budgeting process begins with a yearly plan and then evolves into a monthly review of actual productivity compared with projections. A typical practice budget includes the following categories:

1. Income—hospital care; office practice; laboratory and x-ray; other services.
2. Expenditures—facility/capital equipment; personnel costs; medical and business supplies; maintenance expenses; miscellaneous costs.

At least one physician within the practice should have responsibility to work with the business manager to plan and monitor the practice budget.

COST CONTROL

With the advent of prepaid health plans and with the increased competition for medical services, practices will not have the freedom to increase fees as their expenses rise. The challenge facing medical practices in the age of cost-containment is to operate as efficiently as possible. For example, salaries and administrative costs constitute the largest categories of expense. Periodic review of both the number and roles of office personnel is essential to monitor this expenditure. Redefining job descriptions, consolidating positions, or considering part-time positions are options to explore. Installing office computers, advanced laboratory equipment, and more sophisticated telephone systems as opposed to maintaining manual or outdated operations that appear cheaper, might prove more economical in the long run.

The operating expenses of the practice should be reviewed yearly. You may need to employ an outside consultant or advisor to present an objective picture of how the practice can function more economically.

FINANCIAL ANALYSIS

Financial planning and decision-making requires accurate and timely reports. Two financial statements that analyze practice productivity are the balance sheet and the income statement.

The balance sheet describes the financial position of the practice at any point in time, in terms of available cash, value of equipment, accounts receivable (amount others owe the practice), and any other assets of the practice (see Table 7.4). The balance sheet also reports the liabilities of the practice, accounts payable (creditors of the practice), bank loans, and other debts.

The income statement is a periodic (monthly, quarterly, or yearly) report of the financial outcome in terms of revenue generated and expenditures (see Table 7.5). This statement provides an all-important picture of cash flow, since the income of the physicians and the salaries of the staff will be determined by how much the revenue exceeds the nonwage costs of doing business.

A third statement, the productivity report, provides useful information for each physician about the charges he or she is making, the variety of diagnoses seen, and the demography of the patient

Table 7.4. Components of a Financial Balance Sheet[a]

Assets	Liabilities
Current assets	Current liabilities
Cash	Income taxes
Supplies	Payroll
Accounts receivable	Payroll taxes
Allowance for bad debts	Accounts payable
Fixed assets	Total
Building and land	Long-term debt
Furniture, equipment, fixtures	
Accumulated depreciation	
Total assets	**Total liabilities**

[a]Adapted from Aluise JJ: *The Physician as Manager*, ed 2. New York, Springer-Verlag, 1987, p 78.

Table 7.5. Components of a Medical Practice Income Statement[a]

Income
Collections for professional services
Collections for diagnostic services

Total income
Expenses
Professional salaries
Staff salaries
Wage taxation and insurance
Benefits
Facility rental or mortgage
Supplies
Administration (if by outside contact)
Insurance
Interest expense
Allowance for bad debt (patients for whom no collections can be expected)
Taxation
Depreciation

Total expenses

[a]Adapted from Aluise JJ: *The Physician as Manager*, ed 2. New York, Springer-Verlag, 1987, p 78.

population. Together these three documents constitute the management information system for the practice.

FINANCIAL PROFILE OF A TYPICAL FAMILY PRACTICE

Table 7.6 presents a practice profile of an "average" family physician. This profile may be useful for those who want to compare their actual productivity and workload, and for those who are evaluating the primary care role and responsibilities as a career choice. The most concerning statistic in the profile is the income earned per hour worked, $34.72. Hopefully, with the changes proposed in the revised Medicare Fee Schedules and with physicians expanding their practices into larger groups, the financial return for primary care physicians, particularly family physicians, will be higher.

FINANCIAL ADVISERS

The complexity of medical practices, as a result of changing tax laws, contracts with third parties, and the growth of the practice organization, necessitates that physicians work closely with competent financial advisers. Specific needs for financial counsel are in the areas of incorporation, personal and practice investments, tax liabilities, leases and contracts, benefit plans, and affiliations with third parties. Physicians should select advisers who are willing to educate them as well as perform the financial services. Regular meetings with an accountant, lawyer, insurance representatives, and other appropriate advisers may prevent costly mistakes in both personal and professional financial dealings.

Office Information Systems

Any mechanism that helps you organize your work is a system. Within a medical practice, there are many such systems that help make the office efficient and effective. A patient-scheduling system, for example, is designed to make optimum use of physician and staff time, while minimizing patient waiting. During the last decade, computers have revolutionized many office systems. While today's efficient medical practices do not necessarily use computers, within a few years they will be a staple feature of any doctor's office. Therefore, familiarity with them will be a must. Regardless of whether an office currently has automated or manual systems, there is one key to the success of any system: all personnel, physicians and staff, must be willing to modify their own personal preferences for the benefit of the total practice. Because computerization will be an intricate aspect of offices in the future, its effect on medical practice is discussed here. Then three examples of office systems are reviewed: patient scheduling, medical records, and communication.

The three most prevalent uses of computers in medical practice are (*a*) recording and retrieving patient and clinical information; (*b*) performing financial and administrative functions; and (*c*) accessing medical information data bases. Automated clinical information systems are now available to record physician notes, medical summaries, prescriptions, laboratory and x-ray findings, and health maintenance information. These systems are still in their formative stages, but large group practices are beginning to move toward automating medical information for both patient care and clinical research. Practice management was the initial area of computerization for medical practices. Computerized management systems include billing, bookkeeping, and insurance form preparation, and have expanded into appointment scheduling, word processing, and financial forecasting. Perhaps the most innovative and practical application for the medical office practice is the access to national medical information data bases. Through a computer-telephone device called a modem, a communications program can access in-

Table 7.6. Practice Profile of a Typical Family Physician[a]

Annual practice revenue	$250,000
Annual practice expenses	$150,000 (60%)
Staff payroll	$75,000
Physician net income	$100,000
Employees per physician	3.5
Ambulatory care encounters per year	5,100
Patient care visits (hospital, office, other) per week	140
Office visits per week	110
Professional activities (hours/week)	60
Patient care activities (hours/week)	55
Office hours (hours/week)	35
Weeks worked per year	48
Total professional hours worked per year	2880
Income per hour worked ($100,000 income/2880 hours worked)	$34.72

[a]Based on data from the Medical Group Management Association and the American Medical Association physician surveys.

formation from a variety of sources. The American Medical Association has a medical information system that was designed to enhance physicians' ability to deliver cost-effective, quality care. The system is AMA/NET, which is part of the GTE TELENET Medical Information Network.

PATIENT SCHEDULING

Appointment scheduling policies provide clear guidelines to receptionists regarding new patients, return visits, and special procedures. The appointment system is a contract between patients and the practice, and all parties, especially physicians, should honor this contract. Once a schedule is planned, preferably at least 2 months in advance, changes should be kept to a minimum. This will require vacations and other out-of-office commitments to be planned before the schedule is prepared. If patients are not keeping appointments, appropriate follow-up to determine the cause and to reinforce the importance of respecting the scheduling system is needed. Even though many visits can be scheduled, the practice should always have appointments available for patients' urgent care needs.

MEDICAL RECORDS

Physicians are responsible for documenting personal and medical information during their clinical encounters with patients. The medical-legal implications of medical records and the informational needs of other physicians and staff in a group practice are two important reasons to establish and maintain a top-quality medical records system. Often quality of care and physician competency are judged by reviewing the medical records of a practice. The medical record is the legal property of the physician and/or the practice; however, the patient or the court, under subpoena, has the right to all information in the record.

COMMUNICATIONS

The overall effectiveness of any office practice is tied closely to the various communications systems within the practice. These systems include hardware, such as telephones and word processors, and management features such as meetings. For example, intraoffice communications among staff and physicians are facilitated by having the appropriate equipment, such as multiple telephone lines and intercom equipment at each nursing station. Regular meetings between the staff and physicians provide a structured time to discuss topics pertinent to the delivery of care. Regular meetings should also be scheduled among all physicians in a group practice, and between the physician–medical director and the practice manager to discuss the efficient running of the practice.

Another type of communication involves feedback from patients. This can take the form of periodic surveys to patients about how the practice is operating and may result in valuable suggestions for improvements. Written materials to patients, in the form of letters to new patients, practice newsletters, and health education articles, provide another way for the practice to communicate with its public.

Marketing Health Services

In the past, marketing has taken a low profile in the medical profession because of physicians' unwillingness to advertise themselves and because of their attitude that professional competence and reputation were enough to attract and retain patients. But as the health care field moves from a cottage industry to large-scale corporate organizations, and as competition increases, medical practices will need to market their physicians and their services. Health care marketing can be defined as the process through which patients and physicians exchange services for fair compensation to the mutual benefit of both. As consumers, patients will benefit if their health needs are identified and treated at a reasonable cost. Physicians will benefit if patients use the services they offer, if they receive a fair financial return for their services, and if their work is gratifying.

ETHICS OF MARKETING

The historical code of behavior for physicians stated that advertising or any overt marketing approach was unethical. A commonly heard phrase was "our good medicine will be our marketing program." In 1979 the Federal Trade Commission ordered the United States medical profession, represented by the American Medical Association (AMA), "to cease and desist from restricting, regulating, declaring unethical, or interfering with advertising medical services." This action was followed by the adoption of a new set of principles of medical ethics by the AMA in 1980. These revised standards emphasize the physician's responsibility to provide relevant information to patients and the public. The principles also establish physicians' rights to choose whom they serve and the environment in which they offer their services.

Physicians faced with the dilemma of how to market their services ethically should consider the following questions:

• Are patients' wants and needs clearly understood and being addressed by the practice? How do you know this?
• Has every attempt been made to inform patients about ways to maintain a healthy lifestyle?
• Are patients receiving appropriate medical care regardless of their method of reimbursement or ability to pay?
• Is the practice continuing to improve the medical services offered in terms of quality of care, cost-effectiveness, and patient satisfaction?

Marketing begins with the consumer. If physicians are to market their services ethically, they must be responsive to the changing profile of their consumers and offer the highest quality patient care at the most reasonable cost.

MARKETING STRATEGIES

The competitive environment of health care, along with the trend toward more convenient, affordable medical services necessitates that physicians take a more active approach to marketing their practices. A comprehensive marketing program for a medical practice includes: (a) product considerations, such as the range of services and the differentiation of services to specific consumer segments; (b) pricing policies such as prepaid plans, or industrial contracts; (c) location factors such as accessibility and proximity to other ser-

vices; and (d) promotion efforts such as public relations and patient education. An overview of the four dimensions of a marketing program along with the consumers' perspectives is presented in Figure 7.1.

CONCLUSIONS

The U.S. health care system as late as 25 years ago was inexpensive and relatively simple. In just two decades, it has become a complex, high-technology, and high-finance industry. Physicians have seen their personal judgments restricted by policies and regulations. The cottage-industry mode of operation that was prevalent throughout most of this country's history has evolved into a medical-industrial (pharmaceutical) constellation of enterprises.

Even though physician autonomy has been reduced, there are favorable aspects to these developments. Overall quality of care may be improved. Cross-coverage arrangements provide more free time for the average physician. Entrepreneurism, which in its most basic definition means creating something of value (and receiving rewards when client needs are satisfied) has been preserved. It is quite likely that physicians who work as entrepreneurs and as managers can have a greater impact on medical practice than at any time in the past.

The business of medicine may not be a high priority for medical students and residents during their education and training. As the business of medicine moves into a time of increased competition, cost-containment, and alternative methods of financing, it will be imperative for physicians to incorporate management knowledge and skills into their professional education. Dr. Harold Rypins, a physician-author writing in the middle of this century, stated that the medical profession

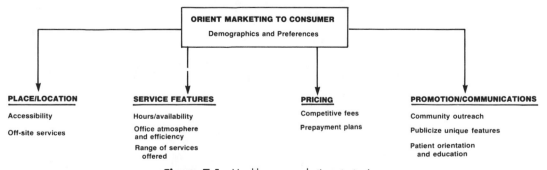

Figure 7.1. Health care marketing strategies.

should recognize the importance of business principles, because a business orientation emphasizes the systems concept. And, if medicine were practiced systematically, the quality of patient care and the quality of the physician's professional life would be greatly enhanced (2).

Now, such changes are occurring. If primary care physicians want to maintain their rightful position as leaders of the community health care system, they should consider implementing as many of the following organizational and management features in their practice as possible:

- Compassionate, communicative staff of physicians and office personnel.
- Regular health team that is held in high regard by the public.
- Accessible location with adequate parking and minimal waiting time.
- Multispecialty professional services including laboratory and x-ray facilities.
- Multiple financial options, including prepayment plans and industrial contracts.
- Inclusion of other health professionals such as family nurse practitioners, nutritionists, counselors, and physical therapists.
- Computerization for efficient financial procedures and to enhance diagnostic and clinical activities.
- Health and wellness programs, within both the practice and community.
- Affiliations with other health care organizations and community agencies.

REFERENCES

1. Bibace R, Beattle KA, Catlin RJ: Psychological aspects of the problem of time in practice management. *Continuing Educ Fam Phys* 18:293–298, 1983.

2. Wolf GD: *The Physician's Business: Practical and Economic Aspects of Medicine*, ed 3. Philadelphia, JB Lippincott, 1949, p xiii.

SUGGESTED READINGS

Aluise JJ: *The Physician and Manager*, ed 2. New York, Springer-Verlag, 1987.

A practical and easy-to-understand guide to the economic and management issues important to physicians and other health care professionals. Contents include marketing, computerization, personnel supervision, financial management, leadership, office systems and communication, and professional relations. Appendices supplement each chapter with further details, guidelines, and examples that are currently in use in community medical practices.

Council on Long Range Planning and Development: The environment of medicine. In *The Report of the Council on Long Range Planning and Development*, ed 4. Chicago, American Medical Association Council, 1985.

This report is published every other year by the AMA Council on Long-Range Planning. According to the 1985 report, some of the most common themes describing the environment of medicine are cost pressures, increasing potential for economic dislocation in the medical care environment; politicization of health policy, and increased influence on medicine by forces in the government and general society.

Longest BB: *Management Practices for the Health Professional*, ed 3. Reston VA, Reston Publishing Company, 1984.

Provides an introduction to organizational theory and management practices as they relate to the organized delivery of medical services. Applies traditional organizational and management concepts to the medical practice setting within the following topics: planning and decision-making tools for practice management, informal aspects of management, coordination and controlling, and managing change.

chapter 8

EXAMINING SMALL CHILDREN
Philip D. Sloane and Simone S. Sommer

Examining children is a skill that takes time to develop. Experience teaches the physician to make a reliable global assessment that the child "looks sick" or "looks well," and to recognize subtle signs that suggest one diagnosis or another. With experience comes comfort in conducting the interview and examination, making it easier to allay anxiety in children and their parents. Nevertheless, even beginning students can use approaches that will generally make such examinations go smoothly and generate the best possible information.

RELIEVING ANXIETY

A child in the physician's office is often anxious. Babies are the exception; they rarely exhibit anxiety and are thus a joy to examine. In toddlers, anxiety manifests itself as a general feeling directed at strange people and strange situations. Once children get beyond their second birthday, they tend to have less general anxiety; instead they fear losing control or remember prior painful or unpleasant experiences in the doctor's office. The parent may also be anxious about the child's physical condition, which the child will often perceive as well.

Helping a child and parent feel comfortable can be challenging. If the physician is anxious (an almost unavoidable situation in medical students and residents doing their first pediatric evaluations), a perceptive child will pick up these feelings. Thus, you are encouraged to try to approach the patient with ease and comfort; be relaxed.

TAILORING YOUR EXAMINATION TO THE AGE OF THE CHILD

Your approach should vary depending on the child's age. Between birth and about 9 months, infants are usually trusting and cooperative. The physician can often readily take, play with, hold,

and examine a child as a parent would. By 6 months, children grab nearly anything with their hands, and it is helpful to have a toy or other object to divert the child's attention from a stethoscope. Beginning at 8 or 9 months, however, children clearly identify physicians as strangers and often become anxious and fearful.

Between 9 months and 2 years, many children will still be calm and cooperative so long as the physician is unhurried, informal, and gentle, speaks softly, and moves slowly. Some children, however, will be anxious and irritable, particularly if they are ill or in pain, and they will not be reassured by a calm, gentle, unhurried approach. Doing your examination with the child in a parent's lap helps; occasionally you will need to hold the child down briefly for one or another part of your examination.

By 24 to 30 months, children begin to respond more rationally to speech and can better control their fears. In these children, negativism and reluctance can often be reduced by having parents discuss the office visit beforehand. They can role-play and even reverse roles so that the child can be "doctor." Then, the nurse can follow up by previewing the procedures that will probably be performed and by explaining everything that will be done. The physician should follow similarly, demonstrating examination techniques on the mother or father or on the child's extremity before moving on to the more sensitive chest, ear, and so on.

A child old enough to sit up often prefers to be examined sitting. Invite the child to sit on the parent's lap or to have a parent hold her/his hand. The pediatric lap examination, in which a child is examined totally in the parent's lap, is ideal for small children and should be learned by all medical students. Older children can be examined on an examining table, but take care not to position yourself between the child and parent(s).

Whatever the child's age, you should attempt to complete the examination without physical restraint. Forcible restraint can terrify children, many of whom perceive a forceful examination as an assault. Giving the child some control of the examination (by choosing where to sit, for example) often enhances cooperation. If the child needs to be restrained, explain gently and lovingly that it is done to help him or her hold still, since such a thing is so hard for one so young to do alone. After the restraining period, the examiner should always give the child some positive feedback.

HISTORY AND INITIAL OBSERVATION

The examination begins with your first look at the child and whoever else is present. Take mental notes of this situation. Note the placement and activity of the child. Is the child clutching a parent? Is the child whining and listless or rummaging through the drawers and office equipment? Attempt to sense the parents' emotional state: Are they anxious, indifferent, angry? It takes time to understand age-appropriate activity; so practice making a mental estimation of the child's age before questioning the parent. Shake the parent's hand and introduce yourself to the child. Younger children will often enjoy having their heads gently stroked, and others will usually welcome an invitation for a handshake or "slap me five" introduction. Very anxious children, however, will prefer that you initially keep a distance.

The examination should follow a thorough but not prolonged history-taking session. Obtain the history while the child is on a parent's lap or playing in the room. Begin with an open-ended inquiry, such as "Tell me what has been happening . . ." or "What is your main concern about . . .(use the child's name as much as possible)." Determine the relationship of the adult to the sick child and inquire into who is the primary caretaker of the child. Occasionally, a grandparent or other relative will bring the child to the office while the primary caretaker is at work, which can make it difficult to take a complete history.

Try to convey to each child that the visit is primarily between the two of you, with the parent as an important coparticipant. Thus, children should be involved in the history from an early age (e.g., "Susie, do your ears hurt? Can you point to which

one?"), and by age 7 or 8 they should provide the primary history, with the parent being turned to only for additional information afterward.

As you approach completion of the history, gradually move closer to the child. Be aware that encroachment on "personal space" can be threatening, and be as reassuring and calm as possible.

ORDER OF THE EXAMINATION

The order of the examination is important, since children often become fussy or impatient. In protesting or anxious infants and children, examine the most relevant part of the body first. In calm children, start by examining areas that involve the least discomfort and manipulation. Thus, the child should be observed, walking if desired, and the extremities, chest, heart, nodes, neck, head, skull, and fontanelles should be examined. It is important to auscultate the chest and heart early in the examination, since far less information can be gathered from a crying child than from one who is quiet. All necessary equipment should be at hand before starting the examination.

The general appearance of the child will have already been observed during the history. Next, examine the skin. Have the parent disrobe the child, including shoes and socks (this can be done while you are taking the history). As you inspect the child, gently stroke the skin for rashes, lymph node enlargement, and areas of tenderness. Examine the head, skull, and extremities first, proceeding to the trunk. Many young children like to search for their belly button, and this can sometimes be done in a playful manner.

Next, examine the chest and heart, starting with the posterior chest and moving anteriorly. Always warm your stethoscope before placing it on the child's chest. In anxious children, allay fears by letting the child hold the stethoscope prior to the examination. If the child is very anxious, first place the stethoscope on the child's hand or foot, or perhaps auscultate the parent or another sibling first. When listening to breath sounds, you can elicit deep inspiration by giving the parent a piece of paper and having the child play a game of blowing the paper over while you auscultate. Another amusing distraction (for children 9 months and older) is having the child "blow out" a pen light.

Next, you will need to choose between two areas that can involve some discomfort, namely the ears/throat/face and the abdominal/genital/hip area. By this point you will have a good idea whether the child will cooperate with these portions of the examination. Recruit nursing assistance to hold the child if you perceive that a struggle will ensue.

Examining the abdominal area first is less traumatic and is usually preferable. If the child is under 4, seat yourself facing the seated parent with your knees touching the parent's knees. Have the child lie with her/his head and upper back supported on the parent's lap and buttocks supported by your knees. If a diaper is present, remove the anterior portion but keep it easily accessible, especially if examining a male baby. Place older children on the examining table, but once again have the parent adjacent and holding the child. Lying down and looking up at a giant adult can be rather intimidating, and therefore a familiar face is reassuring.

First, gently percuss and then palpate the liver and spleen. Then palpate the remainder of the abdomen and the inguinal and genital areas. Optimum relaxation of abdominal muscles can be achieved by holding the child's legs in one hand, rotating the flexed knees in a circle while your free hand gently palpates the abdomen. In males, check for testicular location and tenderness. If a rectal examination is performed, remember to use your little finger and lubrication. Examining the hips for dislocation and subluxation is uncomfortable and often induces crying, so do it near the end of the examination.

Finally, move to the ears, face, and throat. Examine the ears before the mouth; the occasional child who cries during the ear examination will have his or her mouth open and ready for viewing.

Examining the Ears

Careful examination of the ears is critical in evaluating a febrile child. The approach should be systematic, beginning by palpating behind both ears for mastoid tenderness and swelling, and by examining for cervical and preauricular lymph nodes. Next, the ear canal should be examined. Recall that an otoscope has two heads, an open surgical head and a closed diagnostic head. Generally, the diagnostic head should be used, with a rubber bulb and tubing attached for insufflation. To achieve an airtight seal, a small ring of rubber tubing can be cut from the otoscope bulb tubing and slipped over a small speculum tip as seen in Figure 8.1. Always use the biggest speculum possible; it is safer and more comfortable to the child.

In a sick child, one inflamed tympanic membrane will dictate your prescription. Follow-up when the child is feeling well is more important for evaluating both drums, and wax removal is much easier in a healthy child.

Wax can be bothersome and frustrating when you need to view a child's eardrum. Ear wax is either sticky or dry, and the consistency of the wax provides some help in deciding how it should be removed. Occasionally, gentle movement of the ear speculum will cause dry wax to open like a valve and enable you to clearly visualize the eardrum. If wax removal proves to be necessary, a number of tools are available:

- A cotton-tipped swab (Q-tip) or nasopharyngeal swab can be inserted blindly, with care not to insert the tip more than halfway to the drum. Rotate the swab to avoid pushing wax further into the ear.
- A blunt ear curette (wire or plastic loop) can be used under direct observation through the surgical head of an otoscope, and is quite helpful in removing discrete pieces of wax.
- Irrigation with a 5- or 10-ml syringe and tubing cut from a scalp vein intravenous kit can be attempted in any rational and cooperative child. Surprisingly young children, some less than 2 years of age, have been successfully irrigated.
- Suction powerful enough to remove wax is available in many otolaryngologists' offices but rarely in family physicians' offices.

Wax that is sticky and gummy is best removed with a cotton applicator or an ear curette. Dry wax is most amenable to curette removal or to irriga-

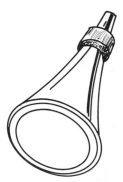

Figure 8.1. Otoscope head with sleeve of rubber-tubing.

tion. If you do not suspect a perforated eardrum, adding a little hydrogen peroxide to the irrigation water will help loosen the cerumen. If the cerumen remains impacted, a few drops of Debrox in the office can occasionally clear the occlusion.

Adequate clearing of the external ear canal can be an arduous process, requiring perseverance and dexterity. You must exercise extreme care, as an inadvertent movement by the child may result in injury. Always protect any instrument from going too far into the ear canal by bracing the hand you hold it with against the child's head. Even without significant injury, bleeding may result that may cause pain to the child, embarrass the physician, and prevent adequate visualization of the eardrum.

Once wax has been cleared, try again to visualize the eardrum. Recall that the ear canal is curved and must be straightened by pulling the pinna backward to visualize the tympanic membrane. Newborns have poorly formed cartilage in the ear canal; thus, the tympanic membrane is often difficult to visualize in infants under 4 months of age. Also, remember that the inner one-third of the ear canal is extremely sensitive to touch; so, be careful not to insert the speculum too far.

For the ear examination, position young infants on their abdomen, with the head turned to one side on the examining table (Fig. 8.2). From about 8 months of age to 2 years, children can be examined seated in a parent's lap, with the parent restraining the child's chest and arms with one arm and steadying the head with the other hand (Fig. 8.3). Older children who cannot be restrained like this should be restrained lying prone with the head turned. This usually takes two adults; one to hold the buttocks and legs and the other to restrain the head and arms. If a child is uncooperative, it is

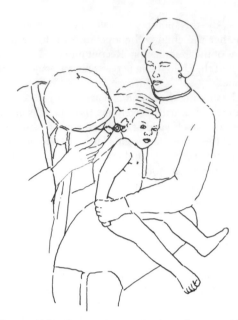

Figure 8.3. Otoscopic examination of young child restrained in parent's lap.

preferable to properly restrain the child than to risk injury during the examination.

Once the tympanic membrane is visualized, it should be systematically examined. First note its color and translucency and look for fluid. The normal color is grayish-pink, which can become injected with infection or crying. The drum is normally translucent but may become opaque with repeated infections. Often, serous otitis media is diagnosed by observing bubbles of air or fluid behind a translucent drum. Next, the contour of the drum should be observed carefully. Fullness usually appears first at the periphery, causing disturbance of the normal light reflex. A grossly bulging or retracted eardrum always has an abnormal or absent light reflex. Finally, pneumatic otoscopy should be performed, observing for mobility of the drum. Lack of mobility is often produced by an inadequate seal of the ear canal, but true abnormalities (bulging or retraction) are the commonest causes of eardrum immobility in a properly performed examination.

CONCLUDING THE EXAMINATION

At the conclusion of the examination, verbally console or reward the child, and acknowledge that the examination is over. Also, acknowledge the parents for assistance and commend them on tech-

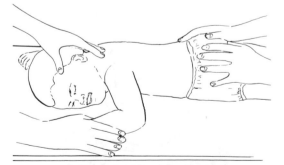

Figure 8.2. Method of restraining an infant for otoscopic examination.

niques that aided your examination. Never mislead a child before the examination is finished by saying to the child that "this is the last thing," and then carrying out many more noxious procedures. Instead, be honest during the examination, and mark the finale.

Once the examination is over and you have made your assessment, clearly outline the positive physical findings and plan with the parents, using principles of effective patient education (see Chapter 17). Be careful to use terms that are familiar to the lay public. Visual aids and printed patient education materials can help parents understand the pathophysiology, severity, treatment, and warning signs associated with their child's illness. If laboratory tests are needed, explain your reasons and the information that will be obtained. If medications are prescribed, write their names and dosage schedule on a piece of paper and/or place explicit directions on the prescription label (for details on prescription writing, see Chapter 12).

Inform the parent and child when you would like the child to return. It is often beneficial to also write this down on the paper with the medication instructions. In addition, outline any important warning signs that you want to be notified about. Then allow the parent to ask questions. At the conclusion of the entire visit, acknowledge the child and inform her/him of your next visit. A reward from the physician, such as a sticker or small toy, is a nice compensation for the child's tribulations.

CONCLUSIONS

Plan ahead, be systematic, and be gentle in examining all young children, especially those who are ill. Elicit the child's and the parents' cooperation as much as possible. Communicate the assessment and plan clearly and concisely. A properly performed physical examination will traumatize a child minimally, while yielding accurate and valuable information for the physician.

chapter 9

CARING FOR THE ADOLESCENT PATIENT

Philip D. Sloane

Adolescence (approximate ages 12 to 20 years) provides a transition from childhood to adulthood. It is a time of rapid physical and psychological change. Among the tasks of adolescence are achievement of physical maturity, development of independence from the family, formation of sexual identity, vocational planning, and identity development. Adolescence is sometimes divided into three stages: *early adolescence* (approximate ages 11 to 14), which corresponds to the junior high years; *middle adolescence* (approximate ages 15 to 17), which corresponds to the high school years; and *late adolescence* (ages 18 to 21), the years immediately following high school, in which individuals attend college and/or enter full-time work.

The adolescent patient provides particular challenges for family physicians. These patients come to physicians' offices relatively infrequently, yet they often have unmet health needs. Because access to health services is often difficult for adolescents, the physician should seek to make the most of each office visit and seek outreach through the schools. Establishing rapport, identifying the patient's real concerns, and carrying out health education are among the most important priorities for each physician-patient encounter.

ADOLESCENTS—AN UNDERSERVED POPULATION

Studies indicate that the U.S. health care system fails to meet the needs of many adolescents. Teenagers are often either unwilling or unable to contact physicians on their own, in part because access to physicians' offices requires initiative, transportation, money, and time away from school. For adolescents who are shy and withdrawn, the task of making these necessary arrangements constitutes a significant barrier to

seeing the physician. In addition, getting to the doctor often requires discussing a potentially sensitive problem with a parent, who makes the appointment, and this itself can be a major barrier to seeking care.

Adolescents often report dissatisfaction about their encounters with physicians. It appears that physicians and adolescents often have divergent opinions about what the *real* health care priorities are for a given encounter. Since adolescents are often not as articulate as adults, physicians should listen especially carefully and allow longer time for adolescent visits. This rarely happens however; one observational study of pediatricians found that they only averaged 7 seconds of anticipatory guidance per patient, and that the typical visit lasted a little over 8 minutes (1).

FAMILY PHYSICIANS AS PROVIDERS OF ADOLESCENT HEALTH CARE

Family and general practitioners see more adolescent patients than any other medical specialty (35% of visits)(2). Pediatricians are second (23% of visits); however, many pediatricians are uncomfortable with such common adolescent health issues as performing a pelvic examination or counseling about contraception (3). The ability to provide continuity of care throughout the entire transition to adulthood, combined with the ability to know other family members, allows family physicians to better understand and serve the needs of their adolescent patients.

Teenagers often prefer a family physician's office to that of a pediatrician, because they are not required to sit in a waiting room full of small children and decorated with "little-kid" motifs. On the other hand, some teenagers—as part of "growing up"—prefer to go to a new physician (e.g., female patients often choose a woman physician), breaking ties with their family physician or pediatrician. What they typically seek, however, is a physician whom they can trust and who treats them with respect.

The most common reasons teenagers see family physicians are acute illnesses and physicals for camp or school. These visits should be viewed as opportunities to make contact about a wide range of health issues and to seek to identify unmet health needs among your adolescent patients. To further gain access to adolescents, one can serve as a team physician for the local high school and/or participate in a school-based clinic.

COMMON HEALTH PROBLEMS OF ADOLESCENTS

The health problems of adolescents include many of the same diseases and problems that affect children and adults. A few medical problems, such as acne and infectious mononucleosis, are particularly prevalent among teenagers. In general, however, the adolescent in the medical office needs health maintenance, advice about minor medical complaints, reassurance, and health education.

Nearly all adolescents have some *acne*, and most are concerned about its effect on their appearance. Many fail to ask their physician for help with their acne, yet wish that the physician would bring the subject up (4). Treatments include regular cleansing, topical keratolytic lotions or gels (benzoyl peroxide or Retin-A), topical antibiotic solutions (clindamycin, erythromycin, or tetracycline), and low-dose systemic antibiotics (tetracycline or erythromycin).

Infectious mononucleosis is another medical illness that is most common in adolescence. Caused by the Epstein-Barr virus, it generally presents with fever, fatigue, and severe tonsillitis. Posterior cervical lymphadenopathy is generally present. There may also be signs of mild hepatitis (anorexia, dark urine, light stools, and right upper quadrant tenderness). Diagnosis is made using an office assay for antibodies (the Mono Spot test), but physicians should be aware that it may take up to 10 days for the test to turn positive. Treatment is generally supportive, but some authorities recommend a short course of systemic steroids if the initial presentation is particularly severe. Complications to be monitored for include splenomegaly (which, if present, should be monitored weekly and should lead to restriction of physical activity) and thrombocytopenia.

PROBLEMS WITH A MAJOR PSYCHOSOCIAL COMPONENT

The biggest health problems of adolescents are psychosocial, arising in response to cultural, family, environmental, and developmental factors. From a national perspective, the magnitude of these problems is immense. Among health problems of adolescents that have a major psychosocial component are pregnancy, substance abuse, sexually transmitted diseases, depression and suicide, accidental injury, eating disorders, and violence. These problems are briefly discussed below; general techniques for prevention are discussed in Chapters 17 and 18.

Accidental Injury. Automobile accidents are the number one killer of adolescents. Half of these deaths are associated with alcohol. Many more would be prevented if teenagers regularly wore seat belts. Motor vehicle injuries are more common among white adolescents than among blacks (5).

Depression and Suicide. Situational depressive symptoms are common in adolescence and can be difficult to separate from clinical depression. A positive family history is an important clue to significant depression. Suicide is actually less common in adolescence than in adulthood, yet it remains one of the leading causes of adolescent death. Impulsive suicide attempts are frequent among adolescents and should be interpreted as serious appeals for help.

Substance Abuse. Most substance abuse begins in adolescence. Among 1987 high school seniors, 29% smoked cigarettes within the past month, 66% had consumed alcohol within the past month, 39% reported engaging in binge drinking, 21% were current marijuana users, 57% reported having tried an illicit substance before graduation, and 3% reported current cocaine use (5). Substance abuse is a major factor in school failure, depression, accidental injuries, sexual promiscuity, and the transmission of AIDS. (See Chapter 37 for further discussion of substance abuse.)

Eating Disorders. Disorders such as anorexia nervosa and bulimia generally have their onset during adolescence. *Anorexia nervosa* is a complex disorder in which patients believe themselves to be fat in spite of significant weight loss due to voluntary food restriction and purging behaviors. Treatment is difficult and generally requires a multidisciplinary team. *Bulimia*, consisting of episodes of binge eating accompanied by self-induced vomiting, is frequent among late-adolescent women.

Clinical clues include wild fluctuations in weight and signs of repeated vomiting (e.g., parotid hypertrophy, dental enamel erosion). Treatment should generally be provided jointly by the family physician and a psychiatrist or psychologist.

Violence. Violence is a part of everyday life for many adolescents. Homicide is the leading cause of death among black males aged 15 to 19. Sexual, physical, and emotional abuse are more common among adolescents than among younger children. The effects of abuse include poor school performance, depression, anxiety, and chronic somatic symptoms such as headaches, abdominal pain, chest tightness, and insomnia (5).

Pregnancy. By age 16, 29% of boys and 17% of girls have had sexual intercourse. These figures rise to 65% of boys and 51% of girls by age 18. About half of adolescents used no contraceptive the first time they had intercourse. It is not surprising, therefore, that 20% of sexually active 15 to 19-year-olds get pregnant. Of these pregnancies, 90% occur in unmarried women, and most are unintended; half are electively terminated, and the remainder are carried to term. In 1987, there were 472,623 births to adolescent mothers. Frequently, the fathers fail to provide emotional or financial support for the child. These teenage mothers are more likely than their peers to drop out of school, to become single parents, and to become dependent on welfare (5).

Sexually Transmitted Diseases (STDs). STDs are contracted by 2.5 million adolescents each year (5). Simple office screening is available for gonorrhea and chlamydia, two common and treatable STDs. Several viral STDs are not curable, notably, genital herpes and diseases caused by the human immunodeficiency virus (HIV), the virus that causes the adult immune deficiency syndrome (AIDS). In the 1990s, HIV infection has begun to spread to increasing numbers of adolescents, including heterosexuals. This is in part because adolescents, more so than adults, tend to see themselves as invulnerable and, therefore, fail to heed advice to limit their number of sexual partners and to use condoms and spermicide. Thus, adolescent education about STDs should be a major focus for physician and public health workers in the 1990s.

APPROACH TO THE ADOLESCENT PATIENT

Establishing rapport with adolescent patients can be challenging. Allow some informal time at the beginning of the visit to chat about relatively impersonal topics, such as school or hobbies. Provide the adolescent with adequate time to explain what she or he would like to accomplish during the visit, and then address each concern seriously. Among the helpful interview techniques with adolescents are open-ended questions, reflection, restatement, summation, and reflection. Some adolescents may not speak easily, and you may need to be very directive and focused in your interview. Be alert for hidden agendas (concerns that are not directly stated).

Continuity of care from childhood allows the family physician, as the patient grows older, to gradually introduce more autonomy into the physician-patient encounter. However, even in the teenage years, when the patient should be seen alone, the physician should maintain strong lines of communication with the parents. Often, parental asides during visits for other problems can alert the physician to potential issues that involve an adolescent family member.

Privacy and Confidentiality

Caring for adolescent patients can lead to dilemmas of confidentiality, because adolescents are in the process of obtaining independence yet are generally still bound to their parents. Your patient's parents may provide transportation, pay for the visit, and accompany the patient; so they may feel that they deserve to know the content and outcome of the encounter. On the other hand, a confidential patient-physician encounter is a critical tenet of effective primary medical care, and there is no doubt that the adolescent—not the parent—is the patient.

No hard-and-fast rules exist about managing confidentiality, but here are a few guidelines:

- Laws vary from state to state regarding the age at which physicians can treat adolescents independent of parental consent.
- Be explicit about confidentiality. Tell both the parent(s) and the adolescent patient that what either shares with you in confidence will be kept in confidence unless you obtain permission to share it with the other. Ideally, this discussion should take place with both parties present, so that there are no misunderstandings.
- By age 12, always see the patient alone for at least a portion of the visit. Some physicians instruct the office nurse to place the adolescent in the room alone. Others allow the parent to be present for a portion of the history, and

then ask the parent to leave for the "physical examination."

- When a parent has come to the office with a teenager, at the end of the visit ask for the patient's permission to discuss your recommendations with the parent. Only in rare situations will the matter be so delicate that the adolescent will object. However, in these situations the patient's wishes should be respected, with the only exception being a situation where someone's health and/or life is threatened.
- Try to maintain openness whenever possible. When adolescents do not want you to share information with their parents (and vice versa), there may be underlying family problems. Be aware that lack of openness when there is conflict between an adolescent and a parent may lead to the physician becoming triangulated (see Chapter 3) to draw attention from family dysfunction.

Assessment of Growth and Development

Adolescence is a time of rapid physical and psychosocial growth. The physical changes of adolescence, which occur over several years, are termed puberty and culminate in physical maturity. These changes include achievement of adult height, development of body hair, and sexual maturation. In girls, puberty begins between ages 9 and 13, with the average age of onset of puberty being 10.5 years. In boys, puberty begins on average about 2 years later, with onset occurring between ages 11 and 15. In girls the first sign of puberty is breast bud development; in boys the first sign is testicular enlargement.

These physical changes should be systematically monitored during adolescent health examinations. The best way to do so is to note and record the patient's sexual maturation using the system developed by Tanner (Figs. 9.1 and 9.2)(5). The Tanner system records the development of secondary sex characteristics on a 5-point scale, with 1 representing preadolescent and 5 representing adult morphology. Tanner staging is useful in evaluating complaints of short stature, in determining whether or not puberty is delayed, and in counseling patients about current and upcoming events (e.g., menses typically occurs at Tanner stage 4).

Discussing Psychosocial Issues

Psychosocial health should also be monitored. To do so involves inquiring about the four major tasks of adolescence: development of independence from the family (with stronger reliance on peers), formation of sexual identity, vocational planning, and development of a positive self-image. Exploring these areas in a limited office visit is tricky and requires being sensitive to the adolescent's degree of comfort and sense of rapport. However, a considerable portion of the office visit should be devoted to these sensitive psychosocial topics.

The most important health issues for adolescents are often very personal ones, such as decisions about sexuality and birth control, relationships with their peers and parents, depression, eating disorders, and substance abuse. As you move onto these topics, start with the less personal (home, school, and friends) and proceed to the more sensitive (drugs, sex, depression). In opening up a new topic, general questions can be helpful. For example, one way to begin a discussion of drug use would be to ask if the patient knows people at school who are using alcohol or drugs.

Physical Examination

The most important thing about physical examinations in adolescents is that most teenagers are easily embarrassed. This is particularly true of the breasts, abdomen, and genitalia. It helps to ask about embarrassment before the examination. It also helps to be extremely careful about gowning and draping the patient so that most of the patient is covered throughout the examination. Finally, giving information (e.g., "talking through" your abdominal examination, or explaining self-examination during the breast examination) can help reduce patient discomfort.

The examination itself is performed in a similar manner to that of other age groups. A few tips to keep in mind are

- Examine the breasts in both sexes, but consider skipping this portion of the examination in early adolescent girls, who tend to be very embarrassed. Adolescent boys often develop some gynecomastia, occasionally with tenderness below the nipple; explaining that this is normal can be reassuring.
- Screen early adolescents for scoliosis (see Chapter 15).
- Routinely check the genitalia in boys as you check for inguinal hernias. This allows you to screen for sexually transmitted diseases (STDs), to point out normal development, and to teach

Stage	Genitalia	Comments
1	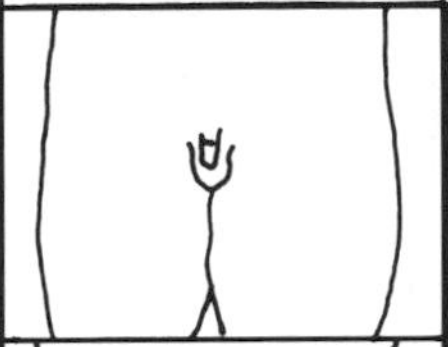	Preadolescent penis and testes; no pubic hair
2	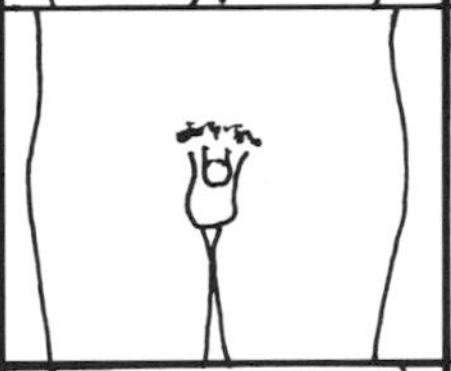	Scant, straight pubic hair; slight penile enlargement; scrotum enlarged and developing texture due to testicular growth; height spurt begins
3	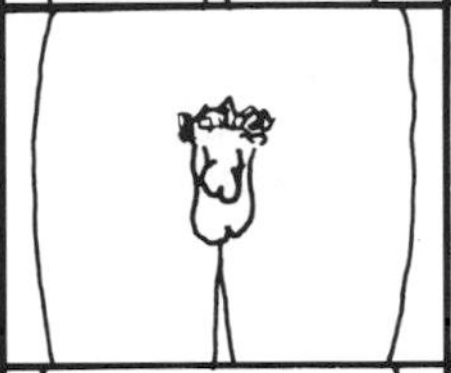	Sparse, darker hair, beginning to curl; Penis longer; testes larger; sperm production has begun
4	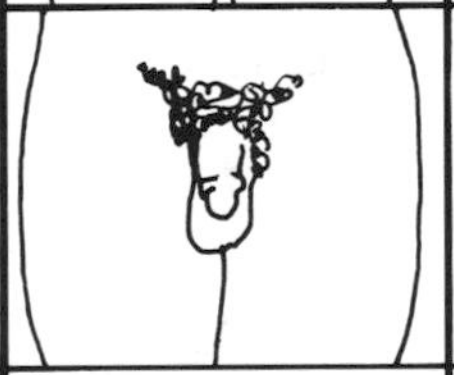	Curly hair covers pubic region; glans and penile shaft increase further in size; testes larger with scrotum darker; adult height generally is obtained.
5	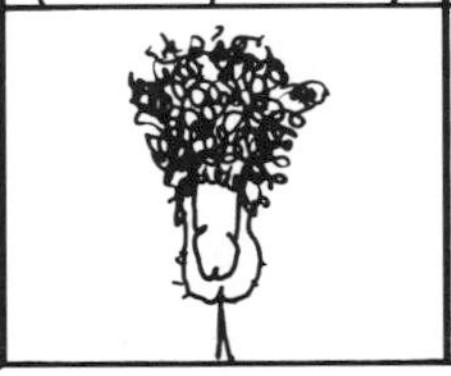	Hair spreading to medial thighs and toward umbilicus; penis and testes are adult in appearance

Figure 9.1. Tanner stages of sexual maturity in boys. (Adapted from Strasburger VC, Brown RT: *Adolescent Medicine: A Practical Guide.* Boston, Little, Brown & Co., 1991.)

testicular self-examination. If your patient develops an erection during the examination, mention that this happens occasionally and not to worry about it.

The *first pelvic examination* should ideally be performed just before a girl becomes sexually active or before she reaches age 18. Beginning in early adolescence, discuss the forthcoming need for a first "pelvic" and explain that you want to see her if she begins thinking about becoming sexually active. In this manner, your patient will have been prepared at previous visits for the first pelvic examination.

The examination itself should be done slowly and with plenty of explanation. If you are a male physician and you have a female partner in your practice, consider asking your patient if she would prefer to have your partner perform the examination. Use a small speculum, unless the patient is sexually active and is relaxed. After taking the Pap test and any appropriate cultures or slides, be sure to arrange a way to communicate the results to the patient. Finally, give positive feedback after the examination is completed.

Closure and Follow-up

At the end of the visit, summarize your impressions and recommendations. Allow time for questions. In outlining your treatment plans, make it clear that you expect the adolescent to be responsible for following up on your recommendations; treat your adolescent patients as adults, and encourage them to accept responsibility like adults.

Stage	Breasts	Pubic Hair	Comments
1	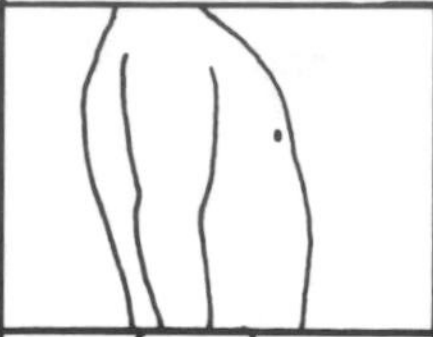	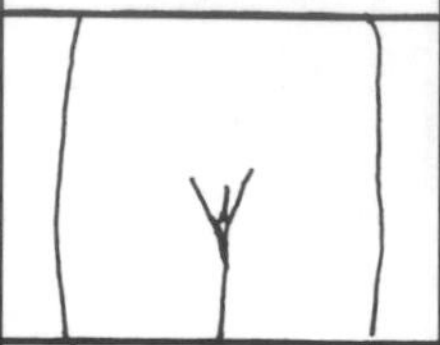	No pubic hair or breast development
2	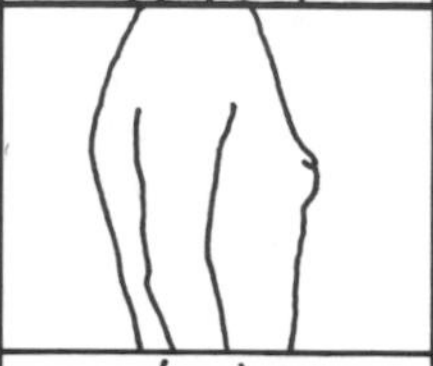	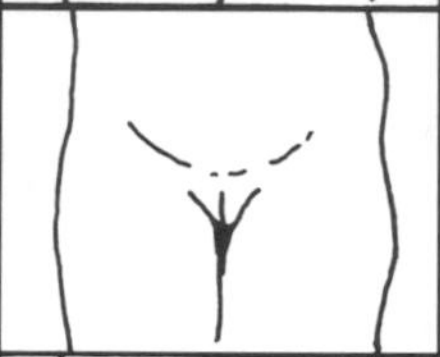	Sparse, straight hair at medial border of labia; breast bud present; growth spurt begins
3	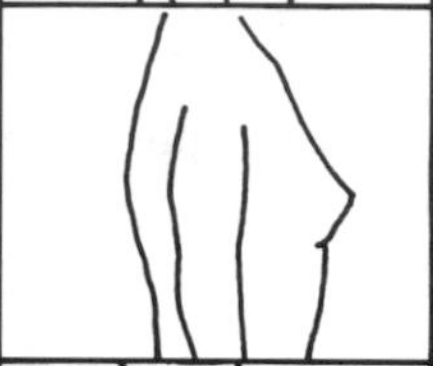	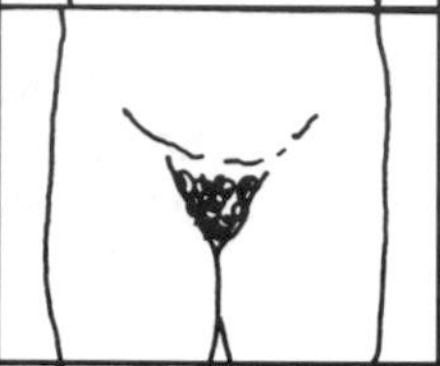	Darker hair, beginning to curl; breast and areola enlarged but with minimal contour
4	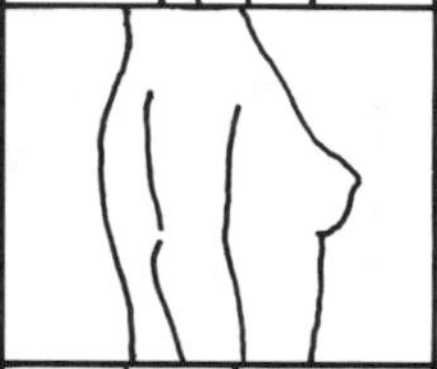	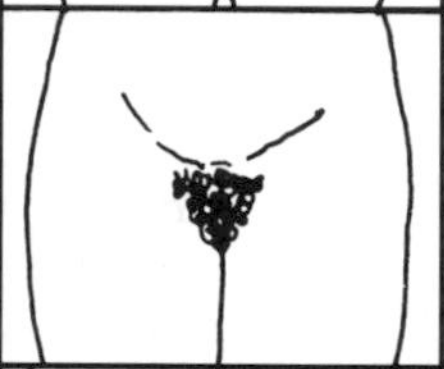	Coarse, curly hair but less than adult; areola and papilla form secondary mound; menarche occurs
5	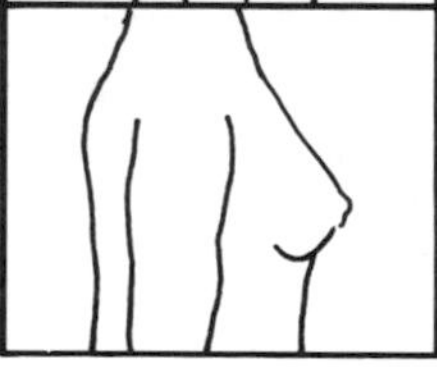	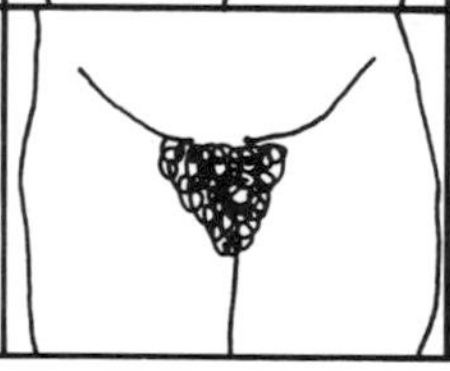	Adult triangle, with hair spreading down medial thighs; nipple projects, mature breast contour

Figure 9.2. Tanner stages of sexual maturity in girls. (Adapted from Strasburger VC, Brown RT: *Adolescent Medicine: A Practical Guide.* Boston, Little, Brown & Co., 1991.)

Ask your patient to schedule a follow-up appointment if one is needed, and invite the patient to phone if she or he has questions. If appropriate, speak with the parents and thank them for bringing the adolescent in. Finally, remember that teenagers especially appreciate a follow-up phone call or card telling them the results of a test or checking up on a problem that was worrying them.

INNOVATIONS IN THE DELIVERY OF SERVICES TO ADOLESCENTS

Because it is widely acknowledged that many adolescents have unmet health needs, a number of new strategies have been developed to better serve these patients. These include adolescent health care clinics, free clinics, comprehensive programs, and school-based health centers.

Adolescent health care clinics are specialty clinics, generally based in hospitals or health maintenance organizations. They typically employ a team, including a physician and a nurse practitioner, and focus primarily on physical (as opposed to psychosocial) health. They commonly serve as training sites for medical students and residents, a practice that has been shown to increase the dissatisfaction of adolescent patients (2).

Free clinics are relatively scarce and rely on volunteer health care providers. They do, however, often provide care in urban areas where services are particularly thin.

Comprehensive programs are also rare, but a few are quite successful. The Door in New York City, for example, employs dozens of professionals and offers medical care, mental health services, social services, drug prescriptions, recreation, legal services, creative arts, and employment training. Only a fifth of its annual budget is provided by fee-for-service and Medicaid; the remainder comes from grants.

School-based clinics in junior highs, middle schools, and high schools may offer the most promising model for reaching underserved adolescents. Such clinics require support from the school administration and the local school board. Start-up funds are typically provided by grants, and continuation requires a creative combination of contributions (e.g., the schools typically provide space and pay utilities, and they occasionally provide a nurse), grants, and fees. School-based clinics tend to be primarily managed by nurse practitioners; physician involvement can be very helpful. Parents must give blanket consent for a student to use the clinic with full assurance of confidentiality; over half of parents typically do so. Among the services offered by such clinics are general primary health care, laboratory work (including pregnancy tests), physical examinations for sports or work, immunizations, chronic illness management, prescriptions, diagnosis and treatment of sexually transmitted diseases, nutrition education, sexuality and pregnancy counseling, mental health counseling, weight reduction programs, family counseling with students and parents, drug and substance abuse programs, and parenting education.

The most common reasons students come to school-based clinics are acute illnesses, injuries, mental health problems, and preventive services.

Reproductive services (contraception, pregnancy testing and counseling, and evaluation of sexually transmitted diseases) are provided in about 12% of visits (2). These services can be controversial, however, and may be met with community resistance if publicized.

CONCLUSIONS

Adolescents are infrequent visitors to the physician's office. Therefore, each contact should be looked upon as a rare and important opportunity to evaluate development and to screen for problems. When seeing adolescent patients, listen for and respond to their own concerns. Allow extra time, if necessary, to explore psychosocial issues such as sexuality and alcohol/drug use. Continuity of care and good communication skills provide the best mechanism for building trust and, consequently, for helping your adolescent patients.

REFERENCES

1. Reisinger KS, Bires JA: Anticipatory guidance in pediatric practice. *Pediatrics* 66:889–892, 1980.
2. U.S. Congress, Office of Technology Assessment: *Adolescent Health—Volume III: Crosscutting Issues in the Delivery of Health and Related Services*, OTA-H-467. Washington, DC, U.S. Government Printing Office, June 1991.
3. Tolmas HC: Adolescent pelvic examination. *Am J Dis Child* 145:1269–1271, 1991.
4. Strasburger VC, Brown RT: *Adolescent Medicine: A Practical Guide.* Boston, Little, Brown & Co., 1991.
5. Gans JE, Blyth DA, Elster AB, Gaveras LL: *America's Adolescents: How Healthy Are They?* Chicago, American Medical Association, 1990.

chapter 10

APPROACH TO THE GERIATRIC PATIENT

Darlyne Menscer and Beatrice B. Leitch

Currently, 15 to 20% of all visits to family physicians are made by people 65 years of age and older. This figure is expected to increase as the proportion of elderly rises. In 1900, only 3.1 million persons, or 4% of the population, were 65 or older. By the year 2000, 38 million persons (13%) will be in this age group, and by 2040 this figure is expected to increase to 55 million (18%). In fact, the age group older than 75 represents the fastest growing segment of the United States population. Life span, defined as the maximum number of years that human beings seem capable of surviving, appears fixed at around 100 years. As a result, society will be comprised of more and more older persons—many of whom will have significant chronic illnesses and functional limitations—but relatively few individuals who will pass the century mark. Providing adequate care for these older Americans may require considerable medical resources. Therefore, it is imperative for tomorrow's physicians to be familiar with the essentials of geriatric medicine.

How is the elderly patient different? What special skills and attitudes are needed when you encounter the elderly patient? We hope that the subsequent sections of this chapter will assist you in answering these questions so that you will be better prepared to manage the care of your elderly patients.

INITIAL ENCOUNTER

Ideally, the initial encounter between a physician and an elderly patient should lay the foundation for a mutually satisfying long-term relationship. Recognize that the elderly patient may have had many interactions with physicians over the years—some pleasant, others not. Put the elderly patient at ease by demonstrating a caring, professional attitude, which should facilitate the development of trust and rapport. Except in a medical emergency, the initial encounter should take place in an unhurried manner. Even so, at the end of the first visit you will probably have an incomplete data base. Subsequent visits will be needed to collect all the pertinent information.

Just as older patients may initially view their new physician with apprehension and uncertainty, physicians too may have preconceived notions of elderly persons. Myths about the elderly include that their medical problems are beyond help; that they are unproductive members of society; that they have lost interest in their own sexuality; and that they are invariably "senile" and noncompliant. Physicians may believe that the vast majority live in nursing homes (actually 95% of the elderly live at home) and may become impatient or even angry with patients who move rather slowly, give rambling answers to questions, and do not hear well. They may be anxious to move on to a "fixable" patient. These attitudes, if present, will likely come across to the elderly patient.

ASSESSING THE GERIATRIC PATIENT

The elderly vary widely—much more so than younger persons. You should anticipate this variability and be prepared to conduct your assessment in a flexible manner, probably over several visits. The assessment includes the traditional clinical approach of history, physical examination, and appropriate laboratory investigation. The history and physical examination should include an assessment of the patient's functional abilities, special needs, and ability to cope in his environment.

History

Early in the encounter, make a general assessment of the patient's ability to communicate, by evaluating hearing, comprehension, mental status, and speech. A general conversation about the reasons for the visit will often reveal major problems. Asking the patient to repeat his date of birth or street address to "update the medical record" (or some other data that the physician can confirm) is an additional way to quickly assess these areas. Such informal methods of screening for communication and mental status problems are ideal for the primary care setting. If problems are identified or suspected, formal testing can be done at a later time. Furthermore, if the patient is felt not to be a reliable informant, a history would need to be obtained from family members or caregivers.

The elderly patient may present with a single chief complaint or a general "I don't feel well." Frequently, your review of systems will reveal multiple problem areas and needs. You should be sure to elicit the patient's agenda and expectations. Some elderly patients will be quite candid and articulate their thoughts; others may require much more time and assistance to verbalize their expectations and needs. If significant problems are reported to you by a family member or health professional but not by the patient, you should consider evaluating the patient for dementia and/or depression.

The past medical history may be extensive and difficult to obtain. Old medical records can be valuable but often are not available. Questionnaires can be used to provide much of the past history, family history, and review of systems; the patient's employment history, including occupational exposures, should also be included. If the patient cannot read and write, well-informed family members or caregivers can assist in completing these forms. Although questionnaires can help to focus the history on significant facts, they should not be used as a substitute for the medical interview.

A crucial component of the history is assessment of *activities of daily living (ADLs)* and *instrumental activities of daily living (IADLs)* (Table 10.1). ADLs and IADLs are crucial to maintaining independence at home, with ADLs being more basic. Studies have shown that loss of independence in ADL and IADL function is directly correlated with the need for family care and with placement in a long-term care facility. Since maintenance of independence is an important aspect of care for older persons, thorough assessment of IADL and ADL function should be an integral part of the geriatric medical examination. In assessing ADLs and IADLs, probably the most revealing information can be obtained

by asking the elderly person, "How do you spend a typical day?" Multiple functional abilities can be assessed from responses to this question. To assess specific ADLs and IADLs, questions such as those listed in Table 10.1 can be used.

Exploring these aspects of daily living is essential to assess the patient's ability to cope in her or his current environment. Problems with such activities as ambulation and toileting provide important information about the influence of chronic diseases such as arthritis, dementia, or cerebrovascular disease on the elderly patient. Also, undiagnosed illness in the elderly frequently presents in nonspecific and insidious ways; therefore, new or increasing difficulties in ADLs and IADLs should be identified and investigated. Finally, you will be able to evaluate patient responses to treatment by noting any changes in functional abilities.

The family history should emphasize the availability and stability of social supports rather than familial diseases. This may clarify for you who the important family members are or have been. It will also provide insight into the elderly patient's experience with chronic disease and death in the family. Many individuals and services can form a network of social support for older persons, including spouse, children, other family members, neighbors, friends, volunteers, social service agencies, home health care agencies, Meals on Wheels, senior citizen centers, adult day care, and churches/synagogues.

When a dependent patient's social support system is limited or fragmented, watch for signs of care giver stress, which may present as subtle abuse or neglect. In addition to overt physical signs, abuse may be manifested as noncompliance with medications, treatments, or follow-up visits; spending the patient's money inappropriately; or preventing the patient from having easy access to eyeglasses, a cane, or a hearing aid. Because abuse and neglect are often hidden, the physician must maintain a high index of suspicion. Ideally, prevention of such problems focuses on identifying and working with caregivers, who are in stressful situations. Encouraging caregivers to explore options outside the family for support helps to relieve the considerable stress of daily responsibilities for an elderly patient.

Lastly, obtain a thorough medication history. Elderly patients are 3 to 7 times more likely than younger patients to suffer a side effect of a medication or drug interaction. Individuals aged 65 and older consume approximately 25% of all prescrip-

Table 10.1. Assessment of Activities of Daily Living and Instrumental Activities of Daily Living

Activities of daily living (ADLs)

Ambulation	How do you get around the house? Any trouble climbing stairs? Any falls? With injury? Do you use an assistive device—i.e., cane, quad cane, or walker?
Eating	Do you eat a special diet or specially prepared foods? Any problems eating or cutting meats? Do you use special instruments to eat?
Bathing	Do you have any problems bathing? Are you able to bathe all parts of your body? Any problems getting in or out of the shower or tub by yourself?
Dressing	Do you have any problems with dressing, such as zippers or tying shoes? Does someone help you dress or select your clothes?
Toileting	Any problems getting on or off the toilet? Is the toilet close to your bedroom? (Inside your house?) Do you use a bedside commode or urinal? Any problems controlling your urine when you cough or sneeze? Any dribbling? Any "accidents" with your urine or bowels?

Instrumental activities of daily living (IADLs)

Transportation	How did you get to the office today? Do you drive? At night? Have you ever used special-transportation vans or buses? Do you have a handicapped license plate?
Money management	How far did you go in school? (Can the patient read and write?) Who pays the bills and manages the money? Do you receive special assistance funds or have Medicare or Medicaid?
Meal preparation	Who prepares the meals? Do you get a delivered meal? Who does the grocery shopping? (Who else lives in the patient's house and is there adequate food for all?)
Housework	Who does the housework? The laundry?
Telephone use	Do you have a telephone? What is the number to call if you had a fire or needed an ambulance? Who in your family would you call for help in an emergency? What is the number?
Medications	What medicines do you take each day? How do you take each? Any nonprescription medicines? Do you use childproof caps? Do you use a medicine box? Who fills it?

tion medications and an even higher proportion of nonprescription drugs. Elderly patients living at home often may take up to 12 medications each day. Thus, all current medications should be reviewed at each visit, including those that are over-the-counter and those prescribed by other physicians. This is best accomplished by asking the patient to bring all medications to each visit and then asking how each medication is taken. If the patient cannot read the labels or if there is a concern that medication errors are likely to occur, medication boxes can be used and filled by family members or home health nurses. For additional details on obtaining a medication history, please see Chapter 12.

Medications are a common cause of symptoms and disability among older persons. For this reason, the physician should always consider whether medication could be responsible for patient symptoms or be contributing to functional difficulties. It is also important to consider whether any medications can be stopped without adverse effects or objections by the patient or family.

Physical Examination

The physical examination of the geriatric patient differs from the traditional physical examination of younger adults. Those aspects which are particularly important for the elderly patient include: (a) mental status; (b) hearing; (c) speech; (d) condition of the teeth and gums; (e) skin; (f) joints; (g) feet; (h) gait; (i) the presence of orthostatic (postural) hypotension; (j) evidence of atherosclerosis: hypertension, bruits, signs of congestive failure, reduced or absent pulses; (k) signs of neoplastic disease (skin and internal organs); and (l) signs of other diseases unique to the elderly, such as temporal arteritis, polymyalgia rheumatica, and benign prostatic hypertrophy.

Like the history, the physical examination of the elderly patient focuses on functional abilities. Observe the patient entering the examining room, noting what assistance, if any, is required. Watch the patient perform tasks such as removing shoes, rising from a chair, and walking in the room. To accommodate patients with physical impairments, compromises in the usual office routine may be needed.

Vital signs are an important part of each visit. If orthostasis is suspected by history, determine the blood pressure and heart rate in both supine and standing positions. When taking a patient's pulse, do so for a full minute to assess for abnormalities in rate and rhythm which may not otherwise be detected. Weight, obtained at each visit, is a good indicator of nutritional status and a useful method of monitoring edema in chronic disease. Many patients who use wheelchairs can stand long enough to be weighed in the office.

Anatomic and physiological changes that commonly occur with aging may be evident on the physical examination. Some of these changes are reduced elasticity and dryness of the skin; rigidity of the blood vessels (producing bruits and elevated systolic blood pressure); reduced muscle bulk and skeletal mass; and diminished or absent deep tendon reflexes. These and other changes can make it difficult for you to distinguish what is benign (and a part of the aging process) from what is pathological (and therefore significant). A summary of these and other aging changes appears in Table 10.2.

Changes in systemic blood pressure with aging deserve special attention. Population studies indicate that the mean systolic blood pressure rises progressively with age, whereas diastolic blood pressure levels off or even falls beyond age 55 to 60. Combined systolic-diastolic hypertension (defined as systolic pressure greater than 160 mm Hg, with diastolic pressure greater than 95 mm Hg) affects approximately one-third of American adults 65 years and older. Pure systolic hypertension (defined as systolic pressure greater than 160 mm Hg with diastolic pressure less than or equal to 90 mm Hg) is fairly unique to the elderly, affecting approximately 10% of those 65 years and older. Although pure *systolic hypertension* increases the risk of stroke and heart disease, treatment is often difficult. The risks of tight control (e.g.,

Table 10.2. Some Normal Body Changes with Aging

Skin	Elasticity decreases, producing wrinkles. Easy bruising occurs, especially in sun-exposed areas. Thinning occurs, especially on extremities, leading to easy tearing with minimal trauma.
Hair	Graying—>50% of Americans have >50% gray hair by age 50. Distribution—thins on scalp, axilla, pubic area, and on upper and lower extremities. Decreased facial hair in men, but women may develop chin and upper lip hair.
Nails	Decreased growth rate.
Body build	Increase in body fat and decrease in body water. Decrease in height caused by intervertebral space narrowing.
Bones	Some demineralization occurs in all elderly but is greater in women and in Caucasians.
Joints	Range of motion decreases somewhat, although exercise may be beneficial. Wearing down of joint surfaces is common, especially in hips, knees, and fingers.
Muscles	Loss of muscle mass and strength is common, but exercise may minimize loss.
Eyes	Thickening of lens (cataracts) is almost universal by the 70s but may not require removal if vision is not impaired for functions important to patient. Lens accommodation decreases (presbyopia) by age 45. The pupil does not admit as much light. Peripheral vision decreases. Tearing decreases, which may cause easy irritation.
Hearing	Age-related hearing loss (presbycusis) affects the inner ear, leading to loss of high-frequency sounds. About 50% of elderly have enough hearing loss to affect communication abilities.
Teeth	Gum disease is more common than decay, but little dental care and absence of fluoridation in their younger years has led to much tooth loss in today's elderly.
Mental function	Stamina and speed decline with age, but judgment and wisdom increase. Mild memory loss (such as names) is common but only progresses if disease is present. Older persons can learn new information, but more slowly than when younger.
Sleep	Stage IV sleep is reduced in comparison with younger adults. Spontaneous awakening occurs more frequently, causing many elderly to sleep shorter periods. Total sleep needed in 24 hours is approximately 1 hour less than for younger adults, but older persons spend more time in bed to acquire that sleep.
Cardiovascular system	Systolic blood pressure increases with age, due to increased peripheral vascular resistance. Diastolic blood pressure increases until about age 55, then plateaus or decreases.
Respiratory system	Decreased pulmonary elasticity and increased airway resistance occurs. There is less ventilation at lung bases and more at the apex.
Digestive system	Reduced gastrointestinal motility causes constipation to be more common.
Urinary system	Glomerular filtration decreases with age. Nocturia is common in both men and women. Incontinence becomes more frequent, but is not a part of normal aging.
Reproductive system	Male: prostate enlargement is virtually universal. Testosterone production decreases, leading to decreased testicular size. Phases of sexual arousal are slower, and refractory time is longer. Female: estrogen production decreases at menopause; therefore, the vaginal lining atrophies and the canal may narrow and shorten. Vaginal secretions become more alkaline.

dizziness and falls) may outweigh the benefits for some patients. However, such treatment has recently been shown to reduce morbidity and mortality in large populations.

Mental status evaluation is another area that requires emphasis in the elderly. The increasing prevalence of Alzheimer's disease and related degenerative brain diseases with advancing age makes screening for early dementia a reasonable goal of primary care practice. Gross cognitive impairments can sometimes be recognized while taking the history. In other instances, however, detailed questioning about memory, orientation, intellectual function, judgment, and affect will be necessary to uncover subtle cognitive dysfunction. Much to the physician's surprise, a pleasant and cooperative, seemingly competent elderly patient may be found to be profoundly disoriented and forgetful on formal mental status testing. There are no clear guidelines about which geriatric patients should receive formal mental status evaluation; however, such testing should be performed on all patients beyond age 80, as well as younger patients in whom cognitive impairment is suspected by informal screening. A number of simple mental status screening instruments are available; one of the most popular is the *mini-mental state* (Fig. 10.1). Family physicians are encouraged to choose one, become familiar with it, and use it consistently in encounters with elderly patients.

Laboratory and Other Special Studies

As with any patient, laboratory studies should be chosen carefully. You should always ask the questions: How will the results of this test alter therapy? Do the potential benefits outweigh the cost and potential risk? Although comprehensive laboratory panels are used frequently for screening purposes, they may not always be cost-effective for the elderly patient, especially if a single abnormal value on a test leads to the "need" for further evaluation.

The results of many laboratory tests performed on elderly patients can be evaluated according to the standards set for younger patients. There are, however, several notable exceptions with which you should be familiar. These include:

- Because of reduced muscle mass, the serum creatinine level underestimates true renal function, which does decline with age. Creatinine clearance must be considered in dosing medications

correctly for the elderly patient. The following formula gives a good estimation of the elderly patient's creatinine clearance (ml/min):

$$\frac{(140 - \text{age}) \times (\text{weight in kg})}{(72) \times (\text{Cr in mg/dl})}$$

- Total iron binding capacity (TIBC) decreases with age; therefore, a serum ferritin level or a bone marrow analysis are better ways to diagnose iron deficiency anemia in the elderly.
- An estimated 10 to 20% of otherwise healthy elderly adults demonstrate autoimmune phenomena such as antinuclear antibodies, thyroid antibodies, positive rheumatoid factor, and positive VDRL.
- Glucose intolerance is common among the elderly. Postprandial serum glucose may be elevated and of little clinical significance. The diagnosis of diabetes mellitus is best made in the elderly patient with a fasting serum glucose determination, using a value of 140 mg/ml as the upper limit of normal. A glycosolated hemoglobin determination will give an estimate of average serum glucose over the previous 1 to 2 months and is a better indicator of glucose control than any single value.

Radiographic studies should be selected with care. The elderly are particularly susceptible to iatrogenic dehydration, for example, as a result of the laxatives and fasting restrictions needed to prepare for contrast studies of the gastrointestinal tract.

ADDRESSING THE PROBLEMS OF THE GERIATRIC PATIENT

A list of problems and needs—possibly quite lengthy—should be generated as you obtain the history, complete the physical examination, and perform any necessary laboratory or radiographic studies. Some problems, such as adverse reactions to drugs, sleep disturbances, muscle and joint pains, and depression, are common among the elderly regardless of their functional status. Patients with significant functional impairments (e.g., strokes, advanced dementia, or severe heart failure) may have common "geriatric" problems such as frequent falls, decubiti, and urinary and/or fecal incontinence.

Regardless of the elderly person's current situation, however, your major objective should be the

Scoring: 1 point per correct answer. Fewer than 24 correct strongly suggests dementia.

		Item	Score
Orientation			
1-5	"What is today's date?" (ask specifically parts omitted)	1. Date	_____
		2. Year	_____
		3. Month	_____
		4. Day of week	_____
		5. Season	_____
6-10	"Can you tell me the name of the place where we are today? What floor are we on? What town are we in? What county are we in? What state are we in?	6. Institution	_____
		7. Floor	_____
		8. Town (city)	_____
		9. County	_____
		10. State	_____
Registration			
11-13	Ask if you may test memory. Use 3 objects: ball, flag, and tree. State them slowly and clearly. Ask for them to be repeated. The first repetition determines the score (0-3), but continue until repeated correctly (maximum 6 tries)	11. "Ball"	_____
		12. "Flag"	_____
		13. "Tree"	_____
Attention and calculation			
14-18	"Begin with 100 and count backwards by 7." Stop after 5 subtractions (65). Score the total number of correct answers. If the subject cannot perform this, ask him to spell "world" backwards, scoring the number of letters in correct order.	14. "93"	_____
		15. "86"	_____
		16. "79"	_____
		17. "72"	_____
		18. "65"	_____
		alt. "dlrow"	_____
Recall			
19-21	"Now recall the 3 words I asked you to remember"	19. "Ball"	_____
		20. "Flag"	_____
		21. "Tree"	_____
Language			
22-23	Naming: Show and ask the names of: wrist watch, pencil	22. Watch	_____
		23. Pencil	_____
24	Repetition: "No ifs, ands, or buts"	24. Repetition	_____
25-27	3-stage command: Give the subject a blank sheet of paper and say "Take the paper in your right hand, fold it in half, and place on the floor"	25. Takes	_____
		26. Folds	_____
		27. Places	_____
28	Reading: Print "close your eyes" in large letters and have the subject read it. Score correct only if eyes close.	28. Reading	_____
29	Spontaneous writing: Ask the subject to write a sentence on a sheet of paper	29. Sensible sentence with subject/verb	_____
30	Copying: "Draw this figure". All 10 angles must be present and 2 intersect	30. Draws pentagons	_____
	TOTAL SCORE		_____

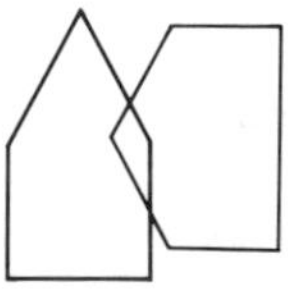

Figure 10.1. A mini-mental status examination. (Modified from Folstein MF, Folstein SE, McHugh PR: "Mini-mental state": a practical method for grading the cognitive state of patients for the clinician. *J Psychiatr Res* 12:189–198, 1975.)

prevention or postponement of functional deterioration. If you work within the conventional "medical model," the problem list may be dominated by components such as "elevated serum cholesterol," "systolic hypertension," and "small left varicocele." Often, however, these problems are of little concern to the patient in comparison with such complaints as constipation, poorly fitting dentures, or the cost of daily medications.

We recommend that your problem list identify three categories of problems: (*a*) medical, including both diagnoses and unexplained findings; (*b*) functional, such as aphasia, incontinence, or impaired gait; and (*c*) psychosocial, such as isolation, poverty, or caregiver stress. Once the patient's problems and needs have been identified, it may be necessary to negotiate with the patient the order in which they should be addressed.

Considerable time and expertise may be required to adequately address the problems of the elderly and to formulate reasonable management plans. It is difficult to explore and address all medical, psychological, social, economic, and family issues during routine office or hospital visits. A complex patient will probably be better managed when the physician works as a part of a team that includes (*a*) other health professionals, such as other physicians, a nurse practitioner, a social worker, home health nurse, dietitian, or clinical pharmacist; (*b*) family members or caregivers; (*c*) neighbors or friends; (*d*) other community resources, such as adult day care staff, Alzheimer's support groups, or Hospice. In the hospital and in specialized geriatric assessment clinics, the multidisciplinary care team is based in the same location and generally meets regularly. In primary care office practice, such teams are less formal and generally communicate by telephone. The physician must actively organize and coordinate such services.

HOME VISITS

Home visits are an essential part of geriatric medicine. More than any other group of patients, the elderly benefit from having a physician who is willing to make house calls. Many patients can benefit from home visits—especially those with multiple medical problems, those with behavioral problems, and those who are homebound because of chronic, debilitating disease. Home health agencies can help monitor such patients, but occasional physician visits are needed for overall assessment or for the management of new problems. A home visit allows the physician to see and understand the realities with which the patient lives. Subsequent office visits may take less time after a home visit, because the physician now knows exactly which questions are most pertinent to ask to assess changes in function. In conducting a home visit, it is important to clarify with the patient and family what can be accomplished, so that unrealistic expectations—such as performing an ECG—are prevented. You will need to rely on your observation and communication skills and the limited equipment in your bag—often only a stethoscope and sphygmomonometer. If appropriate goals are negotiated in advance, however, home visits can be very rewarding and beneficial to both you and your patient. For a more detailed discussion of home visits, please refer to Chapter 6.

HEALTH MAINTENANCE

Although general adult health maintenance is discussed in Chapter 16, there are specific issues to address with the elderly patient. Screening for functional abilities, social support problems, unnecessary medications, and drug interactions should be done at most visits. At least yearly, you should inquire about your patient's habits, including smoking and other tobacco use, alcohol intake, diet, and exercise. Immunizations for influenza, pneumococcal disease, diphtheria, and tetanus should be documented and kept up to date.

Screening for increased serum cholesterol is probably helpful in younger adults, but its usefulness in persons over the age of 70 is uncertain. Regardless, many elderly patients are concerned about their cholesterol and may wish to be treated with diet and even medication. Treating patients who have clear evidence of atherosclerotic disease (such as coronary artery or peripheral vascular disease) may be appropriate at any age. As with all health maintenance issues, discussing the risks and benefits of any intervention with your patient is essential.

For younger women, Pap smears are recommended yearly until three are normal and then every three years thereafter. Screening Pap smears are now covered by Medicare; however, many older women have had few if any pelvic examinations in their lives and may be reluctant to agree to this procedure. Pelvic examinations are needed in the evaluation of incontinence and may reveal vulvar disease and abdominal or pelvic masses of which the patient is unaware. At least one pelvic examination with a Pap smear should be done on all women over 65 who are able to cooperate and for whom it would be reasonable to offer therapy for any discovered abnormalities. If this Pap smear is normal, the need for further Pap smears can be negotiated with your patient, taking into consideration her sexual history and other pertinent factors.

A breast examination by a physician and a mammogram are indicated yearly for all women over the age of 65. However, mammography is probably not appropriate for the patient who has serious medical problems or who would not want therapy for any cancer that might be identified. Flexible sigmoidoscopy is recommended for screening for colon cancer at least every 3 to 5 years, beginning at age 50. This fairly expensive procedure is not yet covered as a screening procedure by most insurers, including Medicare. Flexible sigmoidoscopy also requires considerable patient cooperation and tolerance of some discomfort. Therefore, your patient should be fully informed and agree that the cost is worth the reassurance that a negative test would provide, and that she or he would want further evaluation of polyps or other abnormalities discovered.

An important component of health maintenance for older persons is for the physician to discuss and document how the patient would like to be treated if she or he is incompetent to participate in therapeutic decisions. Older persons generally have given considerable thought to their future and appreciate the opportunity to discuss their wishes and concerns with you as a routine part of their office visits. As of December 1, 1991, with the implementation of the Patient Self Determination Act, all competent adults admitted to hospitals, nursing facilities, home health agencies, Hospice programs, or any facilities that receive Medicare or Medicaid funds will be informed of their right to accept or refuse medical or surgical treatment. They will also be asked if they have an *advance care directive*—usually a living will or health care power of attorney. *Living wills* allow patients to express the desire to not have their lives prolonged by extraordinary means if they are in a terminal or incurable condition and, in some states, if in a persistent vegetative state. In some states (e.g., North Carolina) it is also possible to refuse artificial nutrition and hydration in the situations in which a living will applies. A *health care power of attorney* (HCPOA) is a document that allows patients to choose who should represent them when medical decisions are to be made, if they are ever unable to do so themselves.

When designating power of attorney, patients should explain their wishes to the designated individual, using a written values *statement*.

Advance directives should be discussed with the competent patient before an emergency arises, so that the decisions made later will be consistent with the patient's desires and values. Copies of a living will and/or health care power of attorney should be placed in the patient's chart. Documentation of discussions about the patient's wishes may be useful, even if the patient never completes any advance care directive documents.

LONG-TERM CARE PLACEMENT

Even with a devoted family and excellent home health services, a time may come when the patient's everyday needs can no longer be provided in the home. When this occurs, families and patients generally appreciate having their family physician continue to provide primary care services in the rest home, home for the aged, or nursing home.

CONCLUSIONS

Health in the elderly is defined as the ability to live and function autonomously in society. It is not the absence of disease. Improving and maintaining function, not diagnosing and curing disease, is the primary role of the physician in geriatric care. As such, there are many ethical issues to consider in working with the elderly. Modern medical technology now allows the physician to intervene in many chronic disease processes, but such interventions do not necessarily improve quality of life. In order to appropriately advise and manage the care of your elderly patients, you must examine your own feelings about the aging process and end-of-life issues.

Providing quality care for your elderly patients can be both rewarding and frustrating. You should recognize that it is not always appropriate to "fix" every problem and that the wishes of your patient must always be considered. Comfort may be the most important goal. Lastly, you need not work alone in addressing the problems and needs your assessment has identified. Other members of the health care team should be included to provide the best care possible to your elderly patients.

SUGGESTED READINGS

Abrams WB. *The Merck Manual of Geriatrics*. Rahway, NJ, Merck Sharp and Dohme, 1990.

A concise, inexpensive text with good index for quick reference.

Cassel CK, Riesenberg DE, Sorensen LB, Walsla, JR (eds): *Geriatric Medicine*, 2nd ed. New York, Springer-Verlag, 1990.

A comprehensive text that has information about most geriatric topics.

Ham RJ, Sloane P (eds): *Primary Care Geriatrics*, 2nd ed. Chicago, Mosby-Yearbook, 1992.

A comprehensive yet highly readable introduction to geriatric problems common in family practice and general internal medicine. The text features over 100 case vignettes, which introduce and illustrate major concepts.

Kane RL, Ouslander JG, Abrass IB: *Essentials of Clinical Geriatrics*, 2nd ed. New York, McGraw-Hill, 1989.

A soft-bound, inexpensive text with many helpful tables.

Mace N, Rabins P: *The 36 Hour Day*, rev. ed. Baltimore, John Hopkins University Press, 1991.

A guide for family members caring for demented patients, which has much to teach physicians.

chapter 11

PRIMARY CARE OF THE ATHLETE

K. Bert Fields

Beginning in the 1970s, record numbers of adult athletes chose to participate in sports like swimming, running, tennis, aerobics, cycling, and racquetball. Currently, one in three American adults exercises daily. At the same time, pediatric and adolescent women's sports activity grew dramatically. Boosted by Title 9 legislation, female athletic participation in high school sports increased an astonishing 700% in the 1970s, compared with the previous decade. Now, even after excluding individuals in physical education classes, more than 25 million US children compete in organized athletics. Inevitably these trends are associated with a greater number of athletic injuries.

Family physicians see athletes of all ages for examinations and injury assessment. To perform these tasks effectively, the family physician must understand (*a*) the role of the preparticipation examination, (*b*) how to assess and manage sports injuries, and (*c*) how the sport, training, treatment, and injury rehabilitation interact. This chapter discusses these concepts.

PREPARTICIPATION SPORTS EXAMINATIONS

The main objective of middle and high school preparticipation examinations is to reduce specific risks of athletic competition (rather than to pick up disease). Sports examinations should be conducted as standard doctor-patient visits. Mass examinations with a multistation format do not allow the athlete and doctor to develop rapport. Privacy not only shows respect for the adolescent athlete's dignity but also allows them the opportunity to ask sensitive questions.

History. Studies consistently demonstrate that the clinical history provides the bulk of diagnostic information during preparticipation examinations. Essential information to assess the risk of participating in sports can usually be obtained by asking the questions outlined in Table 11.1.

These questions screen for serious medical conditions that might cause sudden death, such as hypertrophic cardiomyopathy or heat stroke. They also identify athletes at risk for common problems like exercise-induced asthma or an injury that has been inadequately treated. A positive answer to any of these questions should prompt a more thorough inquiry.

Physical Examination. A brief physical examination should assess the three most common abnormal findings that occur on preparticipation examinations. These are elevated blood pressure, heart murmurs, and orthopaedic problems—particularly an abnormal knee examination. Additional evaluation should focus on areas of concern raised during the history, including anatomical areas placed at increased risk by the patient's chosen sport. Laboratory tests such as urinalysis rarely identify athletes who are at increased risk during sports participation and often produce false-positive results.

Recommendations and Follow-up. After the examination, the patient's participation level in the sport is decided. Possibilities include clearance for participation in specific sports; clearance for all sports; reexamination after specific diagnostic testing, rehabilitation, or therapy; or disqualification. Studies demonstrate that only 1% of athletes merit disqualification. Most athletes want and should be offered a second opinion when denied medical clearance.

The physician should provide recommendations for follow-up. Most states mandate yearly preparticipation evaluations. This recommendation allows the physician to review the status of injuries that occurred in the previous year; update

Table 11.1. Key Questions to Ask during a Preparticipation Examination

Question	Risk Area
1. Has anyone in the athlete's family (grandmother, grandfather, mother, father, brother, sister) died suddenly before the age of 50 years?	Cardiovascular
2. Has the athlete ever passed out during exercise or stopped exercising because of dizziness?	Cardiovascular
3. Does the athlete have asthma (wheezing), hay fever, or coughing spells after exercise?	Exercise-induced asthma
4. Has the athlete ever broken a bone, had to wear a cast, or had an injury to any joint?	Musculoskeletal injury
5. Does the athlete have a history of concussion (getting knocked out)?	Neurological injury
6. Has the athlete ever suffered a heat-related illness (heatstroke)?	Heat-related illness
7. Does the athlete have anything he or she wants to discuss with the physician?	Harmful health habits/ sexual activity
8. Does the athlete have any chronic illness or see a physician regularly for any particular problem?	General health screen
9. Does the athlete take any medicine?	General health screen
10. Is the athlete allergic to any medications or to bee stings?	General health screen
11. Does the athlete have only one of any paired organ (eyes, ears, kidneys, testicles, ovaries, etc.)?	General health screen

changes to the health history; continue building rapport with the athlete; and screen again for high-risk behaviors. Physicians should specify on the examination forms that clearance by the doctor is required after any significant injury or new health problem.

IDENTIFYING THE CAUSES OF ATHLETIC INJURIES

Different sports pose variable injury risks. For example, relatively safe activities like archery or table tennis report injury rates of 2 to 5% of participants per season. Distance running, another noncontact sport, necessitates intense training and yields yearly injury rates of 50 to 60%. Full-contact sports like football, wrestling, or rugby lead to seasonal injury rates between 60 and 80%, with as many as 25% of participants experiencing a serious injury. Table 11.2 shows comparative injury rates for different sports.

Since family physicians treat injured athletes in a variety of sports, a general classification system helps orient diagnosis and treatment. The most serious injuries are life-threatening conditions and fortunately are rare. Other classes of injury are macrotrauma and microtrauma. *Macrotrauma* implies a sudden disruption of anatomical structures (e.g., a shoulder dislocation). *Microtrauma* represents the more common form of injury and relates to repetitive minor disruption of an anatomical structure (e.g., Achilles tendonitis). These are overuse injuries, and the doctor can identify a specific cause.

Table 11.2. Comparative Injury Rates in Selected Sports[a]

Sport	Injuries per 100 Participants	
	All Injuries	Lasting >5 days
Baseball (boys)	19	4.5
Basketball (boys)	31	7.4
Football (boys)	81	25.1
Track and field (boys)	33	12.5
Track and field (girls)	35	17.5
Wrestling (boys)	75	26.3

[a]From Sullivan JA, Grana WA: *The Pediatric Athlete*. Park Ridge, IL, Academy of Orthopaedic Surgeons, 1990, p 125. With permission.

Macrotrauma usually represents an injury that requires urgent assessment and treatment. Dislocation of the shoulder joint, for example, is more easily diagnosed and treated before reactive muscle spasm occurs. Early recognition of anterior cruciate ligament injuries of the knee allows protection of a partial tear, thus potentially saving the athlete from major surgical repair should the disruption extend completely through the ligament. Fractures begin healing only after immobilization. Similarly, early splinting, icing, and elevation reduces swelling in an ankle sprain so that functional rehabilitation can begin. Once the macrotrauma is identified, the family physician should initiate treatment or prompt referral.

Microtrauma injuries are nonurgent and allow time for careful assessment by the physician. Treatment focuses on a functional approach aimed at returning the athlete quickly and safely to the sport.

Predisposing Factors

Another element in evaluating a sports injury is determining whether anatomical factors or specific characteristics of a given sport lead to injury. For example, "Little League elbow" is a **sport-specific injury** that occurs only in young pitchers whose medial epicondylar ossification center has not fused. The valgus stress of throwing a curve ball damages the ossification center, causing pain. As a physician, you cannot change the propensity of a growing elbow to suffer injury following repetitive valgus stresses, but you can suggest a modification of activity within the sport so that a prepubertal pitcher can only pitch a certain number of innings per week.

Some injuries occur primarily in a selected group of sports. Patellofemoral stress syndrome (PFSS), for example, ranks among the most common ailments in distance running, biking, and ballet, but rarely occurs in swimming, baseball, or basketball. In this sense, PFSS represents an overuse syndrome primarily occurring in endurance sports. On the other hand, the patient with poor quadriceps alignment has a predisposing anatomical risk that could prompt the development of PFSS in any sport. In general, endurance sports and strength sports show different injury patterns. Similarly, non-weight-bearing sports like swimming, diving, and biking have a lower incidence of impact problems than weight-bearing sports, but they have injuries that are associated with muscular work, such as back strain. Table 11.3 identifies the common injuries in five sports.

Injuries that occur in virtually all sports usually relate to a **weak anatomical area.** Ankle sprains are an excellent example (see Chapter 44 on ankle injuries). They are the most common injury in football, basketball, and soccer. The ankle has limited muscular support to stabilize the bony mortise; therefore, its stability depends on the bony articulation, the joint capsule, and four ligaments. For dorsal and plantar flexion the ankle performs admirably. The deltoid ligament on the medial aspect provides greater support and effectively limits eversion, but the smaller lateral ligaments cannot resist inversion stresses as effectively. Thus, inversion sprains predominate (90% of cases). Ligamentous laxity (which should be looked for during preparticipation examinations) increases the risk of injury.

Table 11.3. Common Injuries in Five Popular Sports

Distance running
Achilles tendonitis
Chondromalacia patella
Metatarsalgia
Plantar fasciitis
Stress fractures
Iliotibial band syndrome
Piriformis syndrome
Posterior tibial tendonitis

Soccer
Skin trauma
Contusions
Lateral ankle sprains
Achilles tendonitis
Meniscus injury (50% of active professional players)
Collateral knee ligament tears
Anterior cruciate tears
Tears of quadriceps, hamstrings, and adductors

Basketball
Skin trauma
Arch strains
Stress fractures
Ankle sprains and fractures
Achilles tendonitis
Contusions
Jumper's knee
Anterior tibialis strain
Iliac crest apophysitis and Osgood-Schlatter disease in
   young adolescents

Tennis
Tendonitis of rotator cuff
Rotator cuff tears (older competitors)
Tennis elbow
"Tennis leg"—rupture of medial head of gastrocnemius or
   plantaris
Strains of upper back
Strain of rectus abdominis
Achilles tendonitis and rupture
Ankle sprains

Baseball
Adult throwers
   Shoulder rotator cuff tendonitis
   Elbow traction spurs
   Rupture of medial collateral ligament
   Ulnar neuropathy
Young throwers
   Little League shoulder
   Little League elbow
   Medial traction spurs
   Ulnar neuropathy
   Osteochondritis dissecans of capitellum
Running/sliding injuries
   Ankle sprains and fractures
   Abrasions and contusions
   Cervical sprains and fractures
   Hamstring strains

Determining the Mechanism of Injury

An understanding of **biomechanics** will often explain the occurrence of a specific injury. Any factor adding stress increases the likelihood of injury. For example, the patella must smoothly glide through the patellar groove thousands of times in an endurance athlete. Even a slight alteration of normal motion, such as occurs in an individual with poor alignment of the quadriceps mechanism (an excessive Q angle) promotes the development of patellofemoral stress syndrome. A weakened joint from prior injury or an ankle that has not regained full proprioception will be at greater risk of serious traumatic injury.

Runners often develop recurrent Achilles tendonitis from excessive speed training or too much training on hills. Why do both of these activities worsen Achilles injuries whereas more mileage at a slower pace may not? The answer lies in the tendency of muscles to tear at the musculotendinous junction during **eccentric contraction.** Eccentric contraction means tightening simultaneously with lengthening. Thus, during hill running the heel of the trail leg drops to meet the surface, maximally stretching the Achilles tendon. The mechanism in speed running is essentially the same, with the foot undergoing maximal dorsiflexion before push-off. Slower running paces and flatter surfaces do not require the same biomechanics.

Understanding the mechanism of injury has greatly improved the treatment for "tennis elbow," for example. Normally the backhand tennis swing should be a continuous motion. Body movement in concert with the racquet motion allows the player to hit the ball with considerable force. The impact caused by collision of the ball and racquet head should transmit linearly up the racquet through the player's arm to the torso, thus dissipating the impact. If the player's arm remains behind the plane of the body, however, the force transmits primarily to the elbow's extensor muscle compartment. Repetitive stress leads to microscopic tears and to lateral epicondylitis. The use of forearm braces, strengthening exercises for the extensor compartment, and antiinflammatory drugs all lessen symptoms while the player corrects the error in backhand form that caused the injury.

ASSESSING THE PATIENT WITH RECURRENT INJURY

When an athletic injury does occur, the physician's role is to assess the possible causes for the injury, make a diagnosis, and recommend remediation. During the assessment, use open-ended, patient-centered questions. This helps develop a trusting relationship with the individual and will facilitate insight into personal problems such as a dysfunctional family, depression, or a character disorder. Often the physician may want to give medical permission not to compete to preserve the emotional stability of the athlete and reduce competitive pressures until the athlete can cope better.

A thorough **training history** will provide clues about whether the oft-injured athlete is a compulsive overworker. Experienced coaches refer to the 50:20:4 rule, which asserts that 50% of athletes who increase their training by 20% or more per week (rather than the recommended 10% or less) will be injured within 4 weeks. Too much training clearly fatigues muscles and places the athlete at increased risk of strains, sprains, and occasionally more serious injury.

Recovery from injury becomes a critical part of the history. Remember that the most common injury is reinjury. If an athlete has previously hurt a joint, ask how it was injured and how long the athlete underwent rehabilitation. Muscle strength protects joints from injury, and unless the athlete has regained 90% or more of normal strength, injury risk is increased.

The term *exercise addiction* refers to an athlete's unwillingness to stop training. Rather than logically reducing training at the time of injury, these athletes may actually increase their efforts. The injury becomes their opponent, and they compete against it, leading to more serious injuries or causing minor problems to become chronic. Until the doctor deals with the addictive influence exercise has on these individuals, treatment of any specific injury often fails.

External and environmental factors can contribute to injury risk and should be explored in the history. The type and condition of protective gear and shoes worn; the specific running or work-out surfaces and field conditions may all contribute to a specific injury. Fatigue occurs more quickly on hot, humid days, and injury risk increases with exhaustion. At the opposite end of the thermometer, muscle warm-up lags on cold days, and strain-type injuries occur more readily.

Psychological assessment of the athlete is also important. Pressure comes from coaches, parents, or athletes themselves. Many changes take place in adolescence, and self-esteem suffers when performance declines. The athlete who judges self-worth by sports performance faces periods of self-recrimination that can lead to depression. Intense individuals may impatiently try to play through an injury, leading to worse problems. Athletes competing to please a parent may not understand that subconsciously they don't want to compete, and injury symptoms become an escape.

Diet history can give important information about the probable cause of certain injuries. Endurance athletes, seeking to remain thin, frequently eat fewer calories than they need. The result is an energy-deprived body in which catabolism can lead to muscle breakdown and impact injury. Poor eating habits, fad diets, and the use of additives such as bee pollen, yeast extracts, and essential amino acids often lead to neglect of nutritional needs. Since many athletes have heard or seen advertisements featuring star performers touting some particular additive or megavitamin, the physician must dispel the notion that a dietary supplement will propel one to champion status. While vegetarian diets can adequately provide all requirements for training, self-planned vegetarian meals may not account for total protein needs. Thus, many athletes benefit from having a nutritionist review and advise them on diet.

Other Risk Factors. Despite the physical demands of sports, athletes often engage in **high-risk health behaviors**. In fact, athletes are just as likely as their peers to engage in alcohol use, unprotected sexual intercourse, driving without a seat belt, and other high-risk behaviors. In addition, certain drugs, such as anabolic steroids, are used by athletes more frequently than by nonathletes in the same age groups. Table 11.4 illustrates reported drug use by college athletes.

Direct observations of increased strength and weight gain, behavioral changes, or school problems may prompt the family physician to ask about drugs such as anabolic steroids, testosterone derivatives, amphetamines, and cocaine. Athletes rarely volunteer information about illicit activity, but, when questioned, often confide in physicians who work closely with their team. Noticing behavioral or physical changes and initiating a discussion are important skills for the physician. Table 11.5 outlines clues for suspecting drug use. Table 11.6 highlights signs and symptoms that may pinpoint anabolic steroid use.

While athletes **smoke cigarettes** less than the general population, some studies show that 6%

still use tobacco through smoking, snuff, or chewing. Athletes who use tobacco products may have started because of peer pressure. Most recognize that these habits negatively affect performance and may respond to the physician's offer to help. Camaraderie with other team members

Table 11.4. Drug Use among 1200 College Athletes[a]

Drug	% Using
Alcohol	62
Marijuana	22
Cocaine	7
Amphetamines	6
Sedatives	2
Anabolic steroids	2
Hallucinogens	1
Heroin	0.1

[a]Adapted from Schneider RC, Kennedy JC, Plant ML: *Sports Injuries: Mechanisms, Prevention and Treatment.* Baltimore, Williams & Wilkins, 1985, pp 632–635.

Table 11.5. Physical Signs and Behavioral Changes Seen in Drug Use

Physical signs
  Unexplained weight loss
  Eye irritation
  Increase in pretraining heart rates (many athletes lose the athletic bradycardia)
  Nasal irritation
  Pupillary contraction
  Needle marks
Behavioral changes
  Decline in school performance
  Nervousness
  Paranoid or suspicious actions
  Changing appetite
  Difficulty sleeping
  Dull affect (loss of normal alertness)
  Practice absence or tardiness
  Continual need for money

Table 11.6. Signs and Symptoms of Anabolic Steroid Use

Fluid retention
Weight gain
Testicular atrophy
Hirsutism
Acne
Deepening voice
Irritability
Aggressiveness
Decreased libido
Increased appetite

can develop into a new peer group that discourages use.

Risky sexual behavior has seldom been discouraged among athletes. The promiscuous behavior of professional athletes and the media portrayal of sexually attractive women flocking to wealthy star athletes contribute to a perception that these behaviors carry few consequences. The recent admission of HIV positivity by one of the nation's most popular athletes helped send a different message. Discussing safe sex practices, including abstinence, with adolescent athletes, who generally feel immortal and have strong emotional and physical drives toward sexual activity, is doubly challenging. More positive role models are needed to underscore the importance of abstinence or safe sex.

The following case illustrates the need to move beyond the musculoskeletal system when assessing an athlete's injuries.

Case Example Kristy

Kristy, a high school senior, frequently came to her family physician for athletic injuries. She was in superb condition, had excellent form, and seemed to most observers the naturally gifted athlete. She had won the state championship in the hurdles and competed successfully in several other races. Her injuries were always ill-defined and, on examination, revealed no physical abnormalities. Typically, she complained of muscle strains and within a day of her visit returned to training.

Intrigued by this successful athlete who seemed to need to seek attention for "injuries," the family doctor attended a couple of Kristy's practices to see if a cause for her recurring injuries emerged. Kristy's father attended every practice session and race. He was vocal, constantly critical and often contradicted suggestions made by coaches. After other athletes went home from practice, he often kept her late to do extra form work, hurdles, or sprint drills. The only time Kristy seemed free of this pressure was when she had some injury.

The family doctor reviewed what he knew about Kristy from her preparticipation examination in the chart and mentally assessed the important factors in understanding athletic injuries.

When the family doctor reviewed Kristy's injury pattern, it became apparent that she presented with an injury on days after she had lost in competition. In contrast, after winning she always said that something hurt but that she could run through it without difficulty. Further information about the family revealed that Kristy's parents had a poor relationship and that family activities centered entirely on the children. Kristy's father had been a high school and college

runner, with only modest success. His involvement in his daughter's career may have reflected some of the frustrations of his own competitive failures. Further complicating the strained family situation was the fact that the coach, who recognized the inappropriateness of her father's intrusion, chose to level most criticisms at Kristy when she complained of injury.

The key to working with Kristy was understanding her stresses and persuading her not to overachieve. When she complained of minor injury it meant that she needed time away from the pressures she faced at practice. Kristy and the family doctor discussed that losing some races was acceptable and that she had to train for herself, not her parents or coach. Gradually she began to assert herself about the type of workouts she would do in practice, and her injuries lessened. She was finally able to say that she really enjoyed running and later attended college on a track scholarship.

EVALUATING ACUTE INJURIES

A family physician best prepares for **life-threatening** conditions by knowing those related to a given sport. A physician covering cross-country track may have to deal with heat stroke or the rarer cardiac arrythmia. The physician for a football team should be prepared to evaluate trauma including head injury, splenic rupture, cervical spine injury, and airway collapse (laryngeal fracture). A knowledge of basic cardiopulmonary resuscitation and a plan for stabilization and transport to a hospital become part of the physician's preparation. Rapid diagnosis and emergency management may save an athlete's life.

In thinking of the mechanics of injury, try to reconstruct exactly what the athlete was doing before the pain began. For example, video analysis of pitching injuries demonstrates that the shoulder must move in conjunction with the torso. When this does not occur, the muscles of the rotator cuff are subject to repetitive microtrauma. With violent throws, shoulder acceleration and deceleration is rapid, and the humeral head moves 2 to 3 cm out of the socket. If sufficient microtrauma to the rotator cuff has occurred, the humeral head is literally thrown through a weakened tendon, causing a rotator cuff tear. In this example, an overuse injury leads to weakness that leads to a major traumatic injury. The key to preventing this injury lies in increasing the strength of the rotator cuff muscles and changing the pitching biomechanics so as not to precipitate the chronic tendonitis. Anatomical characteristics that affect the biomechanics of certain injuries are shown in Table 11.7.

Table 11.7. Anatomical Problems Leading to Injury in Common Sports

Runners
  Alignment problems
  Anatomical changes of the foot
  Functional problems affecting form (e.g., excessive pronation)
  Tightness of hamstrings or Achilles tendon complex
Football
  Muscular weakness (particularly of quadriceps or neck)
  Ligamentous instability of shoulder, ankle, or knee
Baseball
  Rotator cuff weakness
  Limited elbow extension
  Shoulder subluxation
  Ulnar neuropathy
  Tight hamstrings
Basketball
  Pes planus
  Cavus feet
  Long thin metatarsels
  Marfan's syndrome
  Ligamentous laxity
Aerobics (See runners)
  Low back weakness
  Lack of flexibility
Gymnastics
  Patella-femoral tracking problems
  Spondylolisthesis
General
  Obesity
  Visual problems

Focused Clinical Examination

During the physical assessment of a sports injury, an anatomical diagnosis is essential. Inspection helps identify swelling, which occurs in both traumatic and overuse injuries. Palpation demonstrates tenderness, changes in structure, clicking of soft tissue structures, and crepitation during joint motion. Special skills include assessing normal joint motion; estimating strength and flexibility; and performing specific functional testing. Critical errors are avoided by appropriately identifying unstable joints and joint effusions.

Treatment

Four basic principles of first aid comprise immediate care for acute injuries: ice, compression, elevation, and splinting (ICES). Variation in the application of these principles depends on the type of injury and the clinical response.

Application of ice prevents swelling and inflammation, thus speeding the athlete's return to activity. Heat plays little role in acute trauma, but it becomes more important during rehabilitation.

Compression can be done with elastic wraps or more sophisticated air splints. In ankle sprains, placing a horseshoe-shaped felt pad around the malleolus allows the pressure of an Ace wrap to reduce swelling more effectively. Foam rubber, orthopaedic felt, cotton, underwrap, and cast padding are among the supplies that can be adapted to provide better compression and immediate protection.

Elevation reduces swelling by eliminating the effect of gravity on tissue oncotic pressure in an injured extremity. Family physicians advise patients with orthostatic edema to elevate their extremities; however, in most athletic contests the injured player leaves the game, sits on the sidelines, and places the injured extremity in a dependent position. By emphasizing elevation, the family physician may help an injured player return 24 to 48 hours sooner than would otherwise be the case.

Enforced total rest may psychologically or physically devastate an athlete. *Splinting* provides protection for the injured area while the athlete continues to participate or to train. Techniques of splinting for sports differ little from those of general orthopaedics; however, the choice of splint material changes according to the demands of the sport. Functional splinting allows the athlete to substitute protected motion for total rest. For example, a swimmer needs a splint that can tolerate water. Football players with injured fingers require taping or plastic splints, because metal would place opponents at risk of injury. Semirigid splints of plastic or felt for extensor tendinitis of the wrist restrict motion during the healing phase but allow enough wrist function so that training can continue. Many injuries, when appropriately splinted, require minimal rest; so protected training and muscle rehabilitation begin almost immediately.

PREVENTIVE MEASURES

Physicians can stress prevention by attempting to influence the rules and modify training in a sport. As advisers to athletic programs and as team doctors, physicians can emphasize principles of safe training including adequate stretching, warm-up and warm-down periods, and gradual increases in training intensity and volume. Training schedules that rotate hard and easy days and that emphasize different muscle groups on alternate days decrease injury incidence.

In addition, physicians can encourage policies that prevent injuries. For example, the Connecticut Pediatric Society reviewed injuries in Little League football and found that 50% of these occurred on kickoffs and punt returns. With physician encouragement, the state enacted a rule change eliminating these plays in Little League competition, and a dramatic reduction in injuries followed. A similar reduction in injuries occurred after physician efforts encouraged equestrian sports to mandate protective headgear in competition. Prevention remains important in recreational sport as well. Skateboarders and people who use roller blades need protective gear, and most bicycle fatalities could be avoided with universal helmet use.

CONCLUSIONS

The key to success in sports medicine is the continuity that comes from serving as a team physician. The physician can identify high-risk athletes, begin preventive interventions, and more effectively care for injured athletes. Getting to know the athlete allows the doctor to weigh the relative contributions of psychological, physical, and training components to a given injury. The broad training of family physicians prepares them well to provide this type of care for athletes. This is shown by the Olympic Committee's decision to appoint family physicians to head the medical care team for the Olympic games.

SUGGESTED READINGS

Blum RW: Preparation evaluation of the adolescent athlete: timing and content of the examination. *Postgrad Med* 78:52-69, 1985.

Fields KB, Delaney M: Focusing the preparticipation sports examination. *J Fam Pract* 30(3):304–312, 1990.

Garrick JG, Smith NJ: Preparticipation sports assessment. *Pediatrics* 66:803-806, 1980.

Tanji JL: The preparticipation physical examination for sports. *Am Fam Physician* 42(2):397–402, 1990.

The above articles review the essentials of preparticipation examinations for adolescent athletes and the rationale on which recommendations are based.

Clinics in Sports Medicine

This series reviews topics germane to sports medicine and provides comprehensive quarterly reviews of a specific problem.

Bloomfield J, Fricker P, Fitch K (eds.): *Textbook of Science and Medicine in Sport*, Oxford, Blackwell Scientific Publications, 1992.

This is a readable, concise text that combines the scientific basis for sports medicine with a practical review of the common clinical problems.

Kulund DN (ed): *The Injured Athlete*. Philadelphia, JB Lippincott, 1982.

A good general text with fairly comprehensive coverage of most sports medicine topics.

Schneider RC, Kennedy JC, Plant ML: *Sports Injuries: Mechanisms, Prevention and Treatment*. Baltimore, Williams & Wilkins, 1985.

A comprehensive text that reviews both sport-specific and anatomical-specific injuries.

Shahady E, Petrizzi M: *Sports Medicine for Coaches and Trainers*. 2nd ed. Chapel Hill, University of North Carolina Press, 1991.

A review of sports medicine problems seen by team physicians. An excellent beginning text for students and residents.

chapter 12

AMBULATORY DRUG THERAPY

Timothy J. Ives and Geraldine D. Anastasio

A major clinical challenge to family physicians is remaining current on the proper selection and use of an increasing number of medications. This is especially true since family physicians, among all specialists, prescribe the broadest variety of medications. A patient's symptoms may be due to medications prescribed by other physicians or bought over-the-counter (OTC). Therefore the family physician must know the common adverse effects and interactions of all the patient's medications, having ready access to information on rarer effects. The family physician should be able to simplify the patient's medication regimen, by using a single medication to treat more than one disease process, or by using nondrug approaches instead of medication. In this chapter, we discuss both practical and theoretical aspects of ambulatory drug therapy and recommend drug information references.

DRUG INFORMATION RESOURCES

There are two types of drug information reference books—pharmacology textbooks and pharmacotherapeutic textbooks. **Pharmacology texts** organize the information by chemical class; Goodman and Gilman's *Pharmacological Basis of Therapeutics* is the standard example. When seeking information on mechanism of action, dosing, indications, or adverse effects, a pharmacology text provides the best answers. **Pharmacotherapeutic texts** organize the information by disease state. *Applied Therapeutics*, by Koda-Kimble, Young, and Guglielmo is an example. These texts answer the question, Which drug is best to treat a specific disease? The following is an abbreviated list of the most popular drug information resources.

- *Drug Facts & Comparisons* covers all prescription and OTC medications. It is organized by pharmacological system, with some overlap into therapeutic categories. It is simple to use, since the index lists both brand and generic drug names. There are two versions of this text, an annual bound edition and a loose-leaf edition that is updated monthly. This last feature makes it one of the most current sources of new drug information.
- *American Hospital Formulary Service (AHFS) Drug Information* is the best information source on hospital drugs, including infusion protocols for parenterals. Its information on OTC medications is limited. It is published yearly, with quarterly updates, by the American Society of Hospital Pharmacists.
- *Physicians' Desk Reference (PDR)* is printed and distributed by pharmaceutical manufacturers. It is the "Yellow pages" of the drug industry, with only the medications worth "advertising" included. Therefore, it is incomplete. Information is grouped by manufacturers, not by pharmacological or therapeutic classes. Older, generically available prescription medications and OTC medications are frequently not included. The Food and Drug Administration (FDA) regulates the package insert information published in the PDR. Therefore, unapproved indications are not covered.

QUESTIONS TO ASK A PHARMACEUTICAL REPRESENTATIVE

The pharmaceutical industry has an intimate but difficult relationship with the medical profession. It supports a variety of ethical clinical trials of new medications or new formulations of old medications, financially supports continuing medical education, but also offers a variety of inducements to the medical profession to try its products. In the past few years, new codes of conduct for clinicians have been published by the American Medical Association to address issues of unethical inducements to prescribe.

Pharmaceutical representatives are regular visitors to physicians' offices. They want to talk with the physicians and leave samples of their products. Although these samples can be useful to get patients started on therapy or save money for patients, this can be a two-edged sword. The samples are often expensive and the cost of continuing therapy is prohibitive. The following questions are designed to maximize the information you get from representatives.

1. What is your background? Many representatives have baccalaureate and graduate degrees in such diverse fields of study as pharmacy, business, or history.
2. What products does your company have? This will help determine which drug products to discuss.
3. How is this product better than what I already use?
4. What is the FDA rating for this medication? To help you assess the drug's rightful place in your own formulary system, the Food and Drug Administration has a drug classification system to rate a drug's therapeutic potential. The P designation represents the following: a therapeutic advance (because no effective drugs were previously available for the condition), a more effective drug than those already used to treat the condition, or a drug with important advantages (such as convenience or reduced adverse drug effects). The S designation is for drugs that have therapeutic qualities similar to drugs already on the market.
5. What is the drug's adverse effect profile?
6. What is/are the drug's contraindications (i.e., patients or disease states in which not to use the drug)? For example, organisms that are not sensitive, in the case of antimicrobial agents. Can this drug be used safely during pregnancy or lactation?
7. What is the cost to the patient for an average duration of treatment? The actual cost to the patient should be verified by calling a local pharmacy.
8. Do you have scientific and clinical studies to substantiate claims on approved indications?
9. How can I request information from the manufacturer's medical information department on unapproved indications? The FDA regulates

representatives to only discuss approved indications for a drug.

TAKING A MEDICATION HISTORY

A complete medication history provides the physician with the following information. First, it is used to determine if the patient's chief complaint is related to the recent addition or discontinuation of a medication. Second, the success or failure of previous medications can be evaluated. Finally, any adverse medication reactions can be recorded in the medical chart.

The components of a medication history are

1. *Prescription medications* **currently** being taken. Include the dose, the specific dosage regimen, how long the patient has been taking the medication, and for what reason (to assess patient understanding and compliance).
2. *Over-the-counter medications* **currently** being taken. Do not forget vitamin use and contraception methods for both men and women.
3. *Prescription or OTC medications* that were taken previously. This may give you some insight into the patient's past medical history.
4. *Social drug use*
   a) Alcohol: assume that everyone drinks and ask the patient, "How much do you drink?" not "Do you drink?" Ask about past drinking habits. Alcohol products include beer, wine, hard liquor, and moonshine.
   b) Tobacco: ask about cigarette, pipe, cigar, snuff, and chewing tobacco use. If the patient is not currently using any tobacco products, be sure to ask about any previous use.
   c) Caffeine: coffee, tea, cola drinks, many other soft drinks (e.g., Mountain Dew and Mellow Yellow), and chocolate contain caffeine, which can alter sleep habits, cause headaches, contribute to nervousness, or induce cardiac arrhythmias.
   d) Recreational drugs (e.g., marijuana and cocaine): though this is sensitive information, some patients will report use to you. Adverse effects may come from the drug itself or from its abuse in regular, heavy consumption. Addiction and habituation should also be considered.
5. *Home remedies*: remember that one of the primary ingredients in most home remedies is alcohol. Find out why these remedies are used.

6. *Allergies and adverse drug reactions*: is there any history of an allergic reaction to drugs, foods, or the environment? Be sure that the patient (and you) know the difference between an allergy and an adverse reaction.

After compiling the medication history, determine if any adverse drug reactions or interactions might exist, and assess patient compliance with medication regimens. If problems exist, assess whether they are clinically significant and consider altering the drug regimen to prevent adverse effects on the patient.

If a patient has problems complying with the medication regimen, attempt to find out why. Is it forgetfulness, a complicated dosage regimen, lack of knowledge about the disease being treated, or inability to pay for the prescription? Ask patients how often they forget to take their medications, and why. In assessing compliance, think about whether any special dosing devices (e.g., a measuring spoon or oral syringe) would be helpful. Also consider the influence of mental status, eyesight, hearing, dexterity, socioeconomic status, and support systems on the patient's ability to comply with a medication regimen.

PRESCRIPTION WRITING

Before prescribing a medication regimen, determine either through a trial or through a documented history that behavioral and nonpharmacological modalities are not appropriate or that they do not work. Make certain that you are not dealing with a drug-seeking patient. Review the prescription records in the patient's chart and discuss the patient's chemical history before prescribing a controlled drug. If the patient is new or otherwise unknown to you, at a minimum obtain an oral medication history, and discuss the patient's and family's chemical-dependence history. Ask whether the patient is obtaining drugs from other physicians. Check with the dispensing pharmacy if you suspect that a patient is obtaining extra drugs or is "doctor shopping." Pharmacies are able to give a comprehensive profile of what patient prescriptions have been requested over time.

Take the time to explain the relative risks and benefits of the drug, and record in the chart that this was done. When embarking on what appears to be the long-term use of a potentially addictive substance, discuss this with other family members who might be involved. This will require the patient's permission.

Regularly monitor the patient to be sure that the medication provides the intended therapeutic outcome. For prolonged use of drug regimens, monitor the condition itself and any adverse effects of the drug. This is true no matter what type of controlled substance is used or what schedule it belongs to. Drug holidays are appropriate for certain conditions, to assess whether the original symptoms recur (indicating a continuing legitimate need for the drug) or whether withdrawal symptoms occur (indicating drug-dependence).

Regular contact with the patient's family provides valuable information on the patient's response to the therapeutic regimen. The family may be much more accurate and objective than the patient in reporting whether the patient is receiving medications from other sources or is self-medicating with other drugs or alcohol.

Controlled Substances

The FDA assigns controlled substances to "schedules," based on the relative potential for abuse or dependence. *Schedule I* drugs have a high potential for abuse and no currently accepted medical use. Examples include heroin, marijuana, or phencyclidine. *Schedule II* drugs have a high potential for abuse with severe liability to cause physiological or psychological dependence. Examples of schedule II drugs include single-entity opiate agents such as meperidine (Demerol), methadone, codeine (as single entity), morphine, hydromorphone (Dilaudid), or combination opiate products containing oxycodone (Percodan, Percocet, Tylox); stimulants such as dextroamphetamine (Dexedrine) or methylphenidate (Ritalin); and short-acting barbiturates such as secobarbital (Seconal), amobarbital (Amytal), or pentobarbital (Nembutal). These agents cannot be prescribed by telephone except in an emergency (not accepted by all pharmacies). No refills are permitted, and the patient's address and the prescriber's Drug Enforcement Agency (DEA) and telephone numbers are required. No controlled substances, including methadone, can be legally prescribed or dispensed to maintain an outpatient's physical dependence. Such dispensing is legal only through an approved chemical-dependency treatment center.

Schedule III drugs have a lower potential for abuse but may lead to moderate to low physical dependence or high psychological dependence.

Examples include opiates in combination with a nonopiate drug (e.g., hydrocodone in Tussionex or Vicodin).

Schedule IV drugs have a low potential for abuse, but may lead to some physical or psychological dependence. Examples include the synthetic opiates such as propoxyphene (Darvon) or pentazocine (Talwin), opiates in combination with other agents (e.g., codeine and acetaminophen in Tylenol #1, 2, 3, or 4), stimulants such as diethylpropion (Tenuate) or phentermine (Ionamin), benzodiazepines (e.g., Valium, Dalmane, Tranxene, Halcion, Ativan, Serax, Librium, Restoril, etc.), chloral hydrate, and phenobarbital. Schedule III or IV prescriptions are valid for 6 months or 5 refills after the date of issue, whichever comes first.

Schedule V drugs have the lowest potential for abuse and are usually opioid-based products found in combination with other agents. They are primarily used in antitussive preparations (e.g., Robitussin AC or Triaminic Expectorant with Codeine) or in antidiarrheal products (e.g., loperamide (Lomotil). These agents are available by prescription or over-the-counter. All nonscheduled drug prescriptions are valid for one year. Regulations regarding transmission of prescrip-

tions to pharmacies by facsimile machines (i.e., fax) may vary from state to state.

Components of a Properly Written Prescription

The prescription is an important interaction between the patient and the physician. Unless properly written and communicated to both patient and pharmacist, the prescription can contribute to noncompliance and iatrogenic disease. Proper prescriptions must be written legibly. If you have poor handwriting, print or type all prescriptions. Use ink or indelible pencil, particularly when writing for controlled substances. Write only one prescription per order blank as shown in Figure 12.1. The major components of a prescription are:

A. *Date.* This is especially important for schedule II medication prescriptions, which must be filled within 72 hours after writing. Also, prescriptions for schedule III and IV medications cannot be filled or refilled 6 months after writing them.

B. *The patient's name and address.* This information is required on schedule II prescriptions,

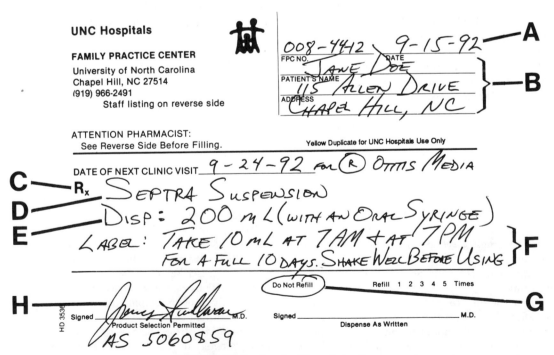

FIGURE 12.1. Standard Prescription Form.

but more importantly, it will avoid potential confusion, especially in families with several people taking medications.

C. *Superscription.* This is designated as the symbol Rx, the abbreviation for recipe (Latin for "take thou").

D. *Inscription.* This is the body of the prescription, containing the name and strength of the drug.

E. *Subscription.* This is the direction to the pharmacist, detailing the amount of the drug to be dispensed, such as "dispense 30 tablets," "dispense 3 months (of oral contraceptives)," or "dispense 120 ml with an oral syringe.

F. *Transcription.* This area contains the directions for the patient. The Latin abbreviation, SIG, has now been replaced by the term "Label." The pharmacist is required to directly transcribe in this space the information the physician has written. To avoid confusion in translating, Latin abbreviations (e.g., BID, AC, QHS) should not be used by physicians even though they seem convenient. Also, avoid medical terms unfamiliar to the patient. The directions cover the amount of drug to be taken, the timing and frequency of dosing, route of administration, and duration of therapy.

Notations such as "take as directed" or "take as necessary" (PRN) are confusing to patients and should be avoided. Directions for use should always begin with a verb such as "take," "apply," or "insert." Use directions that remind the patient of the purpose of the prescription, such as "for pain relief" or "to relieve itching." Other information, such as "shake well before use," "refrigerate," or "take on an empty stomach," is also included here. Pharmacists have auxiliary labels containing this information, which can be attached to the prescription container.

G. *Refill information.* Note this on every prescription you write. Schedule II drugs cannot be refilled, and schedule III and IV prescriptions cannot be refilled more than five times within the 6-month duration. Unless refills are specified, always circle or write "Do Not Refill" to prevent forgeries for extra refills.

H. *Signature.* The physician's personal signature (last name in full) is required, as well as the DEA registry number and practice address.

When noting weights and measures in a prescription, use the metric system. Antiquated terms such as drams, scruples, grains, or even ounces are no longer recommended. A commonly used measure is the teaspoon (5 ml), however, spoon sizes can vary considerably, from 3.5 to 7.5 ml. Calibrated devices, such as measuring spoons and oral syringes, allow for more accurate delivery of the medication and are recommended when prescribing suspensions and liquids.

Physicians can prescribe medications by the trade name or, if desired, by the generic name. Medications that are available generically can be produced and sold by any pharmaceutical company, potentially lowering the cost of the prescription to the patient.

Some drugs, although available generically, should be prescribed by their trade name only. The reasons for this recommendation include variable bioavailability, poor quality control, formulation differences, and a narrow therapeutic index. Drugs with a narrow therapeutic index are usually those monitored by serum drug levels (e.g., digoxin or phenytoin) or those where the specific effect is monitored (e.g., warfarin). Drug classes where a difference in bioavailability has altered the clinical outcome, as documented by case reports, include antiarrhythmic, anticonvulsant, and psychotropic agents. Generic equivalents have also been questioned in the following classes: low-dose oral contraceptives, theophylline, furosemide, and oral anticoagulants. Consider prescribing these by the trade name only. Several drug classes lend themselves to generic substitution. These include antacids, antibiotics, anticholinergic agents, antihistamines, antihypertensive agents, local anesthetics, thiazide diuretics, topical corticosteroids, and vitamins.

GENERAL RECOMMENDATIONS FOR PRESCRIBING

The National Council on Patient Information and Education recommends that all patients be given the following information about their medications: (*a*) the name of the drug, (*b*) its purpose (i.e., the conditions it treats), (*c*) how and when to take the medication (and when to stop taking it), (*d*) what food, beverages, and other drugs to avoid while taking it, (*e*) proper storage, and (*f*) what adverse effects may result (e.g., serious, short-term, or long-term).

Drug therapy is often compromised by a lack of full compliance by the patient. Proper instruction does not guarantee that your patient will take a medication as you prescribe it, but inadequate information virtually guarantees that the patient will not. Thus, clear, comprehensive, and easily understood instructions about the proper use of a medication are essential for good patient compliance.

Medication regimens should be kept simple and associated with a specific daily activity (e.g., taken with breakfast). The importance of contracting with the patient for a therapeutic partnership cannot be overemphasized; make sure you have an agreement with the patient. Make sure that the patient understands the reasons for prescribing the drug. Always be alert to the possibility of noncompliance, and tell patients what to do if doses are missed. To achieve therapeutic goals, use positive feedback and rewards. For example, stickers or small toys are good motivators for children. The physician may need to enlist family support to accomplish the desired outcome.

When available, patient education materials on the medications being prescribed should be given. Pharmacists can also provide these materials when the prescription is dispensed. In addition, using a medication diary or calendar to record daily drug administration will enhance compliance. Other health care personnel (e.g., pharmacists, nurses, physician assistants, and dietitians) can assist with patient education and help eliminate barriers to compliance. Finally, the patient should be encouraged to bring all medications to each office visit, to help you monitor compliance.

Pediatric Prescribing

Unique problems exist during the neonatal period of life. Safe and effective drug therapy during this period is complicated by the immaturity of drug-metabolizing and renal excretory systems. Also, drug activity decreases rapidly as a function of increasing weight and maturing liver cells. Particular drugs should be avoided in certain age groups (e.g., sulfonamides in neonates, tetracycline antibiotics in **all** pediatric groups), and drug effects on growth and development must be considered at all ages.

Factors other than age and size can affect drug response in infants and children. Absorption of oral and parenterally administered drugs is not affected, but percutaneous absorption of topically applied drugs is significantly enhanced, especially in premature infants or children whose skin is burned or excoriated.

Physicians should provide adequate instruction to both the parents and the child, if appropriate, in the correct administration of the medication. Try to avoid prescribing medications during school hours. When prescribing a liquid or suspension, remember that the use of a teaspoon provides an inconsistent and inaccurate method of measurement. Devices such as calibrated droppers, measuring spoons, and oral syringes can assure accurate measurement and delivery of liquid medications and are recommended for use with young children. Additionally, refrigerating liquid medications may improve palatability.

Geriatric Prescribing

Try to manage the patient on as few drugs as possible, including self-prescribed medications (i.e., OTCs). Discontinue medications that are not needed. Monitor the patient frequently for compliance, therapeutic outcome, and toxicity, as older patients are at high risk for adverse effects. Remember that in the elderly, the most treatable medical problem is iatrogenic due to medications (e.g., cimetidine-induced mental confusion). See Chapter 10 for more information on the care of geriatric patients.

Choose a dosage form that can be easily self-administered (e.g., liquids for patients with swallowing problems). If there is any question about drug metabolism or excretion, the rule with geriatric patients is to start low and go slow, beginning at 25 to 50% of the normal adult dose and increasing gradually. Titrate the dose to the clinical response. For drugs or their active metabolites eliminated predominantly by the kidney (e.g., aminoglycoside antibiotics or digoxin), use a formula or nomogram to approximate the age-related decline in renal function, and adjust dosages accordingly. For drugs predominantly eliminated by hepatic metabolism, age-related changes are variable and difficult to predict in the absence of overt liver disease. Serum drug levels can be helpful in monitoring several potentially toxic drugs, such as digoxin, procainamide, quinidine, and theophylline.

Help ensure compliance by asking if the patient has access to a pharmacy, can afford the prescription, and can open the containers. If the patient cannot open the medication vial, request on the prescription that a nonchildproof container be used. Encourage the patient to bring current medications to each office visit. Review the patient's medications at each visit, check the supply, and review dosing instructions. Encourage the return or disposal of old unused medications, as they may confuse the patient.

ADVERSE DRUG REACTIONS

The risk of adverse drug reactions is an inevitable consequence of drug use. Few reactions are life-threatening, but almost all drugs, no matter how skillfully used, can cause serious adverse effects in some patients. Also, the incidence of adverse reactions increases with an increase in the number of drugs prescribed. The risk of a serious reaction is generally acceptable if the disease being treated is serious. The liability of a particular drug to cause adverse reactions, the profile of reactions, and their seriousness dictate both the choice of drugs and the acceptable risks.

Adverse drug reactions can result from inherent risk factors in patient response such as allergy, genetic factors, and physiological variables; from acquired patient risk factors such as disease or intercurrent illness; from problems of drug formulation and administration; or from drug interactions. Important predisposing factors to adverse reactions include use of an excessive amount of drug because of nonindividualized dosing, prolonged or unnecessary drug therapy, very young or old age, a previous history of allergic reaction to drugs, and multiple drug therapy. Disease (especially renal and hepatic) and the drug itself are the most important risk factors for drug reactions.

The physician should weigh the risk of an adverse drug reaction and forewarn the patient about important reactions. The physician is also responsible for recognizing and reporting major adverse drug effects to the Food and Drug Administration and the manufacturer of the product, using an FDA 1639 Adverse Reaction Reporting Form.

To help prevent adverse drug reactions, use drugs with low sensitization potential, when possible. Take a careful medication history, especially with regard to previous adverse/allergic reactions. Try to assure yourself that a reaction, present or previous, is truly an "adverse" one related to the drug; in those cases, quantitate or qualitate the reaction. In rare cases where specific drug treatment is essential in spite of a history of an allergic reaction, skin testing may be advisable.

THERAPEUTIC DRUG MONITORING

Indications for measuring serum drug levels include failure to respond to therapy, the effect of changing metabolic or elimination mechanisms, confirming suspected toxicity, determining patient compliance, optimizing the therapeutic effect with a serum drug concentration in the therapeutic range, monitoring active metabolites, and quantitating suspected drug interactions.

Before ordering serum drug levels, you should be able to answer these questions:

1. What information will be obtained from this analysis?
2. What are the therapeutic and toxic serum concentrations?
3. Does the information to be obtained justify the invasive procedure and its cost?
4. How specific is the assay to be used?
5. How will this information change your treatment plan?

If you have any confusion or uncertainty about the answers to the above questions, a blood sample should not be drawn. Instead, inquire further into the mechanics and interpretation of the proposed serum drug level. Try to decide if such a level is really preferable to monitoring the patient's clinical status alone. In practice, many serum drug levels are determined without a therapeutic rationale.

Every plasma sample drawn for monitoring should be obtained at the time that will provide the most useful information. Before a sample is drawn, steady-state conditions (i.e., 3 to 5 half-lives after initiating therapy or changing the dosage) should be achieved. Ideally, for drugs with short half-lives, such as aminoglycoside antibiotics, peak (after administration and distribution) and trough (just before the next dose) levels should be obtained to get a good idea of the pharmacokinetic profile. For drugs with long half-lives, such as digoxin or phenytoin, a trough level is sufficient. If a patient appears toxic (i.e., you suspect an overdose), get a STAT level. By monitoring serum drug concentrations, physicians can quickly individualize, adjust, and optimize drug therapy in a given patient.

SUGGESTED READINGS

Feldmann EG, Davidson DE (eds): *Handbook of Nonprescription Drugs*, ed 9. Washington, D.C., American Pharmaceutical Association, 1990.

A compendium of almost all OTC medications and patient instruction for the proper use of these products.

Gilman AG, Goodman LS, Gilman A (eds): *The Pharmacological Basis of Therapeutics*, ed 8. New York, Pergamon Press, 1990.

The "bible" of clinical pharmacology for most medical students. Contains practical information on medications as well as background pharmacological data on the agent.

Knoben JE, Anderson PO (eds): *Handbook of Clinical Drug Data*, ed 7. Hamilton, IL, Drug Intelligence Publications, 1992.

Pocket-sized text with readily available clinical information on most medications used in family practice settings.

Koda-Kimble MA, Young L, Guglielmo BJ (eds): *Applied Therapeutics: The Clinical Use of Drugs*, ed 5. Vancouver, Canada, Applied Therapeutics, Inc., 1992.

An excellent and useful case-based approach to pharmacotherapeutics in clinical practices.

McEvoy GK, McQuarrie GM: *American Hospital Formulary Service Drug Information*. Washington, DC, American Society of Hospital Pharmacists, 1992.

Contains information on hospital use of medications (e.g., infusion drip rates).

Olin BR (ed): *Drug Facts and Comparisons*. Philadelphia, JB Lippincott, 1992.

Updated monthly and also available as a yearly bound edition. Best source for recently introduced drugs and general prescribing.

Section II

PREVENTIVE CARE

chapter 13

PREVENTIVE CARE: AN OVERVIEW

Philip D. Sloane and Melissa M. Hicks

Why preventive care? Many persons equate physicians and the health care system with treating disease, not preventing illnesses primarily. Slowly but surely, physicians and their patients are becoming aware of the advantages of preventing disease, of taking positive actions before catastrophic health events occur. The rising cost of health care and the rising numbers of consumers of health care demand a more sensible, proactive approach. Intervening early in a disease by screening, or seeking to prevent a disease through lifestyle changes can be much more satisfying than the usual outcomes of treating end-stage heart disease or lung cancer; particularly when primary prevention (such as smoking cessation) might have been possible for those patients.

Historically, physicians have always played some role in prevention, by encouraging and providing immunizations. It is common knowledge that morbidity and mortality from childhood diseases such as pertussis and diphtheria have been greatly decreased by immunization and that the last case of smallpox worldwide was over 10 years ago, due to a worldwide effort at immunizations. Medicine must now begin to apply this principle to other forms of prevention, not by vaccinations, but by identifying risks, educating people on prevention, and early screening for prevalent diseases.

It is not fun to be sick. Some negative consequences of health problems include

- *Symptoms* such as pain, double vision, numbness, loss of appetite, and insomnia;
- *Signs* such as rash, lump, jaundice, swelling, abnormal stool, or vaginal discharge;
- *Anxiety*, an unpleasant emotion that almost always accompanies symptoms and signs, and which is heightened when chronic illness threatens a patient's livelihood or family relationships;

- *Loss of self image*, which can be very powerful, especially in young and middle-aged persons whose sense of self is wrapped up in work, family, and other productive activities;
- *Financial loss*, which is incurred as a result of medical expenses and time off work.

Treatment usually has its own problems, such as cost, side effects, toxicity, and interference with life routines. Other negative consequences of illness include hospitalization, bed rest, and unavailable positive aspects of life (such as recreation, sex, and food).

Prior experience with illness can help motivate patients both to comply with treatment and to be interested in prevention. This is why middle-aged and older adults, who have more experience with illness in family members and peers, are somewhat more compliant patients than adolescents and are more receptive to prevention. The challenge for physicians (and for society) is to motivate people before the threat of illness is upon them.

This chapter briefly introduces basic concepts of preventive care. Specific information about health maintenance in prenatal care, child care, and adult care is presented in the following chapters in this section. The final two chapters cover health education and health promotion.

SCOPE OF PREVENTION IN FAMILY PRACTICE

We will define "disease prevention" as the process of avoiding target diseases through specific interventions. *Primary prevention* consists of those interventions, such as immunizations, that can completely prevent the disease in individuals at risk. *Secondary prevention* seeks to diagnose disease in its presymptomatic phase or to reduce risk fac-

113

tors in those that have them. Blood pressures and serum cholesterol screening are examples. *Tertiary prevention* is a process for minimizing the effects of diseases once they are present. Examples include programs to rehabilitate athletes after injuries or to maximize function after a stroke. Tertiary prevention will not be addressed in this preventive care section, but the common problems chapters later in this book contain much information about its application in specific disease states.

During recent years, many organizations have produced recommendations for prevention in the primary care office. These tend to consist of extensive lists of tests and investigations, most of which constitute secondary prevention, with recommendations about who should receive which interventions how often. Scientific evaluation of these procedures considers a number of characteristics of the disease and the preventive procedure; these criteria are outlined in Figure 13.1.

Health promotion may be defined as the process of assisting people to attain the optimal health available to them. Since "health" has come to mean merely that no diagnosable disease is present, "wellness" has become a popular term for the highest achievable state of physical, social, and psychological functioning. Figure 13.2 depicts these states on a continuum.

IMPLEMENTING PREVENTION

For the family physician, effective preventive practice involves being familiar with current recommendations, knowing your individual patient, and applying this knowledge in a manner that is efficient and individualized. Putting prevention

into practice requires use of the clinical history and physical examination, appropriate priority setting, spending time educating and counseling patients, and using a prevention-oriented charting system.

To implement prevention in practice, many family physicians find it useful to think and act systematically. One simple system is to use the mnemonic RISE. *R* stands for *risk factor identification*, *I* for *immunization*, *S* for *screening*, and *E* for *education*. Risk factor identification is incorporated into the history and physical examination (e.g., taking a family history), immunizations are regularly updated during either well-patient or acute visits, screening is carried out during the physical examination and using laboratory tests, and education permeates all patient-physician encounters.

Clinical History and Physical Examination

The clinical history most often helps with primary prevention, whereas the physical examina-

1. Does it involve a disease that significantly affects the length or quality of life?
2. Is there an available treatment for the disease that is effective and acceptable to patients?
3. Does early detection and treatment of the disease improve morbidity and mortality?
4. Is the screening procedure effective, acceptable to patients, and reasonably inexpensive?
5. Is the disease common enough to justify the cost of screening entire populations?

Figure 13.1. Five criteria for evaluating a screening procedure.

WELLNESS	ABSENCE OF DISEASE	DISEASED BUT ASYMPTOMATIC	DISEASED AND SYMPTOMATIC (CLINICALLY ILL)	PREMATURE DEATH
Health promotion through self-improvement	Risk factor identification (often referred to as primary prevention)	Early detection through screening (secondary prevention)	Prevention of complications through anticipation of problems and rehabilitation (tertiary prevention)	

Figure 13.2. Health/disease spectrum and preventive/promotive activities.

tion is used primarily for secondary prevention. Historical data pertinent to preventive care needs include

- Dates and results of previous preventive procedures (such as prior immunizations, Pap tests, TB skin tests, mammograms, cholesterol determinations, and blood pressures);
- A careful family history for common and unusual diseases that have a hereditary component;
- A past medical history (allergies, hospitalizations, and prior illness episodes);
- Information about the workplace and living conditions at home;
- Habits such as smoking, exercise, sexual practices, diet, and recreational drug use.

Such data make up much of the traditional history and physical examination; a preventive approach involves not only collecting but also using this information. To gather such preventive data, direct questions should be asked about common conditions (e.g., "Have any of your relatives died of a heart attack or a stroke?"), and open-ended questions should be used to screen for more unusual problems (e.g., "Are there any medical problems that seem to run in your family?" and "Do any of your close relatives have a health problem we haven't already discussed?").

The physical examination is used primarily for early detection of asymptomatic disease. At each patient age, a relatively small number of problems are epidemiologically of highest priority, and an efficient screening physical concentrates on those areas. Therefore, before beginning your physical you should ask yourself, "Which common diseases can be detected early by physical examination of *this* patient, and in which way?"

Much of physical diagnosis is designed to identify disease in patients who already have symptoms, but such measures are often of little use in the asymptomatic patient. In other words, measures that do a good job of diagnosing disease often make poor screening tests, because the predictive value of a positive test result is quite low when the prevalence of disease is low. For example, hearing rales on auscultation of the chest provides valuable diagnostic information in a patient with fever and shortness of breath. But in a healthy, vigorous elderly patient, rales virtually always represent benign conditions—usually either a prior chest infection or simply not having taken a

deep breath recently. Similarly, the neurological examination has many false-positive results in asymptomatic patients and rarely screens for diseases where early treatment improves outcomes; therefore, most of the neurological examination may be omitted in the well-person visit.

A physical examination of a well older man, for example, should at minimum concentrate on:

- Vision and hearing (for cataracts, sensory impairment, vascular changes, and glaucoma screening);
- Cardiovascular examination (for bruits, diminished peripheral pulses, atrial fibrillation, cardiomegaly, aortic stenosis, and peripheral vascular disease);
- Palpation of the thyroid (for nodules and asymptomatic goiter);
- Rectal and prostate examination (for anorectal cancer, prostatic hypertrophy, and prostate cancer);
- Skin (for premalignant and malignant tumors).

Each of the above areas involves conditions that are common and in which physical findings often precede clinical symptoms.

Setting Priorities

The most crucial aspect of preventive primary care practice is taking the time to identify prevention priorities and communicating them to the patient. To select the most important topics for preventive counseling during an office visit, consider the most common causes of death and morbidity. For example, a preparticipation sports examination for a high school boy might productively include vision and hearing screening, testicular examination (with instruction on self-examination), scoliosis screening, a diphtheria-tetanus booster, questions about depression and seat belt use, and counseling about substance abuse and sex. These particular concerns are based on knowledge of cost-effective screening and causes of death (accidents, suicide, and homicide) for that age group.

Case Example

Mr. D.G., a 45-year-old salesman who hasn't been to your office in years, is seen for a sinus infection. Noting that his blood pressure is 150/100, you persuade him to come back for a "physical," and you draw blood for a lipid profile, electrolytes, BUN, and creatinine level. He returns as you requested, and by the end of the visit, you have determined that he smokes 2 packs per day, drinks a six-pack of beer a week, is 75 pounds overweight, eats a high-fat diet, has a cholesterol of 275, has several lipomas on his back, is feeling intense stress at work, is worried about his 16-year-old daughter, probably has mild hypertension, and does not exercise regularly.

Study Questions

- What do you think would happen if, at the end of the visit, you told Mr. D.G. to stop smoking, stop drinking, change his diet, start exercising, and see a psychologist to learn biofeedback for stress reduction?
- From an epidemiological perspective, which *one* behavior would, if changed, cause the greatest reduction in Mr. D.G.'s risk of dying within the next 10 years?
- In setting prevention priorities for Mr. D.G., what single factor is most important?

Case Discussion

Behavioral change is the most powerful preventive health technique, but behavior is difficult to change. Mr. D.G. must have some interest in improving his health, or he would not have agreed to return for a "physical." Epidemiologically, stopping smoking is probably the single most important change he could make, but it may not currently be a priority for him. As his physician, your job is to develop an alliance with him, so that he will see you as helping him rather than judging him.

Your counseling should communicate the dangers associated with his negative health behaviors. It should also motivate him to initiate a process of change and help him see that his situation is not hopeless. You should find things to praise about him and his health. More importantly, you should find out what *his* health priorities are and try to help him achieve them. If he can find an area where he wants to succeed and is able to be successful, he will be more motivated to tackle the "tougher" behavioral changes.

Education and Counseling

Education and counseling occur as part of virtually every physician-patient encounter. Being an effective preventive agent requires developing your communication skills. Patients must be motivated to initiate change; so motivation is your first goal. They then must understand what needs to be done and how to go about doing it. They must take on activities and goals that are doable

and achievable. When your patients fail, you should have ways to keep them motivated to try harder the next time.

The educational process is generally done one-on-one, between physician and patient. There are, however, a variety of adjuncts, from simply writing down your recommendations to referring the patient to a formal program (such as a smoking cessation group). For details on effective patient education, please see Chapter 17.

Prevention-Oriented Office Systems

The physician's office can be organized so that preventive practices are routine. A flow sheet on the chart or a computer reminder system can prompt the appropriate test or intervention at the appropriate time. Delegation of certain tasks to your office staff is effective, provided they have the time and are given explicit guidelines. The fact that blood pressure determination is almost universally performed in ambulatory care underscores how effective prevention can be if it becomes an office routine.

Ideally, preventive systems integrate individualized goals with more general guidelines. For example, a yearly visit for a 40-year-old diabetic woman who smokes might trigger the office staff to perform diphtheria-tetanus immunization, 24-hour creatinine clearance, chest x-ray, maximum expiratory flow rate, urine culture, diet/exercise analysis, and recommendations for dental examination and seat belt use. All this would be obtained or initiated according to protocol by the office staff before the family physician performs an interval history and age/sex/risk-appropriate screening physical examination.

Community Advocacy for Health

Finally, prevention requires "marketing," a distasteful concept to physicians who may not value the potential benefit available to their practice population. In contrast to symptom-based episodic visits, preventive visits are usually made by people in "good health," believing they can feel better, look better, or live longer. That belief is well justified, according to studies of recommended preventive and promotive practices, such as instituting an aerobic exercise program. The question is how to inform members of the community about an available service that will improve their health when they feel well and do not make routine visits. This is the role of marketing.

Some physicians believe that public health education should be a responsibility of the government, mass media, or other organizations. A combination of approaches is most likely to work. Only white, well-educated women are currently well represented as preventive care participants in most practices. Physicians can be active participants in making sure that all demographic and socioeconomic groups obtain preventive care benefits.

Community-oriented health promotion and disease prevention takes the preventive orientation of family practice to its next logical step—community-wide health. Like the individual patient, the community will have particular problems that can be alleviated: e.g., lack of water fluoridation, lack of prenatal care for poor women, high-accident areas, drug abuse, occupational hazards, insufficient activities for the elderly, or environmental pollution. The physician, because of her or his position in the community, can be highly effective in initiating, organizing, leading, and supporting such efforts for change. Chapter 18 discusses further the implementation of community health promotion.

In brief, the community must first recognize the problem. Then it must have a "critical mass" wanting to change the situation. Some family physicians have shown great political sensitivity, skill in creating zeal in others, and patience with the bureaucratic process. Again, the underlying attitude needs to be one of health advocacy.

Acknowledgment. We are indebted to Richard Baker, MD, whose introductory chapter in the first edition of Essentials of Family Medicine *we have drawn on, and who has remained an advocate of health promotion.*

chapter 14

PRENATAL CARE

Margaret R. Helton

The prenatal period offers a unique opportunity for practicing health promotion. At no other time in the human life cycle do patients in good health visit the physician so frequently. It is a time when many women (and couples) are particularly receptive to changing their own health behaviors. Furthermore, the entire process of prenatal care revolves around preventive measures: identifying and managing risk factors, early detection of potential problems, and health education.

For many physicians, prenatal care is one of the most rewarding aspects of family practice, because it is a time during which strong doctor-patient bonds often develop. The continuity of care provided by family physicians allows these bonds to continue postpartum, since the family physician provides ongoing care of the infant and mother after delivery. Continuing to care for the woman, other family members, and the new baby are gratifying aspects of the comprehensive care provided by family physicians. This chapter explores some of the medical and social issues facing family physicians who deliver prenatal care.

PRENATAL CARE IN PERSPECTIVE

High quality prenatal care indisputably lowers maternal, and particularly fetal, mortality rates. In the United States, the maternal mortality rate has decreased from 582/100,000 live births in 1935 to 7.8/100,000 live births in 1985. Most of this decrease is due to innovations in the management of labor and delivery, such as the use of antibiotics, safer blood transfusion capabilities, and the development of safer methods of anesthesia. The independent contribution of prenatal care to this decline in maternal mortality is difficult to assess, since many of the modern advances responsible for better outcomes relate to events occurring at the time of delivery. However, among the aspects of prenatal care that reduce maternal morbidity and mortality are the prevention of pyelonephritis through screening for bacteriuria, better control of diabetes mellitus, and improved detection and control of preeclampsia.

Several lines of evidence link prenatal care with reduced infant mortality rates. In 1940, the infant mortality rate in the United States was 47 per 1000 live births. By 1990, that rate had fallen to 9.1 infant deaths per 1000 live births. Though this is an impressive decline, 20 countries with more than 2,500,000 population had 1989 infant mortality rates less than that of the U.S., led by Japan at 4.4 per 1000 live births. In every European country with an infant mortality rate below the U.S., essentially all pregnant women receive early and adequate prenatal care. In contrast, the U.S. women with the highest infant morality rates receive little or no prenatal care.

In the United States, twice as many African-American mothers receive no or inadequate prenatal care as whites, and the mortality of black infants is twice that of white infants. In institutions where access to prenatal care is equally available to black and white persons, such as in the military, the difference between black and white infant mortality is markedly reduced. Thus, universal prenatal care seems to be a worthy pursuit, since it should contribute to better pregnancy outcomes.

Unfortunately, there have been times when prenatal care, rather than enhancing the pregnancy, brought about just the opposite effect. This occurred when harmful drugs were prescribed for nausea or fluid retention, inappropriate dietary restrictions were advised, or undue anxiety was caused by misguided patient education. "First do no harm," the credo taught to all practitioners of medicine, is aptly applied to prenatal care, especially since most pregnancies will have a healthy outcome anyway. Pregnancy and childbirth are natural processes, not disease states, and should represent joyful and enriching experiences for the woman and her family. The art of prenatal care should promote this experience.

PRENATAL CARE IN THE OFFICE

The goals of prenatal care are comprehensive and aim for three outcomes: a healthy baby and mother, a labor and delivery that go as smoothly as possible, and a smooth adjustment of the mother and family to this life event. The maternal and neonatal mortality rates that have characterized human history are no longer acceptable. Thus, prenatal care must emphasize clinical surveillance of both the mother and her fetus. Such attention should set the stage for a successful labor and delivery.

Ideally, a precondition for all deliveries would be a healthy woman with a reasonable idea of what to expect during labor. Social and psychological support during pregnancy should be an integral part of care during pregnancy and childbirth. Such support reduces anxiety and physical morbidity and increases confidence that the adjustment to motherhood will be successful. The family physician who incorporates this type of care into his or her practice will enjoy satisfied patients.

Pregnancies are conventionally split into three trimesters, each with unique medical and emotional issues. By convention, gestational age is stated as the number of weeks since the last menstrual period (LMP), even though conception does not occur until approximately 2 weeks after that date. Delivery occurs on average at 40 weeks.

Preconception Planning

Ideally a pregnancy is planned or at least wanted, and the prospective mother visits her physician before conception has occurred. At the time of such a visit, the physician can explore and clarify the motives for pregnancy, help the patient maximize her health in anticipation of pregnancy, provide counseling about behaviors and exposures that might jeopardize her or the fetus's health, and explore the motivations for pregnancy.

Among the points that should be covered during prepregnancy counseling are

- *Assessing risk for genetic birth defects*. The relationship between maternal age and Down's syn-

drome should be reviewed, a family history of genetic disease taken, and prenatal screening for neural tube defects reviewed.
- *Attaining physical fitness prior to pregnancy*. Before pregnancy is the time to develop aerobic fitness. Obese patients should be encouraged to lose weight before, not during, pregnancy.
- *Rubella testing and immunization*. Rubella during the first trimester can cause severe congenital anomalies. Ideally, women should be tested for immunity prior to pregnancy and those who are not immune, immunized. If the vaccine is given, woman should use effective birth control for 3 months afterward, since the live virus can theoretically damage a developing fetus.
- *Maternal health behaviors*. These include health habits such as smoking and alcohol use, use (and abuse) of prescription and nonprescription drugs, and sexual promiscuity. All are significant risk factors for maternal and infant mortality.
- *Maternal health problems*. Many chronic illnesses place mothers and their fetuses at increased risk of morbidity and mortality. In some instances (e.g., seizure disorders), medications may constitute an additional risk. In most cases, however, careful medical management will lower the risk of problems. In diabetes mellitus, for example, tight control of the mother's blood sugar will reduce the likelihood of birth defects.
- *Environmental health risks*. Certain occupations pose significant health risks to the mother, either because of exposure to toxins or because of physical stress. These should be identified and discussed in a prepregnancy visit.
- *Prenatal vitamins*. These should be begun prior to pregnancy. There is evidence that folic acid supplementation at 1 mg per day (the standard in prenatal vitamins) reduces the incidence of neural tube defects. Iron and zinc are other important components of prenatal vitamin preparations.
- *Psychosocial risks*. Poor social support and financial stress pose significant risk factors in pregnancy. These should be identified and discussed prepregnancy, if possible.

Table 14.1 summarizes guidelines for a preconception visit. The appointment itself should include time for history taking, a thorough physical examination, education about how to get pregnant and what to do if there are problems getting pregnant, and counseling about the areas outlined above.

Table 14.1. Areas to Assess during a Preconception Visit

General maternal health
  Diabetes mellitus
  Hypertension
  Phenylketonuria (PKU)
  Anemia
  Cardiac, pulmonary, and renal disease
  Epilepsy
Nutrition
High-risk behaviors
  Smoking, alcohol/drug abuse, and sexual promiscuity
Infectious risks
  Human immunodeficiency virus (HIV)
  Hepatitis
  Chlamydia
  Toxoplasmosis
  Syphilis
  Rubella
  Tuberculosis
  Childhood illnesses and immunization history
Genetic counseling
  Age of parents
  Family history of genetic disease
  Family history of malformations
  Previous pregnancy history
  Ethnic risks (Tay-Sachs, sickle cell, cystic fibrosis, thalassemia)
Environmental exposures
  Chemicals
  Drugs
  Radiation
Psychosocial risks
  Personal support
  Marital status
  Housing
  Income
  Education
  Stresses

Diagnosing Pregnancy

The pregnancy tests used today are accurate enough to detect pregnancy before a woman has missed a menstrual period. Signs that the woman herself notices include a missed period, breast tenderness and enlargement, fatigue, and nausea. On physical examination, you should look for uterine enlargement (an accurate method of dating the pregnancy during the first trimester) and dark bluish coloring to the vaginal mucosa and cervix (Chadwick's sign).

First Trimester Prenatal Care

The first trimester (weeks 0–13) is in many ways the most crucial for the developing child. Nearly all organogenesis takes place during these early weeks, making this the period of greatest suscep-

tibility to embryotoxic and teratogenic substances (such as alcohol and many prescription drugs). For the mother, these weeks are often characterized by fatigue, nausea, and the emotional changes that accompany learning of, and adjusting to, the pregnancy. For the physician, initial contacts during the first trimester should help set the stage for a healthy pregnancy.

ESTABLISHING THE EXPECTED DATE OF CONFINEMENT

Because effective detection and management of such problems as intrauterine growth retardation, premature labor, multiple gestation, and postterm pregnancy depends on accurate dating, establishing a reliable expected date of confinement (EDC), or "due date," is important. The simplest method bases your estimated EDC on the date of the last menstrual period, taking into account the reliability of the patient's recall and the length and predictability of her cycles. Nagele's rule estimates the EDC by adding 7 days to the first day of the last normal menstrual period and counting back 3 months. This same principle is embodied in pregnancy wheels (such as those provided by pharmaceutical companies), which are commonly used in office practice to calculate the EDC. Inaccurate dating can result from failure to consider menstrual irregularities, unusual cycle lengths, recent use of oral contraceptives, and the possibility that the presumed last menstrual cycle was really first trimester bleeding or implantation bleeding.

Uterine size, which changes proportionately more from week to week in the first months than at any other time, is another helpful parameter to use in estimating the EDC. During the first trimester, uterine size is detected by bimanual pelvic examination. At 7 weeks, the uterus is the size of a large hen's egg. At 10 weeks, the uterus has grown to the size of an orange. After 12 weeks, the uterus is the size of a grapefruit, and you should feel the upper portion abdominally above the pelvic symphysis. Between 10 and 12 weeks, the fetal heartbeat can first be heard with an ultrasonic Doppler. This milestone should be recorded to add support to other evidence dating the pregnancy.

If there is still doubt about the EDC, ultrasonography performed in the first or second trimester can be helpful. Third trimester sonography is an unreliable predictor of gestational age.

HISTORY AND RISK ASSESSMENT

During the initial patient visit, you should take a thorough medical history. Hypertension, diabetes, and other significant medical diseases can increase the risk of complications during pregnancy. The number of previous pregnancies should be determined and noted using a common shorthand method. As an example of that method, $G_5P_{3-0-1-3}$ would indicate the following: The letter G represents the gravidy of the patient, in other words, how many times she has been pregnant (including this pregnancy). The letter P stands for parity, which is noted using four digits that represent (*a*) the number of term births she has had, (*b*) the number of premature births she has had, (*c*) the number of abortions (spontaneous or elective) she has had, and (*d*) the number of children she currently has living.

An obstetric history must include details of all previous pregnancies—route of delivery, weight and gestation of the newborn, Rhogam administration, and any complications, especially those that resulted in morbidity or fetal mortality. From this historical information, high-risk patients can often be identified. A history of premature delivery, for example, should alert you to the significant risk of recurrence and the need for close surveillance. A history of second trimester losses due to early cervical dilation can signify cervical incompetence, a condition in which the patient may benefit from early placement of a purse-string suture (cerclage). It should also be remembered that women of high parity have an increased risk of placenta previa, puerperal hemorrhage, and multiple gestation.

Risky behaviors should be identified. These include

- Alcohol consumption, which is associated with a variety of congenital malformations and with miscarriage;
- Cigarette smoking, which is related to low infant birth weight;
- Drug use in either the patient or her sexual partners, promiscuity, or relations with bisexual men, all of which are risk factors for the acquired immune deficiency syndrome (AIDS);
- Environmental hazards, including exposure to radiation or potentially teratogenic agents;
- Recent exposure to communicable diseases, particularly rubella or toxoplasmosis;

- A past history of salpingitis or of tubal pregnancy, which may increase the risk of ectopic pregnancy, commonly caused by scarring of the fallopian tubes;
- A past history of herpes, since the infant is at risk for neonatal infection if delivered when the mother has active lesions.

A family history should supplement the personal history and include information on disease, congenital abnormalities, mental retardation, and multiple births in relatives. A social history should describe the patient's level of education, work status, ethnic background, and lifestyle.

PHYSICAL EXAMINATION

The first prenatal visit should include a thorough physical examination, with special attention paid to blood pressure, the size and shape of the uterus and adnexal areas, and the configuration of the bony pelvis. On subsequent visits, examination is generally limited to blood pressure checks, determining uterine size by measuring from the symphysis pubis to the top of the fundus, verifying fetal cardiac activity, and watching for edema. Figure 14.1 is a sample flow sheet for recording prenatal visits.

LABORATORY TESTING

Initial laboratory tests should include hematocrit, syphilis serology, rubella immunity status, hepatitis B surface antigen, urine culture, and a Pap smear. In addition, maternal blood should be typed and checked for antibodies. You should determine if a gonorrhea culture, chlamydia assay, or HIV test are warranted. Table 14.2 lists the routine laboratory tests obtained during prenatal care.

PATIENT EDUCATION AND PSYCHOSOCIAL SUPPORT

First trimester visits occur once a month and set the stage for the ongoing doctor-patient relationship. In your routine visits, you can instruct your patient about symptoms and milestones. Early pregnancy discussions should center on the rapid physical and emotional adjustments demanded of the mother. Education about fatigue, nausea, and ambivalence can be useful. Signs of miscarriage should be discussed at the earliest visit, since nearly all miscarriages occur during the first trimester.

Last menses _____ 8/7/90 _____   EDC ___ 5/15/91 ___
(Circle if reliable)

Comments:

Imprint

Date	Weeks Gest.	Fundal ht	Fetal heart	Presentation	Edema	Blood Pressure	Urine alb/sug	Weight	Next visit	Comments (Nausea/vomiting, headaches, visual disturbances, dysuria, UTI, fever, rash, constipation, bleeding, cramping, vaginal discharge, drugs, special tests)	Resident / Attending
10/2	8	8-10	⊙	—	Ø	110/70	N/N	129	4 wk	New pt. No c/o x̄ nausea	JF
10/30	12	12	⊕ DT	—	Ø	110/78	N/N	131	4 wk	Viable fetus on ultrasound	JF
11/30	16 1/2	16	⊕ DT	—	Ø	108/70	Tr/N	135	4 wk	UTI symptoms resolved	JF
12/27	20	21	⊕ DT	—	Ø	112/68	N/N	139	4 wk	⊕ Fetal movement	JF
1/23	24	24	⊕ FS	—	Ø	120/60	N/N	143	4 wk	Active fetus, no complaints	JF
2/20	28	29	⊕ FS	VTX	Ø	120/68	N/N	146	4 wk	Occasional Braxton-Hicks contr. O'Sullivan test today	JF
3/16	31 1/2	31	⊕ FS	VTX	Tr.	130/72	N/N	151	2 wk	No c/o	SKF
4/3	34	33	⊕ FS	VTX	Tr.	130/76	N/Tr	153	2 wk	Traveling home nxt week, doing well	JF
4/19	36	36	⊕ FS	VTX	Ø	120/70	N/N	154	2 wk	Active fetus	SKF
4/24	37	37	⊕ FS	VTX	Tr.	120/80	N/N	155	1 wk	No complaints x̄ back pain	JF / BG

Figure 14.1. Sample flow sheet for prenatal care.

123

Table 14.2. Routine Laboratory Tests in Prenatal Care

Test	When	Why	Criteria for Abnormality
Hematocrit	1st visit and at 28 weeks	Screen for iron deficiency anemia	≤37 (1st trimester); ≤33 (later pregnancy)
Blood type	1st visit	Determine likelihood of Rh or ABO incompatibility	Rh negative
Antibody screen	1st visit	Determine presence of maternal blood antibodies	Positive
Rubella titer	3 months prior to pregnancy	Test immune status to rubella	titer <1:8
VDRL	1st visit	Screen for maternal syphilis	Positive
Hepatitis B	1st visit	Detect infection or carrier state	Positive
Gonorrhea culture	1st visit	Screen for maternal carrier state	Positive
Pap test	1st visit	Screen for cervical dysplasia	Any dysplasia
Urine culture	1st visit (if high risk, repeat at 28 weeks)	Screen for asymptomatic bacteriuria	Significant growth
Serum α-fetoprotein	16–18 weeks	Screen for neural tube defects (if high) or Down's syndrome (if low)	If outside 95th percentile
O'Sullivan screen	26–28 weeks	Screen for gestational diabetes	Serum glucose >140 mg/dl
Urine dipstick	All visits (proteinuria and glycosuria)	Screen for preeclampsia, likely if ≥2+	Questionable if 1+ for protein and glucose

Good nutrition should be stressed and patients advised that a total pregnancy weight gain should be between 20 and 30 pounds. Calcium intake is important and should be supplemented if the patient is unable to take in 3 to 4 servings of dairy products daily. Prenatal vitamins are usually prescribed; their most important constituents are folic acid and iron.

Many patients and their partners wonder about sexual relations during pregnancy. Unless contraindicated by bleeding or premature labor, intimate relations can continue through the entire pregnancy. In fact, many couples find this period of time to be especially pleasurable.

Other psychosocial issues include a changing body image, a sense of loss of control, fears and fantasies, the father's adjustment, and financial concerns. Advice regarding work and pregnancy (whether it is safe, how long during pregnancy to continue working, and what plans to make for time off after delivery) is usually sought.

Second Trimester Prenatal Care

Between 14 and 26 weeks, a woman really begins to feel pregnant. The common experience of disbelief in early pregnancy is supplanted by an obviously pregnant body and an awareness of fetal movements. Women are socially recognized as being pregnant and start to notice reactions by others. The risk of miscarriage is largely past, nausea has faded, and the uterus is beginning to "show," but it is not yet large enough to significantly reduce mobility. Energy and spirits are often high. The blood pressure drops modestly, a phenomenon that can lead to patient complaints of lightheadedness or fainting.

For the physician, this is an ideal time to get to know the couple better, laying a solid groundwork for working together during labor and delivery. It is an excellent time to schedule a longer visit with both the mother and father, to obtain a genogram, to have each complete a family circle (see Chapter 3), and to discuss family and individual expectations about parenting.

Visits to the doctor normally occur at 4-week intervals throughout the second trimester. During these visits, you should continue to follow the various parameters of pregnancy, as described above. Uterine size from symphysis to fundus is assessed at every visit. Between the 18th and 34th week, the uterine height in centimeters approximates the gestational age in weeks. Discrepancies of several centimeters merit further investigation. At about 20 weeks, you should find the uterus at the umbilicus and should be able to hear the fetal heart with a fetoscope. This specially adapted stethoscope makes use of both air and bone conduction of sound, as you place your skull directly against the receiving portion to enhance sound transmission.

You should ask the woman when she first detected fetal movements. This is known as "quickening" and usually occurs between 16 and 20 weeks. The timing of this sign is too variable to really contribute to the dating of the pregnancy; however, it is a milestone to the woman and you should note it.

These first flickerings of detectable life inside a woman can generate great excitement, as the pregnancy is made real by these movements and by the ever-growing belly. With the belly not yet large enough to interfere with sex, and birth control not an issue, many couples find this to be a time of great intimacy and satisfaction. The second trimester can be a high point psychologically and physically for the expectant mother.

During the second trimester, ultrasound imaging of the fetus is most accurate for dating; this can be added to other dating parameters when data are incomplete or are conflicting. By this time, the baby's sex and overall anatomy can also be accurately assessed by ultrasound.

GENETIC COUNSELING

Congenital malformations occur in about 3% of newborns. Although most of those malformations are minor and do not threaten life, congenital anomalies are now the leading cause of infant mortality in the United States. The most common defects that can be detected through antenatal screening are those caused by neural tube defects, such as anencephaly, and those caused by chromosomal abnormalities, such as Down's syndrome (trisomy 21). Assessment of genetic risks will have begun during the preconception visit or the first prenatal visit, but most of the effort toward early detection of congenital birth defects occurs during the second trimester.

It is now routine to offer neural tube defect screening. This is done by measuring the maternal serum α-fetoprotein (MSAFP) between 16 and 18 weeks gestation. Even if the level is elevated, only a minority of patients will actually have fetal abnormalities. The next step is to repeat the test, as a third of initially elevated results will turn out to be false positives. If the level remains elevated, you should obtain an ultrasound, as inaccurate dating or twin pregnancies are also common causes of abnormal MSAFP results. Ultrasound will also screen for many congenital anomalies, intrauterine growth retardation, or fetal demise, all of which can cause an elevated MSAFP. If the diagnosis is still not clear, amniocentesis to measure the amniotic α-fetoprotein is usually performed.

Screening for Down's syndrome is currently focused largely on older mothers, since the risk of having a baby with a chromosomal abnormality increases with age. Presently, amniocentesis with karyotyping is offered to pregnant women aged 35 and older. The age of 35 is the threshold for routine testing because that is when the risk of the chromosomal abnormalities first approximates the iatrogenic fetal loss rate of amniocentesis (0.5%). However, the vast majority of pregnancies are in younger women; so—although the risk of Down's syndrome is highest in older mothers—80% of children with Down's syndrome are born to mothers under age 35. In an effort to detect these younger mothers whose fetuses have Down's syndrome, screening blood tests are being sought. One approach has been to use the MSAFP, as there is some evidence that low levels of MSAFP are more common in women with Down's syndrome babies. The problem is that this test has very low sensitivity (only about 20 to 30% are detected) and a high false-positive rate, leading to many unnecessary amniocenteses. Use of MSAFP for detection of Down's syndrome remains investigational at this time. Others have suggested routine ultrasonography, as there are characteristic anatomic features in Down's syndrome children that can be detected. However, this has technical limitations and is not yet cost-effective nor reliable enough for routine use.

Genetic screening remains controversial. Some physicians are concerned that the unnecessary amniocenteses and parental anxiety associated with screening do not justify the relatively small number of abnormal fetuses detected. Many parents-to-be, for personal or religious reasons, would not choose to terminate a pregnancy even if a fetal abnormality were detected. For these reasons, you should explain carefully to the expectant mother (or, preferably, to the mother and father together) the benefits and limitations of these screening tests. Allow your patient to make an informed decision about whether to proceed with testing, and document the discussion and decision.

Third Trimester Prenatal Care

For the expectant mother, the third trimester (weeks 27–40) often seems to be in slow motion. Her enlarging abdomen and loosening pelvic synostoses cause increasing discomfort, sleep problems, shortness of breath, urinary frequency, and fatigue. For the physician, this is a time of more intensive medical monitoring, as the incidence of complications (e.g., preeclampsia, maternal hypertension, malposition of the fetus) increases as the patient's due date approaches.

Up to now, the frequency of visits for a healthy woman has been about once monthly. In the last 3 months this increases to every 2 to 3 weeks between 28 and 36 weeks gestation, and weekly during the final month. Obviously, women with obstetric or medical problems require closer surveillance.

Risk assessment is an important component of every visit. The patient should be asked about fetal movements at each visit. Fetal growth is still assessed by measuring the distance in centimeters from the top of the pubic symphysis to the top of the uterine fundus. Fetal position should be determined using abdominal palpation. You should identify whether or not this is a vertex (head first) presentation, a breech, or some other presentation. Ninety-six percent of babies are vertex by the final month of pregnancy. If a breech presentation is detected, you can attempt to turn the baby to vertex (a version). Versions typically have a 50% success rate, with the other half returning to the original breech position.

If the woman has Rh-negative blood, she should receive a Rhogam shot at 28 weeks and another one within 72 hours of giving birth. This immune globulin will prevent Rh sensitization if the baby is Rh-positive. Such sensitization could seriously affect subsequent pregnancies.

Another important parameter to follow is the patient's blood pressure. A rise of 30 mm Hg systolic or 15 mm Hg diastolic heralds the onset of a hypertensive disorder of pregnancy, a potentially life-threatening complication. Edema and proteinuria in addition to the blood pressure rise confirms a diagnosis of preeclampsia and warrants immediate hospitalization, with timely delivery of the endangered fetus.

Although regular screening for glucosuria has occurred at every prenatal visit, urinary screening is an insensitive and nonspecific test for gestational diabetes. The presence of sugar in the urine commonly represents a change in renal threshold rather than hyperglycemia, and glucose intolerance can exist without the appearance of glucose in the urine. At about 26 to 28 weeks, therefore, it is prudent to screen for this complication by checking a serum glucose level on a sample drawn 1 hour after the administration of 50 grams of glucose in a flavored drink (the O'Sullivan test). Levels of 140 mg/dl or greater are abnormal and should be followed with a full oral glucose tolerance test. Risk factors for diabetes include a family history of diabetes; previous delivery of a macrosomic, malformed, or stillborn infant; obesity; and hypertension. Patients at high risk should be screened during the second trimester.

If your patient has a past history of genital herpes, the perineal, vaginal, and cervical region must be inspected weekly during the last month to rule out active lesions that would mandate a cesarean section to lower the risk of congenital herpes in the baby. Those at high risk for sexually transmitted diseases should also have a repeat gonorrhea culture, syphilis serology, hepatitis B screen, and HIV test.

Childbirth education is an important part of third trimester office visits. Once the medical assessment is complete, your attention should turn to the patient and her family's eager anticipation of labor and delivery. This prompts discussions about the varieties of early labor experiences and symptoms that warrant calling the doctor: ruptured membranes, bleeding, decreased fetal movement, and regular contractions. As always, anticipatory guidance about the myriad of sensations of late pregnancy, such as heartburn, leg cramps, backache, and false labor, helps promote patience, understanding, and confidence during the last weeks.

In addition to preparing for the delivery itself, your patient education should focus on caring for the new baby. Breast-feeding should be encouraged through discussion and recommended readings. If the mother-to-be is interested in breast-feeding but is anxious about it, referral to the local chapter of the La Leche League can be helpful. Preparations for the new baby should be reviewed as well, particularly if your patient is having her first child.

Psychosocial issues at this time include discussing dreams and fantasies, support during labor, and "nesting" behavior. Patience must often be advised and empathy expressed, as the last trimester probably will seem the longest.

POSTTERM PREGNANCY

It is difficult to find a more weary and exasperated patient than a woman who has seen her due date come and go. Often, she will come into your office expecting you to do something to get labor started. Hopefully, you will have warned her earlier in the course of prenatal care that delivering 2 weeks past her due date is still within the normal range.

Postterm pregnancy is defined as one that extends more than 42 weeks beyond the last menstrual period. The most common explanation for a postterm pregnancy is incorrect dating of the gestation. The concern with these extended pregnancies is development of oligohydramnios with umbilical cord compression and uteroplacental insufficiency, leading to fetal compromise during labor. Also significant is the fact that 25% of postterm babies weigh more than 4000 grams, resulting in a greater incidence of birth trauma, shoulder dystocia, and cesarean section.

Ideally, you have established an accurate due date as part of your earlier prenatal care. If an accurate due date is unknown, you should review all available data, recognizing that ultrasound is less accurate at this stage. In addition, you must verify fetal health through frequent monitoring as the woman approaches postterm. This monitoring should include (a) an ultrasound study of the baby to assess fetal movement and the amount of amniotic fluid present, and (b) a nonstress test, to verify the baby's cardiac rate and reactivity. Findings of concern may mandate labor induction.

FAMILY PHYSICIAN'S APPROACH TO THE MANAGEMENT OF LABOR

There has been a dramatic increase in childbirth technology over the past two decades. With this has come the assumption that the technological approach espoused by obstetric specialists should constitute the standard of care. The value of "high-tech" labor management in uncomplicated pregnancy has not been demonstrated. Thus, while high-risk pregnancies should receive appropriate intervention and technology, routinely applying these behaviors to normal pregnancies is misguided. It is often up to the family physician to maintain the proper perspective and to resist the obstetrician's tendency to view every pregnancy as a disaster waiting to happen.

The value of a prepared patient and support person in reducing complications of labor cannot be overemphasized. Thus, the time you have spent educating your patient and her support person during prenatal care, and the techniques they have learned in prenatal education classes (which, of course, you have encouraged them to attend) will generally pay great dividends during the stress of labor and delivery.

During labor, the family physician should provide ongoing surveillance of the mother and fetus and provide support to the mother and attending friends and family members. The family doctor should strive to promote personalized care for the woman and her family, even in large institutions with many rules.

Above all, any practitioner delivering babies must learn patience, patience, patience.

FAMILY PHYSICIANS AND OBSTETRIC CONSULTANTS

As generalists, family physicians at times serve their patients best by working with colleagues who have a greater depth of knowledge in a specialized field. Perinatal medicine, like most medical disciplines, has continued to grow and become more specialized. Family doctors are trained to provide independent prenatal and delivery care to low-risk women, identifying and managing emergencies and risk factors as they occur. In the care of complicated patients, family physicians work closely with obstetric colleagues, turning to them for expert opinion about patient management and technical skill for operative maneuvers or deliveries. To clarify their shared responsibility for such patients, family practice and obstetric departments in many hospitals have negotiated a list of high-risk conditions existing during prenatal care or occurring during labor and delivery, which constitute situations where the family doctor is expected to involve obstetric colleagues in the care of the patient. Table 14.3 contains one such list, developed at the University of North Carolina.

When the consultation process works well, the patient benefits from incorporation of specialty expertise while maintaining the trusted continuity relationship with her primary doctor. For such a collaborative effort to benefit the patient, the family physician must be aware of personal limitations, be committed to consultation agreements, communicate the needs and expectations of the consultation directly and clearly, and trust the consultant. The consultant must be responsive to the request for consultation or technical assistance, value the ongoing primary role of the family doctor, respect the long-standing doctor-patient relationship, and be open and di-

Table 14.3. Guidelines for Obstetric Consultation

Major risk factors: obstetric consultation mandatory
- Incompetent cervical os or 2nd trimester spontaneous abortion by history
- Previous or current Rh or other immunization
- Need for amniocentesis (genetic, abnormal α-fetoprotein (AFP), maturity studies)
- Diabetes class B, C, D
- Multiple gestation
- Previous C-section
- Sickle-cell disease or other hemoglobinopathy
- Premature labor
- Preeclampsia
- Significant vaginal bleeding
- Placenta previa
- Postmaturity at 42 weeks
- Previous thromboembolic disease

Other risk factors: consultation should be considered
- Severe anemia <10 g Hb, <30% Hct
- Nonvertex presentation at term
- Previous stillbirth or neonatal death
- Previous premature delivery
- Medical complications (cardiac or renal disease, seizure or bleeding disorder, etc.)
- Obesity >250 lb
- Prepregnancy weight <100 lb
- Recurrent urinary tract infections
- Age >35
- Age <18
- Abnormal uterine growth
- Late prenatal care (after 20 weeks)
- Fetal arrhythmia
- Gestational hypertension, chronic hypertension
- Diabetes class A
- Abnormal AFP
- Inadequate maternal weight gain
- Alcohol or drug abuse
- Multiple spontaneous or elective abortions
- Genital herpes
- Psychosocial complications

rect in negotiating the details of sharing responsibility for patient care.

CONCLUSIONS

Prenatal care serves important functions of medical screening and surveillance. It also offers the opportunity for educating mothers and for planning the birth itself. Countries that provide universal access to prenatal care have lower infant mortality rates than those where access is restricted. As family physicians, we should support efforts to remove the barriers to prenatal care in our communities.

The care of families throughout pregnancy, delivery, and postpartum, and the longitudinal care of families throughout the life cycle, enables family physicians and their patients to view prenatal care as part of an ongoing relationship. This view more closely matches how patients experience their own pregnancies, without artificial punctuation of their lives imposed by a health care system that recognizes pregnancy, newborn care, and adult development as belonging to different specialties.

The goal of healthy babies is shared with other obstetric providers, but as a family doctor you are in a unique position to exert a wide influence over the health of your patient, the newborn, and their family. The provision of excellent prenatal care is but one of the exciting facets of family practice.

SUGGESTED READINGS

Andolsek KM: *Obstetric Care: Standards of Prenatal, Intrapartum, and Postpartum Management*, Philadelphia, Lea & Febiger, 1990.

Written by an academic family physician, this paperback nicely covers obstetric issues.

Chalmers I, Enkin M, Keirse M (eds): *Effective Care in Pregnancy and Childbirth*. Oxford, Oxford Medical Publications, 1989.

A two-volume set, these books offer the most thorough critical review of prenatal care and childbirth practices written to date. Reviews the available literature on practically every aspect of pregnancy and childbirth.

Chamberlain G, Lumley J (eds): *Prepregnancy Care: A Manual for Practice*. New York, Wiley, 1986.

One-of-a-kind guide to physical and mental preparation for pregnancy, considering normal patients and those with preexisting medical problems or pregnancy complications. Thorough literature citations.

Gaskin IM: *Spiritual Midwifery*. Summertown, TN, The Book Publishing Company, 1990.

A fascinating description of birthing experiences and prenatal suggestions to those following alternative practices. Written by a well-known leader in midwifery in the United States.

Kochenour NK: Normal pregnancy and prenatal care. In Scott JR, DiSaia PJ, Hammond CB, Spellacy WN (eds): *Danforth's Obstetrics and Gynecology*. Philadelphia, JB Lippincott, 1990, pp 123–159.

Few major textbooks give careful consideration to normal pregnancy care. This chapter is a better-than-average example.

Myles MF: Examination of the pregnant woman. In *Textbook for Midwives: with Modern·Concepts of Obstetric and Neonatal Care*, ed 9. New York, Churchill Livingstone, 1981, pp 121–148.

British textbook for midwives first published in 1953. This edition is an excellent guide to the physical examination of a pregnant patient. Excellent illustrations.

Niswander KR (ed): *Manual of Obstetrics: Diagnosis and Therapy*, ed 4. Boston, Little, Brown & Co., 1991.

Spiral-bound, problem-oriented manual organized as a series of outlines, designed to be carried around for rapid access to information about diagnosis and management.

chapter 15

WELL CHILD CARE

Lee A. Beatty and J. Lewis Sigmon, Jr.

Well child care is one of the most challenging and rewarding aspects of family practice. In number of office visits alone, it accounts for a large portion of the pediatrics in one's practice. Parents and other caretakers often judge a physician's overall competence by their perceptions of the ability to provide good well child care. Preventive medicine and health promotion practices applied between the ages of birth and 16 years are ways in which family physicians can positively influence the health of future generations.

Well child care can be divided into four areas remembered as the mnemonic, RISE: (*a*) Risk factor identification; (*b*) Immunizations; (*c*) Screening; and (*d*) Education. This chapter contains a discussion of well child care between birth and 16 years of age. It is assumed that well child care is practiced within the context of the family systems approach discussed in Chapter 3.

RISK FACTOR IDENTIFICATION

Risk factor identification for well children is the process of obtaining historical, physical examination, and laboratory data that can place the infant, child, or adolescent into a high-risk group, causing you to modify your management plan. The family history, social history, past history, or review of systems may identify risk factors that would prompt you to provide health maintenance with a particular focus. The interview, screening physical examination, and laboratory tests might alter routine care of the individual child. For example, a child with sickle cell trait or disease in the family would require a screening test for homozygous hemoglobin S. A positive test result would necessitate close follow-up for symptoms, signs, and laboratory testing for hemolytic anemia. Another example is the adolescent girl who is sexually active and should be screened for sexually transmitted diseases (STDs) and for cervical dysplasia at appropriate intervals and have birth control issues discussed.

Risk factors can be ascertained initially from the medical history. Psychosocial information must be sought because risk factors may arise from, or be modified by, overcrowding, poverty, family dysfunction, location of home, community resources, parents' lifestyle (e.g., passive smoking), and so on. Interval well child visits will give you a chance to update risk factors if they are reported in response to questions like, What changed since I last saw you (or 'your child')? How are things at school . . . at home? The problem list should include risk factors and reminders to carry out needed screening tests or education during future visits.

IMMUNIZATIONS

Immunizations have greatly reduced morbidity and mortality from a variety of infectious diseases. Table 15.1 gives recommendations for childhood immunizations by the American Academy of Pediatrics (1). The United States Public Health Service recommendations are similar, with minor variations, particularly around when to administer the MMR booster. There are relative as well as absolute contraindications to certain immunizations, plus alternative schedules for those children deficient in recommended immunizations (1). *Haemophilus* b conjugate vaccines (HbCVs) are available with slightly different recommended routine schedules as noted in Table 15.2 (2). Vaccination against hepatitis B is recommended at 2-, 4- and 6-months by the Public Health Service, and at birth, 1- to 2-months and 16–18 months of age by the American Academy of Pediatrics for routine immunization in childhood as well.

Vaccines have a small but definite risk for adverse reactions. Reactions can range from a mild

Table 15.1. Recommended Immunization Schedule for Healthy Infants and Children[a]

Age	Immunization(s)[b]	Comments
Birth	HBV	
2 months	DTP, HbCV, OPV, HBV	May initiate DTP and OPV as early as 4 weeks
4 months	DTP, HbCV, OPV	
6 months	DTP, HbCV, HBV	Third OPV dose recommended in foreign countries where polio is endemic
15 months	MMR, HbCV	
18 months	DTP, OPV	
4–6 years	DTP, OPV	Generally given before school entry; do not give pertussis vaccine after seventh birthday; some physicians give MMR booster at this time
11–12 years	MMR	Recommendations on MMR boosters are not yet standardized
14–16 years	Td	Repeat every 10 years throughout life

[a]Adapted from Committee on Infectious Diseases, American Academy of Pediatrics: *Report of the Committee on Infectious Diseases,* ed 22. American Academy of Pediatrics, 1991, p 17.
[b]Key: DTP, diphtheria and tetanus toxoids with pertussis vaccine; HbCV, *Haemophilus* b conjugate vaccine; OPV, oral poliovirus vaccine containing attenuated poliovirus types 1, 2, and 3; MMR, live measles, mumps, and rubella viruses as a combined vaccine; Td, adult tetanus toxoid (full dose) and diphtheria toxoid (reduced dose) for adult use; HBV, hepatitis B vaccine.

Table 15.2. Vaccination Schedule for Available *Haemophilus* Vaccines[a]

Vaccine	Age at 1st dose (months)	Primary Series	Booster
HbOC (Lederle-Praxis)	2–6	3 doses, 2 months apart	15 months
	7–11	2 doses, 2 months apart	15 months
	12–14	1 dose	15 months
	15–59	1 dose	None
PRP-OMP (Merck Sharp and Dohme)	2–6	2 doses, 2 months apart	12 months
	7–11	2 doses, 2 months apart	15 months
	12–14	1 dose	15 months
	15–59	1 dose	None
PRP-D (Connaught)	15–59	1 dose	None

[a]From Centers for Disease Control: *Haemphilus* b conjugate vaccines for prevention of *Haemophilus influenzae* type b disease among infants and children two months of age and older. *MMWR* 40(RR-1): 5, 1991.

fever and irritability to anaphylaxis and death. The pertussis vaccine has received some notoriety for adverse reactions (toxic encephalitis). In fact, severe reactions are quite rare and are often misdiagnosed. Thus, the pertussis vaccine's benefits outweigh its risks in most cases. In counseling patients about potential adverse effects, remember that reactions to toxoid vaccines (DTP and HbCV) occur within 48 hours, whereas reactions to live vaccines occur later. In particular, it is wise to warn parents whose children have received the MMR immunization that the child is likely to experience mild rash, arthralgias, and a low-grade fever 8 to 12 days afterward.

Use of live virus immunizations (e.g., measles/mumps/rubella and oral polio vaccine) during pregnancy or in an immunocompromised host carries increased risk for causing clinical disease. Before taking responsibility for immunizing anyone in this litigious society, the health care provider should be familiar with the current relevant vaccine information and be willing and able to convey such information completely, yet understandably, to the child's caretaker. Ideally, this should include written material to take home.

DIAGNOSTIC SCREENING

Screening refers to the process by which one discovers asymptomatic disease. Since the patient has no symptoms, detection occurs by physical examination or laboratory testing. An important role of history taking in this context is to determine risk factors (e.g., family history of ischemic heart disease) so that screening measures can be used more selectively.

Screening Physical Examination

A brief screening examination is usually performed on each well child visit. Not all parts of the examination have equal importance in the asymptomatic child. Therefore, particular attention should be paid to those aspects that have the highest yield of clinically useful data. The following section is a partial list of problems that may have subtle or no symptoms and yet can be discovered by a thorough examination.

GROWTH AND DEVELOPMENT

Poor growth, recognized by an aberrant growth pattern, may be the presenting feature of a variety of disorders such as endocrinopathies and cardiac or renal disorders. Height, weight, and head circumference should be measured during all routine office visits during the first 2 years of life (head circumference is at least 90% complete by 2 years of age). Subsequently, height and weight should be measured on all well child visits through adolescence. Obesity may be documented by plotting a growth curve. The increased morbidity associated with long-term obesity is well documented, which makes recognition and prevention in childhood important.

Development can be monitored by following age-appropriate milestones of intellectual, motor, and social skills (see Suggested Readings). The most common method of assessing development is the Denver developmental screening test (DDST). DDST identifies children who are developing at an unusually slow rate so that appropriate investigation and intervention can be undertaken. Items from the DDST can be integrated with other screening tests, immunizations, and educational reminders to form a health maintenance flowsheet.

CARDIOVASCULAR SCREENING

Childhood hypertension has an incidence of 1.4 to 11%, depending on the age, race, and prevalence of obesity within the population. There is a strong familial pattern often associated with obesity. Blood pressure screening is felt to be appropriate by most experts, who point out the high correlation between childhood and subsequent adult hypertension. Screening should be performed periodically starting at age 3 years. Blood pressure measurements should be taken with the correct cuff size (2/3 of upper arm length). An oversized cuff will give a falsely low reading and an undersized cuff a falsely elevated reading. Remember that normal blood pressure values depend on age. Elevated blood pressure should be confirmed on at least three separate occasions before treatment is started.

Congenital heart disease has an incidence of approximately 1% and accounts for half of all deaths due to congenital defects. Most cases can be detected in the first 6 months of life. Auscultation of the heart and palpation of pulses (including femoral pulses) should be performed in the newborn period and repeated at least twice in the first 6 months.

MUSCULOSKELETAL SCREENING

The incidence of congenital hip disease is 1 to 2 per thousand. It is more common in females, first born, breech births, infants with other congenital postural deformities, growth retardation, oligohydramnios, and in families with a history of the disorder. It is not always possible to make the diagnosis in the neonatal period, either because the examination does not reveal any abnormality or because the dislocation occurs later. Newborns should be screened while in the nursery and during the first 3 months of life, using the Ortolani maneuver. The "classic" signs of dislocation become more common after 6 weeks of age and should be looked for until the child is walking normally. The most important of these signs is limitation of abduction (normal abduction is greater than 75°). Once the child has learned to walk, an abnormal gait may also be a clue to dislocation. Because of the difficulty in detecting congenital hip dislocation in a newborn by clinical examination, ultrasound examinations may become an adjunct screening test.

SCOLIOSIS

The overall incidence of scoliosis varies from 2 to 10% due to the nonstandardized criteria used in defining spinal curvature. Large curves (greater than or equal to 20°) have a much lower incidence (in one study, 0.5% for girls, with an 8:1 female predominance). The average age of onset in girls is 12 to 13 years, and in boys 13 to 14 years, though this varies considerably. The best rule-of-thumb is that the most rapid progression occurs during the peak velocity of the adolescent growth spurt. Screening for scoliosis in girls should be performed between the ages of 10 and 14, and in boys between 12 and 16. Clinical screening can identify the vast majority of large curves, but false positives are common. The test requires inspection of the back in the standing and forward-bending positions as shown in Figure 15.1. Asymmetry of the shoulders, scapulae, or hips is significant. An

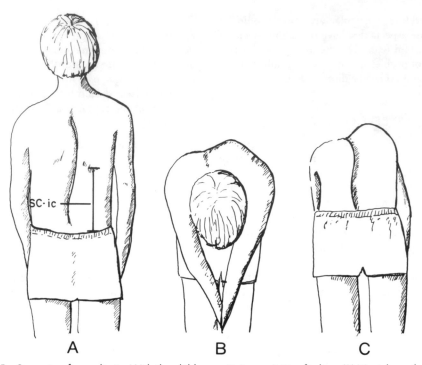

A   B   C

Figure 15.1. Screening for scoliosis. With the child standing (A) look for unlevel shoulders or hips. Measure the distance on each side between the inferior border of each scapula and the posterior superior iliac spine (*SC-ic above*); a difference greater than 2 cm con-stitutes a positive finding. (B) Next, have the child bend forward with arms extended, fingertips interlocked and pointed in the midline. (C) Observing from behind, look for asymmetry of the chest or rib cage. Positive findings should be evaluated radiologically.

asymmetric hump of the lumbar or thoracic paraspinal region noted on forward-bending is also an important finding. The degree of curvature is then determined from a radiograph of the spine.

Children with scoliosis should be followed by an orthopaedist skilled in the management of this disease. Curves less than 20° are generally observed, since fewer than 10% will progress to the treatable range. Curves greater than 20° are observed more closely; more than half will eventually require treatment. Curves greater than 30° usually require bracing, as do curves between 20 and 30° that are rapidly progressing. Bracing does appear to prevent progression in most cases, thus preventing the need for spinal fusion.

HEARING SCREENING

Severe congenital deafness has an incidence of 0.5 to 1 per thousand. The prevalence of some degree of hearing impairment among school age children is 3 to 5%. The vast majority have temporary conductive hearing losses due to middle ear effusion.

Screening tests to detect middle ear disease are much more controversial due to the transient nature of the disorder in most cases and the uncertain morbidity in those that do persist.

Congenital deafness, on the other hand, does require early diagnosis to obtain optimal therapeutic results, as 80% of language growth is achieved by age 3. The high-risk group includes those with other affected family members, a history of bilirubin levels above 20 mg/dl, congenital rubella syndrome, infants with meningitis, infants receiving aminoglycosides, associated anomalies of the ear, nose, or throat, and very low birth weight infants (1500 g or less). Screening office procedures are performed with noisemakers, looking for responses that are appropriate for the age: 4 months—widened eyes, slight turning, listening attitude; 6 months—turning 45°; 8 months—recognizing whether the sound source is above or below. A history should be obtained from parents throughout the first 2 years regarding the child's vocalization, responses to sound, and language development. Noisemaker orientation testing should be performed in 6- to -12 month-old children. Refer all suspected cases to the audiologist early, and all high-risk cases should probably be referred regardless. Hearing can be evaluated in very young children by using brainstem-evoked potential testing.

VISION SCREENING

Vision screening is aimed at detecting five defects: cataracts, ocular tumors, refractive errors, strabismus, and amblyopia. Each of these conditions has a critical detection period for successful intervention. Therefore, for timely and accurate screening, you need to master a routine set of diagnostic techniques that include bilateral red reflex examination, funduscopic examination, corneal light reflex test, cover-uncover test, and visual acuity tests.

The eye examination of the newborn and infant less than 4 months of age focuses on detection of congenital cataracts and ocular tumors, such as retinoblastoma. When performing the red reflex test, you should look for identical, simultaneous red images. Asymmetry in the red reflex indicates either a problem with light transmission through the eye or a retinal defect, and thus should be referred to an ophthalmologist. Assess ocular mobility by observing the child's "tracking" ability while he or she follows an interesting object. Include a funduscopic examination for children ages 3 and older.

Strabismus is a malalignment of the two eyes so that only one eye at a time views the regarded object. It occurs in 2% of children and has a strong family tendency. Strabismus present during binocular vision (both eyes open) is called manifest strabismus or "tropia." Eye deviation present only when binocular vision is interrupted is called latent strabismus or "phoria." The child with either kind of strabismus unconsciously suppresses vision in the affected eye. This condition must be detected early (ideally before 3 years) to obtain maximum benefit from treatment, because development of the visual cortex depends on the eye being actively used. Treatment of strabismus typically consists of patching the unaffected eye (forcing the affected eye's visual image to be used by the visual cortex) or surgery to correct muscle imbalances. Failure to detect strabismus before age 6 can lead to *amblyopia*, a decreased visual acuity of one eye that is uncorrectable with lenses.

The corneal light reflex (Fig. 15.2) detects manifest strabismus (tropia). You should begin this test routinely at age 6 months. Pseudostrabismus, where both eyes falsely appear turned in because of large epicanthal eyelid folds, can be distinguished from true defects with this test. The cover-uncover test (Fig. 15.3) can detect both phorias and tropias. You should begin using this examination for children between 6 and 12 months of age.

Refractive errors, especially if asymmetric, can also lead to amblyopia. Thus you must initiate visual acuity testing as early as possible. When screening infants, direct their gaze to a small attractive object. If occlusion of one eye produces a consistent, reproducible anxious response but occlusion of the other eye does not, this may be a qualitative indication of decreased vision in the eye that can be occluded without the infant's resistance. Allen picture cards are useful in children aged 3 to 4 years, and the standard Snellen chart or more elaborate Titmus tester screens children older than 5 to 6 years of age. You should refer children who have vision worse than 20/40 or who have a two-line or greater difference in visual acu-

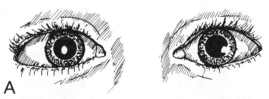

A

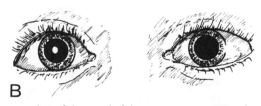

B

Figure 15.2. Infant screening for detection of strabismus using corneal light reflex test. In a darkened room, hold a small flashlight or otoscope in the midline in front of your chin and observe its reflection in the infant's eyes as they fix on it. The reflection should be in the identical location on the cornea of both eyes. A difference between the midpupil of one eye and the outer edge of the pupil of the opposite eye (A) indicates approximately 7° gaze difference (strabismus). A difference between midpupil and the outer edge of the opposite iris (B) indicates about 15° gaze difference. Any noticeable and reproducible difference beyond 6 months of age should be referred to an ophthalmologist.

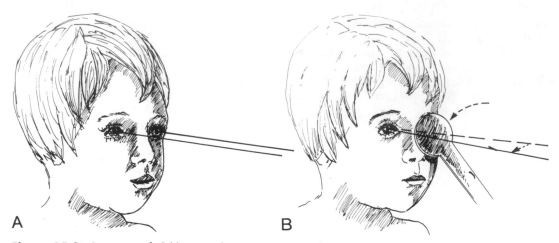

A   B

Figure 15.3. Screening of children aged 1 to 10 years for detection of strabismus: cover test. Have the child fix on a distant object (A). Cover one eye, observing the other. If the other eye jumps to fix on the object when you cover the first, then strabismus is de-tected (B). Next, remove the cover, observing whether the eye that was covered jumps to fix on the object. This indicates a latent (occurring only when the eye cannot fix) strabismus. A positive test result should prompt referral.

ity between eyes. Also, you should refer any child who either you or the parents think has a significant asymmetry of visual acuity, even in the absence of objective findings.

CARIES PREVENTION

Tooth decay is a common dental infection found in children. Its incidence is declining because of simple preventive measures. Baby bottle caries, a condition of rampant tooth decay, can be prevented by not allowing babies to go to sleep bottle-feeding and by weaning from the bottle at an early date—usually around the first birthday. Physicians have an important role in preventive dentistry, because young children rarely visit dentists. Thus, well child care should involve inspection of the teeth and instructions about the importance of regular brushing and (at later ages) flossing. Young children are generally unable to brush their own teeth effectively; so parents should be encouraged to do some or all of each day's brushing themselves.

Fluoride supplementation has also proven a significant deterrent of dental caries. All breast-fed babies should be supplemented with fluoride drops, since fluoride does not enter the breast milk in appreciable amounts. Bottle-fed babies should receive fluoride supplementation if the water supply is not fluoridated. The amount of supplemental oral fluoride prescribed after weaning from the breast depends on the natural or added fluoride content of the water supply plus the individual's total daily volume of water intake from those sources. Local health departments provide information about local water fluoride content. Using such data, fluoride dosage may be individualized to maximize caries prophylaxis and minimize fluorosis (Table 15.3).

Avoidance of tetracycline during pregnancy and childhood up to 8 years of age is important to prevent staining of the child's permanent teeth. Children should begin regular visits to the dentist no later than the second birthday.

Laboratory Screening

Laboratory screening is not necessary on every well child visit. Too often a routine urinalysis and hematocrit are performed, adding unnecessary costs. Other routine studies may provide no significant information and sometimes lead to the vicious cycle of ordering further laboratory tests to disprove the initial abnormal results. On the other hand certain laboratory tests should be routine. The areas most often considered are discussed below.

INBORN ERRORS OF METABOLISM

The incidence of congenital hypothyroidism is approximately one in 4000 to 5000. Profound mental retardation is the inevitable result of not providing

Table 15.3. Fluoride Supplementation Schedule for Infants and Children[a]

Note: Fluoride supplementation should be based on the concentration of fluoride in the water supply and individual's average volume of fluoridated water intake per day. Canned or bottled fluids (e.g., ready-to-feed formulas and sodas) are, in general, not fluoridated. Well water fluoride content varies by geographic site and is often available from local health departments; if not, the water can be tested for fluoride content. The following table is based on 1 part per million (ppm) or 1 mg of fluoride per liter of fluoridated water.

Age (years)	Estimated Daily Intake (ml) of Fluoridated Water	Recommended Daily Fluoride Supplementation (mg)
0–2	None or very little (e.g., breast-fed)	0.25 mg
	>250 ml	None
2–3	≤250 ml	0.50 mg
	250–500 ml	0.25 mg
	>500 ml	None
3–16	≤250 ml	1.00 mg
	250–500 ml	0.75 mg
	500–750 ml	0.50 mg
	750–1000 ml	0.25 mg
	>1000 ml	None

Note: If the patient uses well water or other water with some natural fluoride, then the recommended daily intake of fluoride is as follows:

| Age | Fluoride Concentration in Local Water Supply (ppm) | | |
	≤0.3	0.3–0.7	≥0.7
0–3	0.25	None	None
3–5	0.50	0.25	None
5–14	1.00	0.50	None

| | **Fluoride Preparations** | |
Preparation	Brand Names	Fluoride Content
Liquid	Luride drops	0.125 mg/drop
	Poly-Vi-Flor (or other multivitamin/fluoride combination)	0.25 mg/ml
Chewable tablets	Luride Lozi-Tabs	0.25, 0.5, or 1.0 mg/tab
	Poly-Vi-Flor (or other multivitamin/fluoride combination)	1.0 mg/tab

[a]Adapted from Anastasio GD, Cornell KO, Edwards P, Forston NS, Glazer H (eds): Charlotte, NC, *Carolinas Medical Center Pharmacotherapy Handbook*, 1991–92, p 35.

replacement therapy early in life. Thyroid screening is now routinely done in all 50 states prior to discharge from the nursery. Similarly, the frequency of phenylketonuria (PKU), along with the clearly documented benefit of early detection and treatment, has led to the requirement of screening all term newborns before discharge. Infants discharged at less than 24 hours of age should have the test repeated by 1 week of age. Some states are now screening newborn infants for sickle cell disease and galactosemia. The results of these tests should be made available to the physician within 2 to 3 weeks.

Lack of follow-up on test results is one reason for the occasional case of hypothyroidism or PKU escaping early detection and appropriate management. Other reasons include an inadequate specimen, improper processing of the specimen, and assay error. Therefore, normal results are most as-suring, but they cannot be relied upon absolutely to exclude the diagnosis in an infant with a clinical picture compatible with either of these disorders.

IRON DEFICIENCY

The highest prevalence of iron deficiency in children occurs between 6 and 24 months of age, varying between 1 and 24%, depending on the population studied. Exclusively breast-fed term infants are iron sufficient at age 6 months, but thereafter, they may become iron deficient if not provided with iron-containing foods. Premature infants cannot derive sufficient iron from breast-feeding to meet their increased needs for growth. The Committee on Nutrition of the American Academy of Pediatrics, therefore, recommends iron supplementation in breast-fed babies, starting no later than 4 months of age in term infants and no later than 2 months of age in preterm infants and continuing at least through the first year of life.

There are no highly accurate, simple, laboratory tests to determine tissue iron stores. Several studies have indicated that nonanemic iron-deficient infants (decreased serum ferritin with normal hemoglobin) treated with iron therapy showed improvement in developmental test scores. The implications of this observation are not fully known at present, but it suggests a variety of subtle systemic metabolic disturbances that may result from iron deficiency (3). Neonates should generally be screened, as well as all term infants, at age 9 to 12 months, and all low-birth-weight infants at 6 to 9 months of age. For anemia screening, use a hemoglobin level less than 11.5 g/dl as the cutoff value and follow the response to a trial of iron replacement therapy.

LEAD POISONING

Lead is a ubiquitous by-product of our industrialized society. Lead produces its toxic effects through interference with nerve conduction, hemoglobin synthesis, and vitamin D metabolism. Infants and young children are particularly susceptible to these toxic effects for three reasons: (a) much hand-to-mouth activity (lead paint and lead dust ingestion), (b) vulnerability of the developing nervous system, and (c) high lead-absorption rates compared with older children and adults. Although the major sources of lead (lead-based paint and leaded gasoline) were banned by the mid-1970s, it is estimated that millions of tons of lead persist in the surface soils of urban areas and that about 4 million homes where young children reside have peeling lead paint. Lead solder seals the plumbing of most homes and schools, and lead is an ingredient in many hobby materials such as pottery glazes. Thus, no socioeconomic group or geographic region is spared the potential for lead poisoning.

Since 1985, investigators have found compelling evidence that subtle, but definite, learning deficits occur in children with blood lead levels that were once felt to be safe. In October, 1991, the Centers for Disease Control (CDC) reported that these adverse effects are apparent at blood lead levels as low as 10 µg/dl, less than one-half the threshold level set 6 years earlier. The CDC now proposes universal screening for all children, using a capillary blood lead level test rather than the previously recommended but less sensitive erythrocyte protoporphyrin assay. Since another universal screening test is prohibitively expensive on a national scale and will most likely be phased in over time, the CDC has published new guidelines for identifying, monitoring, and treating children at greatest risk and for eliminating the most threatening lead exposures (4).

TUBERCULOSIS

The prevalence of positive tuberculin tests among those entering school is approximately 0.2%. The Centers for Disease Control and the American Lung Association have recommended discontinuation of routine testing in populations where the prevalence of tuberculin activity is less than 1%. This is based on the fact that most new cases of active tuberculosis are detected by testing contacts of new cases and by screening persons at known high risk. Periodic screening should continue in high risk groups, such as persons who have been in contact with a case, persons from endemic regions of the world (e.g., Mexico or Southeast Asia), and persons residing in communities or residential institutions where the prevalence exceeds that of the general population (possibly including inner city children). Such screening should begin at 12 to 15 months of age and be repeated annually or biannually until school entry. All positive reactions by a multipuncture technique (e.g., Tine test) must be confirmed by an intradermal PPD test.

An alternative point of view is maintained by the American Academy of Pediatrics (AAP), which has noted that the incidence of tuberculosis is increasing in this country. The AAP recommends that a reasonable alternative to no routine testing is to test low-risk children (a) at 12 to 15 months (before or at the time of administration of MMR), (b) before school entry (4 to 6 years), and (c) in adolescence (14 to 16 years). Any child found to have active tuberculosis should be tested for human immunodeficiency virus (HIV) infection.

HEMATURIA, PROTEINURIA, AND GLUCOSURIA

Routine urine dipstick testing of school-aged children will reveal the following approximate prevalence rates: 10% for proteinuria, 4% for hematuria; and 0.4% for glucosuria. It has been demonstrated in several studies that the vast majority of cases of proteinuria and hematuria are transient or intermittent, due to benign responses to activity and upright posture (5). Most cases of glucosuria are caused by a low renal threshold rather than true hyperglycemia. Therefore, routine urine testing is not recommended.

HYPERLIPIDEMIA

Atherosclerotic cardiovascular disease is the leading cause of death in the United States. Risk factors that can be prevented or minimized include hypertension, cigarette smoking, obesity, sedentary lifestyle, and hypercholesterolemia. Long-term studies have not yet been done to conclusively link high cholesterol levels in childhood with coronary artery disease. However, accumulating evidence indicates that atherosclerosis begins in childhood and that lipoprotein abnormalities in children tend to correlate with subsequent adult lipoprotein elevations. Thus, some experts advocate universal cholesterol screening in children after age 2 (which is when dietary fat should be reduced from 50% of total daily calories to the adult ratio of 30% dietary fat).

Universal cholesterol screening in children is quite controversial, however, for the following reasons: lack of standardization and precision of cholesterol screening methods, the necessity of several determinations to identify persistent elevations, lack of consensus on the cholesterol values that predict future disease, the monumental cost of a national screening program, and inadequate information on safe and effective hyperlipidemia treatment for children. As of January, 1989, the Committee of Nutrition of the American Academy of Pediatrics recommends nonfasting cholesterol screening for children more than 2 years of age who have a family history of hyperlipidemia or early myocardial infarction (<50 years of age in men, <60 years in women). If the cholesterol level exceeds 175 mg/dl, periodic fasting lipoprotein profiles should be obtained, and, if persistently elevated, the child should be referred for long-term dietary counseling with an experienced registered dietician. Adding further controversy, recent studies have shown that by screening only the above "high-risk" children, up to 50% of children with elevated cholesterol will not be detected.

SEXUALLY TRANSMITTED DISEASES (STD)

Over a million cases of gonorrhea are reported each year. Chlamydial infections are estimated to be at least twice as prevalent. For asymptomatic, sexually active, nonpregnant female adolescents, the prevalence of *Chlamydia* and gonorrhea has been reported to be 14% and 6%, respectively (6, 7). The asymptomatic carrier state may persist for up to 12 months with gonorrhea, and up to several years with *Chlamydia*. Detection is simple and relatively inexpensive with the direct fluorescent antibody assays for *Chlamydia* and culture media for gonococci.

All sexually active adolescents should be considered for screening, keeping in mind that risk increases with the number of sexual partners. Cultures should be obtained from the endocervical canal in females and the anterior urethra in males. In cases of gonorrhea where no screening for *Chlamydia* was performed, antibiotic regimens should be used which are effective against both organisms, as the coinfection rate in women is at least 25% and in men, 15%. In 1987, reported cases of syphilis rose 25% in the United States, reaching the highest level since 1950. Decreases in cases among homosexual and bisexual men were offset by large increases among women and black and Hispanic heterosexual men. HIV infections, including acquired immunodeficiency syndrome (AIDS), are acquired sexually (both intimate homosexual and heterosexual contact), transplacentally, and through contaminated needles during illicit drug use. Children and adolescents account for a small but growing percentage of AIDS cases in the United States. Adolescent risk factors are similar to those of adults, as the children approach adulthood. Therefore, education about avoidance of risk factors for contracting this virus (e.g., safe sex) must be initiated by the health professional.

EDUCATION DURING WELL CHILD VISITS

Infancy and Early Childhood

Ideally, child care education should begin during the parents' prenatal visits and continue during the newborn hospital stay. The most frequently raised topics during infancy involve "routine care" items such as infant stimulation, feeding, sleeping, crying, skin care, and bowel habits. There are several books on normal development and anticipatory guidance that are useful for both physicians and parents (8–11).

Parents will agree intuitively that stimulation is important to an alert and curious infant. As their physician, you can play a pivotal role in providing ideas and encouragement. Examples of ways to stimulate the child include talking (and later reading), creating a brightly colored environment, periodically changing the location of the bed, rearranging the toys in the crib, hanging attractive mobiles over the crib, dancing and singing with the baby, as well as taking frequent walks and other outdoor activities.

Sleep patterns vary from baby to baby, with the amount of sleep time generally decreasing from birth through the preschool years. You should encourage parents and other caretakers to place the baby on back positions that have been associated with less sudden infant death syndrome (SIDS). To prevent dental caries, a baby should never be put to bed with a bottle of milk or juice. During the first few weeks of life, infants should sleep in the same room as their parents. Sleep location (a crib versus the parents' bed, a separate room versus the parents' room) after the newborn period is controversial, with arguments in favor of all arrangements. The most reasonable option, then, is probably to be flexible in your advice.

All babies cry as their primary way of communicating. Crying may signal hunger, a wet diaper, fever, frustration, anger, pain, or the desire for physical contact. Labeling the child as a "bad baby" or the caretaker as a "bad parent" because the baby is fussy is inappropriate. Daily periods of irritability and crying, usually in the afternoon or early evening, are common. It sometimes reassures parents to point out that the average 6-week-old infant cries 2 to 3 hours a day and that crying may be the baby's only way to "get exercise." Crying and irritability present during much of the baby's waking hours is often referred to as "colic." The cause of this syndrome is unknown, but family turmoil or stress, parental misinterpretation of the baby's crying pattern, heightened sensitivity to natural bowel distention, gastroesophageal reflux, and cow milk intolerance have been incriminated in what is surely a multifactorial process. Holding the crying baby closely, holding the baby more frequently during noncrying times, rubbing and applying gentle warmth to the abdomen, burping more frequently during feeding, relieving stress at home, going for a stroll or ride, swinging the baby in a mechanical device, and attempting a dietary intervention (avoiding cow milk formula in a bottle-fed baby or a trial of maternal milk-free diet in a breast-fed baby) are all techniques that merit individual trials in the colicky infant. Large doses of your empathy and support, combined with a tincture of time, are usually sufficient in this self-

limiting process. Colic usually resolves or improves by 4 months of age.

Children should be dressed appropriately for the environment. If it is warm enough for the parents to wear shorts, so should the baby. Overdressing and overblanketing are common judgment errors and can cause factitious fever and irritability.

Parents currently have the choice of many types of diapers, such as reusable cloth or disposable paper/plastic products. Cost and environmental impact are two important factors for parents to consider when choosing diapers for their child. Cloth diapers are now available with Velcro fasteners instead of safety pins. Frequent diaper changes to assure good perineal hygiene are essential to prevent diaper rash. Contact dermatitis may occur due to fragrances or chemicals in disposable diapers or residual ammonia or detergent in cloth diapers. You should consider these irritants as possible offenders when a diaper rash occurs. Leaving the perineum open to air is excellent therapy for almost all types of diaper rash.

A sponge bath is advised until separation of the umbilical cord (average 10 to 14 days), after which a tub bath using mild nondetergent soap is acceptable. To prevent dry skin, bathing is recommended every other day for babies, rather than daily. Washing the scalp, including the anterior fontanelle area, once or twice a week with a shampoo such as Sebulex can effectively treat the very common seborrhea or "cradle cap." Oils and powders should be avoided to prevent contact dermatitis and ingestion or inhalation of potentially harmful substances. Eucerin or Acid Mantle lotion/cream applied sparingly after bathing treats excessively dry skin.

Between birth and 6 months of age, babies frequently sneeze and have stuffy noses. This does not necessarily mean allergy or upper respiratory infection. Make sure that the caretakers are using clothes that are free of lint and other respiratory irritants. Humidification of the ambient air and the use of normal saline nasal douche (Ocean Mist or Ayr nasal drops) and bulb syringe aspiration alternately in each nostril several times a day treats congestion without the use of systemic medications. Exposure to exhaled cigarette smoke should be avoided, since it is associated with an increased incidence of bronchospasm and otitis media.

The external auditory canals should never be cleaned by the parents. Use of Q-tips may lead to impacted cerumen or even tympanic membrane perforation. Debrox drops instilled in the ear canals once or twice weekly will soften cerumen and facilitate cleaning of the canals by the physician when necessary.

Teething usually begins from 5 to 8 months of age and may cause local discomfort and fussiness, especially when the molars are erupting. Local treatment of the gums with cool liquids, chilled teething rings, and acetaminophen for analgesia should be sufficient symptomatic care. Do not use paregoric for teething, because of its high toxic-to-therapeutic ratio. High fever and profuse diarrhea should not be attributed to teething.

In the United States, 60% of women 18 to 34 years of age with a child less than 1 year of age work outside their home. Thus, giving advice on choosing a facility for child care is an important task for the family physician. In practice, family physicians can help prevent illness and improve community care by serving as medical advisers to local day-care centers. Giving advice on choosing babysitters and educating secondary caretakers, such as grandparents, is an equally essential task. The ideal babysitter is a well-known, reliable adult with prior child care experience. Parents should prepare the babysitter with emergency phone numbers, written parental permission for acute medical/surgical care, and written instructions for feeding, sleep time, and all home exits in case of fire or other emergency.

Injury and Accident Prevention

Accidents remain the leading cause of mortality in children. Thus accident prevention should be a major emphasis at well child visits. Many accidents occur because the child learns a new skill, such as opening doors, for which the parents and other caretakers should have prepared beforehand. You must continue to remind the caretakers of common accidents that correspond to the child's age and stage of development. Table 15.4 lists potential hazards and ways to avoid them.

Motor vehicle safety is important throughout life. A properly approved infant car seat should be used from the day the newborn leaves the hospital until the child is 1 year of age or weighs 20 pounds. A toddler car seat is then used until age 4 years, when the child can switch to a regular seat belt. Advise parents to demonstrate safe driving habits by properly wearing their seat belts.

Trauma prevention with increasing age means education of the caretaker and child about the safe use of toys such as tricycles, bicycles, skateboards, and all types of motorized vehicles. Eighty percent of closed-head injury involving bicycle accidents can be avoided by the use of properly approved (ANSI and Snell certification) bicycle helmets. Backyard trampolines should be specifically discouraged because of their general lack of adult supervision and high rate of fractures and cervical

Table 15.4. Potential Hazards and Ways to Avoid Them

Hazard or Risk	Anticipatory Guidance
Motor vehicle accident (passenger)	Use car seat and seat belt° (age appropriate)
Motor vehicle accident (driver)	Driver education°, use seat belts°, and avoid driving under the influence of drugs and alcohol
Motor vehicle accident (pedestrian or other)	Close supervision near streets and roads, learn traffic safety rules, wear bicycle helmets, avoid all-terrain vehicles, street is not for play
Asphyxiation	Crib bars no more than 2 7/8 inches apart, avoid necklaces in infants and toddlers, avoid toys small enough to fit fully in mouth, avoid easily aspirated foods (popcorn, peanuts, hot dogs), keep plastic bags and balloons out of reach, remove discarded refrigerator doors°
Drowning	Close supervision around water; locked fences for swimming pools° and nearby water; avoid tall, narrow, open 5-gallon containers (toddler drowning!); life jackets worn on boats°
Falls	Keep baby off high surfaces when unattended, use stairwell guards, avoid walkers, carefully supervise gym set play, avoid trampolines
Poisoning	Safe and secure storage of toxic substances, have syrup of ipecac available for emergency use with Poison Control Center phone number handy, childproof medicine containers
Burns	Install smoke detectors and fire extinguishers in home°, practice emergency escape plans regularly, avoid exposed extension cords and overuse of electrical outlets, discourage smoking, set hot water heater to 120°F or less°

°Required by law in some states.

injuries. Any guns in the caretaker's homes should be locked away unloaded, and ammunition should be locked in a separate area, inaccessible to the child. Toy projectiles such as toy guns, BB and pellet guns, and darts should be discouraged as play items. Children should be discouraged from playing with unfamiliar pets, especially dogs, because of potential serious injury.

ADOLESCENTS

Adolescence is a time when health risks are high, as the individual experiments with new, "adult" behaviors. Psychosocial issues and health behaviors are especially important in these patients: sexuality (including contraception and the prevention of sexually transmitted diseases), driving habits (including seat belt use), alcohol and substance abuse, career goals, and self-esteem and self-image. Depression is frequent; so a few screening questions are warranted. When seeing adolescent patients, you should take every opportunity to discuss, and assertively discourage, tobacco use, the major cause of premature death in this country.

Gaining the trust and confidence of your adolescent patients can be challenging (see Chapter 9). All visits by adolescents should include time alone with the physician, so that the adolescent can feel a sense of control and be free to ask questions or raise concerns that may not be mentioned with a parent present. Community involvement, such as volunteering time as high school team physician or attending a school-based clinic, can enhance your credibility with your teenage patients and give you a greater, more gratifying impact on their developing lives.

REFERENCES

1. Active and Passive Immunizations: In *Report of the Committee on Infectious Diseases*, ed 22. Elk Grove Village, IL, American Academy of Pediatrics, 1991, pp 1–66.
2. Centers for Disease Control: *Haemophilus* b conjugate vaccines for prevention of *Haemophilus influenzae* type b disease among infants and children two months of age and older. *MMWR* 40: RR-1: pp 1–7, 1991.
3. Oski FA, Honig AS, Helu B, Howanitz P: Effects of iron therapy on behavioral in nonanemic, iron-deficient infants. *Pediatrics* 71:877–880, 1983.
4. Preventing Lead Poisoning in Young Children. U.S. Department of Health and Human Services/Public Health Service/Centers for Disease Control, October, 1991.
5. Vehaskari VM, Rapola J, Koskimies D, Savilahti E, Vilska J, Hallman N: Microscopic hematuria in school children: epidemiology and clinicopathologic evaluation. *J Pediatr* 95:676–684, 1979.
6. Schachter J, Stoner E, Moncada J: Screening for *Chlamydia* infections in women attending family planning clinics. *West J Med* 138:375–379, 1983.
7. Rettig PJ: *Chlamydia* infection in pediatrics: not for babies only. *J Pediatr* 104:82–83, 1984.
8. Brazelton TB: *Infants and Mothers: Differences in Development*. New York, Delacorte Press, 1969.
9. Brazelton TB: *Toddlers and Parents: A Declaration of Independence*. New York, Delacorte Press, 1974.
10. Ginott HG: *Between Parent and Teenager*. New York, Avon Books, 1969.
11. Arena JM, Bachar M: *Child Safety Is No Accident: A Parents' Handbook of Emergencies*. Durham, NC, Duke University Press, 1978.

SUGGESTED READINGS

Alpert JJ, Guyer B (eds): Injuries and injury prevention *Pediatr Clin North Am* 32(1), 1985.

The first section provides an overview and reviews basic concepts for understanding injuries. The second section reviews recent developments, knowledge, and innovations concerning specific injury types and their prevention. The third section is an update on management of multiple trauma, choking, and poisoning. The last section addresses the principles of injury control: legal, educational, advocacy, and community organizations, as well as providing challenges for future action.

Asher MA: Screening for congenital dislocation of the hip, scoliosis, and other abnormalities affecting the musculoskeletal system. In Staheli LT (ed): Common Orthopedic Problems. *Pediatr Clin North Am* 33(6):1335-1353, 1986.

A nicely illustrated review of examination techniques and office equipment used to screen for these orthopeadic disorders.

Blackman JA (ed): Development and Behavior: The Very Young Child. *Pediatr Clin North Am* 38(6), 1991.

This book discusses child development and behavior from such perspectives as emotional milestones, feeding, language, and child care. It addresses concepts of family-centered care and suggests innovative changes in the roles of health care professionals and parents. Common and glaring pitfalls in developmental diagnosis are presented on the basis of examples from the author's practice.

Christophersen ER, Finney JW, Friman PC (eds): Prevention in primary care. *Pediatr Clin North Am* 33(4), 1986.

Authors with expertise in nutrition, child development, behavioral pediatrics, cardiology, pediatrics, oncology, dentistry, and adolescent medicine review advances in prevention and from their reviews make recommendations about how these advances can be incorporated into primary care practice. Each article includes explicit recommendations for promoting child health and new directions for further scientific inquiry.

Guidelines for Health Supervision, ed 2. Elk Grove Village, IL, American Academy of Pediatrics, 1988.

This is a "cookbook" guideline for conducting well child examinations from the prenatal period through adolescence. Each chapter actually lists the questions to be asked during the interview, the developmental aspects to be assessed, the various anticipatory guidance topics to be discussed, the physical examination highlights, laboratory tests to consider, and the immunizations to give. It does not give the rationale for its recommendations, assuming the clinician already has this knowledge base, but merely serves as a reminder for the busy practitioner.

Report of the Committee on Infectious Diseases. *Redbook*, ed 22. Elk Grove Village, IL, American Academy of Pediatrics, 1991.

This is a comprehensive text of current data relative to the prevention and control of infectious diseases in children. Improved sections in this edition include recommendations for the management of children in day care, tables listing diseases that should be reported to health authorities, and school immunization laws in various states. It is a must for the library of the physicians who care for children.

Rogers PD (ed): Chemical Dependency. *Pediatr Clin North Am* 34(2), 1987.

In addition to discussing specific substances that are frequently abused, such as alcohol, marijuana, hallucinogens, stimulants, narcotics, and tobacco, and their patterns of abuse, pharmacology, and treatment; this book discusses techniques of interviewing the adolescent for substance abuse, specific drug screening techniques, and prevention of adolescent chemical dependency. This rising serious problem among America's youth is extensively reviewed.

Strasburger VC (ed): Adolescent Gynecology. *Pediatr Clin North Am* 36(3), 1989.

This is a comprehensive review of adolescent gynecology from general topics such as sexuality, contraception, and counseling to specific evaluation and treatment of menstrual disorders, STDs, and pelvic pain. There is a nice analysis of the problem of adolescent pregnancy, with review of several prevention programs.

Zuckerman B, Weitzman M, Alpert JJ (eds): Children at Risk: Current Social and Medical Challenges. *Pediatr Clin North Am* 35(6), 1988.

This is an excellent compendium of the biopsychosocial influences on children's health. Issues such as poverty, children's health, foster care, the changing American family, divorce, AIDS, and homelessness, as they relate to the wellness or illness of the child, are discussed. It raises awareness of how important the integration of socioeconomic, behavioral, and medical factors is in the health professionals' role of disease prevention in children!

chapter 16

WELL ADULT CARE

Melissa M. Hicks

Preventive care for adults (aged 17 to 65 for the purposes of most of this chapter) integrates many different aspects of medical care. Preventive, or "well," care relies heavily on the person (patient) and requires an in-depth personal and family history. The clinician must therefore be an expert history-taker and keep accurate records of identified risk factors. Identifying risk factors and designing a plan to decrease and follow these risks are the goals of prevention and the well care visit.

Risk factor identification and early lifestyle modification clearly can make an impact on certain common diseases. Tobacco use, if discontinued, can improve a person's risk profile for cardiac and lung disease. Education about prevention of injuries and counseling patients about the prevention of the spread of sexually transmitted diseases may be of more importance to our patients than any other intervention we can offer.

Recommendations for preventive care vary. There are global recommendations, based on public health and epidemiologic data, and there are the individual opinions and experiences of the physician and the patient. Most of the recommendations in this chapter reflect the more global viewpoint, and there are **many** variations. In general, however, recommendations for preventive care are developed as a result of assessing the most prevalent causes of morbidity and mortality for adults of various age groups, with variation for males and females of these age groups. A screening test is used for general preventive care if it meets the criteria elaborated in Table 13.1 and if the measure itself is reliable. This generally means that the test should identify most of the cases (exhibit high sensitivity) without having too many false positives (moderate specificity). **Most important** to preventive care are the history and the patient's willingness to modify identified risks.

Yearly physical examinations may be unnecessary, especially for young and middle-aged adults. Examinations should differ depending on patient age, sex, and specific **history-related** risks. Counseling and teaching patients about the options of responsible decision-making are much more important than most "routine" physical diagnosis maneuvers. This is particularly true with sexual behaviors and the risks of sexually transmitted diseases (STDs), pregnancy, and HIV disease, and with injury prevention.

To organize your approach to preventive adult care, there is a mnemonic, **RISE**, that may be helpful. **R** is for **risk factor** identification, **I** is for **immunization**, **S** is for **screening**, and **E** is for patient **education**. Each of these areas is important in the assessment and care of the well adult.

RISK FACTOR IDENTIFICATION

Identifying risk factors involves a detailed personal and family history. In taking a personal history, concentrate on habits and hobbies (what they do for fun), the past medical history, and the sexual history (including sexual orientation). The family history should assess psychiatric history, alcohol use, and family violence, as well as medical familial diseases such as diabetes, coronary artery disease, and cancer. An ideal tool in the office or hospital chart is the *genogram*. It provides a concise but in-depth look at medical and social issues that make up the person you are seeing, and it is always there, on the chart. As described in the chapter on families, the genogram can be a dynamic tool for the physician, and it is illustrative to the patient, as well.

In conducting your search for risk factors, think of the major causes of mortality facing the patient now and over her or his lifetime. For example, a 28-year-old man is currently at highest statistical risk of death from automobile accidents, suicide, and homicide. Over a lifetime, his greatest risks include coronary artery disease, cancer (especially lung and colon), stroke, and accidents. With these specific diagnoses in mind, you can direct your evaluation toward inquiry about seat belt use, smoking, stress, alcohol or other drugs, hypertension, and health maintenance habits such as exercise and diet, and review other risk factors from his specific personal and family history. Based on all of this information, you can prioritize any screening and education, while using Tables 16.1 and 16.2 to help with general screening for all female and male adults.

In taking a history, an intake questionnaire for new patients can be a valuable timesaver. This should include an occupational history (hazardous chemicals, noise exposure, etc.), a sexual history as discussed above, and a dietary history.

IMMUNIZATIONS

Around the world, most people now have access to most of the vaccinations considered routine. The major childhood immunizations: diphtheria, tetanus, and pertussis (DPT); *Haemophilus influenzae*; measles, mumps, and rubella (MMR); and oral polio are given to all children in the U.S., with very few exceptions. Adults, however, are much less likely to keep up with recommended vaccinations. For example, a great number of people are unaware of their tetanus immunization status, and most cases of tetanus now occur in inadequately immunized older persons.

The recommended routine immunizations for adults include a diphtheria-tetanus booster every 10 years (Dt). For persons with other underlying illnesses or asplenia, yearly influenza vaccines and a one-time pneumococcal vaccine (pneumovax) are recommended. These two vaccines should be routinely given to persons over the age of 65, to asymptomatic HIV+ patients, and to patients with chronic cardiac or respiratory conditions. Health care workers should consider the yearly influenza vaccination and also the hepatitis B vaccine series (a series of 3). Gay men and others with high-risk behaviors (IV drug use, for example) should also be considered for hepatitis B vaccine if they are not immune.

There are new recommendations now for the measles vaccine because of outbreaks over the past several years, particularly among college-age persons. It is now recommended to revaccinate children with the MMR (measles, mumps, and rubella)

at the time of beginning kindergarten, plus administering a booster when entering college. The pre-college immunization can be waived if the patient was born before 1956, has antibodies demonstrated by laboratory testing, or has had documented physician-diagnosed measles in the past.)

Foreign Travel: Recommendations for Immunizations

Traveling to a different country requires an awareness of local health risks. Of course, the most common cause of morbidity in travel is accidental injury, but there are other preventable causes as well. Several good references are available for guiding you and your patients on the necessary precautions, and most local health departments stay up-to-date on travel recommendations. In addition, the Centers for Disease Control maintains a 24-hour voice information system ((404) 332-4555) with general and area-specific information on diseases and vaccinations, information on food and water precautions, advice on the prevention and treatment of traveler's diarrhea, and other health information.

The main prevention targets for travelers include malaria, cholera, and traveler's diarrhea (caused by many different types of bacteria/protozoa). Most countries expect the basic vaccinations against polio and the usual childhood vaccinations. Some may also recommend

- Gamma globulin, which protects against hepatitis A for about 3 months;
- Malaria oral prophylaxis, which varies depending on whether the region has primaquine-resistant strains;
- Cholera vaccine (in spite of the fact that healthy westerners rarely have major problems, and the disease responds to antibiotics);
- Yellow fever vaccine;
- Typhoid vaccine.

Equatorial countries in particular are prone to malaria, and African and Caribbean areas are also prone to yellow fever, requiring a vaccination. See the reference list for two good resources for you and your patients.

SCREENING FOR ASYMPTOMATIC DISEASE

A large part of the public's concept of the "routine physical" involves screening for diseases that are present but not yet symptomatic (secondary prevention). A mind-boggling array of tests and examinations is available, but with little agreement on who should receive which measures how often. The tables in this chapter were compiled from a review of the major task forces. They should be applied to individual patients based on consideration of other priorities as well, such as your location, the availability of testing, and the probability of disease in this patient. For example, not all men are at risk for HIV; only those with certain high-risk behaviors should be tested.

Tables 16.1 and 16.2 contain recommendations for examinations and screening tests for men and women, as well as some primary prevention recommendations (diet, exercise, immunizations). In using these tables, remember that there is controversy about the timing of many tests. Certain ones, however, have clear importance and fairly clear guidelines. Screening for high blood pressure by routine BP checks every 2 years is a good example of a standard recommendation.

More controversy surrounds the question of screening for colon cancer. The American Cancer Society recommends annual rectal examinations over age 40, annual occult blood screening after age 50, and sigmoidoscopy every 3 to 5 years after age 50. The Canadian Task Force recommends only annual occult blood testing. It is not clear what impact these screens have on the morbidity from colon cancer; so, the US Preventive Services Task Force recommends a very individualized approach, without discouraging screening practices already in place.

PATIENT EDUCATION

The last section of the RISE mnemonic is education of patients. This aspect of prevention uses risk factor identification to tailor education about lifestyle changes. In this area, both public and one-to-one programs have been shown to be effective (1). For example, recent reductions in coronary heart mortality have resulted from public education and from individual counseling about diet and exercise, as well as from better control of hypertension. The value of an individual physician in guiding patients to make lifestyle changes should not be underestimated. Recommendations should be individualized and should direct the individual to community resources such as a weight-loss group or a smoking cessation class. Chapter 17 provides details about educating individual patients in the office.

Some students and practitioners develop a certain therapeutic nihilism about patient education. This attitude results from seeing many patients who do not make the necessary lifestyle changes that would obviously benefit their health. When this occurs, remember that education is only one element needed to produce change. The crucial element is motivation, which comes largely from within the individual, the family, and the social support network. This means that the physician, while responsible for providing the best preventive and educational care possible, is only one factor in determining behavior change. From this perspective, it is often easier to be content with partial results and to be encouraged by the patients who do follow your recommendations.

CASE EXAMPLES

Case 1

A 40-year-old white man comes to your office requesting a physical examination. The only remarkable item in his history is a myocardial infarction in his father at age 50.

Study Question

- Before reading on, think about how you would plan for this patient's preventive care.

Case Discussion

Using the RISE format, you can focus on each element of preventive care for this young man. Risk factors need to be identified. Does he abuse tobacco, alcohol, or drugs? Is there a family history of cancer or a personal history of problems such as elevated cholesterol or blood pressure? Are there sexual or occupational risk factors?

Immunizations must be updated. When was his last diphtheria-tetanus vaccination? Is he in a special risk group that needs the hepatitis vaccine? Is he a health care provider or an asthmatic who should have a flu shot?

He can then be screened by physical examination and laboratory tests, as indicated in Table 16.1 and by your assessment of risk factors.

A large part of this patient's encounter will focus on education, centered on his risk factors and what he can do to minimize them. His plan for preventive care should be amended to take into account any risk factors specific to him. His family history of early coronary artery disease is an indication and likely a motivator for learning about diet, exercise, and weight control. His wife should know CPR techniques.

Table 16.1. Well Adult Female Screening—Compiled Recommendations

	When to Begin	Interval	Special Tools/ Concerns
I. Risk factor identification (history)			
Pregnancy/contraception	Before onset of sexual activity (or by age 18)	Every 1–2 years	
Drug/alcohol/tobacco use	At 1st visit—preferably as a teen	Each visit	MAST; depression scales if history suggestive
CHD risk—family history of cardiac disease & diabetes	1st visit	Ongoing every 4–5 years	Genogram
Cancer risk (breast, colon, ovarian, lung)	Assess with initial family history	Update family history every 4–5 years as necessary	Genogram
Sexual history	1st visit, include sexual orientation/sexual satisfaction	Reassess as needed	
STDs/HIV risk	With above and drug history (use of IV drugs, multiple partners)	Periodically	
Situational/stressors; psychiatric history (e.g., depression)	1st visit	Periodically	Genogram plus family circle
Occupational	1st visit	Periodically	Health questionnaire
II. Immunizations			
Know routine childhood	Check history		Health record
Diphtheria-tetanus	Ten years after last childhood immunization booster	Every 10 years	Flow sheet
Rubella, measles, or MMR	Give measles booster on entering college unless documented immunity or illness	Check *rubella status* at preconception or 1st prenatal visit	• *Do not* give live vaccine during pregnancy; give MMR if born after 1956
Influenza	Age 65 and after; or if chronically ill; health care workers	Every year	
Pneumococcol	Age 65 or after, after splenectomy or chronic illness	One time	Health record or stickers on chart
Hepatitis B	High risk due to IV drug use, sexual behavior, HIV infection, health care workers, family of hepatitis carriers	Series of 3 (one time)	
Others (cholera, hepatitis A, typhoid, yellow fever)	For foreign travel, review health department recommendations for specifics per country	See text	
III. Screening—for disease (secondary prevention)			
Weight	Childhood	Every visit	Compare to national norms
Blood pressure	Childhood	Every 1–2 years if normal, more often if elevated	chart flow sheets if needed
Cholesterol	Age 20–24	Every 4–5 years	
Occult blood	Age 45–50	Yearly per American Cancer Society (USPSTF questions efficacy)	Test has high false positive rate unless patient follows dietary guidelines
Pelvic-bimanual	With Pap smears	Every 2 years; consider yearly after age 50 for ovarian screening	

Table 16.1. *(continued)*

	When to Begin	Interval	Special Tools/ Concerns
Pap smear	At onset of sexual activity or age 18	Every 1–2 years—ACOG says every 1 year; others say every 2 after 2 normal ones	Controversy, i.e. every 1 year or every 2–3 years, also at what age to stop
Breast examination—self breast examination; physician examination	Teach at 1st visit	Efficacy unknown, annually after age 40	See text
Mammogram	Age 40–50 (see text), earlier if family history of premenopausal breast cancer	40 baseline, then every 1–2 years after age 50	
Visual acuity/glaucoma screen	Childhood	If diabetic, recommend optical examination every year; otherwise every 2–5 years	Increase frequency with age
Sigmoidoscopy	Recommended by some at age 50	Every 3–5 years (see text)	Controversial, if family history positive may need colonscopy
Dental screening	Childhood	ADS recommends about every 2 years	
Urine dipstick (for protein, hematuria, asymptomatic bacteriuria)	Age 50 or in pregnancy, possibly also once during adolescence	Yearly	Urine multistick
HIV	Only if high risk	2 times in 6 months	
IV. Education			
Sexual activity and STDs, HIV risk, pregnancy	At or *before* onset of sexual activity (teens)	Review questions with each P.E. visit	Education flow sheet
Diet/nutrition		Every 2–4 years	Review iron and calcium intake
Estrogen therapy, osteoporosis, and cardiac protection	Discuss and provide information at or before menopause (natural or surgical)	Review each visit if *not* using	Also stress calcium and exercise
Exercise	Early	Each visit (every 4 years)	
Injury prevention, seat belts, no drinking while driving	During teens	Each health maintenance visit	
Self-examination: breasts, skin	Some say by age 20	Review every 2–4 years; emphasize by ages 30–35	Screening by examination if positive history
Stressors, relaxation, losses	Age 20	Review with each visit every 2–4 years	Genogram and family circle, relaxation strategies

Obviously this can be too much to discuss in a routine 15-minute office visit. In a family practice setting, these issues and others are usually covered over several visits, often over many years. Scheduling a visit to interpret laboratory data presents another opportunity to discuss preventive health issues.

Case 2

A 67-year-old black woman comes to your office complaining of shoulder pain. A focused history and physical examination reveals fibromyositis with one tender trigger point, which you inject to relieve pain and spasm.

Study Question

• How would you address prevention in this acute visit?

Case Discussion

As a physician, you have two choices with a patient such as this. You can treat the acute problem and

Table 16.2. Well Adult Male Screening—Compiled Recommendations

	When to Begin	Interval	Special Tools/Comments
I. Risk factor identification (history)			
Contraception responsibility	Before onset of sexual activity or age 18	Each visit, every 1–4 years	
Drugs, alcohol, tobacco use; mental health	1st visit	Assess each visit	MAST; depression scales if needed
Coronary artery disease risk; cancer risk (colon, lung, and prostate)	Family history at 1st visit (age of males with MI, etc.)	Ongoing, every 4–5 years	Genogram
Sexual history	1st visit	Reassess as needed	Ask about sexual orientation and sexual satisfaction
Situational Stressors	1st visit	Periodically	Health questionnaire, chemicals, back, hearing, etc.
II. Immunizations			
Obtain records of childhood immunizations	History		Health record
Diphtheria-tetanus	Adulthood, after 14	Every 10 years	Health record
Measles	In childhood: give booster unless documented immunity	On entering college	Health record
Influenza	Age 65 or older, if other underlying illness or health care worker	Every year	Health record or stickers on chart
Pneumococcal vaccine	Asplenia or same as above	One time	Health record
Hepatitis B	High risk may be due to sexual partner(s), sexual practices, exposure to blood products (including certain health care workers), IV drug use	Every year	Health record
Others	See foreign travel text and references		
III. Screening			
Weight	Childhood	Every visit	Compare with national norms
Blood pressure	Childhood (screen history also)	Every 1–2 years if normal, more often if elevated	Normal <140/85, some recommend check at any visit after age 25
Cholesterol (plus counseling about dietary fat)	Age 20–24	Every 5 years if normal; more often; plus HDL/LDL check if elevated	>240 mg/dl is high; 200–239 mg/dl is borderline
Occult blood	Age 45–50	Yearly per American Cancer Society (USPSTF questions efficacy)	Test has high false-positive rate unless patient follows dietary guidelines
Sigmoidoscopy	Age 50	Every 3–5 years (see text)	Controversial; colonscopy & *early* screening for 1st-degree relatives of patients with colon cancer
Rectal and/or PSA for prostate	Age 50 or 60	Controversial	
Vision/glaucoma	Childhood	Every year if diabetic; otherwise every 2–5 years	Increase frequency with age

Table 16.2. (continued)

	When to Begin	Interval	Special Tools/Comments
Dental	Childhood	ADS recommends about every 2 years	
Urine dipstick	Age 60	Yearly	Urine multistick
HIV	*Only* if history suggests		
IV. Education			
Sexual activity risks (STDs, HIV, pregnancy)	Before onset of sexual activity	Review at each "routine" checkup	Discuss responsible decisions, etc.; education flow sheet
Diet/nutrition	When checking cholesterol, weight, and blood pressure	Every 2–4 years	Diet diary, nutrition brochures
Exercise	As above	As above	
Injury prevention	1st visit	Each visit review hobbies & occupation	Discuss seatbelts, drinking, helmets, risk-taking
Self examinations: testicular & skin	Early 20s	Controversial, every 2–4 years	Educate (e.g., sun exposure)
Stressors, losses, changes in life cycle	1st visit	Review every 2–4 years	Relaxation techniques; therapy referral

spend 5 minutes discussing preventive health, or you can recommend a return visit for preventive care. By managing an acute problem, a family physician gains trust and can proceed with caring for the total person. Using the RISE format, a physician can raise some important issues and follow them up when the patient returns to reassess her shoulder problem. By discussing immunizations and cancer screening at the first visit, the patient can be prepared for these interventions during the next visit.

IMPLEMENTING PREVENTIVE CARE

To successfully practice preventive care, you need to include it in your routine care of each patient. Often this is forgotten while attending to an acute problem. But given the right emphasis, preventive care can even be done in an acute setting, which is evident by how well tetanus immunization is updated in emergency rooms. For hospitalized patients it means that each history and physical examination should include a section on health maintenance issues. This is commonplace for all evaluations of pediatric patients and needs to be standardized for all patients.

Outpatients should be taught that they need periodic visits for preventive care instead of annual physical examinations. Their charts can include flow sheets and chart stickers as a conspicuous way to document preventive care issues. Preventive care data must be updated by physicians during each visit, whether or not the stated purpose of the visit is preventive care. Otherwise, most patients will not have these issues addressed.

Many physicians use ancillary personnel to update preventive care flow sheets. A receptionist in a physician's office can be responsible for flagging each chart that does not have a completed age-specific preventive care checklist. Periodic chart audits sometimes uncover neglected preventive care issues. Nursing staff in the office can carry out some preventive care, such as measurement of weight, height, and blood pressure, dietary and exercise assessment, seat belt reminders, and self-examination education. Preventive care can be easily integrated into your office practice by implementing a system that provides periodic updates and reminders to you and your patients.

CHALLENGES IN PREVENTIVE CARE

What are some of the challenges involved in providing preventive care? A critical challenge is determining which interventions are cost-effective and reasonable to include in preventive care. Five criteria assess specific interventions (2). These are outlined on Table 13.1. If a screening intervention satisfies these criteria, it is included in recommendations for preventive care of well adults (3). These criteria assume that there are adequate data about each of the interventions so a decision can be made; sometimes this is not the case. Individual patients may need additions to their flow sheets, depending upon their individual risk factors and your preferences.

Another challenge in preventive care involves motivating patients and physicians. There are several impediments to using preventive care from a patient's view. Preventive care may not be offered or available. Even if it is, patients may refuse it. They may not accept the risks associated with certain procedures. Often patients know of others who experienced adverse reactions to immunizations, such as the swine flu vaccine, and these anecdotal cases serve as strong reinforcement to not receiving any test or procedure unless it is absolutely indicated. Many tests are uncomfortable, such as flexible sigmoidoscopy, rectal examination, and mammography.

Preventive care can be expensive. Since many insurance plans do not cover preventive care, the patient is responsible for the cost. Needless to say, if one has very limited resources, a $100 flexible sigmoidoscopy may not be a high priority. One advantage of some prepaid health insurance plans is that preventive care is covered, and the patient does not directly pay for these services. In fact, such plans benefit financially by preventing illness or reducing its severity.

What are the impediments to screening from a physician's perspective? Preventive care standards are constantly changing. Various organizations provide recommendations, which frequently conflict with each other. For example, published recommendations regarding Pap smears for a specific patient may range from every 6 months to every 5 years depending upon the authority. Furthermore, the "right" answer also depends on individual patient risk factors and personal preferences.

Not all patients come to the doctor specifically for preventive care. For most people, it must be done within the context of acute problems, and because of this, it is frequently forgotten or overlooked. Some physicians feel that there are insufficient data to show that preventive care has a positive effect on morbidity or mortality or that it even saves money. For many practitioners, the problem is one of inertia. We all know that flossing our teeth daily is important and probably prevents periodontal disease, but how many of us do? Preventive care is much the same; it is difficult to perform tasks when the benefits are not readily apparent.

CONCLUSIONS

As with most of medicine, preventive care cannot be learned from one article or one chart. It takes experience in providing preventive care to patients to learn that this approach is more effective than much of modern medicine, which is deeply entangled in end-stage intervention. Preventive care can be effective for patients and physicians, if an organized reminder system and the RISE outline are used in each patient encounter.

Acknowledgment. The author acknowledges the prior work of Richard Baker, M.D., and Kevin Culhane, M.D. Drs. Baker and Culhane authored this chapter in the previous edition, and the current chapter draws extensively from their ideas and words.

REFERENCES

1. Multiple Risk Factor Intervention Trial (MRFIT) Research Group: Risk factor changes and mortality results. *JAMA* 248:1465–1477, 1982.
2. Canadian Task Force on the Periodic Health Examination: The periodic health examination. *Can Med Assoc J* 121:1193–1254, 1979.
3. Frame PS: A critical review of adult health maintenance. Part I: Prevention of atherosclerotic diseases. *J Fam Pract* 22:341–346, 1986.
4. Clinical Guide to Preventive Services. *Report of the U.S. Preventative Services Task Force*. Baltimore, Williams & Wilkins, 1989.
5. Neumann HH: *Foreign Travel & Immunization Guide*, 9th ed. Oradell, NJ, Medical Economic Book, 1990.

SUGGESTED READINGS

Clinical Guide to Preventive Services. *Report of the U.S. Preventative Services Task Force*, Baltimore, Williams & Wilkins, 1989.

An authoritative summary of recommendations by a federal task force.

American Cancer Society: ACS report on the cancer-related health check-up. *CA* 30:194–240, 1980.

The recommended cancer screening in this article is more extensive than the other review articles support, but then ACS recommendations carry considerable weight for clinical practice policies.

Breslow L, Somers AR: The lifetime health-monitoring program: practical approach to preventive medicine. *N Engl J Med* 296:601–608, 1977.

Though this article is somewhat dated, the review of literature and sensible approach to lifetime monitoring, including infants and children, is well worth reading.

Canadian Task Force on the Periodic Health Examination: The periodic health examination. *Can Med Assoc J* 121:1193–1254, 1979.

This long article summarizes a study of the preventive care literature and practice by a large task force of the Canadian Medical Association. An update is due soon.

Frame PS: A critical review of adult health care maintenance part 1–4. *J Fam Pract* 22:341–346, 22:417–422, 22:511–520, 23:29–39, 1986.

These four articles are the most recent of the seminal articles in adult health maintenance. The bibliography in each area; infectious diseases, cancer, atherosclerotic diseases, and metabolic/behavioral/miscellaneous conditions, is extensive. The criteria for inclusion in his protocol for adult health maintenance are very stringent.

chapter 17

PATIENT EDUCATION

John P. Langlois

Patient education is attempted and performed during virtually every clinical encounter in family practice. It ranges from simple to complex: from instructing a patient with an upper respiratory infection to teaching a diabetic to manage and cope with the disease over many years. It covers the range of treatment from preventive medicine to acute illness management. It also covers the entire range of life, as the physician gives both preconception counseling and assists families with terminal care and bereavement.

Patient education involves more than just presentation of information; it is an interactive process that aims at changing knowledge, attitudes, and behavior. To be an effective educator of patients, the family physician must learn and cultivate effective skills and approaches. This chapter introduces basic concepts regarding patient education and helps the physician develop a toolbox of strategies and techniques that can assist patients in complying with medical recommendations.

IMPROVING PATIENT COMPLIANCE

Case 1

An elderly woman presents to the office complaining of vague stomach problems. She has significant congestive heart failure and is told that she has a heart problem. The doctor gives her samples of medication, instructions on how to use them, and an appointment to return the next day.

Upon return, the patient admits to having not taken any of the medication. When asked why, she states, "I came in for my stomach, and until you take care of that, I'm not going to take your heart medicine." When asked what she thought was causing her symptoms, the patient replied, "Someone has put a hex on me and I have snakes in my stomach."

Study Questions

1. What steps can a physician take during an initial office visit to assess barriers to compliance?
2. What educational measures and strategies might have improved the likelihood of patient compliance in this case?

Case Discussion

Failure to listen carefully and to address the patient's concerns leads to dissatisfaction and lack of compliance. Careful assessment and consideration of the patient's needs aids rapport, satisfaction, and compliance.

The above patient's beliefs, no matter how unrealistic they may seem to us, are very real to her. They reflect her cultural background and heritage, which must be respected. Without the information gained by careful assessment of this patient's previous health experience and beliefs, any attempt at treating her symptoms is doomed to fail. Additional data about the patient's health beliefs, lifestyle, habits, education, ability to read, and support system are very useful in developing a sound therapeutic plan.

Reducing Barriers to Noncompliance

The best therapeutic plan is without value if your patient is unable or unwilling to follow it. Between 50 and 92% of patients do not follow prescribed medical regimens (1). Knowledge alone, although important, is not sufficient to insure that the patient will follow the necessary treatment; specific skills and appropriate attitudes are essential. Basic requirements for optimal success are a strong doctor/patient relationship, effective two-way communication, a simple affordable regimen, and clear, concise instructions. Table 17.1 summarizes barriers to compliance and recommends methods of managing them.

Building a solid doctor/patient relationship is the foundation of effective patient education and

155

improved compliance. Patients who are satisfied with this relationship are three times more likely to follow a medical regimen correctly (2). Attentive listening combined with genuine interest, empathy, and concern will foster rapport as well as allow for the accurate assessment of patient needs, attitudes, and beliefs with the result of improved patient satisfaction.

Two-way communication is the foundation of the physician/patient relationship and effective patient education. Physicians should avoid focusing too quickly on what they feel is important while missing the patient's agenda. Patients may be reluctant to state their true reasons for coming to the physician because they are embarrassed or feel that their reasons may not be adequate. The result is a false agenda for the visit. By missing the "hidden agenda" the physician may not deal with the patient's most important issues. Accurate assessment of previous attempts at treatment, prior side effects, fears, concerns, or health beliefs can prevent the repetition of previous mistakes.

Table 17.1. Obstacles to Compliance and Strategies to Overcome Them

Problem Area	Obstacle(s)	Strategies
Relationship	Dissatisfaction	Be courteous and friendly. Show interest, empathy, and concern. Provide opportunities for release of tension (e.g., humor, laughter, permission to express emotions). Listen attentively to the patient. Work with patient to overcome obstacles. Give encouragement, support, and reassurance.
Regimen factors	Complexity, cost, side effects, physical factors (e.g., arthritis, decreased vision, inability to exercise)	Simplify prescription regimen. Tailor regimen to the patient. Counsel about possible side effects. Establish channels for communication of problems that occur at home.
Recall	Inability to remember or recall advice and information	Organize instructions. Provide an adequate amount of relevant information. Instruct in specific skills. Provide opportunity to maintain those skills. Emphasize important points. Summarize major points, perhaps in writing. Supplement discussion with handouts.
Expectations	Patient's concerns or presenting complaints Passive reliance on medical profession Expectation of cure for a chronic disease	Encourage active involvement of the patient. Inform the patient of the diagnosis. Discuss the causes of the problem, its prognosis, and implications. Identify decisions that need to be made. Provide rationale for treatment. Monitor patient's progress or decide how they will monitor their own progress. Identify patient concerns.
Attitudes	Current health beliefs/concepts of health & disease Prior experiences with disease/medications Preexisting knowledge	Explore the patient's knowledge of an issue. Explore the patient's attitudes and beliefs. Share sensitivity to psychosocial issues. Explore patient's attempts and skills in dealing with the issue. Reinforce health behaviors.
Language and communication	Different primary language Medical jargon Decreased hearing Mental incompetence or dementia Illiteracy Poor vision	Communicate in language the patient can understand. Explain findings of examination, tests, and x-rays. Recommend plan to patient. Provide opportunity for patient to ask questions. Explore patient understanding of plan or information. Explore patient's expected adherence/compliance.

A simple, affordable regimen is an ideal to be worked for whenever possible. The simpler a regimen is, the more likely the patient is to comply. For example, in patients with diabetes or congestive heart failure, medication errors were less than 15% when one drug was prescribed, increased to 25% with two or three drugs, and exceeded 35% with a five-drug regimen. Frequency of dosing is also an important factor. Compliance rates vary inversely with the number of daily doses: 30% of patients comply with q.i.d. dosing, 40% with t.i.d. dosing, 70% with b.i.d. dosing, and 93% with once-daily dosing (3). The cost of a regimen is an increasingly significant obstacle for the patient. Often simplicity and cost are in direct opposition, and the patient is in the best position to make the final decision.

The next requirement is clear, concise instruction. The physician must always speak in a language the patient can understand. All too often medical jargon is so confusing that the physician may as well be speaking another language. To improve your communication with patients, you should continually assess your own use of jargon and your patients' level of understanding. Nurses and family will often identify problems with understanding and should be encouraged to tell you about them.

Instruction must be concise and well organized. The more information presented, the smaller the proportion remembered (see Fig. 17.1); almost one-half of information given is forgotten immediately (4). When the most important points are selected, reinforced, and repeated, and comprehension is assessed, compliance is improved.

Many physicians overestimate the time they spend educating their patients. In one study, doctors who felt they had spent about half the visit on patient education actually spent less than 5% (5). Ninety percent of the time no advice was given on how long or how to use the medication (5). Effective teaching of specific knowledge, behaviors, and skills takes time, but it results in improved compliance.

Patient education is not something to be left to the last minute or two of the office visit. The essential functions of establishing rapport, two-way communication, and giving clear and concise instruction are most effective when they are part of the fabric of the visit.

A SYSTEMATIC APPROACH TO EDUCATING PATIENTS

The challenge to physicians is to perform quality, effective education within the real limitations of

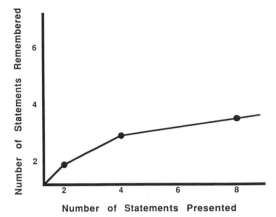

Figure 17.1. "Forgetting curve." Demonstrates that most patients, when interviewed after an office visit, are found to remember no more than three pieces of information presented to them orally by their physician. (Modified from Ley P: Psychological studies of doctor-patient communication. In *Contributions to Medical Psychology*, I. Oxford, Pergamon Press, 1977, pp. 9–42.)

the office , the hospital bedside, the telephone, or the supermarket aisle—wherever the patient is encountered. A "tool box" of patient education skills and strategies, which can be used selectively, is necessary. The most effective technique varies, depending on the patient and on the needed educational function. By being familiar with as many tools as possible, you will be most likely to be effective. Figure 17.2 outlines a systematic approach to patient education. The elements listed on Figure 17.2 are described below; each has been shown to improve compliance (6).

Establish Rapport

The physician-patient rapport needed for successful patient education and therapy begins as soon as your patient enters the office. Staff attitudes and your initial face-to-face contact are crucial. Demonstration of interest, empathy, and concern, combined with a friendly, courteous manner, will go a long way. Attentive listening allows collection of necessary data as well as demonstrating concern and caring. Defusing tense moments with appropriate use of humor, laughter, or permission to express emotions fosters rapport and removes the obstacle to learning that pent-up emotion can present. A style that fosters open communication and demonstrates concern lays a firm base for further interventions.

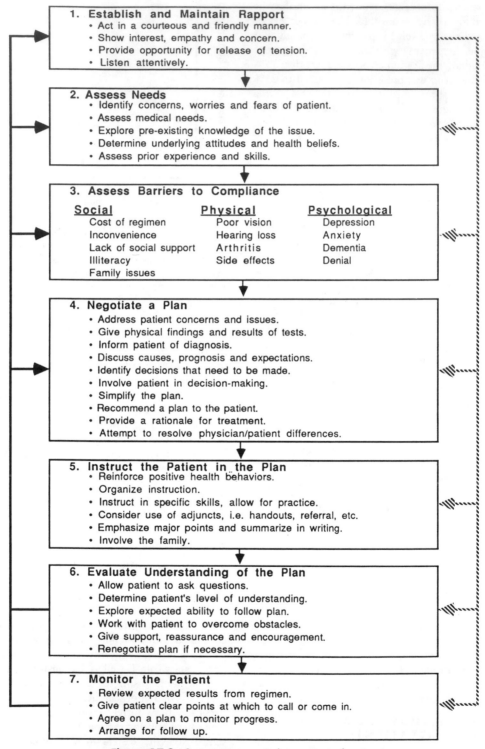

Figure 17.2. Systematic approach to patient education.

Identify Needs

Assessing the needs of the patient is a complex and crucial step. The worries and fears of the patient and the effects of the problem on him/her must be assessed by direct questioning. Similarly, the needs of the physician as the provider of medical care should be weighed in light of the patient's perceived needs. The agenda for the visit must reflect the needs of both if a successful outcome is to occur. Two-way communication, with the physician both addressing the necessary medical issues and meeting patient needs, is necessary.

The physician should also assess the specific educational needs of the patient: What is the patient's preexisting knowledge of this problem? What health beliefs and attitudes will affect the patient's acceptance of your advice? What previous experience does the patient have in dealing with the issue?

Assess Potential Barriers to Compliance

Patient noncompliance with physician recommendations is common and results in significant cost to society. Overall, nearly 50% of patients are estimated to fail to follow medical advice. Failure to comply with primary care therapy can result in more expensive treatment, increased utilization of specialty consultation, and increased testing, as complications develop from lack of effective treatment of the primary problem.

Reasons for noncompliance vary. Lack of knowledge about pathophysiology is a relatively minor factor. More important causes of noncompliance are deficiencies in the physician-patient relationship, problems with the prescribed regimen, miscommunication (or lack of communication) between the physician and patient, and conflicts between the regimen and basic patient values or beliefs (see Table 17.1).

Effective patient education aims at identifying and then reducing potential barriers to patient compliance. The following case example illustrates how, in the context of an acute problem visit, the family physician can identify and deal with compliance issues involving a chronic medical problem.

Case 2

Mr. E.J., a 40-year-old man, presents to the office with tennis elbow. He has an asymptomatic blood pressure elevation of 200/110. After addressing his elbow problem, the physician learns through careful questioning that the patient was diagnosed as having hypertension 2 years ago and β-blocker therapy was started. He developed symptoms of fatigue and sexual dysfunction; so he stopped the medication. He believes that all blood pressure medications cause impotence.

Case Discussion

Although the office nurse pointed out Mr. E.J.'s elevated blood pressure before the doctor entered the room, the physician initially dealt with his presenting complaint. Later in the visit, the patient's experiences with hypertension were explored. His previous health experience, his history of side effects and previous noncompliance, and his health belief that all medications cause impotence, are important data in effectively managing his hypertension. A patient education plan that addresses these issues will be effective in developing a therapeutic alliance between the physician and patient.

Negotiate a Plan

Addressing the patient's concerns and fears, describing findings from the physical examination and other studies, and informing the patient of the diagnosis should be done early in the educational process. The patient who is wondering whether his or her x-ray showed a fracture cannot pay full attention to instructions. A clear explanation of suspected causes and prognosis should follow. This communication sets the stage for the meaningful and informed negotiation of a plan.

The determination of the therapeutic plan should be a cooperative effort by the physician and patient. One regimen may be less expensive but more convenient; another regimen may fit better into the patient's schedule and lifestyle. Active involvement of the patient in decision making improves the likelihood of success. Thus, the physician should present medically acceptable options and identify decisions that need to be made. When medical factors do not contraindicate, the patient's preferences should be respected. Early assessment of acceptability can prevent the frustration of having your plan rejected by the patient after you have already written prescriptions and fully instructed the patient.

When dealing with chronic conditions, negotiation of a management plan is generally an ongoing process. Chronic problems differ from acute ones in that management more often involves long-term behavior changes (e.g., diet, level of exercise, or use of tobacco or alcohol). Thus, your plan will include negotiated behavioral goals, which will be reviewed at the next office visit.

Instruct the Patient in the Plan

Because of the limited amount of information that a person can comprehend and remember after an encounter, an organized approach to patient teaching is crucial. After supporting the positive health behaviors of the patient, you should give clear, concise instructions, focusing on a few major points. Specific skills, such as the use of crutches or back-stretching exercises, need to be demonstrated by the physician (or another health professional) and practiced by the patient. Reinforcing the major point of instruction with repetition and a written reminder aids compliance.

Adjuncts to patient education, such as prepared handouts and videotapes, or referral to professionals such as nutritionists, physical therapists, and diabetes educators can be valuable for common problems (Table 17.2). It is essential, however, that you be thoroughly familiar with the content of education aids you recommend. A handout or class that provides information contradictory to your instructions is harmful to compliance. Patient education aids or referrals should reinforce and build upon the basic education begun in the office. When a pamphlet is read or a referral is complete, the physician will be responsible for continuing the education of the patient.

Evaluate the Understanding of the Plan

This step should occur throughout patient education. Your patient should be encouraged to ask

Table 17.2. Adjuncts to Patient Education

Printed material	Physician-produced handouts
	Preprinted handouts
	Pamphlets
	Drawings or diagrams
	Books (e.g., office lending library)
Other media	Instructional models (e.g., the spine)
	Audiotapes
	Slide/tape presentations
	Videotapes
Computer-assisted	Health-risk assessment
	Nutritional assessment
	Computer-generated handouts
	Instructional programs
Referral	Trained office staff
	Nutritionist
	Physical therapist
	Hospital-based patient educator classes (e.g., childbirth education classes)

questions. Explore whether the patient feels able to follow the plan. Questions like "Does this sound like something you can do?" can uncover potential problems. Complete renegotiation of the plan may be necessary, but this is far superior to covert noncompliance by your patient.

Monitor the Patient

When patients leave the office they are essentially on their own. Support, reassurance, and encouragement are essential to get your patient through the days, weeks, or months before the next visit. Specific criteria for checking in by phone or coming in to the office are to be included. A mechanism for monitoring results by the physician or the patient (e.g., checking blood pressure) should be chosen, and arrangements for necessary follow-up agreed upon. The plan is placed in the patient's record and should be reviewed at the next visit.

Patient accomplishments should be recognized and praised. Little is more damaging to continued compliance than to have a patient achieve a difficult goal and the doctor appear not to notice. Basic aspects of the plan must be reviewed and reinforced routinely, especially in asymptomatic or chronic diseases, such as diabetes and hypertension.

Putting It All Together

A comprehensive strategy has been outlined. At this point, the reader may be wondering how all this can be incorporated effectively into a brief clinical encounter. The following example will demonstrate the selective use of the components of the "tool box" in dealing with a common, acute problem during a brief office visit.

Case 3

A 42-year-old male smoker is waiting in an examination room with the chief complaint of cough. The doctor enters the room, shakes hands, introduces herself, sits close to the patient, and leans forward saying, "How may I help you today?" The patient describes a "cold" beginning 10 days ago which has "settled in my chest." Cough and wheezing keep him up at night. At the suggestion of his wife, he came to the office for "a shot of penicillin to knock it out." Upon closer questioning, the patient states that he is afraid he has pneumonia. He has had to decrease his smoking from two packs per day to one-half pack daily.

After an appropriate problem-oriented history and examination, the physician tells the patient that the history and physical do not indicate a pneumonia and explains the diagnosis of asthmatic bronchitis. The physician explains that a chest x-ray is an option but that the results are unlikely to change the treatment, and the patient chooses not to have an x-ray. The doctor then explains that an antibiotic should help shorten the course of the disease and that certain oral antibiotics will better cover the types of bacteria expected in a smoker than a shot of penicillin. The options presented are an expensive twice-a-day medicine (doxycycline) versus a less costly four-times-a-day regimen that has to be taken on an empty stomach (tetracycline). Since the patient has an insurance plan that pays for most of the cost of any prescription and has a busy schedule, he chooses the simpler regimen. The physician and patient then negotiate what will be the easiest times to take the medication, and the physician emphasizes that all the medication should be taken, to prevent a relapse. They agree that he will ask his wife to help him remember his medication.

Next, the management of the patient's wheezing and cough is discussed. The patient has been unable to use inhalers regularly in the past and so prefers an oral β-agonist for the wheezing. A slow-release, twice-a-day albuterol tablet is recommended, which the patient agrees to take at the same time as the antibiotic.

The physician praises the patient for cutting down on smoking and recommends quitting. Because of stress at work, the patient believes that he is unable to quit now, but he states that he would like to work on this in the future.

While the physician writes down the major points of their discussion, she verifies that the patient is able to state the diagnosis, how he will take the medicine, and possible side effects. The patient is instructed to call if the condition worsens, if intolerable side effects occur, or if he has not started to get better in 3 days.

The patient has no further questions or problems and agrees to return for a follow up visit in 3 weeks to discuss smoking cessation. He receives a pamphlet on quitting smoking as they walk toward the door together. The doctor records the plan in the record, with a note reflecting the patient's interest in smoking cessation.

Case Discussion

All of the components for effective patient education are met in the above case example: establishment of a solid physician/patient relationship, two-way communication, a simple and affordable regimen, and clear, concise instructions. During a 15-minute visit, the physician has established rapport, assessed the medical and perceived needs of the patient, assessed and dealt with barriers to compliance, negotiated an acceptable plan, instructed the patient, evaluated understanding, and arranged recontact and follow-up. In addition, the groundwork has been laid for the next visit. By se-lectively using the needed skills and techniques in an organized manner throughout the visit, the physician has accomplished substantial education and greatly increased the chances for compliance.

CONCLUSIONS

Patient education is performed every day in clinical practice, and all physicians are educators. The word doctor itself comes from the Latin word *docēre*, meaning to teach. Research demonstrates that patients have problems following medical regimens and that improved teaching of patients can improve compliance. This chapter presents a strategy that can be used in every patient encounter.

The basic techniques and strategies outlined here are intended to serve as a framework to which other behavioral, educational, and communication skills are added to create a custom patient education "tool box" for the clinician. The number and complexity of techniques used should vary, depending on the unique challenges of each clinical encounter. Common but complex problems, such as smoking cessation and prenatal education, or chronic conditions, such as diabetes and hypertension, may require a customized approach. The more these tools are used and these skills are perfected, the more effective and satisfying the clinical encounter will be, for both the patient and the physician.

REFERENCES

1. Eraker SA, Kirscht JP, Becker MH: Understanding and improving patient compliance. *Ann Intern Med* 100:258–268, 1984.
2. Geyman JP: How effective is patient education?. *J Fam Pract* 10:973–974, 1980.
3. Ayd FJ: Rational pharmacotherapy: once-a-day drug dosage. *Dis Nerv Syst* 34:371–378, 1973.
4. Ley P: Psychological studies of doctor-patient communication. In *Contributions to Medical Psychology, I.* Oxford, Pergamon Press, 1977, 9–42.
5. Burgess MM: Ethical and economic aspects of noncompliance and overtreatment. *Can Med Assoc J* 141:777–780, 1989.
6. McCann DP, Blossom JH: The physician as patient educator—from theory to practice. *West J Med* 153:44–49, 1990.

SUGGESTED READINGS

Falvo DR: *Effective Patient Education: A Guide to Increased Compliance.* Rockville, MD, Aspen Systems Corporation, 1985.

An in-depth approach to improving compliance through improved patient education.

Fried RA, Iverson DC, Nagle J: *The Clinician's Health Promotion Handbook*. Denver, Mercy Medical Center, 1985.

A practical, "tool box" approach to a number of common clinical problems. Available from the Society of Teachers of Family Medicine, located in Kansas City.

Griffith HW. *Instructions for Patients*, 4th ed. Philadelphia, WB Saunders, 1989.

Collection of preprinted patient education handouts.

Rees AM, Hoffman C: *The Consumer Health Information Sourcebook*, 3rd ed. Phoenix, Oryx Press, 1990.

A comprehensive listing of patient education resources.

Report of the National Task Force on Training Family Physicians in Patient Education. *Patient Education: A Handbook for Teachers*. Kansas City, Society of Teachers of Family Medicine, 1979.

Excellent primer on patient education techniques, with an extensive list of references and resources.

Ureda JR, Taylor RB, Denham JW (eds): *Health Promotion: Principles and Clinical Applications*. East Norwalk, CT, Appleton-Century-Crofts, 1982.

Expands on the patient education techniques and skills needed to promote healthy behaviors and lifestyles.

chapter 18

HEALTH PROMOTION

Adam O. Goldstein

Health, defined as a state of physical and mental well-being, involves far more than the simple absence of disease. Optimal health implies being not only physically well but also satisfied and happy with life itself. Health promotion, then, is the branch of clinical medicine designed to help your patients, their families, and communities achieve optimum levels of good health. Health promotion is also an integral part of daily life, and physicians must remember its place within a societal context of proper housing, good education, and having a meaningful job and relationships.

Increasingly over the past decade, patients have expected their family physicians to treat not only common illnesses, but also to give reliable information and counseling about the prevention of disease. Such concern is justified, considering that almost two-thirds of all Americans who die each year do so prematurely, before the age of 65, and three-quarters of these premature deaths could be prevented by proper attention to preventive health care. Fifty percent of cardiovascular disease and 25% of cancer cases could be eliminated by the application of known health promotion techniques, primarily the elimination of tobacco products. Over the next 20 years, health promotion for women and elderly patients will assume an increasingly important role. You must go beyond your patients' presenting problems and deal with their major risk factors for poor health.

This chapter focuses on the diverse skills you need to effectively assess and counsel your patients for health promotion. Specific interventions discussed in this chapter include

- Physical activity and exercise;
- Nutrition;
- Substance abuse;
- Mental health;
- Violence and injury reduction;
- Community health promotion.

Whether interventions are directed to a patient, a work site, a school, or a community, the key to all successful health promotion is application. Family physicians with good counseling skills use every patient encounter as an opportunity for health promotion. You too can learn to deliver such evaluation, assessment, and initial counseling in 5 minutes or less, incorporating routines into both acute and chronic care visits!

Case 1

A 43-year-old white male construction worker comes into your office for a cough of 2-weeks duration. He has had no fever or weight loss but coughs up a thick green sputum. He has smoked one pack per day of Marlboros for the last 25 years but has no history of chronic medical problems. He is afebrile in the office, has a blood pressure of 140/94, weighs 206 pounds, and has a normal lung examination. You diagnose bronchitis, and place him on a 1-week course of antibiotics.

Study Questions

- Which health promotion issues should you address at this initial visit?
- In what context will you bring up your concerns?
- How will you deliver a succinct and effective counseling message?
- Which issues should you address at a follow-up visit?

Case Discussion

At this visit, you link the bronchitis to his history of smoking. You decide to discuss his motivation to quit smoking, give a short but firm smoking cessation message, and offer a patient education brochure from the Lung Association on smoking cessation techniques. You also perform a quick assessment for underlying alcohol-use problems while informing him that his blood pressure is slightly elevated. You ask to see him back in 1 week to discuss these issues and to recheck his blood pressure. At the follow-up visit, you plan to explore his reactions in more depth and to further assess his own health priorities.

ASSESSMENT FOR HEALTH PROMOTION

When a family physician enters an examination room to talk with a patient, he or she begins thinking not only about the chief complaint but also about whether major risk factors threaten the patient's overall health. While interventions will vary depending on the patient's age, gender, race, socioeconomic status, and prior health habits, physicians should develop standard office procedures for gathering health promotion information on all patients. Methods for gathering general information include health risk appraisal, health maintenance flow sheets, diaries, and physiological testing.

Health Risk Appraisal (HRA). Health risk appraisals are written or computerized quantitative and qualitative assessments of a patient's major risky or unhealthy behaviors. Available for adults and children, HRAs prioritize behavioral modifications that will increase a patient's life span the most. Figure 18.1 provides sample output from a computerized HRA. HRAs are appealing because they allow complete assessment of a patient's health behaviors without a physician interview. However, proper use of HRAs requires a well organized office system and office personnel experienced in their use. An excellent computerized version (Healthy People 4.0) is distributed by the Health Risk Appraisal program of the Carter Center of Emory University (One Copenhill, Atlanta, GA, 30307).

Health Maintenance Flow Sheets. Most family physicians use some sort of flow sheets to guide health promotion assessments. Placed on the front of a patient's chart, a 1-page flow sheet reminds the physician to review and practice health promotion at every patient visit. With each successive patient visit, the flow sheets allow staff or computer-assisted prompts to remind the physician about the patient's major ongoing unhealthy behaviors. An alternative, related assessment tool, the periodic health examination, is discussed more fully in Chapter 16.

When physicians desire more information from patients about specific health behaviors, additional specific health assessment tools are useful, including

Diary Analysis. Three- or 7- day patient diaries can help physicians detect unhealthy eating, exercise, or substance-use patterns. Have the patient keep a detailed record of all behaviors of interest over a specified time period and then return the diary at a follow-up office visit. Such diaries can pinpoint unusual patterns or unsuspected problems. Food diaries help track caloric intake and cholesterol or sodium consumption. Exercise diaries help motivate patients and monitor their progress. When smoking cessation is a goal, a diary can pinpoint when in the day a patient smokes cigarettes and what alternative actions will be most useful.

Physiological Testing. While not a frequently used method, physiological testing can both assess and motivate some patients. Submaximal exercise stress testing will help to formally evaluate a patient's overall level of fitness. Spirometry and pulmonary function tests for patients who smoke may show decreased lung function. Anthropometric measurements through triceps skinfold thickness and midarm muscle circumference may help estimate adipose tissue reserves and lean muscle mass.

HEALTH PROMOTION COUNSELING

Health promotion counseling attempts to give patients the tools for self-empowerment and behavior change. Patients who are motivated for lifestyle change offer the greatest opportunity for effective counseling. Therefore, focus your counseling messages in two domains:

- Motivate patients to seek healthier lifestyles. If motivation is poor, ask the patient, "What will it take for you to want to change?"
- Help motivated patients achieve behavioral change by guiding them as they make detailed behavioral change plans, including resources.

According to behavioral modification theory, several steps can help achieve long-lasting health behavior changes. Patients should

1. Select specific short-term (between 1 and 8 weeks) goals, plus one or more long-term goals, based on their own priorities;

YOUR PERSONAL HEALTH PROFILE

The risk of an average man of your age dying during the next 10 years compared with you is:

Cause of Death	Average	You
Heart attack	4.72%	12.30%
Lung cancer	1.95%	3.88%
Stroke	.65%	1.93%
Emphysema or bronchitis	.52%	.67%
Cirrhosis of the liver	.49%	.49%
Colon cancer	.38%	.38%
All other causes	7.05%	7.05%
Overall risk of death	**15.76%**	**26.71%**

Your actual age is *55*. Your health age is *62*. Your health risk is *above average*.

To improve your health, you can:

Action	% it will lower risk of death in next 10 yrs.
Stop smoking cigarettes	**10.95%**
Lower your blood pressure	**1.61%**
Lower your cholesterol level	**.70%**
Stop alcohol use	**.24%**

If you want to try changing one of these at a time, begin with the ones with the biggest numbers.

If you followed all these suggestions, your new health age would be *53*.

Here are some **good habits** that you already have:

Good physical activity level
Excellent self-reported health
Low violence risk

For more information on good habits and health risk, discuss this appraisal with your *doctor* or another *health professional*.

Figure 18.1. Sample health risk appraisal output for a hypothetical 55-year-old man who smokes cigarettes, drinks alcoholic beverages, and has hypertension and hypercholesterolemia. (Adapted from Ellis LB, Joo HY, Gross CR: Use of computer-based health risk appraisal by older adults. *J Fam Pract*, 33:391, 1991.)

2. Monitor their progress by regular follow-up (encourage patients to seek help whenever their goals seem threatened);
3. Reward themselves in tangible and healthy ways;
4. Encourage family members and friends to give positive reinforcement.

Consider giving all patients a general guideline for successful lifestyle change. Table 18.1 provides one example.

Throughout all your counseling opportunities, remember to use consistent positive reinforcement, both in language and attitudes. Convey positive messages to patients, such as "You are in control of your life" and "You have the ability to change." Appreciate the fact that only a minority of your patients will initially enact behavioral changes in their lives as a result of your efforts. A 30% success rate with behaviors such as smoking cessation or weight loss is excellent! Moreover, some patients will institute health behavior

Table 18.1. Patient Health Behavior Change Guidelines

Your health is important
- You have a responsibility to choose what health habits you want to change.

You can change unhealthy habits to healthy ones
- Choose one specific unhealthy behavior for change.
- Carefully make plans for change: read books, articles, and talk to experts or friends. Anticipate barriers and alternative actions.
- Pick a date for change.
- Reward yourself for short-term success, and maintain your new habit.
- You will eventually succeed.

Steps you can take now
- Do not use tobacco products in any form.
- Exercise regularly, at least four times a week.
- Wear seat belts while driving.
- Never drive after drinking alcohol.
- Practice stress reduction activities on a regular basis.
- Get 7 to 8 hours of sleep every night.
- Practice nonviolence.

changes months to years later because of your prior, brief health promotion message.

BARRIERS TO SUCCESSFUL HEALTH PROMOTION

Patients

It is often a struggle to change good intentions into good health practices. Barriers can include physiological addictions, fear of change, few resources, and poor self-esteem. You should try to identify and deal with barriers up front rather than hoping they will not influence your patient's outcomes. For example, when attempting to persuade a young woman to quit smoking, discuss her fears about weight gain and suggest alternatives such as exercise, meditation, or reading instead of increased eating. Show an overweight and sedentary adult how to increase daily physical activity without major investments of time or money by simply taking stairs instead of elevators and walking faster between routines.

Families

Few health behavior changes affect only the involved patient, and most have strong familial contexts influencing the process. Some behaviors, such as spouse abuse, involve direct insults to health, but frequently remain underdiagnosed by unsuspecting health care professionals. Most familial influence is indirect, such as when alcohol abuse by one family member heightens high stress levels and leads to illness behaviors in other family members. Patients who want to quit smoking have far more success if their spouses are nonsmokers and supportive than if their spouses or other family members smoke. Weight loss for a child or adult frequently depends on solid family support for proper food selection, preparation, and eating habits.

Physicians

Physician barriers include perceived lack of time or remuneration for health promotion, perceived patient disinterest, and poor delivery systems. Recognizing these barriers, insurance companies and government agencies have sought to increase incentives for performing cognitive-based procedures such as health promotion. Physicians also find that they can address many problems by making health promotion a high priority during the office visit. In addition, nurses or other support personnel can implement appropriate health promotion protocols with the patient before the physician comes in the room. Finally, health promotion materials without tobacco or alcohol advertisements can be available to patients in the waiting room.

Physicians must examine their own attitudes and behaviors. A physician who is markedly overweight, never exercises, and gets only 5 or 6 hours of sleep a night may have a difficult time persuading patients to adopt dissimilar, albeit healthier, behaviors.

COMMUNITY HEALTH PROMOTION

Through health promotion, you have the unique ability to become not only a patient advocate, but also a community health promotion specialist. The challenge involves learning how to promote health, a process that is exciting, rewarding, and often fun. The rules are simple:

- Know the leading preventable causes of death in your community (In most communities, the top killers, in descending order, are tobacco, alcohol, violence, and injuries);
- Choose one or two areas as your targets.

There are no other rules. Go for it by unleashing your creative talents and collective energy. Become a *medical activist* for a week, month, or year with targeted community health promotion messages for schoolchildren, teenagers, women, minorities, adults, elderly patients, or whatever groups will benefit the most from your efforts.

An additional assessment method, entitled *community-oriented primary care* (COPC), allows physicians to selectively target the most important perceived and real health problems facing their community. For example, AIDS, teenage pregnancy, and violence may be priorities in an urban area, while injuries and substance abuse may be top priorities for a nearby suburban neighborhood. COPC suggests that physicians collaborate with public health professionals to identify these sentinal health problems, using interviews with a cross-section of community members and review of local health statistics.

After deciding on a program, devise a campaign that will allow you to "sell" good health as accessible, fashionable, and most importantly, fun. Learn which messages work from effective "Madison Avenue" campaigns. For instance, when sponsoring a tobacco or alcohol prevention program for adolescents, consider developing a long-term relationship with a class or school by "adopting" it. Then, through health promotion talks and discussions, teach the youth to become their own "pro-health" advocates. Let them devise creative marketing campaigns against alcohol and tobacco advertising, emphasizing the good looks, sexiness, and success of not using the product. Help the adolescents promote their campaign through newspaper articles, TV interviews, or making their own "rap" health commercials. To reach the entire community, why not work on sponsoring (with a couple of colleagues) a monthly newspaper column or radio talk show?

When "unhealthy" activities occur in your community, do not hesitate to use these events as health education opportunities. For instance, if a beer company sponsors an event for the Special Olympics (with alcohol abuse being the number one cause of mental retardation) or a tobacco company sponsors a music festival (e.g., the Benson and Hedges Blues Festival), organize a group of colleagues to protest such activities and hand out appropriate health education literature.

Professional medical organizations, such as the American Academy of Family Physicians or the American Medical Association, because of their organizational and financial resources, can help support community-wide interventions, particularly legislative efforts to improve health. A food-labeling law, for example, will help consumers make informed food purchasing decisions, and an environmental tobacco-smoke regulation will reduce passive smoke exposure. Encourage your professional associations to pursue such topics if they are currently inactive.

Local medical advocacy coalitions, such as *Doctors Ought to Care* (DOC), specialize in creative health promotion campaigns such as those described above. The most successful campaigns use humor and satire and capitalize on mass media attention to sell good health. By organizing your own DOC group, you will emphasize that your role extends far beyond the office, into the community. As a future community leader, you can make a great difference, as long as you do not underestimate your potential impact and you can have fun!

SPECIFIC HEALTH PROMOTION STRATEGIES

Physical Activity/Exercise

Almost all people can benefit from a regular exercise regimen. The physical and psychological benefits that accrue at all ages include increased longevity, improved mobility, and a greater sense of well-being.

Successful exercise programs include two components: (*a*) aerobic conditioning and (*b*) stretching and proper muscle strengthening. Virtually any exercise that requires individuals to keep their feet moving can provide acceptable aerobic exercise if done regularly (at least three times a week) and for a sufficient amount of time each exercise period (at least 20 minutes). Most patients can incorporate more regular exercise into their daily routines by following a few simple and practical suggestions. Tailored exercise prescriptions will assist such efforts. (See Table 18.2.)

Patients who want to monitor their daily exercise regimens can be taught to take their own pulse after each exercise session. You can calculate a patient's *target exercise heart rate* as follows:

1. Estimate the maximum heart rate in beats per minute by subtracting the patient's age from 220;
2. Have your patient aim to achieve between 60 and 80% of this rate during exercise.

For example, a healthy 26-year-old medical student should achieve a target exercise heart rate ranging from 116 to 155 beats per minute.

Proper stretching is an important adjuvant to exercise programs because it reduces the chance of injury. Advise all patients to include a 5-minute

Table 18.2. Sample Patient Exercise Prescription

Pick an aerobic exercise
• Exercise 3 to 5 days each week for at least 20 minutes each time.
• Jogging or walking 2 miles, biking or swimming 30 minutes, or playing tennis 45 minutes burns equivalent amounts of calories (about 300).
• Exercise at a pace that allows you to maintain a conversation without undue stress.
• Stop exercising or slow down immediately if you feel very tired or begin to have pain.

Perform proper stretching and build up your regimen slowly
• Stretch your muscles every day before going to bed, in the morning, and for 5 minutes before and after exercising.
• Increase your activities slowly over 3 months.

Incorporate exercise into your everyday routines
• Park farther away at work.
• Use stairs whenever possible instead of elevators.
• Pick parking spaces at the mall farther away from entrances.
• Take a 15-minute walk during lunch.

stretching session as a "warm-up" and as a "cool-down" period in all their exercise routines. While the specific muscle groups to be stretched will vary, depending on the exercise, a good general routine includes proper stretching of the Achilles tendon, calf muscles, quadriceps, hamstrings, lower back, arms, shoulders, and neck. Muscle conditioning, through weight lifting or isometric exercises, provides little cardiovascular benefit but plays an important role for certain patients by strengthening key muscle groups. For example, strengthening the paraspinus muscles helps avoid low back pain, and building up the quadriceps helps alleviate stress to the knee.

Some patients require special consideration before starting an exercise regimen. Patients with known heart disease, those with strong cardiovascular risk factors, and certain elderly patients may need screening exercise stress electrocardiograms. Most pregnant patients can safely continue exercise throughout pregnancy but should not initiate a strenuous conditioning program and should avoid overheating themselves. Kegel exercises and stretching are particularly important in pregnant patients.

Nutrition

Our society often appears obsessed with eating patterns. At any time, between 10 and 25% of all patients are on some kind of special diet. The lay press and modern culture strongly contribute to this fascination by linking personal identity with looks or by highlighting unproven, often nonscientific therapies.

Obesity and overeating are our most common nutritional problems, as well as some of the most difficult behaviors to change over the long haul (see Chapter 35 on obesity). Anorexia and bulimia are also common problems, particularly among many adolescent and college females. Certain medical conditions, such as elevated cholesterol levels, may affect up to 40% of the population. Therefore, physician counseling about diets, cholesterol, supplements, or other nutritional concerns may have a large population impact.

Patients who are more than 30% over their ideal body weight may have problems with obesity. To estimate a patient's ideal body weight: For men, start with 106 lbs for the first 60 inches in height and add 6 lbs for each additional inch. For women, start with 100 lbs for the first 60 inches in height and add 5 lbs for each additional inch. Subtract or add 10% for patients with small or large body frames, respectively. Give patients simple dietary advice (see Table 18.3) as well as relevant patient education materials on proper nutrition.

Table 18.3. Tips for a Healthier Diet

Assess
• What is the patient's ideal body weight?
• Is there any history of a lipid disorder?

Questions to ask patients
• Do you think you are underweight, overweight, or about right?
• Do you have any questions about special diets or nutrition?
• What have you eaten during the past 24 hours?
• Do you take vitamin or mineral supplements?

Counseling advice
• Stay within 10% of your ideal body weight.
• Keep the total fat in your diet to less than 30% of your total calories.
• Use monounsaturated fats (olive or peanut oil) or polyunsaturated fats (sunflower or safflower) instead of saturated or hydrogenated ones (coconut, palm, cottonseed).
• Follow a high-fiber diet by eating plenty of fresh fruits, vegetables, cereals, and grains every day.
• Eat less meat and animal products and more whole grains, nuts, and vegetables.
• Limit your use of salt to 5 grams or less per day. Do not salt foods beyond what is used in cooking.
• Eat breakfast every day.
• Read food labels.

Many patients on special diets strongly believe in the value of certain vitamin and mineral supplements. Such patients expect physicians to know basic information about common vitamins and minerals (Table 18.4).

Substance Abuse

One of every three patients abuses some type of drug, most often tobacco, alcohol, and/or prescription medications (narcotics and benzodiazepines most frequently). Despite such high contact with substance abuse, many surveys show that physicians rarely ask patients about such issues, much less offer counseling.

As part of a screening assessment, which serves as a vital sign for all new patients as well as patients that present with diseases linked to substance abuse (e.g., chronic bronchitis, gastritis, ulcer disease, unexplained severe pain), physicians can have a powerful impact on patient's substance use patterns by following several simple rules (1):

1. Anticipate that many patients are likely to have substance abuse problems;

Table 18.4. Vitamins and Minerals: Sources, Benefits and Recommended Adult (nonpregnant) Daily Allowances

Vitamin/Mineral	Sources	Benefits	Deficiency	Recommended Dietary Allowance (RDA)
Vitamin A[a]	Sweet potatoes, carrots, milk	Improved skin resistance to infection; good eyesight	Night blindness, xerophthalmia	1000 µg retinol equivalents (5000 IU)
Vitamin D[a]	Sunlight, dairy products	Strengthens bone development	Rickets	5–10 µg (1000–1200 IU)
Vitamin E[a]	Green leafy vegetables, nuts, whole grains, wheat germ	Oxidative protection of red blood cells	Anemia	8–10 mg (30 IU)
Vitamin K[a]	Green leafy vegetables, tomatoes	Blood clotting cascade	Bleeding diathesis	70–140 µg
Vitamin B₁[b] (thiamine)	Whole grains, vegetables, nuts, wheat germ	Carbohydrate metabolism	Beriberi	1–1.5 mg
Vitamin B₂[b] (riboflavin)	Animal products, mushrooms, broccoli	Protein metabolism, skin and eye protectant	Angular stomatitis/ blepharitis	1.2–1.5 mg
Vitamin B₆[b] (pyridoxine)	Brewers yeast, whole grains, nuts, meat	Helps regulate central nervous system	Peripheral neuropathy	1.7–2 mg
Vitamin B₁₂[b]	Animal products, fish, soybeans	Red blood cell formation	Mental status changes	3 µg
Vitamin C[b]	Broccoli, tomatoes, brussel sprouts, citrus fruits	Resistance to stress; oral hygiene; wound healing	Scurvy	60 mg
Niacin[b]	Nuts, poultry, fish	Cholesterol-lowering agent, coenzyme oxidation reductions	Pellagra	13–16 mg
Calcium	Dairy products	Bone growth	Rickets, osteomalacia	800 mg
Potassium	Tomatoes, citrus fruits	Cellular function	Ileus, muscle weakness	1.8–6 g
Sodium	Most foods	Cellular function	Weakness, confusion	1–3.3 g
Phosphorus	Cereals, dairy products	Cellular function	Mental status changes, osteomalacia	800 mg
Iron	Green leafy vegetables, dried fruits, meat, wheat germ	Red blood cell formation	Anemia	10–18 mg

[a]Fat soluble.
[b]Water soluble.

2. Ask each patient about current or a past history of substance abuse problems;
3. Advise all such patients of the medical problems associated with substance abuse;
4. Assist patients to change their substance abuse behaviors and pick a quit date;
5. Arrange follow-up to enlist support for change.

Specific methods for identifying and treating patients with alcohol and drug addictions can be found in Chapter 37.

Remember that substance abuse affects not only the patient but the entire family as well. Spouses of patients addicted to alcohol may present with vague complaints that will improve once their mate's alcohol problems are discussed. A parent's tobacco addiction often shows up in a child's frequent episodes of otitis media or upper respiratory infection. An adolescent who is abusing drugs may have undergone abuse as a child and/or remains in an hostile home environment. In each of the above cases, failing to consider the familial context of the disease will lead to less than optimal treatment.

Mental Health

At least one of every five adults has dysfunction on one mental health domain or another. Suicide, the end result for millions, kills more Americans each year than all homicides. Good mental health refers not only to freedom from major depression or psychiatric disorders, but more importantly, to the ability to cope effectively with life's daily stresses and to feel good about one's overall physical, social, and spiritual well-being. Personal growth is important, and patients (as well as providers) lead more productive, healthier, and happier lives when they are self-responsible, are basically optimistic, and have meaningful relationships.

As with other health promotion strategies, you must first perform an accurate assessment of your patient's overall mental health. By asking screening questions about sleep, a sense of well-being, patterns of coping with stress, and family dynamics, you will learn to identify patients who are at high risk or who are currently manifesting problems. For example, elderly patients with poor social support networks or those recently widowed may be at high risk for depression or suicide. You may choose to see such patients more frequently in your office or through home visits, thereby establishing yourself as a support .

Table 18.5. Sample Assessment and Counseling Strategies for Good Mental Health

Questions
- How well are you sleeping?
- How well are you satisfied with your relationships?
- What are your current sources of major stress?

Counseling
- Sleep:
  "Try to get 7 to 8 hours of sleep every night."
  "Avoid caffeine, alcohol, or exercise before going to bed."
  "Avoid watching TV in bed."
- Stress reduction:
  "Close your eyes and think of something pleasant as you slowly take 10 slow, long breaths.
  "Let's make a plan now to lessen your most stressful activity."
  "At lunch, eat slowly and enjoy your food. Take a good look around you and laugh with others."

Stress Management. (See Table 18.5.) Stress reduction counseling techniques may play an important role in helping patients cope with daily stressors, and you can incorporate such techniques into your clinical encounter quite easily. Brief, focused, supportive psychotherapy will help your patients better cope with acute situational stressors. Other techniques involve "hands-on" approaches, such as massage and progressive muscle relaxation. For instance, try gently massaging the head and neck of your patients with a muscle tension headache while talking about the current stressors in their lives. Not only will you likely diminish the current intensity of their headache, but you will also be demonstrating an effective technique for the patient to use in future encounters.

In working with patients who feel stressed, emphasize that reducing, not adding, commitments generally lowers stress. Stress reduction techniques must be taught in the context of counseling your patient about reducing conflict in life activities. In your practice, pick two or three stress reduction counseling activities that you can become thoroughly familiar with from the list of such techniques shown in Table 18.6. Have reliable mental health consultants for your more difficult cases.

Sleep. Proper mental health also implies good sleep habits, with studies indicating that most people function best when they average between 7 and 8 hours of sleep a night. Insomnia resulting from situational anxiety, chronic stress, depression, or physical illness is the most common sleep disorder. Poor sleep habits on top of heavy work and family

Table 18.6. Relaxation Techniques

Technique	Qualities
Biofeedback	Effective learning for self-relaxation, but expensive
Exercise	Good for mental and physical health, an active, inexpensive, and underutilized method
Hypnosis	Usually requires referral and can be expensive
Laughter	Effective for short-term, episodic stress reduction
Massage	Optimal method for relieving muscle tension; helps build a trusting relationship; can teach to self-administer
Meditation	Inexpensive, easy to teach, and very effective; useful for brief or extended relaxation periods
Prayer	Very effective for certain individuals; must explore religious beliefs
Progressive muscle relaxation	Easy to learn with taped instructions; good adjunct to sleep
Psychotherapy	Easily incorporated into the clinical encounter by showing empathy and directing the patient toward concrete goal-solving activities
Reading, music	Appropriate for routine, daily use along with other hobbies

and financial responsibilities often lead to poor mental health.

After ruling out medical causes of sleep disturbances, such as sleep apnea or narcolepsy, you can help your patients tremendously by simply helping them redevelop good sleep habits. Improved rest will allow them to better cope with stress. One particularly effective office strategy is to teach your patient the art of progressive muscle relaxation and imaging. Demonstrate the technique over 5 minutes, with the patient lying down in a quiet, dimly lit room, and make a tape of the encounter that can be replayed at home or at work.

Counsel patients with sleep disorders to

- Avoid caffeinated beverages and alcohol within 4 hours of bedtime;
- Choose the same time each night to go to sleep;
- Add a small amount of daily exercise to their lives;
- Avoid using their beds as places for watching television or eating;
- Keep their bedrooms as quiet as possible.

If they have difficulty falling asleep after 30 minutes, advise patients to get out of bed and pursue a relaxing activity for 15 minutes, then retry falling asleep. Hypnotic agents should be reserved for those patients unable to sleep because of severe acute stress, such as the loss of a loved one. Patient charts should reflect the short term (1 to 3 weeks) reason for such use.

Spirituality. For many patients, prayer and religious faith play an important role in coping with stress or uncertainty. Just as medical training today frequently emphasizes technology over talking, societal values often emphasize material goods over spiritual growth. Consequently, you may initially feel uncomfortable asking patients about their religious beliefs or views about God. Therefore, start by asking a broad, nonthreatening opening question such as, "What are your aspirations in life?" or "What do you feel is your purpose in this world?" or "Where do you turn for support in times of trouble?" Your patient's response will guide you to more specific questions about religion, core values, and the relationship between these spiritual values and health. Answers to such personal questions may offer you multiple avenues to help your patients reduce stress, plan on a healthier lifestyle, and place their life in a context that has deep-rooted meaning.

For patients with medical or social problems, the clergy offer a valuable source of consultation and referral. Acknowledging and supporting your patients' spiritual values will often strengthen the doctor-patient relationship, a wonderful therapeutic response in its own right.

Violence and Injuries

Violence and injuries affect almost all Americans at some time or another, with over two million Americans being victims of such acts every year. Violence includes acts of physical or emotional assault, including rape, homicide, and child, spouse, or elder abuse. Injuries are classified as intentional (e.g., assaults) or unintentional (e.g., motor vehicle crashes). Motor vehicle injuries alone are the fourth leading cause of death, and homicide is the leading cause of death for black males between the ages of 15 and 34. Violence and injuries exact tremendous physical, emotional, and financial costs.

Approximately one-half of violent crimes and an equal percentage of unintentional injuries are committed under the influence of alcohol or other drugs. Appropriate physician counseling may help prevent many such deaths and injuries.

To give effective counseling, you should learn the basic epidemiology of violence. For instance, teenage couples with a new child and poor social supports are at higher risk for child abuse. Adolescents have a higher incidence of head injuries if they routinely ride bikes without wearing helmets. Teenage and college women have a higher risk of "date rape." Women presenting to the office or emergency room with a traumatic injury are at increased risk of being in a physically abusive relationship. Young black men should know that their chances of dying in an automobile accident are less than their chances of dying from a gunshot wound.

Armed with such knowledge, physicians can intervene for violence reduction through two simple rules:

1. *Ask* about the occurrence of violence or injuries with your patients;
2. *Counsel* your patients about alternative nonviolent behaviors, acting as their patient advocate or information source for referral where appropriate.

Asking patients about violence in their lives is not easy. Initially, many patients may be reluctant to share such information because of its very private nature, fear of being judged, lack of trust, denial, or fear of increased violence if it is discovered that they have "told." To overcome these barriers, you must establish trust and good communication early in your doctor-patient relationship. Open-ended questions to ask your patients include "Is your current relationship a safe one?, Have you ever been arrested? and Do you own a gun?"

Whatever counseling messages you give should be consistent and clear: Injuries are preventable, violence is wrong, and it is not the victim's fault. Counsel men and women that it is never okay to hit a woman or force her to have intercourse against her will. Teach parents and adolescents to use nonviolent conflict resolution skills through role playing, family conferences, and referrals. Learn your local and statewide regulations about reporting cases of suspected violence. Establish a good working knowledge of the social service agencies that handle particular situations.

Case 2

A 16-year-old black male student comes into your office for a sports physical. He has no history of prior injuries or other medical problems. His weight is 146 lbs, he is 5'10" tall and has a normal physical examination. During your examination, you ask about his health habits and discover that he is a nonsmoker but does drink beer with friends on weekends, that he has had intercourse within the last month without using a condom, and that there is at least one gun in his household.

Case Discussion

While signing the forms for sports participation, you mention that you have several concerns. During the next 5 to 7 minutes, you discuss in a nonjudgmental way the problems associated with drinking alcohol, particularly those related to sports performance and driving with anyone who has been drinking. After inquiring about his knowledge of AIDS, other STDs, condoms, and pregnancy prevention, you give him an educational brochure on AIDS. Finally, you inform him of his higher risk for being involved in a firearm injury and ways to cut down on that risk.

CONCLUSIONS

Health promotion is an ongoing process with no set times or orthodox format for giving counseling messages. Almost all patient encounters, ranging from acute care emergencies to chronic follow-up visits, offer opportunities to improve patient's quality and length of life.

Family physicians and their patients should be able to talk to each other about a wide variety of lifestyle behaviors. The content of such counseling messages will vary depending on the age, sex, race, and priorities of an encounter. You can direct counseling to the patient, their family, or the community itself. With improved control of as few as four or five of the risk factors discussed in this chapter, two-thirds of all premature deaths could be eliminated. The only requirements are that you and your patients genuinely care about leading healthier and happier lives.

Acknowledgment: I would like to thank Richard M. Baker, M.D., for the help and guidance I received from reading his chapter on Health Promotion in the first edition of Essentials of Family Medicine.

REFERENCES
1. Glynn TJ, Manley MW: *How to Help Your Patients Stop Smoking*. A National Cancer Institute manual for physicians. Bethesda, MD: US Dept of Health

and Human Services, Public Health Service, National Institutes of Health. Publication No. 90–3064, November, 1990.

SUGGESTED READINGS

DOC: *News and Views, The Journal of Medical Activism*, 5510 Greenbriar, Suite 235, Houston, TX, 77005, (713) 798-7729.

Published quarterly by DOC, Doctors Ought to Care, this newsletter is an excellent, up-to-date source of innovative health promotion campaigns across the United States and worldwide, particularly focusing on ways to counter the effects of Madison Avenue's tobacco and alcohol advertising campaigns.

Guide to Clinical Preventive Services: An Assessment of the Effectiveness of 169 Interventions. Report of the U.S. Preventive Services Task Force. Baltimore, Williams & Wilkins, 1989.

This book is a landmark document for clinical health promotion activities in the United States. Panels of experts spent 4 years reviewing the body of scientific evidence supporting or refuting clinical preventive interventions. The scientific basis is succinctly reviewed and the recommendations are solid.

Health Affairs: Promoting Health. Summer 1990.

A journal for health professionals interested in policy as well as science, the summer 1990 edition is entirely devoted to innovative, controversial, and current health promotion strategies. The articles, written by well-known leaders in their fields, are succinct and stimulating.

U.S. Department of Health and Human Services: *Healthy People 2000: National Health Promotion and Disease Prevention Objectives*. Public Health Service, DHHS Publication No. (PHS) 91-50212, 1991, pp 90–247.

Healthy People 2000 is a book produced by the Public Health Service to guide national efforts in health promotion through the year 2000. With contributions from hundreds of health professionals with expertise in health promotion, the book is an excellent resource on the current status, strategies, and research needs in the field.

Section III

COMMON PROBLEMS

chapter 19

CLINICAL REASONING IN FAMILY PRACTICE

Peter Curtis, Alan Spanos, and Martha Gerrity

Medical students often feel quite confused as they begin to observe a busy, private medical practice. The doctor's work does not seem to fit the model taught in medical school. Patient management proceeds at an unfamiliarly fast pace, and apparently without need of detailed histories or comprehensive examinations. The doctor seems to be cutting corners all the time, but apparently gets away with it. How is this done?

The answer is, partly, because the doctor knows a lot. But just as important is the fact that the doctor's reasoning differs in some important respects from what the student has so far been taught. Education in medical school is generally designed to teach basic sciences and the mechanisms and management of disease. Students learn that symptoms presented by patients are the *result* of the diseases they have learned about. In primary care, this concept is often reversed. The meaning of symptoms and their patterns, normal and abnormal human behavior, and the effects of lifestyle and environment are important targets of knowledge. Symptoms are often not associated with any particular disease entity. Similarly, clinical reasoning and decision-making styles learned in medical school are often not appropriate for office practice. A major value of a clinical rotation in family practice is to familiarize you with these reasoning processes. In this chapter we examine some key features of clinical reasoning in family practice.

APPROACH TO THE PATIENT IN PRIMARY CARE

Patient-Physician Communication

In primary care, effective clinical reasoning depends on good communication and understanding the biopsychosocial model of disease. Developed by Engel, this model affirms the close relationship of mind, body, and environment in promoting health and causing illness. The family physician evaluates the patient using two paths: (*a*) the biomedical path of symptoms and objective findings and (*b*) the psychosocial path of assessing stressors, family factors, and resources as illustrated in Figure 19.1.

Getting a history that involves both pathways takes skill and experience. One needs to develop and maintain rapport with the patient and often to use the patient-centered approach—using open-ended questions into the patient's concerns and needs for information. In other words, what the patient wants to know and decide is as important as what the doctor wants to find out. Only through these communication techniques will adequate and accurate data be collected as the basis for the clinical reasoning process.

Assembling Information

The breadth of family practice is illustrated in Table 19.1, a typical morning's schedule for a family physician. Note the wide range of problems and patient age groups, and the short time allotted for most visits (except for the well woman check-up and the stroke patient). Each patient needs empathy and understanding, and each visit requires a clinical evaluation and a management decision.

With the exception of some "routine physicals," most patients come to see the family physician because of a problem. They want the problem addressed and solved. However, this "presenting problem" may be complex, multiple, and more confusingly, may not be a "medical" problem at all.

The process of helping the patient with his or her problem involves a number of steps, which constitute a framework for the doctor-patient in-

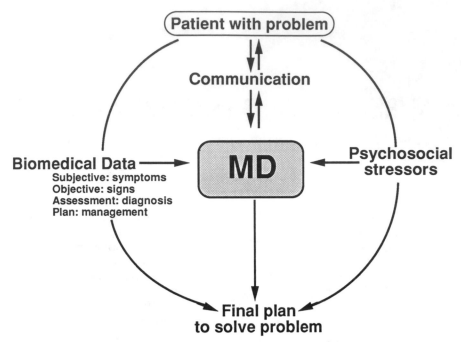

Figure 19.1. Biopsychosocial model of disease.

Table 19.1. Typical Morning Schedule of a Family Physician

	Time	Name of Patient	Age	Problem	Decision
1	8:30 AM	Brett P	11	Hyperactivity. Therapy follow-up	Do nothing new. Continue to monitor. Return 5 months
2	8:45 AM	Amy G	42	Sinus headache. Tired	Treat with decongestants. Return visit to explore stress
3	9:00 AM	Paul J	36	Bleeding. Won't say where	Refer to surgeon. Large hemorrhoids
4	9:15 AM	Jean M	45	Pap and pelvic exam	Arrange mammogram, lipid screen, Pap test
5	9:45 AM	Acute care slot			Return 3 telephone calls to patients
6	10:00 AM	Albert K	69	Stroke; post-hospital discharge	Talk to spouse about prognosis. Arrange home health care
7	10:30 AM	Annie L	2	Routine well child check	No decisions. Remind mother about return checkup
8	10:45 AM	John A	16	Swollen right knee	Refer to orthopaedist. Cartilage tear
9	11:00 AM	Henry J	32	Rash for 3 weeks	Treat with steroid cream
10	11:15 AM	Mary J	26	Vaginal discharge	Treat with antifungal agent
11	11:30 AM	Jean B	40	Urinary infection (?)	Treat with antibiotic, discuss need for IVP
12	11:45 AM	Ruby B	58	Breast cancer follow-up	Arrange hospice care. Modify pain therapy
13	12:00 Noon	Angie M	16	Prenatal visit	Arrange return visit. Arrange for boyfriend to come next time

teraction in the office setting. This framework organizes not only the personal encounter, but also the physician's data collection and decision making.

For the first step, define in your own mind why the patient is making this visit. The reason or rea-sons may be physical, emotional, or social. The patient may have a symptom, but the *problem* may be that the patient or family group may no longer be able to cope with the symptom, with the anxiety it causes, or both. The patient is looking for answers to questions such as: What has happened? Why to me? Why has it happened? Why now? What if we did nothing? and What will happen in the future? Getting at the patient's reason for coming to the physician may be difficult (some people have hidden agendas), but usually a simple question such as, "What made you decide to come to see me today?" is effective.

Your next task is to obtain enough data, from a history and examination (and possibly laboratory tests), to enable you to make a good management decision. Note that a *diagnosis* may not necessarily figure in this process: good management decisions can be made when the diagnosis is not yet known, and perhaps never will be.

This process of assembling information is fairly complex. From the first moment of the encounter, the history and then the physical examination provide cues that trigger hypotheses in your mind. Each cue from the history influences the questions to be asked next, just as each finding in the examination may affect the next step in that examination. Usually, initial hypotheses are based on the recognition of *patterns*, helped by recall of patients with similar patterns. You assemble more data to confirm or rule out these patterns, and each new piece of data may alter the pattern that you are hypothesizing. In addition, immediate and past information about the patient's personal life, illness behavior patterns, beliefs, and family all contribute to the working diagnosis. An example is illustrated in the following case.

Case 1: Sick Child

Mrs. Andrews telephones her family physician about her 1-year-old son Johnny. He is running a fever, sniffling, and coughing, has swollen neck glands, and has had two episodes of mild diarrhea. Instead of proceeding to a detailed history of respiratory, ear, nose and throat, and gastrointestinal systems, the physician asks Mrs. Andrews if Johnny is active (i.e., playing with toys and still taking food). If Johnny is lethargic and not taking food or fluids, he may be seriously ill from viremia, dehydration, or sepsis, and this would generate further questions. If he is active, then the problem is most likely a self-limited illness, and further questions may be more focused.

Mrs. Andrews confirms that Johnny is active, playful, and eating well. The physician, who knows from experience that Mrs. Andrews is a reliable mother, decides that a likely diagnosis is a viral syndrome and the boy does not need to be seen at this point. Observation over the next day or two will be the plan, and the mother is given some simple advice on symptomatic management.

Case Discussion

The whole call probably takes about three minutes. Note that in this case the *main decision* that was made was not what is the definitive diagnosis but does the child need to be seen? And, this decision was made correctly, even when the diagnosis was not clear-cut. In fact, the child can be in the early stages of a pneumonia or other bacterial infection (complicating his virus). Among the key information used by the physician in deciding that the illness was a virus infection and that the child could be managed without an office visit were (*a*) runny nose, cough, and diarrhea (a symptom pattern characteristic of certain viral infections); (*b*) knowledge that a virus producing similar symptoms is present in the community; (*c*) the child's activity level; and (*d*) knowledge that the mother is not overly anxious and that she can be depended on to report back if new symptoms develop.

CLINICAL REASONING STYLES

In the case described above, the physician had a "working" diagnosis of viral syndrome: one illness. However, the working diagnosis may contain one or more hypotheses, which act as blueprints against which the physician tests the "fit" of the data. This fit is based on appropriate and logical relationships of the data, a reasonably simple and single explanation for the majority of the findings, and the degree to which physical and laboratory test results support the findings. In fact, working diagnoses and hypotheses can be developed using different clinical reasoning styles, each having value in different medical settings for different kinds of problems.

What reasoning style was used in the example above? Analysis of medical encounters has revealed four types of clinical reasoning, which have been called "algorithmic," "exhaustive," "heuristic," and "hypothetico-deductive." These are not mutually exclusive; a particular piece of reasoning may involve more than one of the styles. We will briefly describe these four reasoning styles to see which was used in the example.

- **Algorithmic** clinical reasoning proceeds systematically along a series of branching decision paths, using objective data to choose one pathway or another. The method is thorough, time-consuming, and costly. It is most useful for mild to moderately complex medical problems. It can be easily followed and understood by learners. The evaluation of dysuria presented in Chapter 30 uses this style; patients presenting with chest pain in the emergency room can be managed using this reasoning style.

- **Exhaustive** methods gather very comprehensive history and physical examination data and pursue intensive laboratory testing to cover all possibilities. The data are then sifted for abnormal findings. This reasoning style is often the model taught and used in medical schools for inpatient care. It is useful for some unusual and complex medical problems, but is inefficient, time-consuming, and too expensive for most problems seen in the office. Personal clinical experience and prior knowledge of the patient do not play a major role in this reasoning process. More importantly, this method may be hazardous for patients, because it poses real risks of laboratory errors and adverse effects of invasive tests. It is rarely used once a physician is in office practice. An example of its legitimate use might be the assessment of a new elderly patient with multisystem disease.
- **Heuristic (pattern recognition)** seeks to fit the patient's clinical presentation to previously learned patterns of disease using any combination of data from the history and examination. Usually, this quickly limits the working diagnosis to one or two diseases. This method is quick, efficient, and inexpensive, but it requires considerable clinical experience to be successful. It is used extensively by office-based clinicians but has the drawback that some visits may be closed prematurely, missing important problems or cues. Conditions that are often diagnosed using this method include: rashes, bursitis, otitis media, and depression.
- **Hypothetico-deductive** reasoning uses ongoing acquisition of cues to generate hypotheses, prompting further cue collection, with modification of the hypotheses according to the new cues. There is a continual feedback loop. It has been shown that, in a clinical encounter, expert clinicians generate likely diagnoses, on average, within 30 seconds and correct hypotheses within 6 minutes. This is an efficient and low-cost reasoning process, widely applied in office practice. Examples of problems effectively addressed with this reasoning style are fatigue, abdominal pain, and dizziness.

A physician may vary clinical reasoning styles, depending on the environment and patient needs, using pattern recognition with some complaints, hypothetico-deductive methods with others, and algorithmic reasoning when admitting a patient to the hospital.

In the telephone consultation quoted above (case 1), the physician first identified a pattern: that of a 1-year-old with swollen neck glands who is hot, stuffy, coughing, and having loose bowel movements. The pattern resembles that of a mild viral syndrome. Having used the heuristic process to generate a hypothesis, the doctor then uses a hypothetico-deductive style in asking questions to rule out serious disease. The answers help confirm that the pattern originally posited is correct, and this confirmation justifies the resultant management decisions.

In this example, the algorithmic style would have taken very much longer, and might have been used by a novice clinician, or when the physician did not already know the patient and his family. The exhaustive style could not have been applied at all, as it depends on a comprehensive data base, not just a history.

Study Exercise

As an exercise, we suggest you think through case 1 yourself, trying to apply only *one* reasoning style to it: the algorithmic, the heuristic, or the hypothetico-deductive. Do the same with one or two other clinical encounters you have seen in the last few days.

DIAGNOSIS

"Think horses, not zebras."

As part of the reasoning process, you use your knowledge of pathophysiology of disease and draw on the clinical experience of similar cases you have seen and managed. But in addition, your hypotheses are modified by data from the patient's personal characteristics, family, and community. In office practice, these modifiers have a very powerful influence on your diagnostic strategies. The familiar injunction about horses and zebras, given above, would be appropriate almost anywhere on earth: except when on safari in Africa. Within the United States, epidemiologic factors put certain diseases on the differential diagnosis list for certain common symptoms in some communities, which would be unthinkable in others. Examples are Rocky Mountain spotted fever in North Carolina (fever and headache); lead poisoning in the inner cities (exhaustion, muscle cramps); Lyme disease in New England (fever, rash, arthritis).

Epidemiology is the basic science of primary care and provides the background data for developing hypotheses and making diagnoses. Thus, the clinician must be aware of the incidence and prevalence of illness in the community when making diagnostic and treatment decisions. For instance, if 10% of the population in your town has depression, and HIV infection is rare in the community, then patients with weight loss and fatigue are far more likely to have depression than AIDS. The reverse might be true in some other communities.

The best-guess diagnosis of an experienced clinician is the disease the patient is most likely to have, given the clinical and epidemiologic data. Having determined your "best guess," after a focused history and examination, you must decide whether further testing is worthwhile. For instance, a 6-year-old has a sore throat; her brother has a confirmed "strep throat"; and you have heard from a local schoolteacher that "strep throat" is currently prevalent in the child's school. You may proceed to treat with penicillin rather than do a throat culture or rapid strep screen. This is because the likelihood of streptococcal sore throat in this case is so high that it justifies presuming the diagnosis and treating for it. Indeed, this clinical/epidemiologic reasoning may be more accurate than a laboratory test: the usual "rapid strep" tests may *miss* streptococci in more than 10% of cases.

Case 2: Chest Pain

A 49-year-old mechanic who was a smoker and had a family history of coronary artery disease, came to his family physician with nonanginal chest pain (i.e., relieved by antacids). With a normal blood pressure and lipid profile, the likelihood of his having coronary artery disease was calculated to be 14%, based on risk factors and population studies. Since the sensitivity and specificity of a diagnostic exercise tolerance test (ETT) were fairly low for nonanginal pain (54% and 67%, respectively), the family physician did not test for coronary artery disease—the ETT for this clinical picture was not accurate enough, and there was a low probability of disease. Eight years later, the same patient presented with atypical angina and his ECG showed some left ventricular hypertrophy and ST depression in the ventricular leads. This new clinical picture increased the likelihood of coronary artery disease (CAD) to around 59% and the sensitivity/specificity of the exercise tolerance test to 75%. The family physician now had to decide, given the high likelihood of CAD, whether to do an exercise tolerance test or even proceed directly to cardiac catheterization.

Using Probabilities to Make Decisions

Probabilities, like those quoted in case 2, are reasonably well known in the field of coronary artery disease, where there have been numerous epidemiologic studies of risk factors, outcomes of bypass surgery, effectiveness of tests, and so on. But for many other important problems in primary care, there are few data available on which to base decisions for patients. This is one of the great opportunities for research by generalists.

The probability that your patient has a particular disease or problem, and the effectiveness of tests and treatments, will alter your decision thresholds for testing and treating. These thresholds will also be affected by how accurate the tests are, individually or in combination. Excessive reliance on many diagnostic tests may do harm because of the need to follow up false-positive tests. (The probability that a perfectly normal person will have an *abnormal* result is 26% if six tests are done, since "normal" is usually defined as 2 standard deviations about the mean.)

Other factors influencing medical decisions are costs, time, and convenience for the patient as well as any potential adverse effects of the testing or therapy. Finally, and most importantly, the patient's personality, anxieties, and social situation may all bear on the clinical decision. Is this patient well known in the practice for "crying wolf" over minor symptoms? Is the patient the family breadwinner who will lose income while submitting to hospital tests? How high is the patient's need for reassurance that he is not seriously ill? How far does he trust the doctor (unaided by laboratory tests) to provide this reassurance?

"Knowledge" of the patient (as, in case 1, where the doctor knew that Johnny's mother was "reliable") is relevant data you have accumulated from past experience. Thus, when you have long-term continuity with an individual and family, you learn how they deal with stress, what they believe about their health, how they take medications, and how responsible they are. As you weigh up all these factors, you may decide to "underdiagnose" or "overdiagnose" the problem in a way that most benefits the quality of life of your patient.

CLINICAL UNCERTAINTY

In primary care practice, uncertainty "goes with the territory." The clinician is not able to make a specific diagnosis in every case or may need to wait a period of time before the diagnosis becomes clear. Often, clinicians are identifying and treating only symptoms, which may resolve spontaneously before a diagnosis is made. Diagnostic uncertainty comes from three sources: cognitive uncertainty, which is related to the physician's perception of the clinical problem; the feeling state (anxiety, usually) of the clinician; and the variability of the patient's response to communication and therapy.

In resolving uncertainty, *time* is a very powerful diagnostic tool. Its effective use requires considerable skill, however. The physician who is too anxious to await the evolution of a symptom may order unnecessary tests and have the patient return too frequently, at considerable cost. On the other hand, the physician who does not consider more than one hypothesis or who does not ask the patient to return could miss the diagnosis.

Sharing your uncertainty with colleagues and patients, educating patients about possible outcomes, and reassuring them that you will continue to observe them for diagnostic clues, are methods for managing uncertainty. The degree of uncertainty faced by the primary care clinician is greater than that faced by other providers, because of the larger numbers of undifferentiated problems and relative lack of research data. As a result, good communication between the doctor and patient is essential. Management of clinical uncertainty is one of the keys to the craft and science of primary care.

VARIETY OF CLINICAL DECISIONS IN FAMILY PRACTICE

In tertiary level, inpatient care, the vast majority of clinical decisions fall into only three categories: ordering a treatment; ordering a test; or obtaining a consultation. By contrast, in family practice, the variety of potential decisions is much richer. As well as the three just cited, these may involve

- Giving reassurance;
- Dealing with a problem other than the presenting one;
- Checking the patient again;
- Counseling the patient and/or family;
- Collecting data from other sources (family, other physicians, psychotherapists, physical therapists etc.);
- Therapeutic trial;
- Arranging community resources (home nursing, etc.).

It is this wealth of alternatives, presenting themselves in almost every encounter in family practice, that gives this specialty much of its challenge and much of its fascination. These decisions lead to specific plans that may or may not address the original "problem" the patient came with. These plans are made in the context of the potential positive actions that can occur at each visit:

- Management of the presenting problem;
- Enhancement of doctor-patient relationship;
- Modification of help-seeking behaviors;
- Management of continuing problems;
- Opportunistic health promotion;
- Enlargement of the data base on the patient.

In situations where you may be observing experienced office-based clinicians in action, try to identify their clinical reasoning styles and discuss the process with them. They will give you insight into your own thought processes and help you develop your own style of making clinical decisions.

SUGGESTED READINGS

Barrows HS, Norman GR, Neufeld VR, Feightner JW. The clinical reasoning process of randomly selected physicians in general medical practice. *Clin Invest Med* 5:49–55, 1982.

Interesting data on the reasoning process.

Helman CG: *Culture, Health and Illness*, 2nd ed. London, Wright, 1990.

A fine book on cultural aspects of medicine by a family physician.

Kassirer JP, Kopelman RI (eds): *Learning Clinical Reasoning*. Baltimore, Williams & Wilkins, 1991.

All you wanted to know abut the theoretical basis of reasoning and decision analysis, including mathematical modeling.

Marley DS, Mengel MB. Clinical decision making. In Mengel M (ed): *Principles of Clinical Practice*. New York, Plenum, 1991, pp 99–123.

Excellent review of clinical decision making for the primary care physician.

Miller WL. Routine, ceremony, or drama: an exploratory field study of the primary care clinical encounter. *J Fam Pract* 34:289–296, 1992.

Interesting personal paper on the complexities of clinical encounters and the physician patient relationship. Good references for further reading.

Mushlin AI. Uncertain decision making in primary care: causes and solutions. *Primary Care Research : Theory and Methods Conference*. U.S. Department of Health and Human Services Agency for Health Care Policy and Research. September 1991:153-166.

Good short review article.

Neighbour R: *The Inner Consultation*. Boston, MTP Press, 1987.

A fascinating book on history taking and connecting skills. Provides some unusual techniques for learning to interview patients.

Stott NCH, Davis RH. The exceptional potential in each primary care consultation. *J R Coll Gen Pract* 29:201–205, 1979.

Useful conceptual paper on what the office-based physician should do at each visit.

chapter 20

HEADACHE

Gregory Strayhorn

Headache ranks among the top ten reasons for patients' visits to family doctors and represents over ten million visits/year to doctors. Community surveys reveal that 65 to 80% of women and 57 to 75% of men report headaches during any month. The prevalence of headache declines with age, while the frequency of visits to doctors for headaches increases. Although most patients presenting with headaches have no serious underlying medical problem, headache accounts for a large number of days lost from work and for disability, numerous medical tests and prescribed medications, and, not too infrequently, hospitalization.

Most headaches are self-limited and require no medical attention. Patients primarily seek medical attention either because of severity, newness, or chronicity of their headache, or because over-the-counter analgesics have failed to relieve their symptoms. Patients may also visit a doctor when the headache appears to be related to a head injury or to other medical problems. Many patients who consult physicians seek reassurance that a brain tumor or other serious intracranial problem is not present.

Knowing that most headaches are self-limited and benign, but that occasionally very serious problems can present with headache, the family physician frequently must deal with a number of dilemmas:

- Is there an underlying cause for this patient's headache?
- Should medical tests be ordered?
- Is the patient a "drug seeker"?
- Are social and psychological issues involved?
- Will structural abnormalities be missed?
- Will biases about patients with headaches affect the care of this patient?

To deal with these questions, the family physician must develop a sympathetic, systematic, and comprehensive approach to patients with headache. The evaluation should consider both potential underlying medical problems and the patient's social, psychological, and emotional state. Continuity of care should be an important part of the diagnostic and management plans. Observance over time of headache characteristics, precipitating factors, and the patient's response to the headache and to treatment, provides useful information about possible management approaches.

The relationship between the patient and physician plays an important role in the care of patients with chronic or frequently recurring headaches. A trusting and open relationship will facilitate an understanding of the progression of the headache, the response to treatment, the development and prevention of inappropriate coping strategies, the occurrence of new symptoms, and the need for referral.

CAUSES AND CLASSIFICATION OF HEADACHES

Headaches are classified as "primary" or "secondary." Primary headaches generally are not associated with underlying diseases. Secondary headaches are symptoms of an underlying disease or physiological disruption. Table 20.1 lists the differential diagnosis of headache.

There are four basic categories of primary headaches: (*a*) migraine; (*b*) muscle contraction or tension headache; (*c*) cluster headache; and (*d*) miscellaneous headaches associated with environmental, physical, exertional, or psychological precipitants.

The pathophysiology of migraine and cluster headaches was once attributed to intracranial vas-

185

Table 20.1. Causes of Headache

Primary Headaches (no underlying disease present)	Secondary Headaches (reflecting an underlying disease)	
Migraine	Elevated intracranial pressure	Arthritis/joint disease
Common—without aura	Brain tumor	Cervical spondylosis
Classic—with aura	Brain abscess	Osteoarthritis of cervical spine
Migraine variants	Subdural hematoma	Temporomandibular joint syndrome
Ophthalmologic	Cerebral edema	Medications/chemicals
Hemiplegic	Pseudotumor cerebri	Vasodilators
Basilar	Inflammation	Nitrates/nitrites
Muscle contraction/tension headache	Meningitis/encephalitis	Monosodium glutamates
Episodic	Subdural hemorrhage	Withdrawal
Chronic	Temporal arteritis	Caffeine
Cluster headache	Fever	Opiates
Episodic paroxysmal hemicrania variant	Ophthalmologic	Alcohol
	Eye strain	Marijuana
	Acute glaucoma	Miscellaneous headaches and stimuli
	Trigeminal neuralgia	Exertion
	(tic douloureux)	Hypothermia
		Cough
		Sexual activity

cular instability; however, cerebral blood flow studies of patients with migraine headaches generally reveal no vasoconstriction or vasodilation. Now migraine and cluster headaches are thought to be caused by neurotransmitter processes associated with the 5-hydroxytryptamine or serotonergic receptor subtypes in the central nervous system. The various serotonergic receptor subtypes are found in both neuronal and vascular sites, have been associated with the numerous precipitants of migraine headaches, and include vascular, neuronal depolarization, and inflammatory components.

Muscle contraction (tension) headaches continue to be attributed to contraction of scalp, facial, and/or posterior neck muscles; however, EMG studies and blinded studies that elicit scalp tenderness have shown equivocal results. Ischemia resulting from chronically contracted muscles has been suggested to play a role in patients with chronic tension headaches. Serotonin is also implicated in the etiology of tension headaches by its depletion in platelets and impaired binding to lymphocytes and monocytes in patients with this disorder. The role of serotonin may explain why the primary headaches have overlapping precipitants and why many pharmacological agents have some efficacy for each primary headache type.

Causes of secondary headaches are listed in Table 20.1. They include extracranial and intracranial structural abnormalities, infection, inflammatory diseases, trauma, tumors, intracranial bleeding, systemic diseases, drug abuse, environmental exposures, and psychosocial factors. The evaluation of headaches is directed at excluding or establishing a secondary etiology.

EVALUATION OF PATIENTS PRESENTING WITH HEADACHE

History

The patient's history is the most important part of the headache evaluation. Components of the history should include onset, frequency, duration, quality, intensity, location, precipitating and ameliorating factors, associated symptoms, and neurological manifestations. Past and current medication use, allergies, and injuries should be determined. A change in the severity, frequency, location, and quality of headaches with or without focal neurological symptoms may portend a secondary cause.

Family history is important. Migraine headaches tend to run in families, but the relative roles of genetic and environmental factors are hard to disentangle. Learned behavior may play a role in the development and response to headache. A clue to causes of secondary headaches may come from the knowledge of family illnesses such as diabetes mellitus, thyroid diseases, hypertension, infections, and cancer.

It is important to determine social and personal stresses. Inquiries should be made about job, family, and personal relationships. Information on sleep, diet, and exercise habits is important. Consumption of alcohol and caffeinated beverages and use of tobacco products and illicit drugs should be determined. Assessment of patients' emotional and psychological states along with their coping style should be included in the history.

Physical Examination

The principal function of the physical examination is to rule out secondary causes of the patient's headache. Your initial evaluation should record vital signs and pay special attention to the head, neck, and neurological examinations. Palpate and auscultate the head and scalp to identify tenderness, irregularities in shape, and bruits over the orbits and the carotid, temporal, and occipital arteries. Assess for pain with opening and closing the mouth, malocclusions, and temporomandibular tenderness (looking for dental problems and temporomandibular joint disease). Percuss over the frontal and maxillary sinuses looking for tenderness (sinusitis). In occipital headaches, carefully evaluate the cervical spine, assessing mobility through extension, flexion, and rotation; cervical spine disease can lead to headache by causing muscle spasm or occipital nerve radiculopathy. As part of the neurological examination, pay special attention to the cranial nerves, optic nerve, and visual acuity. Muscle strength, sensory perception, and the presence of focal neurological deficits should also be determined.

Since psychological and emotional factors can precipitate or exacerbate headache, psychological assessment should be a part of your evaluation. In chronic headache, standardized psychological tests for anxiety and depression (see Chapter 36) are often indicated.

Laboratory Tests

Laboratory studies should be guided by the findings of the history and physical examination. Examples include the examination of the cerebral spinal fluid (CSF), complete blood count, and blood and CSF cultures (to rule out meningitis and to screen for other infectious causes of headache); the erythrocyte sedimentation rate for patients over 50 years with headache in the temporal region (to rule out temporal arteritis); and electrolytes, glucose, and specific endocrine studies (if a metabolic or endocrine disorder is suspected). Similarly, radiologic procedures such as computerized axial tomography and nuclear magnetic resonance should be used when the history and/or physical examination suggest the possibility of an intracranial lesion.

PRIMARY HEADACHES

Migraine

Typical features of migraine headaches include:

- Location—unilateral, temporal, frontal, temporofrontal, retro-orbital;
- Quality—pulsating, pounding, constant pain, moderate to severe intensity, occurring in distinct episodes;
- Aura—a variety of neurological symptoms that precede the headache onset in many cases;
- Onset—very rapid development of severe headache, with nausea and vomiting typically occurring within the first hour of symptom onset;
- Duration—approximately 4 to 72 hours untreated;
- Associated symptoms—nausea and/or vomiting, photophobia and/or phonophobia.

Migraine is the most frequent primary headache managed in primary care. When the headache is preceded by an aura, *classic migraine* is present. When no distinct aura precedes the headache, *common migraine* is the designation. When neurological symptoms other than headache predominate, the condition is termed *atypical migraine*. Typically, migraine begins during adolescence or early adulthood (before age 30); women are affected more often than men.

Migraine headaches occur in distinct episodes, with the frequency of attacks varying from several times a week to less than once a month. Patients may go for months to years without a headache. Pregnancy has a variable effect on migraine headaches: some women are free of migraines during pregnancy and experience more intense symptoms immediately afterwards; others have more frequent attacks during pregnancy.

Many patients with migraine feel pressure to achieve and can identify stressful situations related to work or school that precipitate headaches. Other triggers include caffeine, nitrates, foods containing tyramine, oral contraceptions, and vasodilators. Noise, light, and sometimes odors exacerbate the pain; so patients typically retreat to a dark, quiet room.

The *common migraine* has no associated aura and is the most prevalent migraine headache (up to 90%). The distribution of pain is similar to that of the classic migraine, but it may vary in location and be bilateral or diffuse. Unlike the common migraine, the *classic migraine* headache is preceded by prodromal neurological or psychological symptoms (the migraine aura). The aura that occurs 2 to 60 minutes prior to the onset of pain may be a visual, motor, or psychic disturbance. Visual auras include scotomata, flashing lights, loss of visual fields, bright colors, geometric shapes (e.g., wavy or jagged lines), altered sizes of objects, and disturbances of central vision. Sensory auras are usually in the form of paresthesias that "march" across the affected body part. Transient monoparesis or hemiparesis may represent the aura phase of migraine but may also develop during the full-blown course of the migraine. As part of the aura, patients may experience difficulty with speech, writing, thinking, and orientation, become amnesic, or display bizarre behavior.

Autonomic dysfunction may accompany a migraine headache. Gastrointestinal tract dysfunction (gastric stasis, vomiting, or diarrhea) may lead to poor absorption and reduce oral medication effectiveness. Patients may experience skin pallor, periorbital discoloration and edema, conjunctival hemorrhage, and frank ecchymoses. Cardiovascular responses vary; they include hypertension, bradycardia with accompanying hypotension, and syncope. Some patients experience a brisk diuresis following a migraine; when combined with vomiting, this may lead to dehydration. Finally, sighing and hyperventilation may cause respiratory alkalosis, leading to peripheral and facial paresthesias and carpopedal spasm.

Variants of migraine are conditions that have neurological or autonomic features as the main symptoms. Such patients sometimes never report headache, although typically they will report migraine-type headaches sometime in the past or mild to severe headaches associated with their other symptoms. Monocular visual loss that is usually ipsilateral to the headache varies from blurred vision to complete transient blindness that lasts several minutes to hours. In rare cases, blindness may be permanent. Ophthalmologic migraine may involve the third, fourth, and sixth cranial nerve, causing ptosis, mydriasis, and ocular muscle dysfunction; symptoms may last for days and (rarely) up to one month. Basilar migraines can present as vertigo, ataxia, bilateral visual disturbance, dysarthria, persistent vomiting, tinnitus, syncopal or drop attacks, and/or paresthesias of the extremities. Finally, hemiplegic migraine may accompany the aura or the full-blown headache and presents with ipsilateral or contralateral weakness. This type of migraine may run in families.

TREATMENT

The treatment of migraine headaches (Table 20.2) is divided into management of the acute attack and prophylaxis to prevent recurrent headaches. Naproxen, aspirin, ergotamine, or Midrin (a combination of isometheptene mucate, acetaminophen, and dicloralphenazone) may be effective during the aura phase or at the onset of the migraine headache and may prevent the progression to a severe and incapacitating headache. Once the full-blown headache develops, these agents are less effective. Dihydroergotamine (DHE), a metabolite of ergotamine, administered parenterally with a phenothiazine antiemetic is very effective in aborting the acute attack. Narcotic analgesics should be used if the above modalities are not affective. Parental analgesics such as meperidine with an antiemetic are preferred over oral analgesics that may be poorly absorbed during the acute attack. Indiscriminate use of narcotic analgesics is frowned upon, however, due to the high potential of abuse.

In patients with frequent headaches, prevention should be your primary goal. Removal of environmental precipitants can be very effective. Psychotherapy to assist patients with developing effective coping strategies is important. In some patients, regular use of aspirin or another nonsteroidal antiinflammatory drug may help prevent headaches. β-Blockers (propranolol is the most widely used) have proven effective for migraine prophylaxis; calcium-channel blockers have not. Antidepressants can also help; amitriptyline is the most widely used, and fluoxetine (Prozac) is gaining prominence. For more refractory migraine sufferers, cyproheptadine and methysergide may be considered. Prolonged use of methysergide can cause retroperitoneal fibrosis; so the drug must be used with caution and limited to 4 to 5 months. Methysergide is contraindicated in patients with severe hypertension,

Table 20.2. Treatment of Headaches

Migraine	Tension/Muscle Contraction	Cluster
Acute		
Aura phase	Aspirin	Inhaled O_2
Naproxin, aspirin	NSAIDs	DHE/antiemetic
Midrin	Acetaminophen	Ergotamine
Ergotamine	Fiorinal	Parental narcotics/antiemetic
Full-blown headache	Midrin	Indomethacin (for episodic paroxys-
Dihydroergotamine (DHE) +	Short course of oral narcotic anal-	mal hemicrania)
phenothiazine antiemetic	gesics	
Torodol + antiemetic	Physical modalities	
Meperidine + antiemetic	Heat, massage, local anesthetic	
	sprays, injection of trigger	
	points, correction of posture	
Preventive		
Removal of environmental	Tricyclic antidepressants	Avoid alcohol and environmental
precipitants	β-Blockers	precipitants
Psychotherapy/biofeedback	NSAIDs	Calcium channel blockers (verapamil)
Nonsteroidal antiinflammatory	Combination of the above	Lithium carbonate
drugs (NSAIDs)	Psychotherapy/biofeedback	Ergotamine in combination with one
β-Blockers (propranolol, Tenormin)	Hospitalization for detoxification of	of the above
	chronic analgesic use and initia-	Methysergide
Antidepressants (amitriptyline,	tion of appropriate therapy	Prednisone
Prozac)		
Avoid narcotic analgesics		
Refractory migraines		
Cyprohetadine		
Methysergide		
Prednisone		

coronary artery and peripheral vascular disease, and cerebral vascular disease. Calcium-channel blockers have not proved effective prophylactic medications for migraine. Sumatriptan, a new 5-hydroxytryptamine-receptor agonist, is under investigation and shows promise for aborting acute migraines, with few side effects.

Cluster Headaches

Typical features of cluster headaches include:

- Location—unilateral and orbital.
- Quality—severe, intense burning, piercing, or stabbing; nonthrobbing.
- Associated symptoms—lacrimation, rhinorrhea, miosis, ptosis, nasal congestion, red eyes, flushed cheeks, bradycardia.
- Frequency—occur in clusters with as many as four to six attacks per day over 2 to 12 weeks. Recurrence often happens at about the same time annually.
- Onset and duration—attacks generally start 2 to 3 hours into sleep and last 30 to 60 minutes.

Cluster headaches are the most severe form of primary headaches. They affect men more frequently than women. Onset is typically between the ages of 20 and 30. The symptoms are well characterized and lead to easy diagnosis.

The symptoms of cluster headaches are consistent with a sudden release of histamine into the bloodstream. Thus, cluster headaches have been referred to as "histamine headaches." However, antihistamines are ineffective in treating this form of headache.

TREATMENT

Treatment of the acute headache (Table 20.2) includes parenteral DHE, ergotamine, narcotic analgesics, and inhaled oxygen, but all may be ineffective. Focus should be on prophylaxis. Prophylactic ergotamine, cyproheptadine, calcium-channel blockers, and lithium carbonate are the first-line agents. Ergotamine in combination with lithium or a calcium-channel blocker may prove effective for prophylaxis. Methysergide can be considered if less benign drugs are ineffective, but it becomes less effective as the patient gets older. Finally, a 10- to 14- day course of prednisone may aid patients who are unresponsive to other regimens.

Cluster headache sufferers are sensitive to alcohol, which should be avoided. A variant of cluster headache, episodic paroxysmal hemicrania, produces up to thirty headaches per day and responds to moderately high doses of indomethacin.

Tension or Muscle Contraction Headache

Typical features of tension or muscle contraction headaches include:

- Location—generally localized to the muscles of the head: the periorbital, temporal, and occipital regions. Thus, tension headaches are typically described as "like a hatband" in distribution. Headaches are typically bilateral and symmetric, but they may be unilateral or localized generally to the occipital and frontal regions.
- Quality—dull, aching, tightness or constricting band around head, tender or sore scalp. The headache typically is mild at first and worsens as the day goes on.
- Frequency—daily or during times of stress.
- Duration—hours to daily. Patients who have a constant headache for days or weeks usually have tension headache (but serious intracranial disease should be considered in the differential diagnosis).
- Aura—none.
- Associated symptoms—nausea and vomiting are rare and if present tend to occur after several hours, when the headache has built up in severity.

Muscle contraction headaches are extremely common. Typically, they begin in early adulthood. They occur more frequently in women than in men, are frequently associated with stressful psychosocial factors, and tend to occur in families. The prevalence of the muscle contraction headache is probably underestimated because many patients treat themselves with over-the-counter analgesics without physician involvement. The muscle contraction headache may be categorized as acute when it occurs on an occasional basis or chronic when patients have no or infrequent pain-free periods.

Unlike migraines, which are prone to occur after a stressful event, the muscle contraction headache tends to begin and intensify during the event. Such patients are frequently anxious and often have multiple unresolved conflicts related to work, personal relationships, and/or family. Patients may frequently be unaware of the conflicts or repress their feelings. Many are depressed.

The pain is described as dull, aching, constant, and nonthrobbing. There is no associated aura or autonomic, or gastrointestinal symptoms. Patients may be generally anxious and experience fatigue and lightheadedness during the headache. The headache usually occurs in the occipital and frontal regions and is bilateral or may be generalized in a band-like distribution around the entire head. Frequently the neck muscles and trapezius may be contracted and tender. Palpable muscle spasm and fibrositic nodules may be apparent. The scalp may be tender when touched and when the hair is combed. Sleep is not affected.

TREATMENT

Most acute muscle contraction headaches only require aspirin, acetaminophen, or a nonsteroidal antiinflammatory drug. More severe headaches may respond to a combination of analgesic with caffeine and the barbiturate butalbital (e.g., Fiorinal) or to Midrin. Rarely, a short course of codeine or propoxyphene is needed, but these should be avoided for chronic treatment, because of their propensity to cause physical and psychological dependency and abuse. Physical modalities such as warm compresses to the neck and forehead or a warm shower, massage, ice, local anesthetic sprays and injection of "trigger points," and the correction of standing, setting, and supine posture may be helpful. Table 20.2 outlines treatment approaches to tension headache.

For patients with frequent or chronic muscle contraction headaches, the goal is to reduce headache severity and to prevent headache onset. Medications have a relatively minor role here. Since many patients have unresolved psychological and emotional conflicts, psychotherapy and counseling should be part of the treatment plan. Regular exercise is also helpful. Biofeedback is more effective than placebo in some patients, but it is very expensive and may not be covered by some insurance. A combination of approaches should be used that includes appropriate drug therapy, insight counseling, short- or long-term psychotherapy, and behavioral modification in an atmosphere that is sympathetic and supportive.

If medications are needed, the tricyclic antidepressants, β-blockers, and nonsteroidal antiinflammatory drugs separately or (rarely) in combination are effective for most patients. The primary effect of the antidepressants may be the alleviation of depression and, secondarily, the headache. Muscle relaxants such as carisoprodol or cyclobenzaprine also may be useful.

Patients with chronic muscle contraction headaches may become refractory to the daily use of analgesics and gradually increase the amount used, causing a rebound phenomenon—the more analgesics the worse the headache. Patients will need detoxification before effective preventive therapy is possible. Because of patients' reluctance to discontinue their analgesics, hospitalization may be necessary for withdrawal and the institution of appropriate prophylactic medication and other therapeutic modalities.

SECONDARY HEADACHES

Secondary headaches have specific causes, many that if treated appropriately, will alleviate the headache. When headache symptoms don't follow the typical pattern of primary headaches, the physician should suspect and search for a secondary cause. Generally, a careful history and physical examination will identify clues to secondary causes of headache. These include:

- A new symptom or change in the usual symptom pattern, especially in children and adolescents;
- New symptoms in patients over 40;
- Symptoms not consistant with those of primary headaches;
- Sudden onset of a severe headache for the first time;
- Presence of symptoms that suggest infection and/or neurological disease;
- Recent history of trauma to the head or neck;
- Use of a drug that is known to cause headaches (caffeine is a common culprit);
- A history of alcohol or drug abuse.

Table 20.1 lists some of the most common causes of secondary headaches with the usual presenting complaints. Findings from the history and physical examination should be the sole guide of the diagnostic evaluation.

HEADACHES IN CHILDREN AND ADOLESCENTS

Headaches are unusual in preadolescent children. They display an equal distribution between boys and girls until about age ten when the prevalence in girls increases over boys. Headache prevalence increases with age. Children with primary headaches tend to have family members with headaches.

Causes of headaches in children are generally the same as in adults: migraine, muscle contraction, and intra/extracranial causes. Sinusitis should always be considered in children with facial pain, with or without fever. The usual causes of sinusitis are infectious, allergic, irritant, or vasomotor. Primary headaches are frequently associated with psychosocial stressors related to home and/or school. These issues should always be explored when evaluating children and adolescents.

Complex migraine and migraine variants are seen in children and adolescents. Hemiplegic and ophthalmoplegic migraines are primarily seen in adolescents. Patients have focal neurological findings that precede, accompany, or follow headaches. Such findings may include hemiparesis or (in ophthalmoplegic migraine) pain localized to the orbit, with partial or complete palsy of the third cranial nerve. Other variants include confusional states with aphasia, nausea, and vomiting. Symptoms localized to the basilar artery are more common in children and include occipital headaches, visual disturbance, ataxia, vertigo and loss of consciousness. When these symptoms first occur, it is important to rule out underlying neurological disorders (e.g., a brain tumor or an intracranial vascular malformation) by undertaking a thorough neurological assessment in consultation with a pediatric neurologist.

A special form of headache is the *somatiform pain disorder*. It is usually associated with dysfunctional coping and depression. These children or adolescents have a fixation on pain without objective physical findings. The headache is vague, frequent, and in many instances continuous. The child may withdraw from normal social activities. This form of headache is most frequently found in dysfunctional families, and therapy should involve the family.

The evaluation of children and adolescents with headaches is similar to that of adults and should be guided by the presenting complaints, symptoms, and the physical examination. Environmental triggers, seasonal variation, exercise, lack of rest, foods, and toxic exposures should be sought. An assessment of family function and adjustment to the social and school environment is paramount.

Management of headaches in children and adolescents requires equal attention to behavioral and psychological approaches and judicious use of medications. Therapy should be family centered, with special attention paid to the development of appropriate coping skills for the patient and family. Once underlying pathological causes of headaches have been ruled out, the child should be approached in a calm, sympathetic, and matter-of-fact manner. Undue attention to the headache (e.g., special privileges) should be avoided. Maintenance of normal daily routines should be encouraged, including regular school attendance and completion of chores. When dealing with their own pain, parents should model this behavior. Severe headaches should be treated with the appropriate medications and rest, with the expectation that normal activities will resume after the headache is controlled.

As in adults, drug therapy of childhood and adolescent headaches involves treating the acute headache and prevention of recurring headaches. Although dependence on "pills" should be avoided, medication in the form of aspirin (in older children), acetaminophen, and ibuprofen should be administered in the early stages of the headache. Use of ergotamines to abort migraine headaches is useful in adolescents, but their effectiveness in children is less apparent. Antiemetics in suppository form should be considered for severe and intractable vomiting; however, brief vomiting may be associated with resolution of the headache.

Prophylactic use of β-blockers is effective in adolescents but has limited or no effectiveness in children. Tricylic antidepressants have not been extensively studied in childhood or adolescents, but they may be effective in adolescents who are depressed. Cyproheptadine and methysergide can be considered in the older adolescent who has frequent migraine headaches that are refractory to other medications. Due to their potential side effects, use should be limited and caution exercised.

Psychological management in the form of biofeedback, cognitive restructuring, and group teaching has proven effective in some settings. A group in Canada has devised a self-help program for children that includes an age-appropriate manual and "minimal therapist contact" by telephone. Stress reduction approaches are very important for muscle contraction headache. Children and adolescents with the somatoform pain disorder and their families will require both long-term family and individual therapy.

CONCLUSIONS

The evaluation and management of patients with headaches requires a comprehensive approach that is guided by the history and physical findings and an appreciation of patients' psychological and social background and their mode of coping with stress situations. The evaluation, diagnosis, and plan of treatment should be guided by information gleaned from this approach. The family physician should strive to establish a supportive and empathetic relationship with the patient. For primary headaches, treatment should focus on minimizing known psychological and environmental precipitants and early ablation of an established headache. A combination of reassurance, education, appropriate medication, and supportive counseling that helps patients develop effective coping strategies will help most primary headache sufferers. If the history and physical findings suggest a secondary headache, the evaluation and management should focus on determining etiology and treatment of the specific cause of the headache.

SUGGESTED READINGS

Diamond S: Headache. *Med Clin North Am* 75(3), 1991.

   An overview of the epidemiology, diagnosis, and management of headaches.

Elkind AH: Muscle contraction headache. Overview and update of a common affliction. *Postgrad Med* 81(8):203–217, 1987.

McGrath PJ, Humphreys P: Recurrent headaches in children and adolescents: diagnosis and treatment. *Pediatrician* 16:71–77, 1989.

An excellent overview of the evaluation, diagnosis, and managment of headache in children. Gives practical guideline for parent's approach to children with headaches.

Mathew NT: Headaches. *Neurol Clin* 8(4), 1990.

Raskin NH: Modern pharmacotherapy of migraine. *Neurol Clin* 8(4), Philadelphia, WB Saunders, 1990, pp 857–865.

An excellent discussion of treating the acute migraine with dihdroergotamine (DHE).

Samuels MA: The splitting headache: listen carefully. *Emerg Med* 23:32–36, 1991.

A succinct expose on the evaluation and treatment of primary headaches that questions the vasospasm/vasodilatation mechanism of migraine headaches.

chapter 21

CHEST PAIN

Joseph R. Shackelford

Chest pain is a common and important symptom. It often does not present as described in textbooks. Chest pain is an unnerving symptom that generally raises one major question in the mind of the patient: Could it be my heart? This fear of death or serious disability, whether openly expressed or not, holds true in our culture for all economic and age groups. Chest pain, therefore, produces considerable anxiety in both patient and physician.

This chapter presents an overview of chest pain as commonly seen in the family physician's office. It will review the causes of chest pain and then discuss the approach to patients presenting with this common symptom.

CAUSES OF CHEST PAIN

Any system of the body may produce chest pain. Common causes of this symptom are listed in Table 21.1. Knowledge of the common and atypical presentations of the major causes of chest pain will help the clinician evaluate each patient efficiently. In most cases, a thorough history, with attention to epidemiologic factors such as age and sex, and a physical examination that focuses on vital signs and the chest will usually yield the correct diagnosis and provide the key to reassurance and effective management of the patient.

Anatomically, chest pain can be caused by problems in the following areas: (*a*) the heart and great vessels, (*b*) the lungs and pleura, (*c*) the musculoskeletal system (including the chest, neck, and back), (*d*) the skin and soft tissues (including breasts), (*e*) the gastrointestinal system, and (*f*) deep thoracic structures.

Heart and Great Vessels

Angina pectoris is anterior chest pain caused by reversible coronary artery insufficiency. It occurs when part of the myocardial muscle is not receiving sufficient oxygen. The pain of angina pectoris is usually precordial, and it may radiate to the neck, jaws, face, and either or both arms. The pain is often described as pressure, heaviness, or squeezing, and the patient sometimes clenches a fist to demonstrate the feeling. Rarely is it burning, never sharp or stabbing. Classical angina is brought on by exercise or emotional stress; variant (Prinzmetal) angina is caused by coronary artery spasm and usually occurs at rest. Classical angina is relieved by physical or emotional rest and responds promptly to sublingual nitroglycerin.

Angina is usually associated with coronary artery atherosclerosis but (rarely) may occur in its absence as a result of hypertrophic cardiomyopathy. Physical findings in angina pectoris are usually normal, but rarely a transient gallop rhythm, paradoxical splitting of the second heart sound or a systolic murmur may be found.

A resting electrocardiogram (ECG) is usually obtained when angina pectoris or myocardial infarction is suspected. Since most patients with angina pectoris are not having pain during an office visit, the office ECG is rarely diagnostic. Such resting ECGs are normal in angina pectoris about half of the time; the remainder show signs of old myocardial damage. The ideal is to obtain an ECG when chest pain is present or when oxygen demands are high, looking for signs of ischemia. This is the basis for the exercise stress test, which uses a bicycle ergometer or mechanical treadmill for graded exercise while an ECG is continuously monitored. The results of the exercise stress test may guide further intervention.

Acute myocardial infarction (MI) results when ischemia persists long enough to permanently damage heart muscle. The pain of MI is similar to that of angina pectoris, only more severe, unremitting

Table 21.1. Causes of Chest Pain

Very common
Angina pectoris
Costochondritis
Contusion of the chest
Dyspepsia (indigestion)
Esophageal spasm
Fracture of rib, clavicle, or shoulder
Gas entrapment syndrome
Hiatal hernia
Intercostal myalgia secondary to viral syndrome
Mastalgia from fibrocystic disease, infection, estrogenic
    hormone medication, pregnancy, or lactation
Myofascial syndromes
Psychogenic chest pain

Common
Acute myocardial infarction
Acute pneumothorax
Acute pleuritis
Axillary adenitis
Herpes zoster or herpes zoster prodrome
Intervertebral disc disease
Peptic esophagitis
Pulmonary embolus

Unusual
Acute pericarditis
Aortic dissection
Cardiac contusion
Expanding thoracic aneurysm
Mitral valve prolapse
Referred pain from abdominal sources
Sternoclavicular arthritis
Subluxed costal cartilage

and generally accompanied by systemic signs such as fatigue, diaphoresis, nausea and/or shortness of breath. In addition, an acute MI may cause bradycardia, tachycardia, hypotension, or any of several dysrhythmias.

The infarction (myocardial necrosis) is completed within 3 to 6 hours of the onset of pain. Therefore, early diagnosis is urgent, since rapid intervention can reduce or reverse ischemic damage. An ECG taken during chest pain will accurately diagnose MI 85% of the time (i.e., the false-negative rate is 15%). Old ECGs for comparison and serial ECGs during the suspected infarction are very helpful for diagnosis. The MB fraction of the creatinine phosphokinase (CPK) enzyme is elevated within 3 hours of the onset of pain and peaks within 12 hours. The MB fraction may be elevated in some myocardial infarctions even when the total CPK remains normal. The level of the CPK-MB permits some assessment of the degree of damage to the myocardium. Eval-

uation of risk factors is especially pertinent in angina pectoris and myocardial infarction because modification can slow or stop disease progression.

Acute pericarditis causes diffuse anterior chest pain, which is usually more intense with inspiration or recumbency. Occasionally the pain is felt mostly in the left trapezius ridge. The most characteristic aspect of pericarditis is that the pain is partially relieved when the patient sits up and leans forward. Acute pericarditis has many causes but most commonly results from a viral infection and is accompanied by a low-grade fever and tachycardia. In most cases, a pericardial friction rub can be heard if listened for repeatedly. ECG changes are usually diagnostic, demonstrating diffuse ST elevation in all leads except AVR, Vl, and/or V4.

Pericarditis can occur 4 to 7 days after a myocardial infarction, particularly a large or transmural infarction. It produces the usual pain and friction rub and is self-limited, but it may be confused with continuing or recurrent ischemic pain. When it occurs some weeks after a myocardial infarction, it is known as Dressler's syndrome and is thought to be autoimmune or viral. The same syndrome may occur 2 to 4 weeks after any operation in which the pericardium was incised.

Mitral valve prolapse may cause sharp precordial pain that is not related to exercise. It is seen predominantly in young females, particularly those who are thin and have a long arm span. Characteristically a "click" and late systolic murmur are present over the mitral valve area. An echocardiogram is necessary to confirm the diagnosis.

Aortic dissection causes severe "tearing" pain that is often posterior in the chest. Typically, the patient has a history of hypertension. Diagnostic clues include reduction, occlusion, or fluctuation of the brachial or carotid pulses and widening of the aorta on chest X-ray.

Cardiac contusion is caused by trauma and can occur during automobile accidents (when the chest hits the steering wheel), contact sports (e.g., football), and fistfights. It causes severe chest pain that is usually masked by musculoskeletal pain. An ECG demonstrates myocardial injury (ST elevation).

Lungs and Pleura

Pleuritis causes chest pain limited to the area in which the pleura is inflamed. It may occur as a result of primary infection, trauma, neoplasm, or from spread of one of these processes from the underlying lung. Pleuritis is usually described as a sharp pain made worse by respiratory or thoracic movements (this is "pleuritic" chest pain). It may cause a feeling of shortness of breath because thoracic movement is restricted by pain.

Primary infection of the pleura (pleurisy) is usually caused by a virus. It may occur in epidemic outbreaks, then labeled "epidemic pleuritis" or Bornholm's disease. This may last several days but carries a benign prognosis. Extension of pneumonia, especially if it begins peripherally (e.g., that caused by *streptococcus pneumoniae*), can cause pleuritis.

Acute pneumothorax can cause chest pain and dyspnea varying from mild to severe, depending primarily on how much of the lung is collapsed. Acute pneumothorax usually occurs in people 20 to 30 years old and favors males 5:1. It often recurs. Most people who have spontaneous pneumothorax are tall and slim. Smoking is a risk factor. Chest x-ray films are generally diagnostic (*if* the physician looks carefully for a pneumothorax).

Pulmonary embolus (PE) can masquerade as nearly any process that causes chest pain. PE may produce only dyspnea, but more typically it is accompanied by mild to severe chest pain, which varies in character from substernal to pleuritic. Pulmonary embolus is usually the result of deep vein thrombosis (DVT) which is often, unfortunately, "silent." Risk factors are a prior pulmonary embolus, a recent surgical operation (or obstetric delivery), prolonged immobilization, marked obesity, thrombophlebitis, and use of exogenous estrogen.

Pulmonary embolus must always be considered in the differential diagnosis of acute chest pain because it is potentially lethal and is often a difficult diagnosis. Beyond the clinical history, your best diagnostic clue is a reduced arterial PO_2. ECG and chest x-ray films are occasionally helpful but are usually normal or nonspecific. A ventilation-perfusion lung scan that is highly suggestive, in the appropriate clinical setting, can be considered diagnostic. Pulmonary angiography is the "gold standard." Early ambulation after injury, illness, or surgical operation is the best prevention. A high index of suspicion must be maintained when risk factors are present.

Musculoskeletal

Contusion of the chest wall, a fracture of ribs, clavicle, or vertebrae; costochondritis; sternoclavicular or shoulder arthritis; or bursitis can all cause chest pain. The clinical history, plus local tenderness on examination, usually provide the most valuable diagnostic data. Intervertebral disc disease or facet joint disease of the cervical or thoracic spine may cause radicular chest pain. Radicular chest pain from cervical facet joints can often be reproduced by pressure over the involved joint(s).

Costochondritis is a very common cause of chest pain. It consists of a mild inflammatory arthritis of the joints between the sternum and selected ribs. Typically, several joints are affected. The patient feels chest pain that is often worse on movement (or, in some cases, respiration). Physical examination is diagnostic; firm pressure on the affected costochondral junctions duplicates the patient's pain. Costochondritis typically lasts between 3 and 6 weeks. Nonsteroidal antiinflammatory drugs such as aspirin, ibuprofen, or naproxen generally provide significant relief.

Skin and Soft Tissue

Inflammation or irritation of soft tissues often presents as "chest pain." Various skin cysts, axillary adenitis, mastalgia from mastitis, fibrocystic disease, and breast abscess are all potential diagnoses. For this reason, a careful examination of the neck, breasts, axilla, and superficial chest will often identify the cause of atypical chest pain.

Herpes zoster is particularly difficult to diagnose when it presents as radicular chest pain. For example, the prodrome of herpes zoster affecting a lower cervical nerve root will cause pain in the chest and the left arm. Zoster pain is severe and precedes the rash by 3 or 4 days. Consequently, more than one patient has been treated to "rule out MI," only to have the characteristic vesicular rash develop later.

Gastrointestinal Disease

Esophageal spasm, peptic esophagitis, hiatal hernia, esophageal rupture, peptic ulcer, gastritis, and pancreatitis may all cause chest pain that can mimic cardiac pain. Gastrointestinal pain is often related to timing or content of meals and is relieved by eructation or antacid medication. It is often confusing for the clinician that the pain of esophageal spasm is relieved by sublingual nitroglycerin, as is angina pectoris.

Ruptured abdominal viscus (peptic ulcer) or diaphragmatic inflammation may cause chest pain.

Another cause is entrapped gas in the splenic flexure of the colon (splenic flexure syndrome).

Other Causes

Chest pain may be caused by mediastinal structures by enlargement (neoplasm), inflammation, or perforation. Mediastinal pain is generally continuous and may vary during respiration. History and chest x-ray films are the most effective diagnostic screening tools.

Anxiety itself can be the primary problem when the complaint is chest pain. When patients are highly anxious, mild musculoskeletal or gastrointestinal symptoms that many people would consider normal can be interpreted as severe.

APPROACH TO THE PATIENT WITH CHEST PAIN

Initial Presentation

Because speed of treatment is a major determinant of survival in myocardial infarction, very rapid access to medical care is crucial for patients with chest pain. In metropolitan areas where rescue services and heartwatch programs have been developed, data show that very early intervention in cardiac chest pain dramatically improves survival. If patients with chest pain do not have a regular physician or if their regular doctor is not available, they often present to the emergency department.

TELEPHONE MANAGEMENT

Many patients with chest pain telephone their own physician's office, home, or answering service. They want to talk to the doctor for reassurance and advice. Telephone calls about chest pain put all the family physician's telephone management skills on trial. The actual reason for a call (stress, for example) may differ radically from the initial stated reason of "chest pain." We have all seen or heard of the patient who has chest pain on the anniversary of "Uncle Bill's" heart attack.

Salient points of the history and risk factors can be obtained briefly on the telephone. Most chest pain patients eventually see the doctor; the goal of telephone encounters is not to make a specific diagnosis but to determine a management plan (i.e., how urgently the patient should be seen).

Since telephone calls to the doctor first go through a receptionist and then a nurse, it is important to have clearly established protocols for handling these patients. For example, a family physician could define a chest pain call that should be put through immediately as "Any continuous chest pain not resulting from trauma and lasting more than 10 minutes in a person over 35 years of age." Also, patients should be asked about their sense of urgency by the office staff, and this should be passed on to the physician. After office hours, the physician may be contacted directly or through an answering service as in the following example of a call at 9 PM on a Saturday night.

Case 1: Telephone Call

Ms. Mary D., age 27, calls because of midsternal chest pain and concern about heart disease. She describes the pain as dull, becoming sharp when she moves her arms or takes a deep breath. She has lost about 25 pounds in the last year as a result of a diet and exercise program. On further questioning, she says that her father-in-law had a stroke 4 weeks ago and an aunt died of lung cancer 6 months ago. Her father has untreated hypertension.

Case Discussion

In making decisions during this telephone encounter, the physician recognizes the low probability of serious heart or lung disease in a young woman. Aggravation of the pain by arm movement suggests that the cause is probably musculoskeletal. A few additional questions confirm that the patient does not have any systemic symptoms and, other than the pain, feels fine.

Having made a tentative diagnosis of musculoskeletal chest pain, the physician concludes that the most urgent issue for this caller is anxiety about the meaning of her symptom, given a background of recent family health problems. The physician, therefore, counsels Ms. D. on the phone, arranges early follow-up in the office, but does not see the patient that night.

History

When obtaining a history in patients with chest pain, first ask about the *pain*. Since the sensation of pain means different things to different people, it is best to have the patient describe the pain in her or his own words. Pain may be described as aching, burning, throbbing, stabbing or knifelike, pinching, squeezing, or heavy.

Bonica identifies three categories of chest pain: visceral, deep somatic, and referred(1). *Visceral (central) chest pain* is unfocused, not easily localized, dull, aching, and diffuse. It is often associated with nausea, vomiting, and autonomic disturbances such as sweating, hypotension, and bradycardia. When visceral pain is present, the myocardium, trachea and bronchi, pericardium, pulmonary arteries, or aorta are involved, in approximately that order of frequency. *Deep somatic chest pain* is described as dull and aching, is quite well localized, and is often referred to the chest wall from deeper structures. It is associated with reflex muscle activity and sympathetic hyperactivity. This pain comes from a pleural, orthopaedic, or neurological source within the chest. *Referred pain* is described as is poorly localized, and is associated with muscle pain and tenderness.

Other characteristics of the pain that should be discerned are its location, intensity, variation over time, and associated symptoms. The pain may be located anywhere in the chest and may radiate to the upper extremities, neck, jaws, face, abdomen, or elsewhere in the chest. Intensity is often rated on a scale of 1 to 10. Precipitating events, such as exercise, movement of the trunk or arms, or emotional stress, and relieving measures such as a change in position, eructation, or medication, should be noted. Associated symptoms, such as shortness of breath, cough, and nausea, should be identified.

Next, ask about risk factors such as smoking (a risk factor for angina pectoris, myocardial infarction, spontaneous pneumothorax, and peptic ulcer) and precipitants such as trauma. Advanced age and male gender are risk factors for angina pectoris and myocardial infarction, as are diabetes mellitus, obesity, hypertension, sedentary lifestyle and increased blood cholesterol. Recent surgical operation, prolonged immobilization, obesity, varicose veins and estrogen use may all increase the risk of pulmonary embolus.

Physical Examination

The examination should be guided by the history. Certainly, the heart, lungs, and chest wall should be examined carefully in any patient with chest pain. In most cases, the abdomen and neck should be examined as well. The following case illustrates the importance of an adequate examination in the clinical evaluation of chest pain.

Case 2: Missed Diagnosis

A 22-year-old basketball player falls in a game and develops left anterior chest pain. He is brought to the emergency room and seen by a resident. The patient has some difficulty in getting his breath. Examination of the heart and lungs is normal. There is some tenderness of the muscles over the upper chest wall, but this is not proportionate to his severe pain.

An electrocardiogram, chest x-ray, and full admission panel are obtained, all normal. At that point, the attending physician evaluates the patient and, on examining the neck, reproduces the patient's pain with palpation over the left 5th and 6th cervical facet joints, extension of the neck, and turning the head.

Case Discussion

This is referred chest pain. The basketball player "cricked" his neck in the game. The resident, worried about serious diseases, pulled the diagnostic trigger too early, without a careful examination. He also did not pay enough attention to the patient's age and the circumstances of the onset of pain, to assess the probabilities of diagnosis in a young adult.

Office Laboratory

Most family physicians have office equipment that will aid in diagnosing and providing emergency treatment for chest pain. The ECG is helpful in suspected angina pectoris, myocardial infarction, pericarditis, or pulmonary embolus. A chest x-ray can give useful information in rib, shoulder, clavicle, and vertebral fracture or spinal disease but not in soft tissue pain. The chest x-ray is often diagnostic in pneumothorax and pneumonia and may give valuable information about mediastinal structures or suspected pulmonary embolus. Simple laboratory tests such as the CBC and stool guaiac can provide clues to infection and gastrointestinal bleeding, which may be associated with problems that can cause chest pain.

Spirograms and pulse oximeters give clues to respiratory and vascular problems that may bear on chest pain. More family physicians are now doing exercise stress testing in the evaluation of chest pain and/or coronary artery reserve.

When managing chest pain patients, it is important for physicians and ancillary office personnel to know the location and working order of resuscitative equipment. This, as well as knowledge of basic cardiopulmonary resuscitation (CPR), should be evaluated on a regular schedule.

Communicating with the Patient

Since chest pain induces so much anxiety, the physician must explain the diagnosis or potential diagnoses to the patient, whether on the telephone or in person. Medical jargon and technical words or initials must be avoided or explained carefully. The physician must, in a clear and nondescending manner, be sure that the patient *truly* understands the issues. While the patient is in the office, simple pictures can be drawn for explanation or handouts can be used. In addition, the physician should have access to anatomical models to explain the situation to the patient.

CONCLUSIONS

In this brief introduction to chest pain, no effort has been made to explore the sophisticated, high technology tools that are now part of the diagnostic armamentarium. The usefulness of such tests as Holter monitoring, myocardial imaging, and cardiac catheterization is limited to relatively few primary care patients with chest pain, since most do not have life-threatening disease. Many sophisticated techniques are not readily available to the family doctor who is charged with the care of the inner city, suburban, small town, and rural populations. The time-honored methods of history, physical examination, and a few office tools (especially ECG, chest x-ray, and treadmill test) will usually suffice to diagnose most cases of chest pain.

REFERENCES

1. Bonica JJ, Hammermeister KE, Pope JE, Sola AE. Section C: pain in the chest. In Bonica JJ (ed): *The Management of Pain*, Vol. 2. Philadelphia, Lea & Febiger, 1990, pp 959–1045.

SUGGESTED READINGS

Evans CH, Karunaratne HB: Exercise stress testing for the family physician: Part 1. Performing the test. *Am Fam Physician* 45:121–132, 1992.

Presents the practical aspects of performing exercise stress testing in the family physician's office. Includes discussion of equipment, indications, hazards, and protocols.

Guerci AD, Weisfeldt ML: Clinical management of acute myocardial infarction. *Hosp Pract* 24:67–80, 1989.

Presents recommended management of myocardial infarction in the CCU, based on studies up to this time. Covers variations relating to age of patient, location of infarct, and ECG findings.

Mark DB, Shaw L, Harrell FE, et al.: Prognostic value of a treadmill exercise score in outpatients with suspected coronary artery disease. *N Engl J Med* 325:849–853, 1991.

Presents a large case series of treadmill testing in outpatients.

Plotnick GD, Fisher ML. Risk satisfaction: a cost effective approach to the treatment of patients with chest pain. *Arch Intern Med* 145: 41–42, 1985.

Evaluates different strategies for the management of chest pain, discussing the relative merit of enzyme determination and observation over a relatively short period of time.

chapter 22

FEVER IN INFANTS AND PRESCHOOL CHILDREN

Philip D. Sloane

Fever in children is the most common reason for after-hours phone calls to family physicians, and febrile illness is the commonest reason children are taken to pediatricians (other than well child care).

Although respiratory or other symptoms usually accompany fever in children, it is the fever that often prompts the parents to seek help. Fever is a subject of considerable misunderstanding in the general public. First, not all temperature elevations constitute fever. Vigorous activity and overwarming of an infant can increase core body temperature to the febrile range. Second, there is diurnal variation in temperature, with higher temperatures recorded in late afternoon and early evening. Third, rectal temperatures tend to be close to 1°F higher than oral temperatures.

Most physicians define fever as a rectal temperature of 101°F (38.3°C) or higher, or an oral temperature of 100°F (37.8°C) or higher. Dangerously high temperatures, termed hyperpyrexia, occur above 106°F (41.1°C) and are associated with increased ambient temperature or abnormal inability to dissipate heat. Fever this high is very rare indeed. Below this temperature, fever poses no direct threat to the health of an ill child, but it may be a clue to a serious underlying illness.

The physician's primary concern is to identify those children whose symptoms result from a life-threatening bacterial illness, such as pneumonia, meningitis, or bacteremia. These severe bacterial infections represent about 10% of febrile illnesses in infants less than 2 months old, and up to 5% of similar episodes in children 3 months to 2 years. They are more common in poor communities, in infants and children who look sick, and when physical examination fails to reveal signs of focal infec-

tion. Table 22.1 lists the frequency of diagnosis for infectious diseases during the first year of life.

ISSUES IN DIAGNOSIS

On the Telephone. Since fever in young children generally presents over the telephone, the family physician's first task is to determine whether and when the patient should be examined. Many factors should enter into that decision, including the reliability and anxiety of the parents, the prior health history of the child, and the clinical features identifiable by phone. In general, children that are under age 2, have higher temperatures, do not have symptoms suggesting an upper respiratory infection (nasal congestion, sneezing, cough), and appear "ill" should be seen. In case of doubt when dealing with telephone questions about febrile children, always err on the side of seeing the patient.

Taking a History. The history should be brief and focused. Ask about appetite, sleeping, fussiness, and activity (Has the child been playing as usual?). Ask if there has been any vomiting, diarrhea, coughing, sneezing, or pulling at the ears. Try to determine if dehydration is likely, by asking specifically about fluid intake and the frequency of urination. Find out who else at home has been sick. Listen carefully to the parents; they know the child best.

Be sure to find out the actual reason for having the child seen. This may be different from the chief complaint. For instance, a mother may identify fever as the chief complaint, but her concern may be fear of meningitis.

Ruling out Life-threatening Disease. During the office visit, one of your main tasks will be to estimate the likelihood that the child's problem is a life-threatening one. These problems generally fall into two categories: (*a*) bacteremia and (*b*) dehydration.

Bacteremia is relatively common in young children. It always precedes the development of sepsis or meningitis, and it frequently accompanies bacterial pneumonia. Its incidence is probably about 1% of all febrile children, but its likelihood increases if (*a*) there is no evidence of an upper respiratory infection, (*b*) the child is under two years old, (*c*) the temperature is above 39°C, or (*d*) the child "looks ill."

Dehydration can generally be suspected by a history of poor fluid intake and reduced urinary output. Remember that less than 24 hours without fluid intake can lead to significant dehydration in young infants. On physical examination, dehydra-

tion manifests itself as dry mucous membranes, sunken fontanelles and eyes, absent tears, and reduced skin turgor on the chest, abdomen, and thighs. If the child was weighed at a recent office visit, it is easy to estimate the degree of dehydration based on weight loss.

Studies of febrile children confirm that an experienced physician's overall impression (Does this child look "sick?") is an excellent predictor of bacteremia and of other life-threatening conditions (2). In making your own overall assessment, look for decreased activity, diminished response to stimuli, lack of purposeful eye movements (such as fixing on the observer or looking around the room), poor tone, and sleepiness. You may find the acute illness observation score (AIOS) to be helpful in guiding your observations. The AIOS (Table 22.2) scores six variables on a 5-point scale,

Table 22.1. Most Frequent Diagnoses in Infants with Fever

Age ≤2 Months[a]		Age ≤1 Year[b]	
Diagnosis	% of Cases	Diagnosis	% of Cases
1. Nonspecific viral illness	36.7	1. Upper respiratory infection	38.6
2. Upper respiratory infection	24.8	2. Otitis media	32.9
3. Viral gastroenteritis	9.4	3. Nonspecific viral illness	15.9
4. Aseptic meningitis	8.5	4. Gastroenteritis	11.4
5. Otitis media	6.7	5. Pneumonia	1.6
6. Pneumonia	3.1	6. Bronchiolitis	1.2
7. Sepsis/meningitis	2.7	7. Croup	1.2
8. Bacterial gastroenteritis	2.7	8. Chicken pox	1.2
9. Other bacterial infections	2.7	9. Roseola	1.2
10. Urinary tract infection	1.7	10. Streptococcal pharyngitis	1.2

[a]Data from Kimmel SR, Gemmill DW: The young child with fever. *Am Fam Physician* 37:196–206, 1988.
[b]Data from Hoekelman RA: Infectious illness during the first year of life. *Pediatrics* 59:119–121, 1977.

Table 22.2. Acute Illness Observation Scale[a]

Item	Normal = 1	Moderate = 3	Severe = 5
Quality of cry	Strong	Whimper/sob	Weak, moaning, or high-pitched
Amount of crying when with parents	Brief, can be consoled	Cries on and off	Cries continuously or hardly responds
Color	Pink	Pale or blue extremities	Pale, cyanotic, mottled, or ashen
Wakefulness	If awake, stays alert; awakens from sleep quickly when stimulated	Closes eyes during wakeful periods; awakens with prolonged stimulation	Minimally or not arousable
Hydration	Normal	Skin and eyes normal, slightly dry mouth	Poor skin turgor, dry mucous membranes, sunken eyes or fontanelle
Response to social overtures	Smiles or is alert (if ≤2 months)	Smiles or is briefly alert	No smile, anxious face, dull expression, or is not alert (if ≤2 months)

[a]Developed by McCarthy et al. Adapted from Kruse J: Fever in children. *Am Fam Physician* 37:127–135, 1988.

thus generating a total score between 6 and 30. In a study using the AIOS, serious underlying disease was identified in 92% of children with an AIOS score of at least 16, in 26.2% with a score of 11 to 15, and in only 2.7% with a score of 10 or less (1).

Making a Specific Diagnosis. As you evaluate a feverish child, try to see if the clinical picture supports a specific diagnosis. In doing so, be guided by your knowledge of what diagnoses are common (Table 22.1) and how they present, and by your estimation of the likelihood of life-threatening disease. Look for a source of infection in the nose, throat, ears, and chest. Do not forget urinary tract infection as another possibility. If the infant or child is vomiting, do not assume that the problem is purely gastrointestinal; pneumonia, otitis media, and meningitis, as well as abdominal disease, often present with vomiting.

Because young children often cannot use words to describe how they feel, the physical examination is particularly important in making a diagnosis. In examining febrile children, note the following:

- Examining the ears is often difficult, but is crucial. Unfortunately, absolute diagnostic criteria for otitis media do not exist. Bulging and lack of movement of the eardrum are probably the most reliable signs. Redness, changes in the light reflex, and dullness of the eardrum can be caused by crying or by previous ear infections.
- Rhinitis usually (but not always) indicates an upper respiratory infection. In children under 3 years old, it can be the presenting sign of streptoccal disease, and at any age, a foreign body in the nose can cause one-sided foul-smelling nasal discharge. Purulent rhinitis is of no value in differentiating viral from bacterial respiratory infections; most viral colds begin with serous drainage and develop a thicker, more purulent discharge after a few days. A prolonged "cold" is suggestive of allergic rhinitis, particularly if the secretions remain serous. In this situation, ask about a family history of allergy and about recurrent seasonal rhinitis in the patient. Collect a nasal smear for an eosinophil count. Examine conjunctivae and pharyngeal and nasal mucosae for signs of allergy.
- Tender, swollen anterior cervical lymph nodes suggest streptococcal pharyngitis. Nontender cervical nodes may occur in many viral and allergic diseases. Enlarged posterior cervical nodes or occipital nodes, in the absence of scalp disease, are usually caused by viral infection.

- Elevated respiratory rate accompanied by fever and cough should make you think of lower respiratory disease. If wheezing is present, bronchitis or bronchiolitis is likely. If the child looks "sick," consider bacterial pneumonia.

Laboratory studies are often unnecessary in evaluating a febrile child. The most common test is probably the rapid strep test (see Chapter 24, Sore Throat), which is used to identify streptococcal disease. The white blood count is often used to identify patients with a high probability of bacterial illness. Other studies of value in selected patients include urinalysis and culture (remember, however, that a few white blood cells in the urine can be found in almost any febrile illness), blood culture, chest x-ray, and lumbar puncture.

When You Cannot Identify a Source for the Fever. This is a difficult and controversial area. The issue is how far to go to rule out bacteremia and meningitis. Studies indicate that age 2 years or under, a fever of $39°C$ or higher, and a white blood count over 15,000 often accompany occult bacteremia; this information may help augment your overall clinical impression of how ill the child appears.

One approach that has gained favor in children who have high fevers yet do not appear septic is to obtain one or two blood cultures and to treat with antibiotics on an outpatient basis while awaiting the culture results. In the past, oral amoxicillin was used, but it does not appear to eradicate bacteremia or reduce the rate of meningitis (2); therefore, intramuscular ceftriaxone has gained favor as the treatment of choice for this strategy.

Children under 2 Months of Age. Children less than 2 months old comprise a special situation. They are less capable of mounting a febrile response to infection, and they are more susceptible to bacteremia. In the past, all infants under 2 or 3 months of age who had *any* fever were hospitalized for a "sepsis workup." They received a lumbar puncture, spinal fluid cultures, a urine culture, and blood cultures and were placed on antibiotics until the culture results were known. More recently, however, it has become apparent that the risk of complications from hospitalization is high (around 20%) and the risk of meningitis is low (less than 5%). Therefore, more conservative management strategies are now becoming common (3, 4).

One reasonable approach might be to divide these patients based on the overall clinical impression. Those who appear "sick" should be hospitalized for a traditional sepsis evaluation. Those who appear well can be managed more conservatively. In borderline cases, the following factors suggest infants at low risk for serious bacterial infection: age ≥1 month, temperature ≤39° C, and a white blood count <15,000 (5). Identification of a likely cause for the infection (e.g., a red ear or a recent immunization) would favor conservative management. Careful follow-up is extremely important in any infant who is not hospitalized.

Providing Adequate Follow-up. At the end of your visit, carefully instruct the parents about what to do, when to return, and what signs to look for that would prompt a telephone call or revisit. Remember that any illness may initially appear mild, only to worsen later. Therefore, when you send a child home with a diagnosis of viral illness, encourage the parents to call back if new signs or symptoms occur. The case is not resolved until the child is well again.

COMMON DIAGNOSES

This section discusses the clinical patterns of a number of common illnesses presenting with fever, and highlights features of rarer entities with significant morbidity.

Uncomplicated Upper Respiratory Infection (Common Cold)

The common cold is a viral infection that involves mainly the nasal mucosa but can include any respiratory epithelium. Over 300 types of viruses have been implicated, with rhinoviruses the most common cause. Once an individual has had a cold from one particular virus, he or she has lifelong immunity. This is the main reason why the incidence of colds is highest in childhood and decreases with age. Thus, preschool children may have up to 12 colds per year, while adults average only 2 to 3. The incubation period is usually 2 or 3 days, with the average duration of symptoms being 3 to 5 days. Colds are spread primarily by hand-to-face contact, not, as previously thought, by respiratory droplets. Children with the common cold usually appear relatively well and continue to play, eat, and be active in spite of respiratory signs.

Otitis Media

This disease involves infection of fluid and epithelial tissue in the middle ear. The underlying problem is eustachian tube dysfunction, which prevents ventilation of the middle ear and subsequent fluid drainage into the pharynx. Normally, the respiratory columnar epithelium that lines the middle ear cavity secretes small amounts of mucus, which is continuously drained via the eustachian tube to the pharynx. Upper respiratory infections often increase the volume of secretions in the middle ear and also obstruct one or both eustachian tubes. Thus, otitis media typically occurs in children who have had a cold for several days.

A child with an upper respiratory infection first develops fluid (retained secretions) in one or both ears. This condition is termed serous otitis media. It produces a sense of fullness or pressure in the ears, mild fussiness and irritability, and occasionally a low-grade fever. Subsequently, the fluid can become infected, and purulent (acute) otitis media results. In acute otitis media, the inflammatory process in the closed middle ear space distends the eardrum. The severe pain associated with infection in a closed space causes children with otitis media to cry and be irritable. Thus, acute otitis media is a likely diagnosis when parents call about a febrile infant who has remained fretful and cried all night. Around 50% of otitis media episodes are associated with upper respiratory infections, often developing when the cold appears to be improving. Bacteria are implicated in approximately two-thirds of cases, with *Haemophilus influenzae* (types B and untypable) and *Streptococcus pneumoniae* the most common isolates.

Miscellaneous Viral Infections

Fever with no localizing signs often signals a viral infection. Coxsackie, ECHO, herpesvirus type 6, and parainfluenza viruses have been implicated most often. A dry cough with muscle aches, malaise, headache, and a sore throat, particularly occurring in epidemic pattern, suggests influenza.

Roseola is a syndrome of very high fever (up to 105°F) in infants who appear remarkably well and have no localized physical findings. After 3 days of fever, the affected child quickly defervesces, then develops a characteristic fine papular rash. Herpesvirus type 6 has been implicated as the cause of roseola.

Croup

Croup is a viral infection that affects the lower pharynx and larynx. It causes laryngitis in adults. In young children, because the airway is smaller, it results in stridor with cough and can lead to respiratory compromise. The expression "croupy cough" is often used by parents to describe a barking cough without stridor, usually due to bronchitis. This expression is misleading because the characteristic sign of croup is inspiratory stridor, not the cough. The illness itself generally has an onset over 24 to 48 hours but can develop quite abruptly. Children usually recover with rest, liquids, and inhalation of steam or humidified air, but occasionally severe obstruction requires hospitalization and tracheal intubation. Croup typically occurs in children under age 4.

Epiglottitis

A similar but rare illness that occurs mainly in children age 4 to 7 is acute epiglottitis, a life-threatening illness characterized by high fever, inspiratory stridor, drooling, and impending respiratory obstruction. Epiglottitis is caused by *H. influenzae*, progresses rapidly, and is a medical emergency. Avoid examining the pharynx in children with stridor unless intubation is possible immediately.

Acute Chest Infections: Bronchitis, Bronchiolitis, and Pneumonia

Basically, there are two general types of chest infection: those affecting the airways (bronchi and bronchioles) and those affecting the lung parenchyma. Bronchitis is characterized by rhonchi, and bronchiolitis is characterized by wheezes; both may develop during or following upper respiratory infections. Affected children usually are not seriously ill. Some children wheeze during recurrent respiratory illnesses; this tendency may later progress into asthma, but often does not.

Respiratory syncytial virus (RSV) causes relatively severe lower respiratory infections in infants. A rapid antibody test is available to identify the viral antigen in respiratory secretions; a positive test result helps identify the specific diagnosis in a child hospitalized for lower respiratory disease.

Children with fever, cough, tachypnea, and general malaise should be suspected of having pneumonia. Listen carefully for rales. If pneumonia is suspected, especially in infants, get a chest x-ray and check for signs of consolidation. Both viral and bacterial pneumonias occur in children, and their differentiation may be difficult. Bacterial pneumonia in children is often accompanied by bacteremia; it must be aggressively treated.

Meningitis

Meningitis is a major fear of both parents and physicians when a child presents with a fever. The cardinal features of bacterial meningitis—high fever, irritability, photophobia, vomiting, lethargy, and neck stiffness—are often not present in infants. The disease frequently begins with respiratory symptoms, mild fever, and irritability, and progresses rapidly. Always suspect meningitis when clinical signs suggestive of bacteremia are present. The possibility of progression from a minor URI to meningitis is a major reason for encouraging parents to call or return if a child worsens. Careful follow-up of undiagnosed fevers may require daily visits or phone calls.

Bacteremia

Bacteremia is possible in any child with an undifferentiated febrile illness. As noted previously, it is more common in infants under 2 years old and is more likely if the fever is high, the white blood cell count is elevated, and the child appears "ill." In newborns (up to 8 weeks of age), the most common pathogens are *Escherichia coli* and group B streptococci. Between 3 months and 3 years the most common pathogens are *S. pneumoniae* and *H. influenzae*. Children over 3 years of age have a very low likelihood of bacteremia; when they are bacteremic, the most common organisms are *S. pneumoniae* and *N. meningitidis*.

If a febrile child with bacteremia is sent home without antibiotic treatment, the chance of spontaneous resolution is around 65%. The remainder of these children will have persistent fever (35%) and are at high risk for persistent bacteremia (12%) and meningitis (7%). *S. pneumoniae* is most likely to resolve spontaneously; *H. influenzae* and *Neisseria meningitidis* are more likely to lead to meningitis (6).

Immunization Reactions

Many children become febrile after a routine immunization. The DPT (diphtheria-pertussis-tetanus) often causes soreness at the injection site (usually the anterior thigh) and a fever that peaks 12 to 48 hours after the immunization. The MMR (measles-mumps-rubella) may cause a less impressive febrile reaction shortly after the immunization. In addition, the MMR induces a mild infection with an incubation period of about 10 days. Thus, many children develop a low-grade fever, rhinitis, conjunctivitis, and occasionally a maculopapular rash 7 to 14 days after receiving the MMR. These symptoms represent a mild measles-like infection produced by the live attenuated virus in the vaccine.

Sinusitis

Sinusitis does occur in childhood, though not as often as in adults. Radiographically, air can be seen in the ethmoid and maxillary sinuses during the first year of life, in the frontal sinuses by age 6, and in the sphenoid sinuses by age 9. Children with respiratory symptoms, rhinitis, and headache should have the frontal and maxillary sinuses percussed for tenderness. Older children with persistant headache and fever following an upper respiratory infection are particularly likely to have sinusitis.

Other Infectious Diseases

The likely causes of fever may include infectious diseases more prevalent during certain times of the year or in certain geographical locations (such as Rocky Mountain spotted fever or Lyme disease).

THERAPEUTIC CONSIDERATIONS

This discussion will focus on the most common therapeutic decisions facing the family physician dealing with febrile children with respiratory symptoms.

Treating the Common Cold

A wide variety of treatment approaches to the common cold have been tried, but no treatment has been shown to result in significant differences in complication rates. Generally, the treatment of choice is to do as little as possible, since most children recover with simple measures such as warm drinks and humidified air. Infants, who are obligate nose breathers for the first few months of life, will occasionally develop respiratory difficulty from nasal secretions. Parents of infants with colds should thus be advised to (*a*) use a nasal syringe ("bulb syringe") to remove secretions and (*b*) use saline nose drops to loosen thick or dried secretions. Elevating the head of the crib or bed may help infants breathe more easily. Do not use a pillow under babies.

Decongestants, antihistamines, and combination antihistamine-decongestants are often used to treat children with colds. Many are available with-

out a prescription. These agents appear to diminish nasal secretions, but there is no evidence that they prevent complications such as otitis media. Side effects are common. Adults react predictably to these medications (decongestants cause tachycardia and irritability; antihistamines cause drowsiness); but children can respond either way to either type of medication.

Decongestants (α-adrenergic agents that shrink swollen nasal mucosa by acting as vasoconstrictors) have few systemic effects when used topically as drops or sprays. Topical decongestants should not be used for more than 3 days, however, because rebound nasal congestion occurs with more extended treatment. Antihistamines dry nasal secretions; they tend to be better for allergic rhinitis than for the common cold. Vitamin C is often used, but there is no conclusive evidence that it reduces the incidence of colds or lessens the duration of cold symptoms.

Otitis Media

Over half the cases of acute middle ear disease have a bacterial component. Nevertheless, many cases of otitis media will resolve without antibiotics (7). Most physicians prefer to use antibiotics whenever otitis media is diagnosed, however. Ampicillin (or amoxicillin) is usually the drug of choice in communities where *H. influenzae* is not resistant to ampicillin. In areas where a significant percentage of *H. influenzae* isolates are resistant to ampicillin, other treatment options can be used: trimethaprim-sulfamethoxazole (Bactrim or Septra), erythromycin-sulfisoxazole (Pediazole), cefaclor (Ceclor), and amoxicillin/clavulinate potassium (Augmentin) are the most popular alternative drugs.

Decongestants and antihistamines have not been demonstrated in controlled trials to hasten the resolution of otitis media. Nevertheless, some physicians believe that they aid in opening the eustachian tube and prescribe these drugs. If this is indeed true, then the optimal time to use these agents would be when Eustachian tube dysfunction and serous otitis media are present, a situation that typically arises after a child has had an upper respiratory infection for a few days.

Follow-up of otitis media is important to ensure resolution of both the acute infection and the middle ear effusion. Any child who remains febrile 48 hours after being placed on antibiotics should be reevaluated for the possibility of infection with a resistant organism. Children who respond to treatment should be rechecked when they finish their antibiotic course (10 days) and then monthly until both ears are clear of fluid and demonstrate normal movement of the tympanic membrane to pneumatic otoscopy. Middle ear effusions often resolve slowly, with 50% of effusions cleared within 4 weeks and 90% cleared by 3 months after infection. Risk factors for persistent effusion are a past history of nasal discharge and living in a home where individuals smoke. Referral to an otolaryngologist is indicated if an effusion does not clear in about 3 months.

Persistent middle ear effusion is the major indication for placement of middle ear ventilating tubes, which are small plastic tubes that maintain a patent opening through the eardrum and thus allow the middle ear to be ventilated and drain externally. These tubes are designed to be expelled after a few months, by which time the middle ear will generally be healed. Occasionally, ventilating tubes are used to treat repeated episodes of otitis media without persistent middle ear effusion, although their value in this situation is debatable. Low-dose antibiotic prophylaxis may be as effective as surgical tube placement in preventing recurrences. Frequent infections or chronic serous otitis media cause delayed verbal development in some children.

Cough—to Treat or Not to Treat?

Persistent cough is the most common reason why patients with colds make a second visit to the physician's office. Although a cough can represent bronchitis, pneumonia, or asthma, the most common situation is a benign, persistent cough that lasts for weeks after the resolution of a cold.

Most coughs will gradually resolve without treatment. Nearly all coughs are productive and thus aid in preventing pneumonia by clearing respiratory secretions. These post-URI or postbronchitis coughs often bother the parents more than the child, because the child's coughing spells awaken mom and dad. Prescribing cough suppressants is rarely indicated in young children.

Treating Fever

Many parents worry needlessly that fever might cause their children serious injury, especially brain damage. The fact that fever may represent an infection-fighting strategy of the body (many viruses and bacteria grow less effectively at elevated temperatures) is unknown to most of the public. When you, as a physician, talk to parents of febrile children, keep in mind that the temperature elevation itself may be a major source of anxiety. Seek to reassure parents that fever alone is not harmful, but recognize and appreciate that

---

Table 22.3. Guidelines for the Treatment of Fever in Children

1. Remember, and reassure parents, that fever is a normal response to infection. Fever reduction is only indicated if (a) the child is uncomfortable and/or not taking fluids well; (b) there is a history of febrile seizures; or (c) the fever is above 40.1°C (104°F).
2. Acetaminophen is the treatment of choice for fever. Recommended doses are as follows:

Age	Weight (lbs)	Recommended dose every 4 hours (mg)[a]
0–3 months	6–11	40
4–12 months	12–17	80
13–24 months	18–23	120
2–3 years	24–35	160
4–5 years	36–47	240

[a]Acetaminophen dosages are standardized among all major brands, including Tempra, Tylenol, and Panadol. The standard doses are

Drops	80 mg/dropper; 40 mg/half-dropper
Syrup (elixir)	160 mg/tsp (5 ml)
Chewable tablets	80 mg/tablet

An easy way to remember this is 10 to 15 mg/kg/dose every 4 to 6 hours.
3. Sponging with tepid water should be discouraged except as an emergency measure to reduce very high temperatures (≥41°C). It does lower temperature effectively, but it increases the metabolic rate and tends to lead to "rebound" temperature elevation when it is discontinued.
4. Encourage parents to allow a child to sleep rather than to awaken the child to medicate with acetaminophen or to take the temperature.

your reassurances may not be enough and that parents may need specific instructions on fever control. Always question parents about what they have done to help fever. Some parents may have piled on blankets, or they may have given large doses of antipyretics.

Parents of children with recurrent febrile seizures (between 2 and 5% of children will have one febrile seizure before age 7) are advised to treat all fevers, even if the child is acting well. One should note, however, that no evidence shows that this treatment reduces the incidence of seizures. In fact, half of febrile seizures occur before the parents are aware a child is febrile.

In children not subject to febrile seizures, the only reason for treating fever is to make the child feel better. Children who are achy and miserable or who will not drink because of fever probably benefit from fever reduction. Because Reye's syndrome in children has been linked to aspirin use during certain viral infections (influenza and varicella), physicians should recommend only acetaminophen for febrile children. Table 22.3 provides guidelines for fever management in infants and young children.

REFERENCES

1. Kimmel SR, Gemmill DW: The young child with fever. *Am Fam Physician* 37:196–206, 1988.
2. Fleisher GR: Management of children with occult bacteremia who are treated in the emergency department. *Rev Infect Dis* 13(suppl 2):S156–159, 1991.
3. Gehlbach SH: Fever in children younger than three months of age: a pooled analysis. *J Fam Pract* 27:305–312, 1988.
4. Baraff LJ, Oslund SA, Schriger DL, Stephen ML: Probability of bacterial infections in febrile infants less than three months of age: a meta-analysis. *Pediatr Infect Dis J* 11:257–264, 1992.
5. Dagan R, Powell KR, Hall CB, Menegus MA: Identification of infants unlikely to have serious bacterial infection although hospitalized for suspected sepsis. *J Pediatr* 107:855–860, 1985.
6. Baraff LJ, Lee SI: Fever without source: management of children 3 to 36 months of age. *Pediatr Infect Dis J* 11:146–151, 1992.
7. Van Buchem FL, Peeters MF, Van'T Hof MA: Acute otitis media: a new treatment strategy. *Br Med J* 290:1033–1037, 1985.

SUGGESTED READINGS

Kimmel SR, Gemmill DW: The young child with fever. *Am Fam Physician* 37:196–206, 1988.

An excellent review.

Kruse J: Fever in children. *Am Fam Physician* 37:127–135, 1988.

Gives a thorough discussion of the issues around treatment versus nontreatment of fever in children.

Lieu TA, Schwartz JS, Jaffe DM, Fleisher GR: Strategies for diagnosis and treatment of children at risk for occult bacteremia: clinical effectiveness and cost-effectiveness. *J Pediatr* 118:21–29, 1991.

Evaluates the benefits, complications, and costs of six management strategies for febrile children at risk for occult bacteremia, using decision analysis methods.

chapter 23

RESPIRATORY TRACT INFECTIONS

Gregory Strayhorn and Philip D. Sloane

Infections of the respiratory tract are the leading cause of illness among children and adults. Upper respiratory tract infections are the most common acute problem seen by family physicians and cause the most days lost from work. This chapter reviews the common infections of the upper and lower respiratory tract.

APPROACH TO DIAGNOSIS

The respiratory epithelium, along with the skin and the lining of the gastrointestinal tract, comprises a major interface between the human body and the external environment. The high frequency of respiratory infections probably results in part from the fact that the upper respiratory tract is designed to warm and humidify the air. This warm, humid environment is relatively hospitable to the growth of viruses and bacteria.

While respiratory infections are common, our body defenses usually keep them localized and self-limited. There are, however, many local and systemic complications of respiratory infections that should be watched for and, when possible, prevented and treated. Therefore, accurate diagnosis and appropriate management of respiratory infections is important.

Clinical History

The respiratory tract includes the mucosal surfaces of the nose, paranasal sinuses, pharynx, eustachian tube, middle ear, epiglottis, larynx, trachea, bronchi, bronchioles, and alveoli. Clinically, we usually differentiate between the *upper respiratory tract*, which comprises all respiratory structures above the larynx, and the *lower respiratory tract*, which consists of the larynx, trachea, and pulmonary structures. Each of these areas, when infected, presents with a different clinical syndrome.

In evaluating patients with respiratory tract symptoms, it is generally possible to identify a probable location of the problem based on the character of the symptoms. Table 23.1 summarizes the common signs and symptoms of respiratory tract disease by anatomical location. Each of the common symptoms of respiratory disease is discussed briefly below.

Fever is a nonspecific sign. However, both the height of the fever and the pattern of its development can give clues to diagnosis. For example, upper respiratory infections ("colds") generally cause little or no fever. A patient with rhinitis and a low grade fever who, after several days, develops a high fever, probably has a secondary bacterial infection.

Rhinitis signifies a disease of the nose or paranasal sinuses. The disease could be either infectious or noninfectious, since nasal respiratory epithelia produce mucus in response to any insult. Thus, hay fever (an allergy to airborne allergens), a foreign body in the nose, the common cold, and sinusitis can all present with rhinitis. Some physicians differentiate between purulent and mucoid rhinitis, suggesting that purulent drainage implies a bacterial etiology. This generalization does not always hold true in practice however; it is typical for the common cold to begin with a mucoid rhinitis, which thickens after a few days.

Headache can arise from many nonrespiratory structures. Frontal headache, particularly if it is worsened by leaning over, suggests sinusitis. Facial pain is another symptom of paranasal sinus disease, since portions of the sinuses and the skin of the face are both supplied by the trigeminal nerve. Pain in the upper teeth can result from infection in the maxillary sinus, since the superior alveolar nerve passes through that sinus. (For a detailed discussion of headache, see Chapter 20.)

Table 23.1. Presenting Signs and Symptoms of Respiratory Infections

Anatomic Site	Typical Presenting Signs and Symptoms	Common Diagnoses
Nose	Sneezing, rhinitis, nasal stuffiness, mild headache; fever (rare)	Common cold
Paranasal sinuses	Headache (either frontal or on top of the head), facial pain, dental pain; nasal discharge, fever; tenderness on percussion over the affected sinus	Sinusitis
Pharynx	Sore throat; swollen anterior cervical lymph nodes; redness, swelling, and exudate on examination; fever	Pharyngitis
Middle ear/eustachian tube	Earache, ear stuffiness, hearing loss, fever; bulging and loss of normal landmarks of tympanic membrane	Otitis media
Epiglottis	Abrupt onset of high fever, chills, sore throat, loss of voice, stridor, drooling	Epiglottitis
Larynx	Inspiratory stridor (children); hoarseness or loss of voice (adults); mild fever	Laryngitis
Trachea	Cough, low-grade fever (most infections are viral), tenderness on palpation of the trachea	Tracheitis
Bronchi	Cough, sputum production, wheezes and rhonchi, low-grade fever	Bronchitis
Bronchioles	Cough, dyspnea, wheezing, fever	Bronchiolitis
Alveoli	Cough, fever, dyspnea, chest pain, chills	Pneumonia

Sore throat suggests pharyngitis. To review this symptom and its differential diagnosis, see Chapter 24.

Earache can be caused by a variety of problems, some of which are respiratory in origin. In office practice, acute ear pain is common, and the differential diagnosis is often between otitis externa and otitis media. As will be discussed below, the physical examination usually provides the key to differentiating between these two common causes of ear pain.

Ear pain can also be referred. It is not unusual for patients with pharyngitis to refer pain to the ear, for example, because the pharynx and portions of the external and middle ear are supplied by the vagus nerve. Other diseases that can present as ear pain include inflammation of the preauricular or postauricular regional lymph nodes (usually secondary to a skin infection on the scalp or face), parotitis, and temporomandibular joint disorders.

Cough is the cardinal symptom of lower respiratory tract disease (see Table 23.1). Any inflammatory disorder of the trachea, bronchi, bronchioles, or alveoli can cause cough. In part, this is because cough is the body's mechanism for clearing secretions from the tracheobronchial tree, and lower respiratory infections often increase mucus (sputum) production. Cough can occur in the absence of sputum production, too, probably because the cough reflex is activated by any irritation of the trachea or bronchi. Influenza, mycoplasma, and viral infections are typified by nonproductive ("dry") cough. Degree of cough provides little indication of disease severity; many viral respiratory infections cause severe, persistent cough even when they are largely healed.

Dyspnea is generally a sign that pulmonary gas exchange (and, consequently, blood oxygenation) is inadequate. Cardiac and respiratory disorders are the most common causes of dyspnea. Some respiratory infections (e.g., bronchitis) do *not* cause dyspnea because gas exchange in the lungs remains unimpaired. The general rule is that the more severe the dyspnea, the more severe the pathology.

Hoarseness generally indicates narrowing of the airway in the region of the larynx. Typically, the cause is inflammation of the vocal cords due to laryngitis. In small children, narrowing of the same air passage leads to *stridor*.

Chest pain is not usually caused by respiratory infection. Cough can lead to chest pain by straining or otherwise injuring the muscles and bones of the chest wall, or by irritating an inflamed trachea or bronchi. Pleuritic chest pain can be caused by pneumonia adjacent to the pleura. In general, however, the differential diagnosis of chest pain extends beyond respiratory disease. (For a detailed discussion of chest pain, see Chapter 21.)

Physical Examination

In patients with respiratory tract disease, a careful physical examination often establishes the diagnosis. Therefore, students of family medicine should become skilled in physical examination of the respiratory system. Elements of the respiratory examination include:

- Ability to interpret cues from inspection of the patient and vital signs;
- Percussion and transillumination of the paranasal sinuses;
- Visualization of the nasal cavity using an otoscope;
- Examination of the mouth and throat;
- Physical examination of the ear, including use of the otoscope and the insufflator bulb;
- A technique of office laryngoscopy;
- Palpation of the structures of the anterior neck;
- Inspection, palpation, percussion, and auscultation of the chest.

Physical findings provide the key to resolving several common diagnostic dilemmas involving respiratory infections. These include:

- *Differentiating otitis media from otitis externa.* When a patient presents with ear pain, the physical examination usually provides your diagnosis. A diagnosis of otitis externa is supported by (*a*) tenderness of the ear canal on movement of the pinna or gentle insertion of the otoscope speculum, and (*b*) an inflamed external canal, often covered by friable cerumen. Otitis media is the diagnosis if the external canal is normal and the tympanic membrane is bulging and red, with distorted or absent landmarks.
- *Differentiating sinusitis from the common cold.* Patients frequently present to primary care physicians with rhinitis and low-grade fever, wondering if they have a "sinus infection." Physical examination can help identify paranasal sinus disease, in that (*a*) frontal and maxillary sinus infections are generally accompanied by tenderness to percussion over the involved sinus, and occasionally by edema of the skin over the sinus, and (*b*) occasionally, purulent drainage can be seen entering the nose on one side only in a region that corresponds to the drainage of one or more of the major sinuses (e.g., between the upper and middle turbinates).
- *Differentiating bronchitis from pneumonia.* The two most common lower respiratory tract infections, bronchitis and pneumonia, can be most reliably distinguished based on the physical examination. Cough, malaise, and fever are common presenting complaints of both diseases.

Physical findings consistent with bronchitis include absent or low-grade fever, a normal respiratory rate (unless the patient has chronic lung disease), and rhonchi and wheezes on auscultation. In pneumonia, dyspnea and an elevated respiratory rate are common, moderate to high fever is generally present, localized inspiratory rales can be heard on auscultation, and dullness to percussion over the affected area is occasionally present.

Laboratory and X-Ray

The laboratory is used sparingly in the evaluation of respiratory infections in family practice, because it is generally not very helpful. Cultures are unreliable, x-rays are often unnecessary, and empirical treatment is often the most cost-effective strategy.

The most common test is the rapid strep test (see Chapter 24), which can identify streptococcal pharyngitis. The white blood count is frequently used to help the clinician determine the probability that a bacterial or viral etiology is present. In patients with suspected pneumonia, a sputum Gram's stain is often used to identify the probable organism, but many infections are treated empirically, based on epidemiology and the clinical picture.

Radiologic studies are an important adjunct. The chest x-ray will occasionally identify a pneumonia (e.g., mycoplasma) that is not readily apparent on physical examination. For this reason, chest x-ray films should be obtained on all patients with lower respiratory symptoms in whom you suspect but cannot clinically diagnose pneumonia. Another common situation in which chest x-ray films are ordered is to rule out occult disease (e.g., a foreign body, a mediastinal mass, or a pulmonary infiltrate) in the patient who has a persistent cough.

X-ray films of the paranasal sinuses can be helpful in diagnosing chronic sinusitis; acute sinusitis is generally identified based on the history and the physical examination. X-ray films of the lateral neck are also occasionally ordered, because they can often differentiate laryngeal edema (croup) from epiglottitis in children with fever and stridor.

ISSUES IN MANAGEMENT

The management of specific infections is discussed later in this chapter. A few important general issues are presented here.

Patient Expectations

Your patient may present with a minor respiratory infection, but the *actual reason for coming (ARC)* may be something very different. A common ARC is the need for a written work excuse from a physician. Anxiety, depression, or stressful situations (e.g., marital discord) can underlie a seemingly minor medical complaint. Thus, uncovering the patient's concerns is often as important as making the diagnosis.

Demands for antibiotics in the treatment of apparent viral infections are common. Such demands usually occur either because a previous physician was liberal with antibiotics or because the patient had a personal experience in which antibiotics appeared to terminate a prolonged respiratory infection. When you work with patients who demand antibiotics, remember that antibiotics *do* work for many respiratory pathogens, particularly mycoplasma, which can present as "cold" symptoms. Also be aware that your ability to change a patient's opinion is directly related to how well she or he knows and trusts you. Sometimes, agreeing that you'll prescribe an antibiotic if the patient is not better in a few days can prevent unnecessary antibiotic use.

Telephone Management

People with respiratory infections frequently telephone their physician. Usually, the decision that needs to be made is whether to reassure the patient over the phone or to request an office visit. Here are a few general principles:

- Know what infections are prevalent in your community.
- Fever, malaise, and other constitutional symptoms suggest a more severe infection.
- Since the likelihood of bacterial infection is highest in young children (see Chapter 22) and in the very old, these groups should be seen most frequently.
- Printed patient education materials about common respiratory complaints can be helpful in reducing telephone calls and office visits. Your office staff should be similarly educated, since they screen calls.
- If the patient has a typical "cold," telephone reassurance is generally all that is needed, but be sure to probe for hidden concerns.
- In speaking with patients with cold symptoms, be aware that worsening of symptoms several days after the onset of illness suggests a secondary bacterial infection (e.g., otitis media or sinusitis).
- Some patients call because they want to know whether or not they have a "strep" throat. Most offices allow such patients to have a rapid strep test or a throat culture performed (for details, see Chapter 24) without seeing the physician. If your office has such a policy, be sure that the nurse who performs the culture instructs each patient to return for a formal physician visit if the sore throat persists for longer than 3 or 4 days, if symptoms become very severe, or if breathing difficulty develops.

When the Physician Has a Respiratory Infection

Should physicians work when they have respiratory infections? If so, what precautions should they take to avoid infecting their patients?

Often, the medical profession mistakenly praises the physician who continues to work in spite of fatigue or illness. In fact, patients rarely suffer because a physician takes care of his or her own illness. Minor respiratory infections are problematic, however, because the individual has little difficulty working while ill.

If you do work with a minor respiratory illness, be especially careful to wash your hands between patients and to clean your stethoscope with alcohol between patients. Avoid seeing immunocompromised patients, infants under a year of age, and the very old. Consider taking medication yourself that decreases respiratory secretions, because this may reduce contagion.

Epidemics

Most common respiratory infections are viral and are contagious. As a result, respiratory infections often occur in epidemics, particularly where people live closely together. When an epidemic occurs, or the risk of one is high, the family physician should work to institute preventive measures. Such preventive measures can be designed to (*a*) reduce contagion (e.g., hand washing), (*b*) identify and treat cases early (e.g., streptococcal pharyngitis during an epidemic of scarlet fever), or (*c*) enhance herd immunity (e.g., influenza vaccine). Common respiratory epidemics that can be targeted for preventive measures include upper respiratory infections in day-care centers; streptococcal pharyngitis in elementary schools, mycoplasma among military recruits, and influenza among nursing home patients.

COMMON INFECTIONS ENCOUNTERED IN THE FAMILY PRACTICE OFFICE

Upper Respiratory Infections

THE COMMON COLD

The common cold is the leading upper respiratory tract infection in both adults and children. Adults average two to four colds per year with the incidence rising in the fall, peaking in the winter, and declining significantly in the early to late spring. Children on average have between six to ten colds per year and are a major reservoir of cold viruses, as evidenced by an increased incidence of colds among adults who have children in their household. The rhinovirus, with more than 100 antigenic serotypes, is responsible for 25 to 40% of colds. The corona virus, parainfluenza virus, respiratory syncytial virus, influenza virus, adenovirus, and enteroviruses cause another 10 to 40% of infections. Less commonly, *Mycoplasma pneumoniae* and other agents may cause cold symptoms.

Cold viruses enter the body via the nose and attach to the respiratory epithelium, causing edema, hyperemia of mucous membranes and increased nasal secretions, which contain the virus. Transmission primarily occurs by hand contact with the infectious agent, which can survive on objects or on the skin of infected individuals. Transmission by respiratory droplets from sneezing and coughing has not been experimentally substantiated. Symptoms usually develop within 2 days after exposure, with a range of 1 to 6 days.

The diagnosis of the common cold is based on a mild clinical presentation and the absence of pronounced constitutional symptoms. Usual symptoms include sneezing, nasal congestion, and a watery nasal discharge that becomes thick and yellow after several days. Some patients complain of malaise, headache, muscle aches, chilliness, and burning eyes. If present, fever seldom exceeds 102º F. A scratchy or sore throat with pain occasionally referred to the ear, a nonproductive cough, and (less frequently) hoarseness are common associated symptoms. Impaired taste and smell along with pressure in sinuses and ears may also be present. Symptoms peak by the second or third day and subside within 7 days. Cough may persist for days to weeks after the resolution of other symptoms, particularly in young children and in smokers.

Physical findings include mildly swollen and erythematous nasal and pharyngeal mucosa without exudate, nasal passage occlusion, postnasal discharge, and enlarged posterior pharyngeal lymphoid tissue. Cervical lymph nodes may or may not be enlarged and tender. Tympanic membrane dysfunction with transient impaired hearing may accompany eustachian tube obstruction secondary to mucosal edema.

Secondary bacterial infections can occur as complications of the common cold. These secondary infections include acute otitis media, sinusitis, tonsillitis, pharyngitis, cervical adenitis, laryngitis, tracheobronchitis, bronchiolitis, and pneumonia. They usually present between 3 and 10 days after onset of cold symptoms as an increase in fever (above 102°), localized pain, and/or pronounced cough.

Anterior nosebleeds occasionally occur as complications of the common cold. They develop because increased nasal secretions lead to alternate wetting and drying of the mucosa overlying Hasselbach's plexus. This causes cracking of the mucosa, exposing one or more small blood vessels. Frequent nose blowing and wiping can traumatize the area, increasing the likelihood of a bleed. Pinching the nostrils for 5 to 10 minutes usually stops nosebleeds associated with the common cold. Gentle topical application of petroleum base products can often prevent recurrences by protecting the mucosa from drying.

Treatment of the uncomplicated common cold is for symptom relief. Management of colds in children is discussed in Chapter 22. In treating adults, oral pseudoephedrine 60 mg every 6 hours singularly or in combination with an antihistamine is more effective in relieving nasal congestion than placebo or antihistamines alone. Antihistamines may cause drowsiness and should be avoided in situations that require alertness. Phenylpropanolamine is frequently found in over-the-counter preparations, but it must be used judiciously or not at all in hypertensive patients because it tends to elevate blood pressure.

Topical nasal decongestants may avoid the systemic effects of oral decongestants/antihistamines but should be limited to 3 days of use because of their potential to cause rebound persistent congestion. Although evidence is inconclusive, topical nasal decongestion may prevent secondary sinus or ear infections. Decongestants also may reduce transmission of the virus by decreasing nasal secretions that contain shedding virus. Xylometazoline hydrochloride (Otrivin), 0.05% spray or drops is preferred because of its prolonged duration of action, allowing an every 8-to-10-hour application of two to three sprays or drops. Topical nasal decongestants are not recommended for small children; however, saline nasal drops and suction with a bulb syringe may be effective in alleviating nasal congestion. Drinking warm liquids and inhalation of steam or cold water vapor from a vaporizer offer some relief.

Antibiotics do not have a role in treating the common cold and should be used only in the case of secondary bacterial infections.

Cough in young children should generally not be treated (see Chapter 22). Persistent cough in older children and adults may be relieved with products containing dextromethorphan in an equivalent dose of 10 to 20 mg every 6 hours for adults; 5 mg q.i.d. for children 3 to 6 years and 10 mg q.i.d. for children over 6. For severe coughs, codeine 30 mg every 6 hours is recommended, but it should be used with caution and use should not be prolonged because of the potential of abuse and constipation. Expectorants are no longer recommended because they have not been shown to relieve symptoms. Mild sore throat can be relieved with lozenges, sprays, or gargles that contain topical anesthetics such as benzocaine or phenol. Gargles with warm salt water (1 teaspoon in 1 quart of water) may be as effective. Antiseptic mouthwashes are generally not beneficial.

Fever and muscle aches are usually relieved with aspirin or acetaminophen in doses of 650 to 975 mg every 4 to 6 hours for adults and acetaminophen 10 to 12 mg/kg every 3 to 4 hours for children. Because of its association with Reye's syndrome, aspirin should not be used in children.

There are well over 200 available over-the-counter cold and antitussive preparations, of which 75% have subtherapeutic doses of active ingredients or contain compounds that either are clinically unacceptable or may adversely affect existing clinical conditions. When recommending these products, physicians should be aware of the ingredients and instruct the patient on the appropriate dose.

Prevention of the common cold is generally focused on limiting transmission by frequent hand washing, use of disposable tissues, and limiting human contact with symptomatic individuals during the peak of nasal discharge. Studies on the preventive effects of vitamin C have failed to demonstrate efficacy. Vaccines are impractical due to the multiple serotypes of the rhinovirus and the multiple viruses that can cause the common cold.

PHARYNGITIS

Pharyngitis is most frequently caused by viruses, some which may mimic bacterial infections. Diagnosis is made by the presenting symptoms and if necessary appropriate laboratory tests to rule out specific bacterial infections. Adenovirus infections typically present with sore throat, conjunctivitis, fever, and often rhinitis; the infection usually lasts around 5 days. Adenovirus infections occur primarily during summer months; transmission has been associated with contaminated swimming pools. Coxsackie virus causes herpangina, an acute pharyngitis with small, tender blisters (vesicles) on the soft palate, uvula, and tonsilar pillars that rupture and leave a shallow, grayish ulcer with an erythematous halo. Outbreaks are prevalent in summer months. Occasionally the herpes simplex virus causes a similar clinical syndrome. Distinguishing features are that herpes ulcers are fewer and larger, and that coxsackie infections are often accompanied by ulcerations of the hands and feet ("hand, foot, and mouth disease") and by abdominal symptoms (vomiting, pain, and/or diarrhea). Infectious mononucleosis frequently presents with pharyngitis, tonsilar exudate, fever, prominent lymphadenopathy, and fatigue. Treatment for viral infections is symptomatic.

Of bacterial infections, streptococcal pharyngitis is by far the most common. It classically presents with severe sore throat, tonsilar or pharyngeal exudate, anterior cervical adenopathy, fever to 104° F, lethargy, myalgias, and anorexia; however, 40% of patients have symptoms indistinguishable from the common cold. It is most prevalent between the ages of 5 to 17 years. The importance of diagnosis and treating this infection is to prevent the severe complications of rheumatic fever and glomerulonephritis, and the local suppurative complications of peritonsillar and retropharyngeal abscess, cervical lymphadenitis, otitis media, and septicemia. Rarer bacterial causes of pharyngitis include group G streptococci, *Neisseria gonorrhoeae*, anaerobic and spirochetal organisms (Vincent's angina), *Staphylococcus aureus*, and, rarely, diphtheria. In adolescents and young adults, mycoplasma infections can also cause pharyngitis.

For details on the diagnosis and management of patients with sore throat, see Chapter 24.

SINUSITIS

Sinusitis in adults may be classified as acute, subacute, or chronic, based on the length of symptoms (less than 3 weeks, 3 weeks to 3 months, and longer than 3 months, respectively). The typical presentation of *acute sinusitis* includes:

- Pain located over the affected sinus, which increases as the day progresses and with bending;
- Pain may be referred to structures contiguous to the affected sinuses (see Table 23.2), presenting as headache;
- Nasal congestion, often with purulent nasal discharge;
- Fever;
- Symptom onset 3 to 10 days into a "cold."

However, these symptoms are not specific to sinusitis, and many cases of sinusitis do not present classically.

Sinusitis in children presents with cold symptoms lasting longer than 10 days, nasal discharge, and a daytime cough. Children may also present acutely with high fever, periorbital swelling, facial pain, headache, and copious purulent nasal discharge. Since frontal sinuses are not fully formed in childhood until about the age of 10 years, frontal sinusitis is not present in young children.

Physical examination in both children and adults will generally reveal tenderness over the affected sinus, edematous nasal mucosa, and a nasal discharge that may or may not be purulent. Transillumination may aid in diagnosis for frontal and maxillary sinusitis. In a dark room, placement of the transilluminator over the lower orbital rim will direct light through the ipsilateral maxillary sinus and cause a glow on the hard palate that can be seen through the open mouth. Failure to transmit

Table 23.2. Location of Referred Pain in Sinusitis

Sinus Involved	Location of the Pain
Maxillary	Cheek and upper teeth
Ethmoid	Behind (deep to) the nose and eyes
Frontal	Forehead
Sphenoid	Occiput or top of the head

a glow suggest sinusitis. Placement of the transilluminator at the medial superior orbital rim directed cephalad will illuminate the anterior wall of the frontal sinus: no illumination suggests frontal sinusitis.

Cultures of nasal discharge do not reliably aid in the diagnosis of sinusitis since the results do not correlate with culture of material directly aspirated from the affected sinus. Although expensive, x-ray films of the sinuses provide the best evidence for sinusitis, revealing air fluid levels, opacification, and thickening of the mucosa. Due to their expense, x-ray films should be reserved for failure of response to appropriate treatment, chronic sinusitis, and patients who are at high risk of complications from sinusitis, such as diabetics and the immunocompromised.

Haemophilus influenzae, *Streptococcus pneumoniae*, and anaerobes are the most frequent bacterial pathogens found. Less prevalent are *Branhamella catarrhalis*, group A streptococci, *Neisseria* species, and *Staphylococcus aureus*. Viruses, with the rhinovirus most predominant, cause acute sinusitis in up to 15% of cases. Fungi may be found in immunocompromised patients.

Treatment consists of antibiotics for at least 2 weeks and decongestants. Choice of antibiotics is not clear-cut, due to the many possible pathogens and the unreliability of cultures. Both *H. influenzae* and *Moraxella catarrhalis* may produce β-lactamase, which should be consider when selecting an antibiotic. Common first-line agents for adults include ampicillin 500 mg q.i.d.; amoxicillin 250 to 500 mg t.i.d.; trimethoprim-sulfamethoxazole two tablets b.i.d.; doxycycline, 200 initially and 100 mg b.i.d.; and cefaclor 250 mg q.i.d.. All are equally effective in adults. Ampicillin, 50 mg/kg q.i.d., amoxicillin, 40 mg/kg t.i.d., trimethoprim(TMP)-sulfamethoxazole(SMZ) based on 8 mg/kg TMP or 40 mg/kg SMZ b.i.d., and the β-lactamase-resistant antibiotics, cefaclor, 40 mg/kg t.i.d., erythromycin (EM)-sulfisoxazole (SSZ), based on 40 mg/kg EM or 120 mg/kg SSZ, and amoxicillin-clavulanate, based on the amoxicillin component, are appropriate for children. Adults or children with severe sinus pain, facial cellulitis, and fever may require hospitalization, parenteral antibiotics, and direct drainage of the sinuses. Referral to the otolaryngologist should occur for treatment failures, chronic infection, or the suspicion of complications. Three- to 4-day use of topical sympathomimetic decongestants in spray or drops, inhalation of steam, and oral analgesics offer symptomatic relief.

Otitis Media

Otitis media, because it occurs most frequently in young children, is discussed in detail in Chapter 22. It also occurs in older children and in adults, although less frequently, presenting as acute ear pain with or without decreased hearing. Direct observation of the tympanic membrane is required to make the diagnosis. A pneumatic otoscope is recommended that will allow direct visualization and determination of the mobility of the tympanic membrane. Removal of cerumen may be necessary to visualize the tympanic membrane. Classically, the tympanic membrane is red, bulging, opaque and immobile, and the bony structures are obscured. The appearance is not always so dramatic, however, and the diagnosis may be based on less prominent changes in the appearance of the tympanic membrane and the loss of its mobility. The impedance tympanometer is sensitive and reliable in determining the presence of middle ear fluid and is frequently used in office practice.

Antibiotics may not significantly change the clinical course of uncomplicated otitis media, but they do help reduce recurrences and prevent suppurative complications, such as chronic otitis media, cholesteatoma, and mastoiditis. Penicillin is preferred in adults. As alternatives, the antibiotics listed for sinusitis are effective. Be aware, however, that trimethoprim-sulfamethoxazole (TMP-SMZ) may not eliminate *S. pneumoniae* and that cefaclor and amoxicillin-clavulanate are expensive. Oral and nasal decongestants are controversial. Auralgan has limited usefulness as a topical anesthetic. Acetaminophen in children and/or aspirin in adults provides effective analgesia for mild to moderate pain; narcotics may be necessary for up to 48 hours to relieve severe pain.

Lower Respiratory Infections

Most lower respiratory tract infections (LRIs) in children between the ages of 2 months and 12 years are caused by viruses, including the respiratory syncytial virus, parainfluenza viruses, and the adenovirus. Viruses remain common as pathogens in adolescents and young adults, but *Mycoplasma pneumoniae* emerges as a prominent pathogen in this age group.

In adults, viral respiratory infections are less frequent than in children but remain common. Bacterial causes are relatively more frequent, and *Mycoplasma* is a common cause of pneumonia and bronchitis. In the elderly, Gram-negative organisms and *Legionella* become prominent as causes of LRIs. Smokers have a particularly high incidence of lower respiratory tract disease, presumably because the protective mucociliary system is damaged. They are often colonized with Gram-negative organisms such as *Klebsiella pneumoniae*, which explains why these organisms are more frequent LRI pathogens in smokers.

CROUP

Croup, seen in children between 3 months and 3 years of age, is generally caused by the parainfluenza virus. It presents with inspiratory stridor and a characteristic barking cough, a low-grade fever, and coryza. The infection is generally self-limited and is helped by humidification. Decongestants may also be of some value. In older children, it must be differentiated from epiglottitis, a severe illness that presents acutely with stridor and fever and is cause by *H. influenzae*.

LARYNGITIS

Laryngitis is the adult counterpart of croup. In adults, because the airway is larger, hoarseness is the only symptom produced by the laryngeal edema, and respiratory compromise does not occur. A viral illness usually preceded by pharyngitis and/or rhinitis, laryngitis is self-limited. Treatment is with acetaminophen, aspirin, or ibuprofen, with humidification, and with warm liquids. Resting the vocal cords speeds resolution of the hoarseness.

BRONCHIOLITIS

Acute bronchiolitis is a distinct syndrome occurring in infants under 2 years with a peak incidence at 6 months of age. It is usually caused by the respiratory syncytial virus (RSV), although other viruses can occasionally be responsible. Typically, a minor respiratory illness in an older family member is passed to the infant, leading to bronchiolitis. The severity of symptoms results from the fact that the infant's bronchiolar airway is so small that wall edema caused by the infection significantly reduces airflow.

Bronchiolitis begins as an upper respiratory infection, but soon the patient develops a cough, audible wheezing, irritability, listlessness, dyspnea, and cyanosis. Chest x-ray films may reveal either atelectasis or hyperinflation, or both. Untreated, infants with bronchiolitis can die from hypoxemia, dehydration, or apnea. Fewer than 1% of affected infants die, however. Most recover but suffer recurrent wheezing episodes, usually precipitated by viral infections, for 5 to 10 years following the infection.

Respiratory syncytial virus (RSV) is the most important respiratory tract pathogen in early childhood. It is the most common cause of bronchiolitis and pneumonia in children under 1 year of age. An antiviral agent, ribavirin, is effective against RSV, particularly if used early in the infection. Rapid antibody kits for RSV, similar to the rapid strep test kits, are now available; these can help identify infants who may merit hospitalization because of increased risk for severe lower respiratory disease.

BRONCHITIS

Bronchitis is seen at all ages beyond 6 months. In children, it is usually the result of a viral infection that initially affected the nasopharynx and progressed to involve the trachea and bronchi. Symptoms include low-grade fever (≤101°F), mild cough, wheezing, rhonchi, and, occasionally, rales.

In adults, acute bronchitis is the most frequent lower respiratory infection. It is most prevalent in winter and is primarily caused by the rhinovirus, coronavirus, adenovirus, or influenza virus. The typical presentation includes:

- Being preceded by an upper respiratory tract infection;
- An initially nonproductive cough that becomes productive of mucopurulent sputum;
- Substernal chest pain brought on by coughing, deep breathing, and movement;
- Absent or mild fever.

Physical findings are rare, but auscultation of the lungs may reveal rhonchi or wheezes that shift with cough.

Treatment should be symptomatic. Antitussives should be used sparingly for cough (see section on the common cold) and acetaminophen for fever. Antibiotics are used to treat bronchitis in smokers, since they are often colonized with pathogenic bacteria. Erythromycin, amoxicillin, and trimethoprim-sulfamethoxazole are commonly used antibiotics. Complete smoking cessation may be necessary to clear the cough in smokers.

Chronic bronchitis is seen primarily in older adults with a history of smoking and/or exposure to air pollutants. It results from permanent inflammatory changes in the lower respiratory tract. Superimposed infection occurs frequently and presents as increased sputum production, cough, wheezing, and respiratory distress. *S. pneumoniae, H. influenzae*, α-hemolytic streptococci, and *Moraxella catarrhalis* are common pathogens. Antibiotics are generally indicated, with the recommended agents being the same as those used in acute bronchitis. Adequate hydration, supplemental oxygen, and bronchodilation are important.

INFLUENZA

Several related viruses cause the "flu." Classic epidemic influenza is caused by influenza virus type A (80% of epidemics) or influenza virus type B (20% of epidemics). Its onset is abrupt, with severe myalgias, prominent headache, a nonproductive cough, and fever in the range of 102 to 103° F. The illness is generally self-limited and subsides within a few days. In some individuals, however, pneumonia results. This pneumonia can be either caused by the influenza virus or by a secondary bacterial pathogen, most commonly either *H. influenzae, S. pneumoniae*, or *S. aureus*.

Influenza should be prevented in high-risk patients (adults with chronic pulmonary or cardiovascular diseases, nursing home residents, age greater than 65, diabetes, renal or marrow dysfunction, and the immunocompromised). Flu shots are made available annually in October or November, and each family practice should have a plan for getting as many patients as possible immunized. Early use of amantadine 200 mg per day during an acute infection with influenza A may be beneficial. Supportive care consists of rest, liquids, and acetaminophen.

PNEUMONIA

Children. Most pneumonias in children are viral and require symptomatic treatment. Predominant bacterial pathogens vary by age:

- In the newborn, *E. coli, Staphylococcus aureus*, group B streptococci, and *Chlamydia* are the most common pathogens;
- Between 3 months and 8 years of age, *S. pneumoniae* and *H. influenzae* predominate;
- In older children, *Mycoplasma pneumonia, S. pneumoniae, and N. meningitidis* are common pathogens.

Antibiotics should be selected accordingly.

Clinical symptoms and laboratory findings that suggest bacterial pneumonia include sudden onset, high fever (>102°F), tachypnea, tachycardia, cough, consolidation on x-ray films, leukocytosis, and, in older children, chest pain, sputum production, and shaking chills. Symptoms associated with viral pneumonias and *Mycoplasma pneumoniae* are gradual onset, prominent nonproductive cough, and low-grade fever without significant laboratory findings.

Adults. Pneumonia in adults presents in two general ways, as "typical" pneumonia and as "atypical" pneumonia. Table 23.3 outlines the differences between these pneumonia syndromes. In general, atypical pneumonias are milder and slower in onset, whereas typical pneumonias are more severe and abrupt in onset. Most pneumonias in adults under age 40 are atypical, with *Mycoplasma pneumoniae* being the predominant pathogen. As adults become older, and as the prevalence of chronic disease rises, the relative frequency of typical pneumonias rises. The diagnosis of pneumonia is based on a history consistent with the disease and demonstration of either (*a*) rales or signs of consolidation on physical examination, or (*b*) an infiltrate on chest x-ray films.

S. pneumoniae is the most common community-acquired pneumonia. It is rapid in onset ("typical"), presenting with shaking chills or rigor, high fever, a cough producing rusty blood-tinged sputum, pleuritic chest pain, and dyspnea. Occasionally, it can present as upper abdominal pain accompanied by fever and chills. Auscultatory examination of the chest may reveal signs of consolidation and/or a friction rub. Chest x-ray films will show a lobar consolidation with or without effusion. There is prominent leukocytosis.

Mycoplasma pneumonia tends to occur in epidemics in late summer and early fall among closed groups such as families, college students, summer camps, and military recruits. It presents with a dry hacking cough, low-grade fever, headache, sore throat, and myalgias. Patients usually do not appear very ill and are ambulatory. Physical findings may be nonspecific, but in advanced cases, rales and signs of consolidation will be evident. A chest x-ray film usually looks worse than the patient appears, revealing one or more infiltrates. Rash, otitis media, and joint symptoms may be present. There is not a prominent leukocytosis. Cold agglutinins may be present, but are positive in only about half of cases.

In office practice, pneumonia in otherwise healthy adults without respiratory compromise can be managed on an outpatient basis with appropriate antibiotics, hydration, and symptom relief. Patients with chronic illness or debilitating or immunocompromised conditions generally require hospitalization, more aggressive management, and a search for less common pathogens.

Ideally, a sputum should be obtained and Gram-stained to help guide therapy. (Sputum cultures are unreliable and are not worth obtaining in the office setting.) If the patient has typical pneumonia and the sputum shows polymorphonuclear leukocytes (PMNs) and Gram-positive streptococci, *S. pneumoniae* is very likely to be the causative pathogen, and penicillin is the drug of choice. If the patient's sputum shows many PMNs and Gram-negative organisms, then a second-generation cephalosporin is the best choice for outpatient treatment.

In practice, many uncomplicated community-acquired pneumonias are treated empirically, either because the patient cannot produce sputum or because the Gram's stain is nondiagnostic. In such cases, antibiotic choice is based on epidemiology and the clinical presentation. Table 23.4 provides a guide to empiric outpatient treatment of such

Table 23.3. Characteristics of "Typical" and "Atypical" Pneumonias[a]

Characteristic	"Typical" Pneumonia	"Atypical" Pneumonia
Onset	Rapid	Gradual
Chills	Common	Rare
Cough	Productive	Nonproductive
Pleuritic pain	Common	Rare
Fever	>38.9° C (102° F)	<38.9° C (102° F)
Usual distribution	One lobe or segment	Multiple lobes or segments
Most common pathogen	*Streptococcus pneumoniae*	*Mycoplasma pneumoniae*

[a]Adapted from Rodnick JE, Gude JK: Diagnosis and antibiotic treatment of community-acquired pneumonia. *West J Med* 154: 405–409, 1991.

Table 23.4. Selecting an Antibiotic for Empiric Treatment of Adults with Community-Acquired Pneumonia[a] (when a sputum Gram's stain is unavailable or is not helpful)

If the patient is...	The most likely organism is...	Other likely pathogens include...	The antibiotic(s) of choice include...
A healthy adult			
with "typical" pneumonia	*Streptococcus pneumoniae*	*Hemophilus influenzae*	Penicillin, ampicillin, or amoxicillin; a second-generation cephalosporin
with "atypical" pneumonia	*Mycoplasma pneumoniae*	Viruses	Erythromycin or doxycycline
A geriatric patient			
without suspected aspiration	*S. pneumoniae*	*H. influenzae*, mixed flora, *Legionella*	A second-generation cephalosporin, trimethoprim-sulfamethoxazole
with suspected aspiration	Oral anaerobes	*Bacteroides*, mixed flora, *Staphylococcus aureus*	Penicillin, clindamycin
A smoker or with chronic lung disease	*S. pneumoniae*	*H. influenzae*, *Moraxella catarrhalis*	A second-generation cephalosporin, trimethoprim-sulfamethoxazole

[a]Sources: Mcfarlane JT: Treatment of lower respiratory infections. *Lancet* II:1446–1449, 1987; Norman DC: Pneumonia in the elderly: empiric antimicrobial therapy. *Geriatrics* 46:26–32, 1991; Perlman PE, Ginn DR: Respiratory infections in ambulatory adults: choosing the best treatment. *Postgrad Med* 87:175–184, 1990; and Rodnick JE, Gude JK: Diagnosis and antibiotic treatment of community-acquired pneumonia. *West J Med* 154:405–409, 1991.

patients who are not severely ill; those who are very sick should be hospitalized and potentially treated with other agents.

An important treatment decision is whether or not to manage the patient with pneumonia at home. Patients who can take medication and fluids by mouth, who have a family member or other caretaker to look after them, and who are not gravely ill can be considered for home treatment. Easy access to the physician and the patient's ability to comply with the prescribed regimen (and follow-up) are other factors favoring outpatient treatment.

Follow-up is important in pneumonia. Patients can fail to respond to antibiotics because of noncompliance or because the pathogenic organism was not susceptible to the drug used. Occasionally, tuberculosis will present as pneumonia and will only be identified when the patient does not get better. Complications such as parapneumonic effusions, empyema, and secondary infections can occur. Finally, pneumonia can be the presentation of carcinoma of the lung.

For these reasons, patients with pneumonia should return frequently for reassessment until they are clinically better. All patients over 40 should have a follow-up chest x-ray in 3 to 6 weeks to confirm resolution of the infiltrate. If the patient has not previously received one, a pneumococcal vaccine should be administered as soon as he or she has recovered from the pneumonia.

SUGGESTED READINGS

Bucker PC (ed): *Primary Care Clinics in Office Practice.* 17(4), 1990.

Volume on infectious diseases in office practice with chapters written by primary care physicians. Excellent overview of common pediatric and adult infectious diseases in office practice.

Dornbrand L, Hoole AJ, Fletcher R, Pickard, CG (eds): *Manual of Clinical Problems in Adult Ambulatory Care*, ed 1. Boston, Little, Brown, & Co., 1985.

Book presents brief chapters on common problems seen in the ambulatory setting, including chapters on common upper and lower respiratory infections.

Dornbrand L, Hoole AJ, Fletcher R, Pickard CG (eds): *Manual of Clinical Problems in Adult Ambulatory Care*, ed 2. Boston, Little, Brown, and Co., 1992.

Updated version of the first edition, with new chapters on sore throat and the common cold. The sore throat chapter presents a simple algorithm to estimate the probability of streptococcal pharyngitis and when to treat.

Mcfarlane JT: Treatment of lower respiratory infections. *Lancet* II:1446–1449, 1987.

An excellent review of the microbiology and treatment of lower respiratory tract disease in adults.

Parry MF, Neu HC. Infectious diseases: respiratory tract infections. In Rakel RE (ed): *Textbook of Family Practice*, ed 3. Philadelphia, WB Saunders, 1984, pp 497–502.

Concise overview of lower respiratory tract infections in children and adults.

Rodnick JE, Gude JK: Diagnosis and antibiotic treatment of community-acquired pneumonia. *West J Med* 154:405–409, 1991.

A practical discussion of the approach to pneumonia in an urban family practice department.

chapter 24

SORE THROAT

Thomas A. Cable

"Sore throat" is a symptom: pain in the throat. "Pharyngitis" is a diagnosis: inflammation of the pharynx. Sore throat is usually due to pharyngitis, and pharyngitis is usually due to local infection of the pharynx. But remember there are other possibilities: Sometimes sore throat is not due to pharyngitis. Other causes include referred pain, drying of the pharyngeal epithelium from mouth breathing, and chemical irritation from smoking or other toxic inhalation. Keep these distinctions in mind as you read this chapter.

HISTORY

Confirm that the patient does indeed have a sore throat rather than neck pain. Are there other symptoms? Ask specifically about fever, nasal discharge or stuffiness, ear pain or stuffiness, and cough. How long have symptoms been present, and do people at home or work have similar symptoms? Is this a recurrent problem? A more detailed history is required if symptoms are chronic or recurrent, see "Diagnostic Considerations."

EXAMINATION

Ask the patient to point with one finger to the most painful area. Is it midline or unilateral, high or low? Can the patient breathe through the nose? Percuss the sinuses for tenderness, and examine the ears. Palpate the neck for enlarged glands, noting their position and whether or not they are tender. Now examine the oral cavity and pharynx. Are there ulcers in the mouth or pharynx? Are the fauces, tonsils, or posterior pharyngeal wall red or swollen? Is there exudate on the tonsils, or trails of mucus (postnasal drip) on the pharynx?

Further examination is warranted if specific clues are present, as noted below. Note that the complaint of sore throat in a young child *always*

mandates a general assessment of how sick the child is (see Chapter 22).

DIAGNOSTIC CONSIDERATIONS

Distinguishing between viral pharyngitis and pharyngitis due to group A β-hemolytic streptococcus (GABHS) is often the main issue for the physician (and for well-informed patients). A history of associated cough, runny nose, and hoarseness points to viral pharyngitis; absence of these symptoms increases the probability of GABHS. GABHS pharyngitis is most common in children between the ages of 5 and 15, and rare in patients under age 3 or over 30. It is more prevalent in the winter and spring and in lower socioeconomic groups, where crowded living conditions may be a factor. Specific clinical findings associated with an increased likelihood of GABHS are: fever greater than 101°F and tender anterior cervical adenopathy. The fine, raised rash of scarlet fever, like sandpaper to the touch and typically present on the trunk and arms, accompanies streptococcal pharyngitis only rarely, but when present is virtually pathognomonic.

Streptococcal infection is confirmed by routine throat culture or a rapid test for streptococcal antigen, which can be performed while the patient is still in the office. Neither of these tests, however, proves conclusively that streptococcus is the cause of the pharyngitis, as asymptomatic carriage of this organism occurs in around 15% of the population, and both tests have a false-negative rate around 10%. The implications of this are discussed later in this chapter.

Peritonsillar and retropharyngeal abscesses occasionally complicate streptococcal pharyngitis and produce obvious asymmetry on inspection. If the patient is drooling and has pain on opening the mouth for examination, then an abscess should be strongly suspected. Epiglottitis is another diagnosis that, while rare, must not be forgotten. It, too, presents with fever, sore throat, and drooling (due to trouble swallowing). Children under 8 are most often affected. Onset is rapid, typically over a few hours. Difficulty breathing suggests imminent respiratory arrest.

Many viruses can cause pharyngitis, usually as part of a more widespread infection, with nasal symptoms often predominating over the sore throat. Coxsackie virus and herpes simplex type I both cause shallow, red, painful ulcers on the posterior palate or fauces.

Infectious mononucleosis can produce severe pharyngitis and tonsillitis. It should be suspected when an adolescent or young adult with pharyngitis is noted to have bilateral enlarged *posterior* cervical nodes, especially if there is a history of recent exposure. Other clues are generalized adenopathy, fatigue, splenomegaly, and a rash. The full clinical picture of infectious mononucleosis may develop only gradually if at all. Often, the condition is diagnosed only when the patient returns a week or so after an initial visit, complaining of persistent fever, anorexia (due to mild hepatitis), or extreme fatigue. These complaints, in a patient who originally presented with sore throat, should prompt testing for the disease even if none of the confirmatory signs are present. Either a Monospot test or microscopic examination of a blood smear for atypical lymphocytes can confirm the diagnosis.

Influenza is common in the winter, usually occurring in epidemics. Typically, its sore throat is mild and transitory; fever, chills, and a dry cough are prominent complaints. Influenza causes fewer nasal symptoms and much more fatigue than other viral upper respiratory infections.

Gonococcal pharyngitis may be asymptomatic or cause a painful throat. Because gonococcal pharyngitis has no distinctive physical signs, it should be considered in any patient with recent symptoms suggesting sexually transmitted disease. (Remember to be sensitive and nonjudgmental as you take the sexual history.) Certain groups are especially at risk because of their sexual behavior; for instance, in some college undergraduate populations the incidence of gonococcal pharyngitis approaches that of strep throat. When gonococcal pharyngitis is suspected, perform a throat culture on Thayer-Martin medium.

Seasonal respiratory allergies (hayfever, sneezing, itchy eyes) may cause sore throat as a result of postnasal drip or excessive mouth breathing with drying of the pharyngeal mucous membranes.

Sore throat may accompany other illnesses such as otitis media or sinusitis, hence the importance of examining the ears and checking for sinus tenderness. Chemical irritation from cigarette smoke or environmental agents should be considered if the complaint is chronic or recurrent. Cancer of the pharynx or tongue may present as a persistent sore throat. Other less common causes of sore throat include candidiasis, thyroiditis, dental problems, retropharyngeal abscess, leukemia, and even myocardial ischemia. Diphtheria is a medical and public health emergency; fortunately, it is now extremely rare. It is characterized by sore throat with a high fever and a confluent pharyngeal exudate (pseudomembrane). Pointers to these conditions will usually arise on the initial history and examination.

THERAPEUTIC CONSIDERATIONS

A few causes of sore throat are medical emergencies. Impending airway obstruction from epiglottitis, retropharyngeal abscess, or extreme tonsillar enlargement due to tonsillitis or infectious mononucleosis requires quick diagnosis and appropriate therapy to stabilize the patient. Most other causes of sore throat are nonemergent.

Therapeutic measures for sore throat are both general and specific. General measures include gargling with warm water (salted or not) and/or Benadryl Elixir. The latter antihistamine, used topically for its anesthetic effect, should be gargled for 3 to 4 minutes and is much more palatable than topical viscous xylocaine. Throat lozenges and sprays are available without prescription and provide temporary relief. With prolonged use, however, some patients can become sensitized to these agents and actually experience sore throat from overuse. Specific therapy for infectious pharyngitis is ideally directed toward the causative agent. No specific treatment is yet available for the great majority of viruses causing sore throat; the exception is influenza type A, for which amantadine is available.

Severe symptoms of infectious mononucleosis, especially copious pharyngeal secretions, may be helped by a short course of steroids, a time-honored but controversial therapy. Many college infirmary physicians note that steroid treatment leads to faster recovery, with less time lost from classes (1).

Since antigen testing kits now make it possible to identify GABHS with reasonable accuracy while the patient is still in the office, the physician is no longer obliged to decide on presumptive treatment, based on the clinical presentation, or on delaying treatment until a culture result is available. Treatment of all patients with sore throat and a positive GABHS test, however, inevitably leads to some unnecessary treatment in those cases where the streptococcus is merely a commensal, and not causing pharyngitis. This state of affairs will continue until we have tests that rapidly distinguish between colonization and infection of the pharynx.

Penicillin is the drug of choice for the treatment of GABHS. The route of administration depends primarily on the likelihood that your patient will comply with oral treatment. A 10-day course of oral penicillin or, in the penicillin-allergic individual, erythromycin, is usually appropriate. Early treatment, continued for a full course, results in rapid improvement of symptoms, reduces the spread of infection, and lowers the likelihood of both nonsuppurative (rheumatic fever) and suppurative (peritonsillar abscess) complications. Patients who are likely to be noncompliant should be considered for injectable penicillin (a single dose of benzathine penicillin). The two disadvantages of this route should be remembered, however. First, the injection is painful and the pain may persist for several days. Second, a life-threatening anaphylactic reaction to a penicillin injection is sometimes a patient's first manifestation of penicillin allergy. Deaths from this cause continue to be reported, whereas death due to oral penicillin is almost unknown.

The treatment of gonococcal pharyngitis is subject to frequent updated recommendations from the Centers for Disease Control (CDC), based on research on new antibiotics and changing patterns of bacterial resistance. The physician should therefore check the latest CDC guidelines on this topic.

REFERENCE

1. Collins M, Fleisher G, Kreisberg J, Fager S: Role of steroids in the treatment of infectious mononucleosis in the ambulatory college student. *J Am Coll Health* 33:101–105, 1984.

SUGGESTED READINGS

Centor RM, Ruoff GE, Selner JC: Sore throat: streptococcal or not? *Patient Care* 21:28–44, 1987.

Up-to-date review article with pragmatic flowsheet for diagnosing the cause of pharyngitis. Available rapid screening tests for group A streptococcus are listed with known specificity and sensitivity.

DeNeef P: Selective testing for streptococcal pharyngitis in adults. *J Fam Pract* 25:347–353, 1987.

An analysis of the clinical strategies for testing adult patients for streptococcal pharyngitis.

Dillon HC: Streptococcal pharyngitis in the 1980s. *Pediatr Infect Dis J* 6:123–130, 1987.

A review article on streptococcal pharyngitis, including pathophysiology, differential diagnosis, tests, and treatment.

Lieu TA, Fleisher GR, Schwartz JS: Cost-effectiveness of rapid latex agglutination testing and throat culture for streptococcal pharyngitis. *Pediatrics* 85:246–256, 1990.

Discusses the recent change in practice patterns in which rapid testing for streptococcal antigens has largely replaced throat cultures.

chapter 25

ABDOMINAL AND PELVIC PAIN

William A. Hensel and Mary N. Hall

Abdominal pain ranks among the top 15 presenting symptoms in primary care. Its diagnosis is often difficult and one of the major challenges in clinical medicine. Lower abdominal pain in women (i.e., pelvic pain) is an especially important and difficult diagnostic challenge. The causes of abdominal pain vary from those requiring immediate intervention to prevent a fatal outcome to those in which neither diagnosis nor treatment presents any urgency. A diagnosis may not be possible at the first visit; however, a decision on how urgently to proceed with the problem must be made at that time.

On the initial visit of patients with abdominal pain, the family physician must decide, provisionally, into which of the following four categories the problem falls:

- An acute, life-threatening illness requiring immediate intervention;
- A subacute but progressive and serious illness that demands timely recognition;
- A chronic illness that merits a workup at the patient's and physician's convenience;
- A self-limited illness that will require no further investigations.

Each of these problem categories are illustrated below and discussed in detail later in the chapter.

PATIENT EVALUATION

Acute, Potentially Life-threatening Process

Case 1.1

Mr. M.R. is a 32-year-old insurance salesman with 6 hours of abdominal symptoms. Initially he noted the onset of vague discomfort in his midabdomen, followed by anorexia, and eventually, nausea. The nausea increased, and he began to notice a low-grade fever. Within 5 hours after onset, the pain had worsened and shifted to his right lower quadrant. Physical examination showed markedly diminished bowel sounds and right lower quadrant guarding, with localized tenderness and rebound pain at McBurney's point.

Case 1.2

Miss L.S. is a 15-year-old girl, followed in this practice since she was child. She presents with a 1-week history of vague, bilateral lower abdominal pain that began after a particularly heavy menstrual period. These symptoms have worsened over the past week and are exacerbated with movement. She has a 2-day history of nausea and low-grade fever, and she vomited once this morning. She has also noted a yellow vaginal discharge. On physical examination, her patient's temperature is 100.4°F and her pulse is 94. There is bilateral lower abdominal tenderness with minimal guarding and no rebound. The pelvic examination shows a yellow cervical discharge and tenderness with motion of the cervix. The adnexa are tender bilaterally, and no masses are appreciated.

Subacute but Progressive and Medically Serious Process

Case 2.1

Mrs. L. R. is a 60-year-old woman with a 20-year history of diabetes mellitus who presents with a 4-month history of abdominal pain. At first, the pain appeared to be primarily epigastric. She treated herself with antacids for a week and seemed to improve. A few weeks later, however, she noted that she frequently got a distended feeling after meals, and that this feeling of fullness took several hours to go away. This was occasionally accompanied by a discomfort in her abdomen. In addition, she reports a 5-pound weight loss and a decrease in the caliber of her stools. Abdominal examination shows normal bowel sounds, no masses, and a stool that is negative for occult blood.

Chronic Yet Medically Important Process

Case 3.1

Mrs. E.G. presents with a 2-month history of intermittent abdominal pain. The pain is burning, located in the upper half of the abdomen, and appears worse before meals and late at night. Meals tend to improve these symptoms, although certain foods—such as cabbage, onions, and spicy foods—aggravate the pain. Ten years ago, she was diagnosed as having peptic ulcer disease and took antacids for about 6 months. Since then she has had several episodes of similar discomfort, which went away in a month or two on antacids. Recently she has had to fill in for her supervisor at work, who quit unexpectedly; this has resulted in unusual stress. She also has a 14-year-old daughter who is argumentative and who "hangs out with the wrong crowd," creating conflict at home. There is no history of melena or vomiting.

Case 3.2

Mrs. J.S. is a 34-year-old G_0P_0 married woman with a 4- to 5-year history of pelvic pain. This midline low abdominal pain begins 1-week prior to her menses and can be quite disabling, keeping her from her usual occupation as a nurse. This pain is referred to the low back and rectum. She experiences dyspareunia with deep penetration. She reports having suffered from mild to moderate dysmenorrhea since menarche. She has no prior history of gynecologic illnesses or surgery and has used no birth control for 2 years.

Self-limited Illness That Will Require No Further Investigations

Case 4.1

Mr. A.G. is a 23-year-old medical student with a 4-year history of intermittent abdominal pain. The pain is crampy and occurs in episodes lasting hours to days, separated by weeks or months when he is asymptomatic. Emotional stress and certain foods (spicy meals, cabbage, and green peppers, by history) bring on the pain, which is occasionally followed or accompanied by diarrhea without blood or visible mucus. His general health is excellent. Physical examination is normal.

CLINICAL HISTORY

The history of a patient who presents with pain should explore seven different aspects of that pain: quality, quantity, location and radiation, duration and timing, remissions and exacerbations, setting, and associated signs and symptoms. Each of these seven aspects of pain is important and potentially crucial in determining the cause of abdominal pain. Pain localization merits special consideration, as it immediately helps focus the rest of the history and examination.

Epigastric pain usually originates from one of the structures derived from the embryologic foregut; i.e., esophagus, stomach, duodenum, liver, gallbladder, pancreas, and spleen. However, pneumonia and inferior wall myocardial infarction can also present as epigastric pain. Early pathology involving these organs may present with a vague epigastric discomfort. As the disease progresses, symptoms typical for the specific disease entity appear. For example, a patient with pancreatitis may initially complain of a vague epigastric pain. Later the same patient will give the classic description of a severe, unrelenting epigastric pain that bores straight through to the back. Liver and gallbladder pain usually localize to the right upper quadrant, splenic pain to the left.

Periumbilical pain usually originates from those structures derived from the embryologic midgut, i.e., jejunum, ileum, appendix, and ascending colon. Inflammation, ischemia, spasm, or abnormal distension of these structures all present with periumbilical pain.

Infraumbilical (lower abdominal) pain generally originates either from (*a*) those structures derived from the embryologic hindgut; i.e., the descending colon, sigmoid colon, and rectum; or (*b*) midline genitourinary structures; i.e., bladder, uterus, and prostate. Men and women present very different diagnostic considerations in lower abdominal pain. Since urinary tract infections are less common in men and since the testes and epididymides are outside the abdominal cavity, the anatomical considerations of the causes of abdominal pain in men are more limited, with pathology of the prostate being the only special consideration. Causes are more complicated in women because the reproductive structures are intraabdominal, and pathology, especially infection, of the genitourinary tract is far more common.

Lateralized pain can have many causes. Local inflammation of either the skin or peritoneum causes pain at the point of irritation. Irritation of the posterior peritoneum lateralizes less precisely than that of the anterior peritoneum. Acute appendicitis is an excellent example of this distinction. An inflamed appendix irritating the anterior peritoneum gives classic right lower quadrant pain. A retrocecal appendix that irritates the posterior peritoneum causes vague right-sided pain. Pain arising in paired organs is lateralized; the main ones to be considered are the kidneys, ureters, fallopian tubes, and gonads.

Generalized pain originates from diffuse inflammation of the gastrointestinal (GI) tract, peritoneum, or abdominal wall. Diffuse peritoneal irritation from either bacterial infection or blood in the peritoneal cavity gives generalized pain, as does viral gastroenteritis involving the entire alimentary canal. Generalized pain can be confused with more localized pain in patients who have difficulty communicating. For instance, a young child when asked, "Where do you hurt?" might reply "all over." Further questions such as "Show me where you hurt most?" or "Does it hurt more above or below your belly-button?" will often more accurately locate the pain.

Screening questions that cover the respiratory, cardiac, gastrointestinal, genitourinary, and musculoskeletal systems are often necessary to pin down a precise diagnosis. A thorough (and nonjudgmental) sexual history is needed to identify risk factors for pregnancy (intrauterine or ectopic), sexually transmitted diseases, and birth control use (i.e., use of an IUD places the woman at higher risk for PID, while barrier methods are protective). It is advisable to conduct at least this portion of the history without a parent, partner, or other friend or family present, to obtain the most accurate information possible. If you develop the habit of seeing preadolescent children without a parent or guardian present, the patient and family will be accustomed to this habit before you are likely to need to take a sexual history.

The psychological history should be carefully assessed. Psychosexual concerns may need to be explored, since abdominal pain is a common presenting symptom in patients with sexual problems, sexual trauma, or abuse. Also, somatizing patients (see Chapter 38) often present with abdominal pain or some form of gastrointestinal distress.

Finally, assessing the urgency of the clinical condition by history is essential. Possible red flags in the history that suggest a life-threatening condition are listed in Table 25.1. The potential mechanisms of death are exsanguination, overwhelming sepsis, and profound volume depletion. Patients at special risk for life-threatening illnesses are those with chronic medical problems (e.g., diabetes mellitus), the immunocompromised, the very young, and the very old.

PHYSICAL EXAMINATION

The dual task of both finding the cause of the abdominal pain and assessing the urgency of the presentation continues into the physical examination. The vital signs and general appearance of the patient are especially important in assessing the severity of the problem. Fever usually implies infection, but note that in the elderly, sepsis may present as hypothermia instead. Tachycardia, while nonspecific, may be important as a signal of volume-depletion or sepsis. Supine hypotension occurs only in profoundly volume-depleted or septic patients. Postural hypotension is a more sensitive indicator of volume depletion; a persistent rise in pulse rate on standing is even more sensitive. Tachypnea may be a clue to sepsis, acidosis, or pneumonia. The heart and lungs should always be examined when the complaint is abdominal pain, as should the skin. The physician's global assessment that the patient has a "toxic appearance" or is a "sick kid" is an important and perhaps critical observation.

When starting the abdominal examination, have the patient point to the painful area. Focal pain, as from abdominal wall lesions or focal peritoneal irritation, can often be localized with one finger. Visceral pain is usually indicated with a spread palm.

A thorough abdominal examination includes inspection, auscultation, percussion, and palpation. Palpation is especially important, with focal tenderness or rebound tenderness being two crucial findings. Always start with gentle, light palpation and progress to deeper palpation. Focal

Table 25.1. "Red Flag" Symptoms and Signs of Abdominal Emergencies

Symptoms	Hematemesis
	Rectal bleeding or melena
	Progressive abdominal distention
	Progressive intractable vomiting
	Prostration
	Light-headedness on standing
	Acute onset of pain
	Pain progresses in intensity over hours
Signs	Shock
	Fever
	Orthostatic hypotension
	Rebound tenderness
	Severe tenderness
	Leukocytosis and granulocytosis
	Decreased urine output

tenderness, like the location of pain discussed in the history, implicates certain organs as the source of pathology.

Sometimes the examination will pinpoint the patient's pain more precisely than did the history. For example, a patient with gallbladder pathology may perceive only epigastric discomfort but on examination have focal tenderness in the right upper quadrant and a positive Murphy's sign. Focal tenderness may point to a specific diagnosis as, for example, costovertebral angle tenderness usually implies pyelonephritis. At other times it is another useful but nonspecific finding (e.g., epigastric tenderness has many possible causes).

Rebound tenderness and involuntary guarding specifically imply peritoneal irritation. Some causes are potentially life-threatening, so urgent assessment is needed for all patients with rebound tenderness. Peritoneal irritation may be focal as in nonruptured appendicitis, or general as in bacterial peritonitis. Blood is an irritant in the peritoneal cavity; hemorrhage, as in ruptured ectopic pregnancy, should be considered in the diagnostic evaluation of patients with rebound tenderness.

Pelvic and rectal examinations are important in the workup of patients with abdominal pain. (Remember to introduce these examinations in a sensitive manner, especially to a young patient who may not have prior experience). Both examinations can demonstrate abnormal masses and focal tenderness (e.g., cervical and uterine tenderness in cases of pelvic inflammatory disease), as well as vaginal or rectal bleeding or discharge. The rectal examination also allows the opportunity to test stool for occult blood.

LABORATORY ASSESSMENT

Urinalysis, complete blood count (CBC), and urine pregnancy test (UCG) are immediately available in most family physicians' offices to aid in the initial workup of patients presenting with abdominal pain. The urinalysis is an excellent screen for such conditions as cystitis, pyelonephritis, and renal calculi. In women who are obese, menstruating, or who have a vaginal discharge, catheterization may be needed to yield interpretable results. Appropriate cultures of the urine and cervix can be obtained on the initial visit, but the results will not be immediately available.

The CBC is helpful in diagnosing hemorrhage and infection. Chronic blood loss often results in a low hemoglobin level. The hemoglobin level may

be deceptively normal in acute blood loss, however. The white blood cell count (WBC) and differential are often helpful in diagnoses. For instance, moderate leukocytosis with granulocytosis supports the diagnosis of appendicitis rather than viral gastroenteritis. Note, however, that leukocytosis by itself is highly nonspecific. Noninfectious physiological stresses can produce a leukemoid reaction. Also, severe intraabdominal infections are sometimes unaccompanied by any abnormalities of the white count; so physicians should be cautious about relying too heavily on this single piece of information.

Tubal pregnancy and other pregnancy complications should be considered in all women of childbearing age who present with abdominal pain. Consider getting a UCG on any such patient in whom the diagnosis is not clear from the history and examination, whether or not the possibility of pregnancy is acknowledged by the patient. Be cautious about obtaining x-ray films in patients who may be pregnant.

Imaging techniques should be used selectively and critically in patients with abdominal pain. Plain abdominal x-ray films should be ordered to seek specific signs whose presence is already suspected, such as air under a diaphragm or a stone in the ureter, not as a general screening test. The mere presence of severe abdominal pain is not an indication for an x-ray film. Note that imaging by ultrasound reveals many structures not shown by plain x-ray films, and has the advantage of being safe in pregnancy.

The history, physical examination, and tests detailed above are nearly always sufficient to enable the physician to make the initial, critical decision: whether to send the patient home or to admit the patient for observation.

DEVELOPING A DIFFERENTIAL DIAGNOSIS

As you gather information from the history, physical examination, and the laboratory, you should be developing and refining a differential diagnosis. Because the possibilities are numerous, you must constantly review and reevaluate the possible diagnosis. Table 25.2 lists important causes of abdominal pain.

In developing your differential diagnosis, try to identify what organ seems to be involved. Often, your physical examination will isolate an area that clearly appears tender and contains only one or

Table 25.2. Some Important Causes of Abdominal Pain

Gastrointestinal causes
  Hepatic: trauma, abscess, hepatitis° passive congestion°
  Biliary: acute cholecystitis°, ascending cholangitis, biliary colic
  Stomach: peptic ulcer disease°, tumor, obstruction, gastritis caused by alcohol or medications°
  Duodenal: peptic ulcer disease°, obstruction, rupture secondary to blunt trauma
  Jejunal or ileal: viral gastroenteritis°, giardiasis°, obstruction, Crohn's disease, infarction, intussusception
  Colon: irritable bowel syndrome°, obstruction, diverticulitis°, carcinoma, ulcerative colitis, volvulus, infection, appendicitis°
  Mesenteric: mesenteric lymphadenitis, mesenteric thrombosis
  Pancreatic: acute or chronic pancreatitis, neoplasm

Musculoskeletal causes
  Spine: radiculitis from arthritis, fracture, osteomyelitis
  Muscular: hernia°, hematoma, strain°, wound abscess

Thoracic causes
  Cardiac: myocardial infarction (especially if it involves the inferior wall), angina, pericarditis
  Pulmonary: pneumonia, pleurisy, pulmonary embolism

Psychogenic causes
  Depression, hypochondriasis, anxiety, school phobia, sexual dysfunction, other somatizing patients (see Chapter 38)

Neurogenic causes
  Tabes dorsalis, herpes zoster, causalgia

Vascular causes
  Aorta: aneurysm, dissection, rupture
  Spleen: infarction, rupture secondary to trauma

Urinary tract causes
  Kidney: tumor, pyelonephritis°, perinephric abscess
  Ureter: stone°
  Bladder: urinary tract infection°, distension secondary to outlet obstruction°, rupture secondary to trauma

Dermatologic causes
  Herpes zoster, cellulitis, trauma

Genital causes
  Male: prostatitis, contusion or torsion of testes
  Female:
    Ovary: cyst°, torsion, tumor
    Fallopian tube: ectopic pregnancy, tubovarian abscess, pelvic inflammatory disease°
    Uterus: pelvic inflammatory disease°, torsion of fibroid, dysmenorrhea°, mittelschmerz°

Other causes
  Uremia, porphyria, lead poisoning, black widow spider bite

°A common cause in primary care settings.

two structures. Do remember, however, that the abdominal wall musculature and ribs can also lead to abdominal pain. Also recognize that referred pain is common in visceral structures, although tenderness is rarely referred.

In addition, carefully review the history because you may be observing an evolving condition. For example, sudden sharp pain in the pelvis, which becomes more generalized, could indicate rupture of an ectopic pregnancy or an ovarian cyst. On the other hand, an appendicitis that ruptures is generally reported as pain that gets better for a period of time. Keep in mind that the common causes of chronic pain differ from those whose time course is acute. Causes of chronic abdominal pain are listed in Table 25.3.

From what you can learn about the anatomical location of the problem, about the time course of the illness, and about the likely causes, given the patient's age and past history, your differential diagnosis will take shape. Always look carefully for surgical problems (e.g., ectopic pregnancy, appen-

Table 25.3. Causes of Chronic or Recurrent Abdominal Pain

Relatively common
  Peptic ulcer disease
  Irritable bowel syndrome
  Recurrent urinary tract infections
  Recurrent pelvic inflammatory disease
  Cholelithiasis (prior to cholecystectomy)
  Ovarian cyst
  Endometriosis
  Adhesions[a]

Relatively rare
  Crohn's disease
  Ulcerative colitis
  Chronic pancreatitis
  Chronic or recurrent hepatitis
  Malabsorption syndromes
  Diverticulitis
  Parasitic diseases
  Porphyria
  Sickle cell anemia
  Nephrolithiasis or ureterolithiasis

[a]It remains controversial as to whether adhesions cause pain. The authors believe they are a cause of pain, but would urge caution in applying this diagnosis.

dicitis, colon cancer), because these often do not present in the classical way and can be overlooked unless specifically considered.

For patients with clinical problems that suggest potential acute and/or life-threatening illnesses, appropriate specialists should be involved at the earliest possible moment. Depending on the precise nature of the illness, consultation or referral to a general surgeon, gynecologist, urologist, or gastroenterologist may be necessary. Each of these specialists offers unique procedural skills and cognitive knowledge that may be needed in caring for certain patients. A consultant involved early has the opportunity to help coordinate and expedite patient management and observe the patient's signs and symptoms as they evolve over time.

CASE DISCUSSION

Case 1.1. Acute Appendicitis
Acute appendicitis usually begins with obstruction of the appendix by fecal material or with inflammatory swelling of its walls. This inflammation and obstruction of the appendix causes distension. As the appendix is embryologically a midgut structure, its distension produces poorly localized, periumbilical pain. Anorexia, vomiting, low-grade fever, and a moderately elevated white count with a left shift are typically present. On examination at this stage, re-

bound tenderness is absent, but the patient may have focal periumbilical or right lower quadrant tenderness.

As the inflammation progresses to involve the serosal surface of the appendix, focal peritoneal irritation occurs. Physical findings depend on the anatomical location of the appendix. An inflamed anterior appendix gives classic right lower quadrant pain with rebound tenderness. If the appendix is posterior (retrocecal),there may be no rebound tenderness, but there may be a positive psoas sign (pain on hip extension due to irritation of the psoas by the overlying appendix) or exquisite tenderness on deep rectal examination. Loss of appetite and vomiting are almost universal at this stage.

If the appendicitis continues untreated, the inflamed appendix will rupture, contaminating the abdominal cavity. Rupture may briefly relieve some of the patient's pain as the distended appendix decompresses. Pain quickly returns, however, as peritoneal infection and inflammation ensue. If the omentum walls off the infection, focal peritoneal findings persist. If the infection is not quickly walled off, generalized peritonitis with generalized rebound tenderness occurs. The patient now has evidence of systemic toxicity, and the diagnosis of an acute abdomen, requiring immediate hospitalization, is obvious.

Case 1.2. Pelvic Inflammatory Disease
Pelvic inflammatory disease (PID) usually refers to an ascending infection of the uterus, fallopian tubes, and broad ligaments. The diagnosis of acute PID can be difficult and must be differentiated from other causes of acute pelvic pain, such as ectopic pregnancy, acute appendicitis, urinary tract infections, and complications of ovarian cysts. Acute PID is almost exclusively a disease of sexually-active women. Important risk factors include; age between 15 and 25 years, a previous history of PID, the use of an intrauterine device, multiple sex partners, or a male partner with symptoms of urethritis. The risk of acute PID is decreased in patients on oral contraceptives as well as those using barrier methods of contraception.

Acute PID typically presents as vague, dull midline abdominal pain caused by endometritis or bilateral lower abdominal and pelvic pain caused by salpingitis. The onset of gonoccocal PID is typically more acute than that of chlamydial PID, although both are often associated with an abnormally heavy menses. Patients may also present with generalized abdominal pain caused by peritonitis or right upper quadrant pain caused by perihepatitis. The pain may be associated with nausea, vomiting, or abnormal vaginal bleeding or discharge.

On physical examination, evidence of a fever and orthostatic changes must be noted. Look for peritoneal signs on abdominal examination. Mucopurulent cervical discharge and cervicitis are common findings on pelvic examination. Cervical motion tenderness (Chandelier sign) is common, but not specific for pelvic inflammatory disease. Bimanual examination will often show uterine fundal tenderness, secondary to endometritis, and adnexal tenderness, secondary to salpingitis, which is usually but not always bilateral. A patient with an adnexal mass or fullness must be further evaluated, with ultrasound. Many women with acute PID will have an elevated white count on CBC, or an elevated erythrocyte sedimentation rate, but the absence of these findings should not rule out acute PID. Microscopic examination of a saline wet mount preparation showing inflammatory cells will also support the diagnosis. A Gram's stained smear of endocervical secretions may show Gram-negative intracellular diplococci, strongly suggesting, but not diagnostic of, a gonococcal infection.

Once a diagnosis of acute pelvic inflammatory disease has been made, treatment should be instituted immediately, without waiting for the return of cultures. The most common etiologic organisms are *Neisseria gonorrhoeae* and *Chlamydia trachomatis*, but treatment must also cover anerobic organisms, Gram-negative enteric pathogens, and genital mycoplasmas. Pregnancy must first be ruled out, and then the decision of whether or not to hospitalize must be made. If the patient is afebrile and can take p.o. medications and fluids, outpatient management is appropriate. The current Centers for Disease Control guidelines advise treatment with Ceftriaxone 250 mg IM (single dose) followed by doxycycline 100 mg b.i.d. for 14 days. Indications to hospitalize include noncompliance as an outpatient, pregnancy, peritonitis, suspected pelvic abscess, temperature greater than 38°C, or failure to respond as an outpatient in 72 hours. These patients and those with underlying medical problems are especially susceptible to sepsis and rarely, death. If hospitalized, treat with Cefoxitin and doxycycline or clindamcyin and gentamicin.

It is essential that the patient receive education in the prevention of sexually transmitted disease and in contraception. It is also imperative that the partner(s) be treated, and that the patient be told to return if symptoms do not improve over the next few days, otherwise within 1 to 2 weeks for repeat cultures.

This case demonstrates the importance of establishing a confidential, nonjudgmental relationship with the young patient with pelvic pain. A trusting environment will enable the physician to obtain information about the patient's sexual activity, birth control use, prior history of gynecologic illness, as well as discerning a history of sexual abuse. This can be an emotionally charged experience for the young patient, especially if this is her first pelvic examination. The timely diagnosis and management of PID is essential, to avoid the long-term complications of chronic pelvic pain and infertility.

Case 2.1. Carcinoma of the Colon

Cancer of the colon is largely a silent disease in its early stages, and by the time abdominal pain develops the disease is often advanced. Pain tends to develop when constriction of the bowel opening makes it difficult for stool to pass through. A gradual partial bowel obstruction develops, characterized by bloating and abdominal discomfort. Other presenting symptoms include weight loss, tiredness due to anemia, and visible blood in stool. Prevention and early detection are the current best hope for decreasing morbidity and mortality from this disease. There is evidence that risk factor modification by eating a low-fat high-fiber diet is prudent for decreasing colon and rectal cancer risk. Both sigmoidoscopy and occult blood testing of stool are recommended as routine screening measures for carcinoma of the colon. This recommendation by the American Cancer Society is not universally accepted.

Prevention and early detection can result in surgical cure. Unfortunately, cancers detected by the time they become symptomatic have poor survival rates. Comprehensive and continuous care, especially in the asymptomatic or minimally symptomatic patient, is the best hope for decreasing the morbidity and mortality of colon and rectal cancer.

Case 3.1. Peptic Ulcer Disease

An acutely bleeding gastric or duodenal ulcer may cause life-threatening exsanguination. This dramatic presentation is uncommon. Far more often patients present with a group of symptoms that are generally termed dyspeptic or acid-related. These symptoms may include:

- A burning or gnawing epigastric discomfort that is relieved by food or antacids;
- Symptoms increasing with an empty stomach or the ingestion of GI irritants such as aspirin, alcohol, or coffee;
- Pain most often severe in the late afternoon or late at night.

Often symptoms are insidious in onset and progressive over weeks or months.

These characteristic dyspepsic symptoms usually suggest the diagnosis of "peptic disease." Peptic disease is common, with duodenal ulcers having a population prevalence of 6 to 15%. Ulcers are a recurrent problem, with 60% of healed duodenal ulcers recurring after 1 year, and 80 to 90% after 2 years. Many external factors such as medications, alcohol, tobacco, stress, and diet can affect the frequency and severity of the patient's illness.

Diagnosis of peptic disease often does not require diagnostic testing. The majority of such patients who present early will not have ulcers evident on upper gastrointestinal x-ray examinations. Instead, they will have gastritis, esophagitis, or duodenitis. Such conditions can be diagnosed by gastrointestinal endoscopy, but they are better off being treated presumptively if the history is suggestive. Place such patients on antacids, H2-blocking agents, or both, and reevaluate them in 2 to 4 weeks. If their symptoms are gone, tapering the medication over weeks to months is all that is needed. In those whose symptoms do not resolve, x-ray or endoscopy evaluation must be considered. As part of the initial workup, however, do obtain three stool specimens for occult blood and check for anemia.

Appropriate care of this common, chronic problem should be multifaceted to be effective. Appropriate diet modification, including abstinence from alcohol and tobacco, is important. Cautioning the patient about medications such as aspirin and nonsteroidal antiinflammatory drugs is necessary. The physician should explain the role that stress plays in the illness and offer either stress reduction or lifestyle modification strategies. Prophylactic regimens such as long-term H2-blockade will reduce recurrences. Finally, prompt recognition and early treatment of recurrences are needed to prevent life-threatening complications.

Of patients with peptic symptoms seen in primary care, most have gastritis, esophagitis, or duodenitis rather than a frank peptic ulcer. The exact diagnosis is unimportant as long as the patient improves with treatment; so, many family physicians treat such patients based on the history and physical (including a stool for occult blood) and perhaps a serum hemoglobin or hematocrit. Only those who fail to respond to therapy within about 4 weeks receive endoscopy or upper gastrointestinal radiography.

Case 3.2 Endometriosis

Endometriosis is characterized by the development of ectopic endometrial tissue outside the uterus. Although it is a chronic, nonprogressive disease, it is an important cause of chronic pain and infertility. Endometriosis occurs most commonly between the ages of 30 and 40 but can exist at any age after menarche and before menopause. It has been estimated to occur in 5 to 15% of women of reproductive age in the general population and in 30 to 50% of women undergoing surgery for infertility. It most often presents as chronic pelvic pain occurring just prior to and during the menses. Other symptoms include dyspareunia, pain with defecation, and infertility. There is little correlation between the severity of pain symptoms and the extent of disease.

Physical examination may show a fixed uterus, tender nodularity along the uterosacral ligaments or enlarged cystic ovaries. The diagnosis is confirmed by direct visualization, usually diagnostic laparoscopy. Treatment is determined by the patient's

degree of pain, desire for fertility, extent of disease, and results of previous therapy. Treatment options include observation (of mild disease with no associated pain or infertility), hormonal suppressive therapy (moderate disease), conservative surgery (if fertility is desired), or total hysterectomy and bilateral salpingo-oophorectomy.

Evaluation of chronic pelvic pain can be quite challenging for the physician. A complete and careful medical, social, and sexual history with an excellent physical examination is of primary importance. The laparoscopic examination is most important in women with pelvic pain in the same location for at least 6 months. About one-third of these women will have a normal pelvis, one-third will have endometriosis, and one-third will have adhesions. The correlation of these findings with the degree of pain and the response of the pain to treatment is not clear. Several studies report a history of major psychosexual trauma (i.e., rape, incest, childhood sexual abuse) in 20 to 48% of women with chronic pelvic pain.

In women with chronic pelvic pain, an organic cause is often not determined, and if it is, therapy does not often effect resolution of the pain. An integrated approach from the beginning, which includes attention to psychosocial and sexual factors as well as a careful physical evaluation, has been shown to be more effective in reduction of pain than a traditional solely medical approach. Patients with a history of major psychosexual trauma must be referred for appropriate therapy.

Case 4. Irritable Bowel Syndrome

Irritable bowel syndrome (IBS) is an excellent example of a chronic, benign condition in which medical urgency is not a factor in the diagnostic and treatment decision making. IBS is common, with an estimated prevalence of 32% in the general population (1). IBS is a heterogeneous group of disorders that can present with esophageal, gastric, or colonic symptoms. Various synonyms have arisen, such as spastic colon or irritable colon. Typical symptoms are (a) abdominal pain, either cramps or a feeling of distension, usually relieved by defecation; and (b) episodes of frequent, loose bowel movements, sometimes alternating with periods of constipation, and including passage of mucus with the stool. On examination, the descending colon may be palpable and tender, or there may be no abnormal findings at all. In a young person, such a clinical picture is very unlikely to signal serious disease; presumptive diagnosis of IBS may be made and an appropriate treatment plan begun. Only if the patient does not respond, or if new symptoms develop, do laboratory tests or special procedures such as sigmoidoscopy need to be performed. Often the decision to perform such tests does not follow from the physician's concern to rule out other diagnoses, but on the patient's need for reassurance of the absence of serious disease.

Management of IBS involves educating the patient to self-manage the symptoms and to observe what the particular precipitating and relieving factors are in his or her own case. The symptomatic management is by dietary modifications, which varies in effectiveness from one patient to another, and the cautious use of antispasmodics during severe exacerbations. Stress plays an important role in flare-ups of IBS. Psychosocial factors causing exacerbations of symptoms, such as job or family conflict, must be identified and dealt with. Over time, the recurrence of symptoms may signal deeper issues such as depression, unresolved grief, or family dysfunction, which are more important to attend to than the abdominal symptoms. Patients respond well to this comprehensive and continuous approach to their medical care. Patients are rarely completely cured, but over time symptoms are markedly reduced, and the patient deals more appropriately and effectively with the symptoms when they do appear.

CONCLUSIONS

Abdominal pain is a common presenting symptom in ambulatory patients. As with most medical problems, a thorough history and physical examination is the first and most important step in formulating a diagnostic and therapeutic plan. A few common office laboratory tests are helpful in the initial evaluation. Physicians should be vigilant about signs and symptoms that suggest possible acute/life-threatening illnesses. Patients with nonurgent problems require a timely and cost-effective treatment. For patients with chronic or recurrent problems, the principles of comprehensive and continuous care should be followed.

REFERENCE

1. McLeod ME: Irritable bowel syndrome. *NC Med J* 47:245, 1986.

SUGGESTED READINGS

Braunwald E, Isselbacher KJ, Petersdorf RG, Wilson JD, Martin JB, Fauci AS: *Harrison's Principles of Internal Medicine*, ed 11. New York, McGraw-Hill, 1987, pp 23–26, 1223–1384.

Pages 23-26 provide a good general description of the evaluation of abdominal pain. Pages 1223-1384 provide more in-depth descriptions of the individual diseases.

DeGowin EL: DeGowin and DeGowin's *Bedside Diagnostic Examination*, ed 5. New York, Macmillan, 1987.

This physical diagnosis text exhaustively lists historical and physical findings in patients with abdominal complaints. An excellent reference text for referring to the physical findings of specific diseases.

Guyton AC: *Textbook of Medical Physiology*, ed 8. Philadelphia, WB Saunders, 1991.

A good discussion of the physiological pain sensors in and about the abdomen.

Kresch AJ, Seifer DB, Sach LB, et al.: Laparoscopy in 100 women with chronic pelvic pain. *Obstet Gynecol* 64(5):672–674, 1984.

McLeod ME: Irritable bowel syndrome. *NC Med J* 47:245–248, 1986.

An excellent summary of irritable bowel syndrome, which is probably the most common cause of abdominal complaints in the family physician's office.

McWhinney IR: Problem-solving and decision making in family practice. *Can Fam Physician* 25:1473–1477, 1979.

A good discussion of the decision logic involved in caring for patients in an ambulatory setting. This decision analysis involves not just abdominal pain, but any of the clinical decisions made in ambulatory care.

Quan M: Diagnosis of acute pelvic pain. *J Fam Pract* 35:422–432, 1992.

A good review article on diagnosis of acute pelvic pain.

Roseff SJ, Murphy AA: Laparoscopy in the diagnosis and therapy of chronic pelvic pain. *Clin Obstet Gynecol* 33(1):137-144, 1990.

Rakel RE: *Textbook of Family Practice*, ed 3. Philadelphia, WB Saunders, 1984, pp 998–1035.

Taylor RB: *Family Medicine: Principles and Practice*, ed 3. New York, Springer-Verlag, 1988, pp 1446–1453.

Rakel's and Taylor's textbooks are the most widely accepted general texts for family practice. They both have excellent discussions of the diagnosis and treatment of abdominal pain. The discussion in Rakel is more extensive.

chapter 26

DIZZINESS

Philip D. Sloane and John Dallara

Dizziness is one of those vague symptoms that makes family physicians anxious. This anxiety arises because in dizzy patients a specific diagnosis is difficult to make and serious problems hard to rule out. Usually, dizziness has a benign cause, but it occasionally represents a life-threatening, progressive, and treatable process. Because it has many different possible causes spanning a spectrum from the self-limited to the life-threatening, dizziness represents a diagnostic and therapeutic challenge. However, familiarity with common diagnoses and the use of a systematic evaluation can make this symptom less anxiety-provoking for the family physician.

The spectrum of problems presenting with dizziness depends largely on the practice setting and the age of the patient. Data from community surveys suggest that dizziness significant enough to result in a physician visit or which interferes with daily life has occurred in approximately one-third of all individuals by age 65 and nearly half of all individuals by about age 80. The frequency of dizziness increases with age, as does the likelihood that it represents a disabling progressive disease. According to the National Ambulatory Medical Care Survey, dizziness is the third most common complaint of patients 65 and older in family physicians' offices (1), and it is the most common presenting complaint of patients aged 75 and older (2). Among patients with dizziness coming for routine visits to the offices of primary care physicians, chronic, non-life-threatening problems predominate. Among patients in acute settings, such as after-hours visits to family physicians, acute care ambulatory clinics, and emergency departments, the frequency of more life-threatening disorders is higher (although still representing fewer than 10% of all cases of dizziness).

Many referral specialists see dizzy patients, since dizziness can represent an underlying disorder of any number of body systems. The perspectives of such specialties as cardiology, neurology, and otolaryngology are helpful in understanding the range of diagnostic possibilities, but each specialist tends to overestimate the commonness of certain causes within his or her field and to overstate the need for early technological intervention. The natural history of dizziness in primary care is not well described, but more often than not, a complaint of dizziness should not cause undue alarm and haste on the part of the physician. Generally, the family physician can take a less aggressive approach, once the office evaluation has excluded rapidly progressing, life-threatening causes of dizziness.

MECHANISMS OF DIZZINESS

Dizziness is a subjective feeling experienced by the patient. It cannot be measured or quantitated, except by the patient's self report. Other words used to describe dizziness include giddiness, lightheadedness, "swimmy-headedness," falling sensation, a sense of imbalance, and vertigo. The various sensations that patients label as "dizziness" can arise from a variety of mechanisms. In general, dizziness results when there is an imbalance between the body's sensory input regarding position and movement and the brain's ability to sort out the information it receives. Dizziness can result from an isolated problem (one diagnosis) or from multiple factors.

Classically, dizziness occurs when there has been a disturbance in one of the three principal body systems that maintain equilibrium: the vestibular apparatus, the proprioceptive fibers, and the ocular system. The *vestibular system*, consisting of the semicircular canals, the saccule, and the utricle in the inner ear, their associated nuclei and connecting fibers, and the central portion of the cerebellum, provides the brain with sensory information on body position and rotation. Typically, a disruption in this system causes a sensation of spinning or of angular displacement, which we refer to as vertigo. Dysfunction of *proprioceptive fibers* in the facet joints of the neck, in the ankles, and in other bony joints, will interfere with the body's ability to judge its own position, leading to a variety of sensations, most prominent of which is disequilibrium. Many disturbances of the *ocular system* can lead to dizziness. A common example is the lightheadedness or disequilibrium that one gets when wearing new eyeglasses for the first time. Visual problems often contribute to dizziness, because the eyes can often be used to compensate (through visual fixation on stationary objects) when other systems (e.g., vestibular) are impaired.

Problems with other body systems can also result in dizziness. Loss of blood flow to the *cerebral cortex* typically results in a feeling of lightheadedness. Dysfunction of the *cerebellar cortex* and its connections causes a variety of sensations, which are generally associated with balance and coordination problems. Dizziness can also result from *peripheral nerve* dysfunction, usually only in the presence of multiple neuropathies or in concert with problems in other body systems. Finally *psychiatric and emotional* problems can present with dizziness through less well understood mechanisms.

One useful way to approach dizziness is to use the classification system developed by Drachman and Hart (3). That system seeks to categorize a patient's dizziness as vertigo, presyncopal lightheadedness, disequilibrium, or other. *Vertigo* is a sensation that the environment is spinning or of movement; this type of dizziness generally arises from disturbances of the vestibular system or of the middle ear. *Presyncopal lightheadedness* is the type of dizziness that makes one feel as though one were about to faint. It typically results from diminished circulation to the cerebral cortex and implies a cardiovascular cause such as postural hypotension or a cardiac arrhythmia. *Disequilibrium* is a dizziness sensation in which imbalance predominates; neurological and multisensory causes most often produce this sensation. *Other* sensations cannot be attributed to a single mechanism, but psychological causes (such as anxiety) do frequently cause dizziness sensations that are difficult to describe.

Unfortunately, the subtypes of dizziness that we have just described do not work as reliably in practice as one would like. Many patients, particularly the elderly, have difficulty describing their sensations or describe a combination of symptoms. Furthermore, terms such as vertigo, disequilibrium, or dizziness carry different meanings from patient to patient, and even from doctor to doctor. For example, the term vertigo is used in medical textbooks to describe a rotatory dizziness, with either the environment or the individual appearing to spin. Authors have generally described a narrower differential diagnosis for "vertigo" than for "dizziness," and the distinction is often useful. However, in practice it is often difficult to be sure whether the patient is describing "true vertigo" or some other sensation. Also, in clinical practice the classical causes of "vertigo" sometimes present with the patient complaining of another sensation, such as imbalance or nausea. Thus, the separation of dizziness complaints into pathophysiological types must be approached with caution.

Epidemiology of Dizziness

The possible causes of dizziness are numerous; Table 26.1 summarizes many of the causes that primary care physicians will encounter. Table 26.1 includes symbols that identify causes that are particularly common in young, middle-aged, and geriatric patients. It must be emphasized, however, that reliable epidemiologic data from the primary care setting are largely absent from the medical literature. Instead, family physicians must base their estimates on the likelihood of diagnoses largely on experience and on inferences drawn from studies performed in other settings.

One of the best-known studies from specialty settings was conducted in a dizziness clinic jointly run by the neurology and otolaryngology departments at Northwestern University (3). That clinic largely treated patients with chronic dizziness and, therefore, only partially represents what is seen in primary care. Each patient received a detailed evaluation, including a battery of physical, diagnostic, biochemical, and occasionally more technological tests. In that study, anxiety and hyperventilation were the most common causes of dizziness in young adults, and vestibular problems most common in the middle-aged. In addition, the authors popularized the concept

Table 26.1. Reported Causes of Dizziness

Systemic viral infection
#*+Influenza
  Gastroenteritis
  Upper respiratory infection
#*+Other viral infections
Bacterial infection
  Otitis media
  +Sinusitis
  Syphilis
  Arachnoiditis/meningitis
Drug toxicity and poisonings
#*+Medications: phenytoin, barbiturates, aminoglycosides,
    quinine, cocaine, nitroglycerin, sedative/hypnotics,
    antidepressants, antihypertensives
  Vitamin A toxicity
  Carbon monoxide
  #Alcohol
  Lead, arsenic
Metabolic problems
  Diabetes mellitus
  Thiamine/niacin deficiency
  Hypothyroidism
  Hypoglycemia
  Azotemia
  Hyperparathyroidism
Central nervous system—neurological
  Traumatic head injury
  Seizure (temporal lobe, partial complex, petit mal)
  Parkinson's disease
  Multiple sclerosis
  Cerebellar degeneration
  Subdural hematoma
  Acoustic neuroma
  Cerebellar tumors
  Other mass lesions (meningioma, metastatic tumors,
    arachnoid cyst)
Central nervous system—vascular
#*Migraine
+Vertebrobasilar insufficiency
+Stroke (several syndromes)
  Cerebral aneurysm

Peripheral neurological disease
+Cervical vertigo
  Peripheral neuropathy
+Multiple sensory deficits
  Syringobulbia
Psychological conditions
#Hyperventilation
#*Anxiety (including panic disorder)
#*+Depression
  Excessive awareness of normal sensations
    (somatization)
Cardiac disease
  Myocardial infarction
  Arrhythmia
  Congestive heart failure
  Hypertrophic subaortic stenosis
  Valvular disease
Otologic diseases
*+Neurolabyrinthitis
  Ménière's disease
  Semicircular canal hemorrhage
  Perilymphatic fistula
  Postural vertigo
*+Benign paroxysmal positional vertigo
#*Serous otitis media/sinusitis
  Cerumen impacted against tympanic
    smembrane
*+Labyrinthine disease (unspecified)
Ocular disturbances
  Post cataracts
  New bifocals
  Extraocular muscle imbalance (diplopia)
  Refractory disturbances
  Abnormal optokinetic stimulation
Other
  Hypertension
  Cough syncope
  Sarcoidosis
  Cogan's syndrome
  Paget's disease
  Bell's palsy

aKey—Common causes in: #young adults; *middle-aged adults; +geriatric patients.

that partial deficits in more than one sensory system could result in dizziness, especially in the elderly. They called this syndrome *multiple sensory deficits* and suggested that it was quite common in the elderly.

Three studies from emergency departments shed light on more acute causes of dizziness. One study reported 46 different diagnoses causing weakness and dizziness in 106 patients (91% of which were dizzy) (4). The common diagnoses in that study included medications, viral illness, depression, anxiety, and labyrinthine vertigo. Another emergency department study looked at 121 patients with dizziness. The most common final

diagnoses included acute neurolabyrinthitis (13 patients), viral illness (11 patients), other peripheral vestibular problems (13 patients), and anemia (9 patients) (5). The third study reported 125 patients, identifying peripheral vestibular disorders (54 patients), cardiovascular causes (27 patients), and unknown causes (13 patients) as the most prevalent final diagnoses (6). More than one cause of dizziness was identified in 23 patients (18%).

The largest case series from a neurological consultation service suggests that psychogenic causes are common. That study reported 400 consecutive inpatients or outpatients referred for neurological consultation because of dizziness. About 25% of these were thought to have psychogenic causes. Among the others, the most common diagnoses were miscellaneous peripheral vestibular problems (154 patients) and vertigo arising from the brainstem and cerebellum (52 cases, most of which were due to vascular insufficiency or multiple sclerosis). There were nine central nervous system tumors in this series (7).

One published report from primary care offices utilized data from the National Ambulatory Medical Care Survey (8). That study confirmed that dizziness is common in primary care offices, that its frequency increases with patient age, and that it is more prevalent in women. It also demonstrated that 95% of patients were managed without referral. The unique epidemiology of the primary care office is exemplified by comparing hospitalization rates between the primary care office and the emergency department. Between 15 and 20% of emergency department patients with dizziness are reported to be admitted to the hospital; in contrast, fewer than 2% of primary care office patients with the same complaint are hospitalized (5, 6, 8).

Upon reviewing the available literature on causes of dizziness, several themes are apparent. First, many diagnoses, particularly those in the peripheral vestibular system, have overlapping categories and labels. Making a distinction between viral labyrinthitis, vestibular neuritis, miscellaneous peripheral syndromes, and even Ménière's disease is fuzzy and controversial. A number of other diagnoses are reported with widely different frequencies. In particular, hypertension, cerebral vascular insufficiency, and multiple sensory deficits are either overdiagnosed or underdiagnosed as causes of dizziness, depending on which author you read. All of which is to emphasize that the diagnosis of dizziness is often imprecise, no matter what the setting. In family practice, this imprecision should be accepted, and careful follow-up used to reassess your initial diagnosis.

It is clear that the majority of cases of dizziness seen in family practice are self-limited and benign, and that for many patients treatment is supportive rather than curative. There are, however, a large number of conditions that are life-threatening: acute hemorrhage, myocardial infarction, pneumonia and other systemic infections, aortic stenosis, cardiac arrhythmias, brain tumors, drug adverse effects, depression, neurosyphilis, and

stroke. Furthermore, the list of curable or highly treatable causes of dizziness is impressive, including: anemia, arrhythmias, cervical vertigo, cerumen against the tympanic membrane, otitis media, systemic infections, valvular and ischemic cardiac disease, migraine, neurosyphilis, perilymphatic fistula, subclavian steal, hypovolemia, adrenal insufficiency, diabetes and other metabolic problems, toxicity (e.g., vitamin A), drug adverse effects, anxiety, and depression.

APPROACH TO THE DIZZY PATIENT

The family physician can generally make a provisional diagnosis with a thorough history, physical examination, and a few selected tests. Often, the patient presents with a classical history, and the physical examination supports the diagnosis. When a specific diagnosis is not apparent, a general classification scheme can greatly assist in patient management by narrowing the range of possibilites.

Thus, the first tier of decision making is recognition of certain *classical syndromes*. Of the numerous syndromes that can be diagnosed during the history and physical, three are discussed here, benign paroxysmal positional vertigo, anxiety, and acute neurolabyrinthitis.

Benign Paroxysmal Positional Vertigo. Caused by loose otoconia or other anatomical disturbances in the vestibular end organ, this common cause of dizziness in middle-aged and older adults is characterized by sudden bursts of vertigo upon changes in body position or on head turning. Typically, the vertigo develops a few seconds after the movement and subsides within 30 seconds. Benign paroxysmal positional vertigo usually begins abruptly, with attacks becoming milder and less frequent as the weeks go by.

Anxiety. Two types of anxious patients present with dizziness. Young adults, who hyperventilate (often unknowingly) as part of general anxiety problems, present with a history of dizziness and recent life stress. Middle-aged and older adults, in whom dizziness is one of many symptoms and persists for years, often have underlying depression, consider themselves nervous, and complain of dizziness as part of an overall somatization syndrome.

Acute Neurolabyrinthitis. Sudden onset of vertigo, nausea, nystagmus, and vomiting characterizes this condition. The underlying pathology is partial or complete destruction of the vestibular and/or auditory components of the eighth nerve, either by a viral infection or by vascular occlusion. Some physicians call this condition *acute labyrinthitis* if hearing loss and tinnitus are present, and *vestibular neuronitis* if hearing is spared. Quite severe at onset, symptoms typically resolve within days to weeks but may persist longer in the elderly. Other causes of dizziness that can be diagnosed by the history and physical include viral infections, postural hypotension due to medication, serous otitis media, and cerumen against the tympanic membrane.

In the absence of a clearcut diagnosis, we have found it useful to employ a classification scheme that breaks the causes of dizziness into major categories based on the principal underlying cause of the symptoms (Table 26.2). For example, *central nervous system* causes of dizziness include a brainstem transient ischemic attack, a cerebellar lesion, migraine, a tumor, or a subdural hematoma. *Cardiovascular* causes range from a low-output state due to myocardial infarction to other less serious causes such as a simple faint. *Otologic causes* generally involve the vestibular system, the labyrinth, or the middle ear. *Peripheral nervous system* causes include autonomic and peripheral neuropathies, as well as disorders of proprioception. Dizziness due to *psychiatric* causes and *medications/toxins/drugs* is self-explanatory. It is worth noting, however, that modest elevations of carbon monoxide can cause dizziness. *Systemic medical illness* causes dizziness through volume depletion (viral infections or gastrointestinal bleeding), reduced cerebral oxygenation (chronic anemia), specific metabolic abnormalities (hypoglycemia), or vasodilation (pneumonia).

This pathophysiological scheme is obviously imperfect and, in some cases, arbitrary. It is extremely valuable, however, as a means of organizing the clinical evaluation and making therapeutic decisions. For example, if a patient's history is confusing, you may find it useful to redirect the interview by performing a review of systems that aims at covering the major categories outlined in Table 26.2. Similarly, the areas to emphasize in a physical examination can be generated by reviewing these diagnostic categories. Furthermore, a provisional diagnosis that either includes or excludes certain categories is often helpful in planning what to do next. For example, knowing that a patient with chronic dizziness likely has some unspecified otologic problem is more helpful than just saying that the diagnosis is unknown, since such conditions rarely reflect a progressive, life-threatening disease. In contrast, new-onset cardiovascular dizziness that does not have an identifiable cause would suggest the need for further testing.

Taking a History in the Dizzy Patient

Even in the most complex patients, a careful history is the most important factor in making a diagnosis (9). Since many diagnoses do not have a clinical sign or laboratory test that confirms them with absolute certainty, you must proceed carefully, being always willing to reevaluate and reconsider when new information arises or if the patient does not improve.

First, learn about the character of the dizziness itself. Try to find out if it can be categorized as true vertigo (a definite feeling by the patient

Table 26.2. Classification Scheme of Dizziness Complaints

Pathophysiological Category	Typical Symptoms and Signs
Systemic medical illness	Lightheadedness on standing, recent onset, accompanied by fever and fatigue
Toxic/metabolic (including medications)	May produce a variety of dizziness sensations; temporal relationship between dizziness and exposure or ingestion
Central nervous system	Imbalance or mild vertigo; associated neurological symptoms (e.g., diplopia); abnormal neurological examination; vertical nystagmus
Peripheral nervous system	Imbalance; symptoms generally occur only when standing; positive Romberg's sign; gradual onset
Psychological	Vague lightheadedness; mood disturbance; associated symptoms such as headache, muscle aches; history of prior episodes
Cardiac	Presyncopal lightheadedness occurring either in distinct episodes or upon assuming upright position
Otologic	Vertigo (often severe); horizontal or rotatory nystagmus
Ocular	Mild dizziness; associated with visual changes; worse with eyes open; absence of nystagmus

that the room is going around). If so, vestibular, eighth nerve, cerebellar, or brain stem causes are likely. Remember, however, that these causes can be present without producing classical vertigo symptoms. If your patient's dizziness is a light-headedness that makes him or her feel like fainting, think about causes that would temporarily impair cerebral perfusion, such as postural hypotension, a cardiac arrhythmia, or hyperventilation. All other types of dizziness are usually not specific enough to help narrow a differential diagnosis.

In addition to characterizing the dizziness, find out how long it has persisted, and whether or not it occurs in attacks, with freedom from dizziness between attacks. Then ask about the following activities to see whether they provoke or worsen the patient's dizziness:

- Standing up—think postural hypotension or medical illnesses that cause volume depletion;
- Rolling over in bed or bending over and straightening up—think otologic disease, particularly benign paroxysmal positional vertigo;
- Missing a meal—think of hypoglycemia;
- Urinating—think vasovagal mechanism (micturition syncope);
- Head turning—think cervical spine disease or vestibular problems;
- Coughing, sneezing, or straining—think of perilymphatic fistula, a treatable condition in which a small leak in the round window or oval window permits periodic leakage of fluid from the inner ear into the middle ear;
- Looking up—think cervical spine or basilar artery disease;
- Emotional upset—think of psychological causes such as depression, anxiety, or hyperventilation.

In taking the history, inquire about general health problems that predispose to certain causes of dizziness. Be sure to ask about the following:

- High blood pressure—disputed as a cause of dizziness, it is a risk factor for vascular disease and for drug-induced dizziness;
- Neck pain or stiffness—suggesting cervical spine disease;
- Hearing and/or visual problems—suggesting disturbances of these important sensory areas;
- Depression, nervousness, or anxiety—all known causes of dizziness;

- Medication use—particularly new medications, a common cause of dizziness;
- Head injury—dizziness frequently arises and persists following head injuries.

Also, ask what was happening when the dizziness began. Ask the patient specifically about exposure to a loud noise or blow to the head. This suggests traumatic vestibular injury. Ask if the patient had flu-like symptoms or a cold 1 to 2 weeks beforehand. This is often associated with viral labyrinthitis or vestibular neuronitis. For women, ask about ovulation or menstruation, which sometimes causes dizziness.

Finally, a systems review is important to identify symptoms that are concurrent with the dizziness. Particular symptoms to ask about include

- Cranial nerve abnormalities—suggestive of central nervous system disease;
- Numbness or tingling around the mouth or in the hands—a symptom that often accompanies hyperventilation;
- Balance problems—which could suggest vestibular disease, cerebellar/brain stem problems, or generalized weakness;
- Loss of consciousness—which suggests a cardiovascular cause such as an arrhythmia, or other causes of syncope (e.g., seizure);
- A pounding or rapid heartbeat—suggesting anxiety or an arrythmia;
- Headache—suggesting migraine, viral syndrome, central nervous system infection, sinusitis or (occasionally) a transient ischemic attack;
- Stuffiness, fullness, or pressure in the ears—suggesting otitis media or Ménière's disease;
- Hearing trouble or tinnitus—suggesting a lesion that affects both the vestibular and auditory components of the eighth cranial nerve.

Physical Examination and Laboratory

Having completed your history and developed a list of diagnostic considerations, the next step is to perform a focused physical examination. What maneuvers you do will be dictated by the history. For example, a patient with a sudden onset of dizziness, ear stuffiness, and upper respiratory symptoms should have an ear examination to look for otitis media. If this is confirmed, no further examination is necessary. On the other hand, many patients require a more extensive evaluation to look for specific physical findings linked to suspected diagnoses.

A general examination of the dizzy patient should focus on the cardiovascular, neurological, and otologic systems. Vital signs, especially postural changes in blood pressure, should be obtained in most cases, particularly if a cardiovascular cause is suspected or if the patient complains of symptoms associated with changing to the upright position. Other areas to cover in the physical examination may include hearing and vision; signs of systemic disease (pallor, wasting, and weight loss); the cervical spine; and emotional and mental status.

In addition, a number of provocative maneuvers can be performed to bring on dizziness by duplicating its cause. They should be used selectively, but they can be quite helpful if they replicate the patient's symptoms. The most important maneuvers include

- **Lying, sitting, and standing blood pressure and pulse.** This tests for postural hypotension. Most authors recommend taking the standing blood pressure and pulse 2 minutes after the patient arises.
- **Forced hyperventilation.** In anxious patients, this will often duplicate their dizziness symptoms. A number of methods are available to make the patient hyperventilate. We recommend coaching the patient to take 50 deep, moderately rapid breaths over the space of about 2 minutes.
- **Maneuvers for paroxysmal positional vertigo.** In the office, you can test each semicircular canal individually by setting its endolymph into rapid motion using the maneuver in Figure 26.1. To correctly perform this test, the patient must have his head turned 30° to the right or left, depending on the side you are testing. Support the patient's head, and be especially cautious in older patients with cervical spine disease.

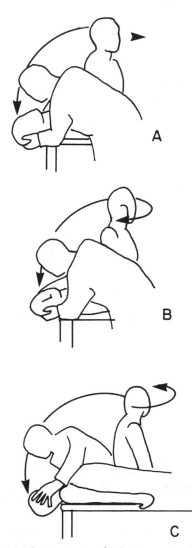

Figure 26.1. Testing for benign paroxysmal positional vertigo. From a sitting position, rapidly take the patient to the head-hanging position shown here, 30° below the level of the table. Perform this test, going from sitting to head hanging, in each of the following head positions: (*A*) turned 30° to the right, and (*B*) turned 30° to the left. Observe the patient for vertigo and nystagmus beginning within a few seconds of the rapid position change.

In most dizzy patients, the laboratory will be of little value. Patients who appear to have metabolic abnormalities or fatigue should be checked for anemia and have a standard biochemical profile (calcium, BUN, creatinine, and electrolytes). Syphilis is a rare but known cause of dizziness, so a VDRL is occasionally useful to rule it out. If thyroid disease is suspected, thyroid function tests are indicated. An electrocardiogram will document cardiac arrhythmias that are noted on physical examination.

More sophisticated testing that can be ordered in specific cases includes electronystagmography, Holter monitoring, audiometry, brain CT or MRI scanning, and electroencephalography. These tests are rarely required for primary care patients. If you are thinking of such tests, you should consider a consultation to the appropriate specialist.

ISSUES IN TREATMENT

Developing a management plan for patients with dizziness depends largely on the severity of the problem and the certainty of your diagnosis. Some patients can be diagnosed rapidly and confidently in the family practice office. Others clearly require other testing and/or specialty consultation. Many will have less-specific dizziness syndromes and require therapeutic trials and observation. As you develop a management approach to your patient, remember that some causes of dizziness can be cured. If you keep these causes in mind during your evaluation and review them periodically, a progressive problem that was not evident initially will be diagnosed. Many of the more common and important curable causes of dizziness were presented earlier in our discussion of epidemiology. Most of these can be suspected or ruled out by your history and physical, but they should be reassessed as possibilities whenever a patient develops new symptoms or fails to improve. When a specific diagnosis, such as a drug side effect, appears responsible, the underlying cause should be treated.

Treatment of an acute dizziness attack depends on the suspected cause. For example, disorders of the otologic apparatus, such as neurolabyrinthitis, can be treated supportively with medications. Popular choices include meclizine (an antihistamine), in doses of 25 to 50 mg three or four times a day, and diazepam (which decreases brainstem response to vestibular stimuli) in a dose of 2.5 to 5.0 mg t.i.d. For other causes of acute dizziness, the underlying condition has a specific treatment; antibiotics for sinusitis is one example. Benign paroxysmal positional vertigo (BPPV) is noteworthy because these patients appear to respond to specific exercises aimed at reproducing their symptoms. Exercises for BPPV involve repeatedly performing the exact motion that leads to dizziness, thereby training the brain to no longer respond to the stimulus.

Patients with chronic dizziness or in whom the diagnosis cannot be reliably made are managed differently. In these patients, the focus is on relief of symptoms, on psychological support, and on the prevention of secondary disability due to physical deconditioning. Many patients with chronic dizziness need to be managed this way, particularly older persons with conditions such as multiple neurosensory deficits, imbalance secondary to stroke, or idiopathic postural dizziness. Medications can be cautiously tried in these patients, but generally they worsen rather than improve the patient's symptoms and functional ability.

CONCLUSIONS

Dizziness is a common condition with an extensive differential diagnosis. It can arise by a wide variety of mechanisms, some of which are poorly understood. Its epidemiology is incompletely described, but it is clear that studies from specialty settings have only limited relevance to primary care. In the evaluation of these patients, the family physician should concentrate on obtaining a good history and physical, seeking to identify specific disease entities when possible, and classifying other patients by the suspected pathophysiology. Using a systematic approach that may require multiple visits, dizziness can nearly always be managed to the satisfaction of both patient and physician. As in other complex areas of medicine, major pitfalls to be avoided include arriving at a diagnosis without gathering enough data and failing to provide adequate follow-up.

REFERENCES

1. National Center for Health Statistics: Patterns of ambulatory care in internal medicine: The National Ambulatory Medical Care Survey. *Vital Health Stat* Vol. 13;No. 80. Washington DC, Government Printing Office, 1984.
2. National Center for Health Statistics: Office-based ambulatory care for patients 75 years old and over: National Ambulatory Medical Care Survey, 1980 and 1981. *Nat Cent Health Stat Adv Data* No. 110, U.S. Department of Health and Human Services, Public Health Service, Washington DC, 1985, p 6.
3. Drachman DA, Hart CW: An approach to the dizzy patient. *Neurology*, 22:323–334, 1972.
4. Skiendzielewski JJ, Mantyak G: The weak and dizzy patient. *Ann Emerg Med* 9:353–356, 1980.
5. Madlon-Kay DJ: Evaluation and outcome of the dizzy patient. *J Fam Pract* 21:109–113, 1985.
6. Herr RD, Zun L, Mathews JJ: A directed approach to the dizzy patient. *Ann Emerg Med* 18:664–672, 1989.

7. Macrae D: The neurologic aspects of vertigo: analysis of 400 cases. *Calif Med* 92:255–259, 1960.
8. Sloane PD: Dizziness in primary care: results from the national ambulatory medical care survey. *J Fam Pract* 29:33–38, 1989.
9. Sloane PD, Baloh RW: Persistent dizziness in geriatric patients. *J Am Geriatr Soc* 37:1031–1038, 1989.

SUGGESTED READINGS

Baloh RW, Honrubia V: *Clinical Neurophysiology of the Vestibular System*, ed 2. Philadelphia, FA Davis, 1990.

While this text provides more neurophysiological data than are needed by the average primary care physician, Chapter 4 provides an excellent primer on evaluation of the dizzy patient, with an emphasis on chronic dizziness.

Brandt T: *Vertigo: Its Multisensory Syndromes*. London, Springer-Verlag, 1991.

Oriented toward otologic and neurological causes of dizziness, this detailed clinical text was written by one of the leading experts in the field and describes with clarity a wide range of dizziness syndromes.

chapter 27

HYPERTENSION

Warren P. Newton and Timothy J. Ives

Hypertension is a major public health problem, so every family physician should be familiar with its detection and management. According to national estimates, approximately 60 million Americans have hypertension, defined as a systolic pressure over 140 mm Hg and/or a diastolic pressure over 90 mm Hg, and/or current treatment. The prevalence increases greatly with age, changing from 15.2% of 18- to 24-year-old individuals to 60.2% for ages 65 to 74 years. For all ages, about two-thirds of hypertension falls into the categories of mild hypertension (diastolic pressures from 90 mm Hg to 104 mm Hg) or isolated systolic hypertension (systolic above 140 mm Hg, diastolic below 90 mm Hg). Unfortunately, however, only about half of all hypertensive patients are aware of the problem, and only 11% are being treated adequately.

The importance of hypertension is that it is the first manifestation of a chronic progressive process that may end in stroke or renal failure and contributes powerfully to coronary artery disease. Moreover, treatment dramatically lowers end-organ complications. Nationally, the incidence of strokes has dropped by 45% in the last 15 years, and mortality from coronary heart disease has also declined significantly. Both changes are in part attributable to better detection and control of hypertension.

The major responsibility for detecting and treating hypertension does not rest with special hypertension clinics or programs, but rather with family physicians who see patients in their own communities. This chapter focuses on family physicians and what they should know about hypertension: making the diagnosis, the initial evaluation, nondrug and drug therapy, and long-term management.

MAKING THE DIAGNOSIS

The first step toward treating hypertension is looking for it. Every family physician should have a strategy for detecting hypertension in his or her patient population. Most physicians screen for hypertension "opportunistically," in that patients presenting to the office for any reason have their blood pressure measured. This approach is similar to that used for rubella vaccination in women of childbearing years. It works well for those patients who come to the physician several times a year. Some groups, however, such as middle-aged males, underserved populations, and teenagers, do not go to the doctor regularly and may require special efforts with mailings, health fairs, or work site screening. Identification of patients with special needs is easier in practices where the physicians have defined panels of patients, such as in health maintenance organizations or in small communities.

How blood pressure is measured is crucial. Occasionally, a patient's blood pressure will be elevated by apprehension or previous activity, so make an effort to have your patient relaxed and at rest when you make the measurement. Tobacco, caffeine, or decongestant therapy use within 1 hour of measurement may give spuriously high blood pressure readings. The air bladder portion of the cuff should encircle 80% of the arm, and a wider cuff should be used for obese or thick arms. Too small a cuff will falsely elevate the readings by as much as 10 to 15 mm Hg. In contrast, a tight sleeve or other constriction of the upper arm may increase arterial blood turbulence and lower blood pressure readings. The cuff should be inflated to the pressure at which the radial pulse disappears so that the auscultatory gap does not confuse the systolic reading. Finally, the diastolic pressure should be noted at the disappearance of the sounds, not muffling, because disappearance is a more reliable criterion for diagnosis and most studies of treatment have used it.

Once you have detected the patient with an elevated blood pressure, keep in mind that the final diagnosis of hypertension is a *clinical* one—a function of risk factors, the impact of the diagnosis on the patient, and the actual blood pressure. A single blood pressure reading of 140/100 mm Hg should not sentence your patient to a lifetime of therapy and increased life insurance premiums! A single, greatly elevated blood pressure reading (systolic greater than 210 mm Hg and/or diastolic greater than 115) is adequate to make the diagnosis of hypertension. For patients with somewhat elevated blood pressure (systolic greater than 140 mm Hg and/or diastolic greater than 90), however, an average of three readings over at least 6 weeks should be used. If the average systolic pressure is greater than 140 mm Hg and/or the average diastolic is greater than 90, the diagnosis should be made.

The term "isolated systolic hypertension" refers to a systolic blood pressure above 140 mm Hg when the diastolic blood pressure is less than 90. In practice, the weight of tradition has used the diastolic blood pressure to distinguish severity of hypertension, although longitudinal work shows systolic blood pressure may be a better predictor of future morbidity and mortality. The term *mild* hypertension is used for diastolic pressures between 90 and 105 mm Hg, while *moderate* and *severe* refer to diastolic pressures between 105 and 115 mm Hg, and over 115, respectively.

INITIAL EVALUATION

Once you have diagnosed a patient as hypertensive, your initial visits should focus on looking for primary causes of hypertension, baseline screening for end-organ damage, screening for other cardiovascular risk factors, and beginning the education of the patient and the family. Often, several appointments will be required to accomplish these goals.

The first question is whether there is a primary cause for the elevated blood pressure. The major primary causes of hypertension are chronic renal disease, use of oral contraceptives, renovascular hypertension, hyperaldosteronism, and pheochromocytoma. While not commonly considered in studies of primary causes of hypertension, heavy alcohol use may also result in hypertension.

All patients should be asked about the history of their hypertension-associated symptoms, response to pharmacotherapy, and change over time, as well as alcohol use and contraceptive history. The physical examination should screen for cushingoid features, the diastolic abdominal bruit suggestive of renovascular hypertension, and the diminished femoral pulses with hypertension in the arms that suggest coarctation of the aorta. There are no firm rules about additional tests. Most physicians do obtain serum potassium and creatinine levels, to screen for hyperaldosteronism and chronic renal disease, respectively. As recently as 10 years ago, it was fashionable to undertake an extensive workup; increasingly, it has been recognized that curable hypertension is rare (less than 1% in unselected patients). Therefore, further workup is now indicated in the patient under 25 or those in whom a primary disease is suspected on clinical grounds, such as malignant course, change of responsiveness to therapy, lability, or physical findings.

Assessment of end-organ damage should be done to establish a baseline for future comparison and to guide the aggressiveness of treatment. Cardiovascular examination should include noting the cardiac size, the presence of an S_3 sound or other signs of cardiac failure, decreased pulses, and carotid bruits. Neurological examination should look for changes suggestive of a prior cerebrovascular accident (CVA) and use fundoscopic examination for evidence of hypertensive retinopathy. Laboratory tests should include a urinalysis to identify proteinuria and hematuria, serum BUN, and creatinine to assess renal function, and an ECG to check for left ventricular hypertrophy and ST changes. If clinical suspicion of left ventricular hypertrophy is high, an echocardiogram or chest x-ray may be appropriate.

Your evaluation should also include assessing for other cardiac risk factors that interact with hypertension to increase the rate of atherosclerosis. You should elicit a smoking history and family history of early cardiac disease. Obtain a fasting blood glucose level and a lipid panel to detect silent diabetes mellitus and hyperlipidemia. Sedentary lifestyle, obesity, and type A behavior pattern are other risk factors that should be assessed.

The final component of the initial patient evaluation is patient education. By taking time for a thorough history and physical examination, you underscore the importance of the hypertension and begin to teach the patient how lifestyle influences the problem. Over the long term, your effectiveness in managing the hypertensive patient depends on your ability to educate both your patient and the family. The first visits set the tone.

TREATMENT

After the initial evaluation, you should take time to develop an individualized treatment plan that contains elements of both drug and nondrug therapy. A period of observation on nondrug therapy alone is very valuable, and it may be continued for up to several months if the patient is compliant with the regimen. Always keep in mind that the overall goal of treatment is improving the long-term survival and quality of life, rather than quickly lowering the blood pressure to a normal range.

Almost all patients with moderate to severe hypertension benefit from pharmacotherapy. The risk of strokes and other sequelae in these groups is so great that some minor adverse effects may be worth tolerating. For patients with mild hypertension, however, the overall benefit of treatment is less clear. These patients do have an increased risk of strokes and the other sequelae of hypertension, and they may have an increased risk for a progressive increase in blood pressure, but the adverse drug effects may counterbalance the benefit of pharmacotherapy. Nondrug modalities are relatively more attractive in this group.

Evidence shows that treating isolated systolic hypertension in the elderly patient can reduce the incidence of strokes, although the adverse effects of some medications may be greater in this population. Nondrug therapy may be a reasonable place to start.

Nondrug Therapy

Nondrug therapies—exercise, weight loss, stress reduction, and dietary changes—should be considered for every patient with hypertension. There is good evidence that these therapies alone are often effective in treating mild hypertension and may be useful in combination with medication for patients with moderate or severe hypertension. In general, nondrug therapies have fewer adverse effects and are cheaper; however, they are not a panacea. In most cases, the proper use of a nonpharmacological modality, such as an exercise prescription or a weight loss program, requires a great deal of commitment by both physician and patient. Furthermore, some therapies, such as biofeedback, may be very expensive. More information is presented in Chapters 17 and 18, which discuss behavioral changes and lifestyle modification.

Exercise. Certain patients, especially those less than 40 years old with mild hypertension, may benefit from an exercise program. Blood pressure has been shown to be lowered in normal adults by 10 to 15 mm Hg for 4 to 6 hours after exercise. Other benefits of an exercise program include reducing life stress through improved psychological health, helping weight loss, and increasing serum HDL levels. Exercise is an appropriate first step for most hypertensive patients. An example of an initial, minimal exercise regimen would be walking for 30 minutes three or four times a week.

Weight Loss. There is a strong correlation between obesity and hypertension, especially in people with centrally dependent body fat. Weight loss and subsequent maintenance of weight within 20% of a person's ideal body weight can lower blood pressure. If a weight loss program is prescribed, a simple instruction like "you should try to lose some weight" is not sufficient. The physician should specify a target weight, coordinate a dietary intervention, such as a 1500-calorie diet, give an exercise prescription, and use frequent follow-up office visits or local community groups such as Weight Watchers to help the patient lose weight.

Stress Reduction. Stress reduction strategies have been shown to lower blood pressure over several months, although long-term effects are unknown. Techniques used include meditation, biofeedback, and patient education about stress and coping mechanisms.

Dietary Changes. A variety of dietary interventions have been used to treat hypertension, with mixed results. Many studies have suggested a correlation between salt intake and hypertension, and, consequently, many physicians prescribe a salt-restricted diet. In practice, however, both accurate assessment of sodium intake and dietary intervention are very difficult. Severe restriction (less than 500 mg of sodium per day) is impossible in most cases. Moderate restriction (2 g of sodium per day, or no added salt with avoidance of high sodium products) has less therapeutic benefit. If salt restriction is to be used as part of therapy for hypertension, the physician must commit to regular dietary follow-up or refer the patient to someone who can provide these services.

Potassium or calcium supplementation may also be useful in some cases. When patients with hypokalemia due to diuretic use are supplemented with potassium, a fall in blood pressure ensues. Patients should therefore be counseled to eat foods rich in potassium, such as bananas, citrus juices, and leafy vegetables. In addition, calcium supplements (e.g., Tums, Rolaids) reduce blood pressure in selected patients. Presently, calcium supplementation is attractive in situations where there is another indication, as in the perimenopausal woman at risk for osteoporosis.

Antihypertensive Medication

In the early to mid-1970s, drug selection was a relatively simple matter. The stepped-care model considered thiazide diuretics as initial agents. For patients with hypertension uncontrolled by a diuretic alone, a centrally acting agent was used (e.g., β-blockers, clonidine, methyldopa). Peripheral vasodilators (e.g., hydralazine or prazosin) were used as third-line agents. This approach seemed reasonable, as about 40% of patients achieved good control with a diuretic alone. For those cases requiring more than one agent, a diuretic provided a valuable adjunct.

In the last 10 years, the rationale for using the stepped-care model has been challenged on the basis of emerging information: (*a*) thiazide diuretics produce adverse effects in many patients (e.g., hypokalemia, elevations in serum lipids and glucose levels), (*b*) for certain subgroups of patients, other classes of agents are more effective than diuretic therapy, (*c*) new and more effective agents with specific hypotensive activities continue to be released onto the market, and (*d*) there may be limits to the degree of treatment desired in individuals with hypertension. Currently, instead of the simple stepped-care formula, initial drug selection has moved to individualization, taking into account the patient's demographic characteristics, adverse drug effects, medical history, frequency of dosage, and cost. Table 27.1 lists the major types of medications. Issues to consider when selecting an antihypertensive agent, either as monotherapy or as an adjunct, include patient subgroups within a hypertensive population, coexisting medical problems, lifestyle, dosing frequency, and cost.

Patient Population. Thiazide diuretics and calcium channel blockers seem to be more effective for African-American and elderly populations. In contrast, β-blockers and angiotensin converting enzyme (ACE) inhibitors may be more effective for Caucasian and younger patients.

The end point of therapy may be modified, especially in older patients. For example, older

Table 27.1. Characteristics of Antihypertensive Medications

Drug	Major Disadvantages	Dosing Regimen	Generic Availability
ACE inhibitors (e.g., captopril, enalapril, fosinopril, lisinopril)	Rash, transient loss of taste, drug fever, proteinuria, cough	q.d. to t.i.d.	No
Calcium channel blockers (e.g., diltiazem, nifedipine, verapamil)	Constipation, dizziness	q.d. to t.i.d.	Yes (for some agents)
Thiazide diuretics (e.g., hydrocholorothiazide)	Hypokalemia, hyperuricemia, hyperglycemia, elevation of LDL	q.d.	Yes
α₁-Blockers (e.g., doxazosin, prazosin, terazosin)	Dizziness, headache, lethargy, syncope	b.i.d. to t.i.d.	Yes (for some agents)
β-Blockers (e.g., atenolol, metoprolol, propranolol)	Mood changes/depression, heart block, nightmares and sleep disturbances, increased bronchospasm, decreased cardiac output, tolerance to exercise	q.d. to b.i.d.	Yes (for some agents)
Clonidine (available in both oral tablets and transdermal patches)	Mood changes/depression, sedation, hypertensive crisis with rapid withdrawal	q.d. to b.i.d	Yes
Reserpine (Serpasil)	Mood changes/depression, sexual dysfunction (both male and female), nasal stuffiness, peptic ulceration	q.d.	Yes

persons with isolated systolic hypertension must be treated very cautiously to prevent postural syncope and falls. Also, some studies suggest that patients with multi-infarct dementia benefit from diastolic blood pressures somewhat higher than usual (i.e., around 85 to 95).

Coexistent Medical Problems. In patients with diabetes mellitus, β-blockers may mask hypoglycemic symptoms, and both thiazide diuretics and β-blockers may worsen glucose control. An ACE inhibitor or calcium channel blocker may be preferred. In patients with asthma or chronic obstructive lung disease, β-blockers may trigger bronchospasm. In patients with cardiac arrhythmias or those receiving digitalis, hypokalemia induced by thiazide diuretics may lead to serious arrhythmias.

Cardiac conduction delay may be worsened by β blockers or calcium channel blockers, and in these cases, an ACE inhibitor may prove to be of benefit. Renal insufficiency may be exacerbated by ACE inhibitors; choose an agent carefully, based upon the potential agent's pharmacological profile and route(s) of metabolism and excretion. Patients with depression or sleep disorders may be adversely affected by all sympathomimetic blocking agents, including clonidine, β-blockers, methyldopa, and reserpine.

Patient Lifestyle. Sexual dysfunction has been ascribed to all of the antihypertensive medications, particularly centrally acting agents and thiazide diuretics. Whether any of these adverse effects force a change in the drug regimen depends upon the severity of symptoms and the importance to the patient. Sedation produced by clonidine or methyldopa may impair the manual coordination required at work by some patients; similarly, β-blockers can make aerobic conditioning more difficult and so are less attractive for patients with occupations that require strenuous physical activity or those in athletic training. ACE inhibitors (e.g., captopril, enalapril) or β-blockers (e.g., prazosin) may be preferred in these cases.

Dosage Frequency. Therapeutic regimens should be as simple as possible. Dosing frequency is more important than the total number of medications used. If possible, prescribe a medication that may be taken once daily (e.g., atenolol, metoprolol, enalapril, verapamil, nifedipine, prazosin, clonidine, thiazide or combination diuretics, reserpine) or twice daily (e.g., methyldopa). Older antihypertensive agents have been reformulated into products that can be taken on a once-daily (or less)

basis. These agents include diltiazem, verapamil, nifedipine, metoprolol, or propranolol (sustained-release tablets or capsule) or clonidine (transdermal patch applied weekly). Remember that improvements in formulation also incur an added cost to the patient for these agents.

Cost. Think in terms of monthly cost of the medication to the patient. Newer agents such as ACE inhibitors are effective but are currently much more expensive than older agents, primarily due to the lack of generic products available for substitution. Generic products, if available and of adequate quality, can save the patient up to twenty-fold (e.g., $5.00 vs $100.00/month).

After you have chosen a medication and started treatment, take care to bring the blood pressure down slowly. Lowering the blood pressure too rapidly can result in deleterious adverse effects, such as postural hypotension, syncope, or other cardiac events, and is a common cause of noncompliance and failed pharmacotherapy. Keep in mind that treatment is usually not urgent and the overall goal is to prevent long-term complications. If control is not achieved after an adequate trial of a particular medication, consider substituting agents rather than adding another agent. Many patients will have a better response to a different type of agent.

LONG-TERM MANAGEMENT

Initially, the patient should be seen every 1 to 2 weeks until the blood pressure is stabilized. Then, gradually decrease the frequency of visits to every 3 months for 1 year, and finally, every 6 to 12 months. Ideally, patients should have their blood pressures checked occasionally between visits, either at work or at home. Reliable home blood pressure monitoring devices are readily available, and after you have determined that both the machine and the patient's measurement technique are acceptable, this will provide an excellent source of ongoing data. Patients should be told to always bring their medications with them to each visit for review.

In addition to reviewing medications and possible adverse effects, each visit should include, at the very least, a blood pressure measurement and an interval history. A detailed examination should be performed annually, to detect evidence of end-organ damage. Urinalysis, serum potassium and creatinine levels, ECG, and chest x-ray may also be screened every 2 to 3 years, or more frequently if indicated; patients taking a diuretic should have their serum potassium checked every 3 to 12 months. A flow sheet in the patient's chart will allow you to easily monitor the patient's blood pressure, physical findings, laboratory studies, and prescribed treatments over time.

There are several ways to assess patient compliance with the treatment plan. Talking with the family is often useful, as is counting the pills the patient brings to the office visit. Other tests of compliance include checking a serum uric acid level, which is almost always elevated in patients taking diuretics, or following the pulse rate of patients taking β-blockers. Finally, calling the patient's pharmacy may reveal how many times the prescription has been refilled.

Continuous 24-hour ambulatory monitoring of blood pressure is rapidly becoming available in the United States and may be helpful in managing hypertensive patients who are difficult to control. With a good monitor and use of the proper technique, ambulatory monitoring is quite accurate, but the prognostic significance of 24-hour blood pressure readings remains unclear. Like many of the new technologies, the value of ambulatory monitoring in ongoing clinical practice is yet to be proved. Over time, the key issues in the management of hypertension are patient education and patient involvement in personal care. As hypertension is a silent "disease" (actually it is more correct to call it a risk factor), treatment does not usually make the patient feel better. The physician's task is to diagnose hypertension and then to educate the patient and family about its significance. Often the physician must persuade the patient to make major changes in lifestyle or to take medication that may be expensive or have unpleasant side effects for the rest of the patient's life. In this regard, it is important to encourage the patient's sense of responsibility for monitoring and treatment. Regular blood pressure measurements at home or work provide direct reinforcement for continuing a diet or exercise program or taking medication. How well the physician educates and helps the patient maintain a normal blood pressure determines the success of the treatment plan at 5, 10, and 15 years.

CONCLUSIONS

Hypertension has become more easily and effectively treated, and its improved detection and management have had excellent results in lowering the incidence of stroke and ischemic heart disease. Nondrug and newer pharmacotherapies have proven useful in providing better cooperation by patients and fewer side effects. Patient self-care over time is the key to successful management.

SUGGESTED READINGS

Chockalingam A, Abbott D, Bass M, et al: Recommendations of the Canadian Consensus Conference on Non-pharmacological Approaches to the Management of High Blood Pressure. *Can Med Assn J* 1990; 142:1397-1409.

An excellent introduction to nondrug option in treating hypertension.

Farnett L, Mulrow CD, Linn WD, et al.: The J-curve phenomenon and the treatment of hypertension. *JAMA* 1991;265:489-495.

A good introduction to the issue of what the target blood pressure ought to be.

Hart JT: *Hypertension.* New York, Churchill Livingstone, 1980.

Well-written and opinionated, it provides an excellent synthesis from the point of view of the primary care practitioner.

Laupacis A, Sackett DL, Roberts RS: An assessment of clinically useful measures of the consequences of treatment. *N Engl J Med* 1988;318:1728-1733.

An excellent introduction to "number needed to treat" techniques that are helpful in expressing the benefits and risks of treating mild hypertension.

Law MR, Frost CD, Wald NJ: By how much does dietary salt reduction lower blood pressure? III—Analysis of data from trials of salt reduction. *Br Med J* 1991;302(6780):819-824.

A meta-analysis of trials of salt reduction, contrasting clinical and public health measures.

Multiple Risk Factor Intervention Trial Research Group: Mortality after 10 1/2 years for hypertensive participants in the Multiple Risk Factor Intervention Trial. *Circulation* 1990;82:1616-1628.

A study that suggests that a multifactorial approach to the management of hypertension can provide long-term benefits to the patient.

National High Blood Pressure Education Coordinating Committee: National High Blood Pressure Education Program Working Group Report on Ambulatory Blood Pressure Monitoring. *Arch Intern Med* 1990;150:2270-2280.

An introduction to the pitfalls and promise of ambulatory blood pressure monitoring.

The Treatment of Mild Hypertension Research Group: The Treatment of Mild Hypertension Study: a randomized, placebo-controlled trial of a nutritional-hygienic regimen along with various drug monotherapies. *Arch Intern Med* 1991;151:1413-1423.

Programs that emphasize weight loss, dietary interventions, and behavioral modification provide an effective first-step treatment of mild hypertension.

chapter 28

DIABETES MELLITUS

Samuel G. Weir, Timothy J. Ives, and Paul F. Dunn

The ongoing care of patients with diabetes mellitus can be a challenging and rewarding experience; unfortunately, for some physicians it can also be difficult and frustrating. It is impossible for one individual from any medical specialty or subspecialty to command all of the expertise that these patients require; a team approach is essential. The goal of this chapter is to provide a general approach to the primary care of patients with diabetes.

EPIDEMIOLOGY AND PATHOPHYSIOLOGY

Diabetes mellitus is one of the most prevalent chronic diseases; in 1987, there were 6.8 million persons in the United States with diabetes. It accelerates atherosclerosis in major blood vessels, making it an important risk factor for ischemic heart disease, peripheral vascular disease, and stroke. These *macrovascular* complications are the major cause of death among persons with diabetes (1). Women with diabetes lose their "gender longevity advantage" by virtue of their disease and have nearly the same cardiovascular disease rates as men (2). Diabetes is the leading cause of lower extremity amputations in the U.S., with diabetic patients being at 15 times greater risk than nondiabetic patients (1).

In addition to these macrovascular complications, diabetes mellitus also affects small blood vessels. These *microvascular* complications include chronic renal disease and blindness. In 1986, 27,919 diabetics were treated with dialysis or transplantation for end-stage renal disease; this comprised one-third of all cases of end-stage renal disease in this country (1). African-American women are at greatest risk of this complication. Diabetic retinopathy is the most frequent cause of new blindness in American adults (3).

A heterogeneous disease, diabetes mellitus has distinct clinical types. Listed here in order of descending prevalence, they are: *non-insulin-dependent diabetes mellitus* (NIDDM), *insulin-dependent diabetes mellitus* (IDDM), *glucose intolerance of pregnancy* (GIP, previously known as gestational diabetes), and *maturity-onset diabetes of the young* (MODY). In addition, the "gray zone" between normal glucose tolerance and frank diabetes mellitus is termed *impaired glucose tolerance* (IGT). This chapter focuses on NIDDM, the most common type seen in office practice, with secondary attention given to IDDM.

Non-insulin-dependent Diabetes Mellitus (NIDDM)

The unique and somewhat puzzling feature of *non-insulin-dependent-diabetes mellitus* (NIDDM) is that it is a genetic disease that presents in middle-aged or geriatric populations. Twin studies demonstrate a greater than 90% concordance among twin pairs in the expression of NIDDM. NIDDM is rare in persons less than age 30, and if it does present in this age group, it is termed *maturity-onset diabetes of youth* (MODY). Incidence of NIDDM increases with increasing age. Certain racial groups are at increased risk for NIDDM; in the U.S., these groups include native Americans, African-Americans, and Mexican-Americans.

In addition, important environmental factors contribute to NIDDM. Sedentary lifestyle and obesity both increase the risk of NIDDM. Finally, both impaired glucose tolerance and glucose intolerance of pregnancy are risk factors for subsequent NIDDM.

The inherited trait in NIDDM is almost certainly a form of insulin resistance. The metabolic site of this insulin resistance is in the muscle cell's

253

ability to store glucose as glycogen. Patients with NIDDM have less efficient nonoxidative metabolism (i.e., storage) of glucose within their muscle cells. This trait may have a survival advantage in an environment of frequent feast-famine cycles; unfortunately, in the current environment of feast-feast-feast, it may lead to NIDDM in those with less pancreatic reserve.

Insulin-dependent Diabetes Mellitus (IDDM)

Insulin-dependent diabetes mellitus (IDDM) occurs primarily in children and young adults. It is more common in those with certain HLA types and is the result of autoimmune destruction of the beta cells of the pancreas. Currently, this genetic susceptibility is thought to be activated by viral infections (e.g., Coxsackie viruses) that trigger the autoimmune destructive process. The usual abrupt clinical onset of IDDM as diabetic ketoacidosis (DKA) is preceded by a more gradual loss of beta cell function over several months. As a result of this autoimmune destruction of beta cells, these patients are insulin deficient and require multiple insulin injections (usually at least twice a day) to survive.

DIAGNOSIS

Clinical Presentation

NIDDM has mild, nonspecific symptoms of gradual onset. As a result, the disease often goes undetected for years. It has been estimated that the average case of NIDDM has been present for more than 5 years prior to detection. Therefore, practitioners should foster a high index of suspicion for the disease among patients with one or more risk factors. Signs and symptoms that should alert the clinician to possible NIDDM include:

General: weight loss, fatigue, chronic malaise, gradually increasing thirst;
Dermatologic: recurrent fungal infections (vaginal, dermatophytic, intertrigo, etc.), slow healing of skin injuries;
Ophthalmologic: recent visual changes (often requiring a change in refractive correction), blurred vision (caused by osmotic and fluid changes in the lens due to hyperglycemia);
Dental: periodontal disease;
Urinary: nocturia and polyuria;
Neurological: burning, tingling, numbness in feet and/or hands.

Less commonly, and most often in geriatric populations, NIDDM presents acutely as nonketotic, hyperosmolar, hyperglycemic coma, with confusion, lethargy, prostration, malaise, and occasionally coma. Such patients have profound dehydration and weight loss. Hyperglycemia is marked (as high as 2000 mg/dl or higher!), with hyperosmolality and little or no ketosis.

In contrast, IDDM typically presents acutely as diabetic ketoacidosis (DKA). These patients, usually children or adolescents, describe a rapid onset of some or all of the classic symptoms of diabetes: polyuria, polydipsia, polyphagia (the "polys"), weight loss, and fatigue. The seasonal incidence of IDDM parallels that of viral infections, with more cases presenting in winter and early spring.

Diagnostic Criteria

When the history or physical examination raises the question of diabetes, plasma glucose (not capillary blood glucose) measurement is indicated. The criteria for diagnosis of diabetes mellitus in the nonpregnant adult are:

* A random plasma glucose level greater than or equal to 200 mg/dl plus the classic symptoms, or
* Two or more fasting plasma glucose levels of 140 mg/dl or more.

If the fasting plasma glucose level is between 115 and 140 mg/dl, then oral glucose tolerance testing (OGTT) is indicated. The OGTT consists of the oral consumption of a 75-gram oral glucose load, with plasma glucose measured beforehand (fasting) and at 30 minutes, 1 hour, and 2 hours after the patient drinks the solution. To diagnose diabetes using the OGTT, the 2-hour and at least one other measurement must equal or exceed 200 mg/dl on at least two separate oral glucose tolerance tests.

The physician is responsible for making a thoughtful and careful diagnosis and for communicating the diagnosis in a way that the patient can understand. The diagnosis of diabetes mellitus should not be made prematurely; it labels a patient in employment and insurance circles as being at high risk for cardiovascular and other diseases. On the other hand, it is inappropriate to tell patients that they have "just a touch of sugar."

EVALUATION OF THE NEWLY DIAGNOSED DIABETIC

The diagnosis of diabetes mellitus prompts a comprehensive initial evaluation. With NIDDM, the most appropriate strategy is to briefly discuss the diagnosis and initial therapy with the patient and to schedule a return visit as soon as possible for a full evaluation. This initial medical evaluation has three goals:

1. Assessment of duration of diabetes prior to discovery;
2. Assessment of associated risk factors for macrovascular and microvascular disease;
3. Assessment of any current complications.

In addition, each newly diagnosed patient deserves thorough *education* about the disease, its behavioral treatment, and the signs and symptoms of hypoglycemia, hyperglycemia, and common complications. Most often, this is done by a member of the physician's staff, preferably one who is a certified diabetes educator.

History

A careful history of prior symptoms of diabetes should be taken. Patients with newly discovered NIDDM are often able to recall months or even years of previous nocturia, visual difficulties or recurrent candidal vaginitis before the discovery of their disease. Ask all patients about their family history of diabetes and its complications. This underscores the complications for which they are at risk and brings out their previous experience with diabetes.

It is equally important to ask about their response to the news of the diagnosis. Were they surprised? afraid? angry? depressed? Just as terminally ill patients go through emotional adjustments to the news of their diagnosis, so do newly diagnosed patients with diabetes. It is important to assess the emotional response of the patient and the family and, where appropriate, to help them toward acceptance of the diagnosis. We are careful to speak of "patients with diabetes" rather than "diabetics" because we want our patients to know they have a disease but that diabetes does not define their identity.

Evaluation of risk factors for vascular complications should include careful questioning of smoking habits, previous blood pressures, previous lipid measurements, and family history of cardiovascular disease. Assessment of current complications can begin with history items aimed at discovering visual difficulties, problems with periodontal disease, cardiovascular history, history of sexual dysfunction, and problems with peripheral neuropathy. Prior ophthalmologic, dental, or podiatric care should be noted. A recent epidemiologic study found that the simple question, "Have you in the last 6 months had any burning, numbness, or tingling in your toes or feet while at rest?" is a valuable predictor of the presence of peripheral neuropathy.

Physical Examination

The initial physical examination should be similarly comprehensive. Pay particular attention to the blood pressure, weight, and height. (Body mass index is calculated as follows: weight (kg)/height $(m)^2$; those with values less than 27 are not considered to be obese, above 27, they are.)

A pulse that has not recovered within 30 seconds after standing from a supine position is a sensitive indicator of autonomic neuropathy. Examination of the eyes (dilated), dentition, heart and peripheral pulses, feet and legs, and the peripheral neurological system should be meticulously documented at the initial evaluation, because these organs are the targets of microvascular disease.

All patients with NIDDM should be examined by an ophthalmologist as part of the initial workup and annually thereafter.

Laboratory Workup

A glycated hemoglobin test will document level of glycemic control in the immediate 3 months prior to diagnosis. Serum protein and creatinine determinations on a 24-hour urine collection can document the presence or absence of nephropathy. A fasting lipid profile should also be obtained.

The spot urine albumin to creatinine ratio helps to detect patients at high risk for diabetic nephropathy. This represents a significant improvement over the 24-hour collection and may prove to be the screening test of choice.

MANAGEMENT OF THE PATIENT OVER TIME

Physicians expect much from their patients with diabetes. These patients are expected to have at their fingertips knowledge of the signs and treatment of hypoglycemia. They are asked to modify their eating habits in ways that are strikingly different from the habits of their family and friends. They are encouraged to perform at levels of physical activity that are often higher than those of their family and friends. Patients receiving insulin therapy are expected to inject themselves up to four times a day. Many are asked to draw their own capillary blood, test it for glucose, record the results, and adjust their activity, diet, or dosage of medication based on the results three or four times a day! Finally, these patients are asked to maintain these complex new behaviors, not for a period of several weeks or months, but indefinitely!

Unfortunately, when patients have trouble with these difficult behavioral changes, they are often labeled as "noncompliant" or "difficult." At a time when the patient is already keenly aware of his or her failure with a nearly impossible task, many physicians express their frustration, either explicitly or implicitly, adding to a patient's sense of failure and further lowering an already compromised self-esteem. It is no wonder that many diabetic patients also struggle with depression.

If patients and their family members are to make these difficult behavioral changes, they must have an understanding and empathic physician who will not abandon them when they fail. These changes in lifestyle require instruction, encouragement, and reinforcement. In the office setting, these crucial activities are often best accomplished by a health care team consisting of a health educator (this can be a nurse), a dietician, and a physician.

Patients vary in their levels of intellectual functioning, social support, daily routines, and socioeconomic status. At the time of diagnosis and initial evaluation, many patients will require intensive, daily visits; others will require only one or two initial visits. All patients will require periodic updates in their knowledge and their individual behavioral treatment plan.

To help patients adhere to behavioral changes, a clear and understandable rationale for the desired behavior must be provided, and specific behavioral goals must be negotiated. This is one instance where a continuous relationship with a family physician is crucial. Primary care physicians can feed back current status, review behavioral goals, and encourage new goals and the continued work that these changes require.

Goals of Ongoing Diabetes Care

As the primary care physician of a patient with diabetes, you should work with the patient to achieve a level of blood glucose that is normal as much of the time as possible, while avoiding severe hypoglycemic episodes. There are two reasons for this overall goal.

First, the patient will feel better. You can explain to these patients that they can look forward to sleep that is uninterrupted by nocturia, vision that is clear, and enough energy to complete their daily activities. Normalizing blood glucose concentrations improves quality of life for these patients.

Second, patients will reduce their risk of microvascular complications. Fasting blood glucose levels below 180 mg/dl and glycated hemoglobin values below 10% are associated with a decreased incidence of retinopathy, nephropathy, and neuropathy (1). Sustained levels in these ranges will lead to a decreased rate of progression as well as possible improvements in peripheral and autonomic neuropathy.

Many variables affect blood glucose levels among patients with diabetes, ranging from biologic to psychosocial. Commonly encountered biologic factors include level of physical activity, infection, surgery, hormonal changes (especially the menstrual cycle), other medications, meal timing, composition, and fiber consumption. Psychosocial factors range from personal stress and emotional problems, to nonsupportive home environments. Whether biologic or psychosocial, these factors can be managed with an emphasis on patient behaviors.

In addition to normalizing blood glucose values, patients should be helped to achieve normal values of total cholesterol, HDL cholesterol, and triglycerides. A properly designed diet and an individualized activity level for each patient contribute greatly in bringing these abnormalities back into an acceptable range.

Although patients with NIDDM are often overweight, weight loss (or a particular target weight) is seldom made an explicit goal of treatment. The patient's progress toward behavioral goals is of greater importance. Weight loss in these patients can be very difficult to achieve and may prove even more difficult once normalization of blood glucose has begun. The goal is to provide a successful experience that the patient will be able to savor. We define success in behavioral terms:

starting a walking program or changing to a liquid margarine. Patients may not have such a powerful success experience with an explicit weight reduction goal.

Prevention of Complications

One of the major goals of diabetic care is tertiary prevention. This important activity begins at the initial evaluation, but should be included in any continuity care plan for these high-risk patients.

Because cigarette smoking is an important risk factor for both macrovascular and microvascular complications, smoking cessation is an important part of prevention. If the patient is physically addicted to nicotine, nicotine patches can help ease withdrawal during the initial weeks. Formal group smoking-cessation programs may be useful if the patient is unable to quit alone.

Hypertension should also be controlled aggressively, especially in patients with evidence of early nephropathy. In these patients, maintaining blood pressures of 130–135/80–85 mm Hg has been shown to slow the progression of nephropathy.

Aspirin (40 to 80 mg/day) should be recommended for most diabetic patients as a preventive strategy to reduce the incidence of macrovascular disease. Normalization of serum lipids will also help to prevent macrovascular disease. The most common lipid abnormality seen with NIDDM is a pattern of elevated triglycerides, decreased HDL cholesterol and mild to moderately elevated LDL cholesterol (type IV hyperlipidemia). As activity increases and eating habits are modified, these risk factors will likely improve, but repeated monitoring and drug intervention may be necessary.

Patient education is an important component of any strategy for prevention of diabetes-associated complications. Amputation rates can be reduced significantly by educating patients in proper foot care. Any complex or chronic foot problem should be referred to a podiatrist or orthopaedist with an interest in diabetic foot care.

In addition to these efforts at tertiary prevention, the family physician is in the unique role to practice primary prevention among family members of patients with NIDDM (who are at high risk of developing the disease themselves). Increased activity (e.g., aerobic exercise, walking, stretching, gardening) reduces the risk of subsequent NIDDM; it should be routinely recommended for all siblings and children of patients with NIDDM, especially those who are obese (4). An example of an initial exercise regimen would be walking for 30 minutes three or four times a week.

Exercise

Regular physical activity helps to overcome insulin resistance by depleting muscle glycogen and inducing more glucose storage. Its practical value can be demonstrated with a treadmill session in the office or, more commonly, a 15- to 20-minute walk. Capillary glucose is measured before and after 20 minutes of activity to demonstrate a significant drop in the patient's blood glucose.

Walking, stretching, calisthenics, and swimming are excellent activities. For older patients or those not in good physical condition, exercise should begin slowly and only after an evaluation of their cardiovascular status with a formal exercise tolerance test.

There are two possible complications of exercise that are unique to diabetes. First, patients taking insulin or oral hypoglycemic agents should be warned about hypoglycemia during or after exercise. They should be instructed to have a form of glucose or sucrose available (e.g., Life-Saver candies) should hypoglycemic symptoms develop. Second, in IDDM patients who have little or no insulin in their systems (i.e., no injection within 12 hours), preexercise glucose values greater than 250 mg/dl combined with exercise can result in hyperglycemia and ketosis.

Diet

Dietary education of patients with NIDDM should focus on four general principles:

1. Get most of your calories from complex carbohydrates, avoiding simple sugars.
2. Eat a diet that is low in fat and that favors unsaturated fats.
3. Control your weight.
4. If you are on insulin, synchronize your meals with the peak action of your insulin.

Dietary guidelines for diabetics are provided in Table 28.1. Avoidance of simple carbohydrates (e.g., sugar in any form: candy, cookies, pastries, pies, cakes, regular soft drinks, in iced tea or coffee, etc.) and the encouragement of complex carbohydrates and high fiber (e.g., pasta, grains, whole-grain breads, fruits, vegetables) will reduce insulin resistance and, calorie for calorie, improve serum glucose levels. Low fat consumption, favoring polyunsaturated and monounsaturated fats (e.g., canola oil or olive oil), will reduce insulin resistance and help normalize plasma lipid values. Weight control increases insulin sensitivity; it applies especially to the 80 to 90% of NIDDM patients who are overweight. The dietary guidelines published by the American Diabetes Association (see Table 28.1) should be reviewed with patients.

The final principle applies to patients maintained on insulin therapy, especially IDDM patients: the number of calories consumed should remain fairly constant from day to day, and the timing of meals (or snacks) should correspond to the times when the action of insulin, either regular or long-acting, is at its peak. Individuals taking multiple daily injections of regular insulin or those on an insulin infusion device have greater flexibility in the timing of meals.

These dietary principles can be highlighted and reinforced by the physician, but they also need to be supplemented by detailed suggestions for behavioral change by a dietician who will individualize meal plans to the patient's own cultural and family food heritage. Dietary changes can rarely be made en masse; instead, your goal should be incremental change. Setting one to three goals at each office visit is reasonable.

Table 28.1. American Diabetes Association Dietary Guidelines

Nutrient	Recommended Distribution of Calories (%)
Carbohydrates	55–60
Protein	15–20
Fat (total)	<30
Saturated fat	<10
Polyunsaturated	<10
Monounsaturated	10–15

	Recommended Daily Intake
Protein	0.8 g/kg of ideal body weight
Fiber	35–40 g/day, with 50% coming from soluble fibers such as dried beans, lentils, oats, guar gum
Cholesterol	<300 mg/day
Sodium	<3000 mg/day

Pharmacotherapy

ORAL HYPOGLYCEMIC AGENTS

For many patients, behavioral management alone will not be enough. Fasting plasma glucose levels will remain above 180 mg/dl, and symptoms such as nocturia or vulvar candidiasis will remain. For these patients or those with fasting glucose levels consistently greater than 200 mg/dl, an oral hypoglycemic agent is recommended to supplement the behavioral methods outlined above. Oral hypoglycemic agents vary in relative potency, duration of action, metabolism and excretion, and adverse effects. The family physician should become familiar with several of these agents (Table 28.2) to accurately monitor efficacy and select the best regimen for the individual patient.

Several general principles guide the use of these agents. First, choose an agent with a relatively short half-life, especially in the elderly, as the most common adverse effect seen with the use of these agents is hypoglycemia. With longer-acting agents (e.g., chlorpropamide), this unfortunate adverse effect can become prolonged and requires hospitalization. Second, the first-generation agents are now available generically and are much less expensive than their newer counterparts. For patients with limited finances, these agents are still the drugs of choice. Third, start with a low dose, administered 30 minutes prior to the morning meal, with dosage increases every 5 to 7 days. More rapid dosage adjustments are inappropriate and may lead to hypoglycemia after a "steady-state" has been reached. Fourth, when splitting these agents into a twice-daily regimen, give the second dose 30 minutes before the largest meal of the day, usually dinner. Finally, the dosage of these agents may be reduced or the agent may be discontinued in some patients who become more active and change their eating habits.

INSULIN

Patients who fail behavioral management alone or in combination with oral hypoglycemic agents will require insulin. Many patients fear injecting themselves and face the prospect of using insulin with trepidation. You will need to reassure such patients that being on insulin will probably not be nearly as bad as they fear, while insisting that insulin will make them feel better and will lower their risk of complications. If a patient is going to need insulin, this should be discussed for one or

Table 28.2. Oral Hypoglycemic Agents

Drug	Daily Dose (mg)	t½ (hr)	Metabolism/Excretion	Duration of Action (hr)	Equivalent Dose (mg)	Cost (30-day supply)
Acetohexamide	250–1500 in 1–2 doses	1.6 (1–2.5) Metabolite: 5.3 (2–12)	*Active* liver metabolites	12–18	500	$9.33
Chlorpropamide	100–750 in 1 daily dose	25–62 (av = 34)	70% hepatic metabolism, 30% excreted unchanged via renal elimination (tubular secretion)	24–72	250	$4.58
Tolazamide	100–1000 in 1–2 doses	7	Metabolized to *active* and inactive products; renal excretion (tubular secretion)	10–24	250	$18.38
Tolbutamide	500–2000 (3000) in 2–4 doses	7 (4–24)	Metabolized to inactive products	6–12	1000	$6.38
Glipizide	2.5–40 in 1-2 doses	6	Converted to inactive metabolites (90% liver/10% kidney)	8–12	5	$22.66
Glyburide	1.25–20 in 1–2 doses	10	Converted to inactive metabolites (50% liver/50% kidney)	10–22	5	$29.26

two clinic visits before actually beginning insulin therapy, to allow the patient to get used to the idea.

Although insulin therapy is often thought of as the "last resort" in patients with NIDDM who fail the other modalities (i.e., exercise, dietary management, and weight control), it may be appropriate to use a short course of insulin therapy during times of acute stress, when rapid normalization of blood glucose is required: initial diagnosis, surgery, infection, etc. The recent development of human insulins via recombinant DNA technology has made this short-term, intermittent use of insulin practical by significantly reducing the risk of developing antiinsulin antibodies and subsequent insulin allergy.

Measuring C-peptide, a marker of endogenous insulin secretion, helps to determine whether the patient really requires insulin therapy or if further behavioral interventions or the use of another oral hypoglycemic agent is required. Patients with an intermediate C-peptide level may require concurrent therapy with an oral agent and insulin (i.e., a BIDS regimen: *B*edtime *I*nsulin and *D*aytime *S*ulfonylurea).

Rational therapy with exogenous insulin requires some knowledge of the physiology of endogenous insulin secretion. Endogenous insulin secretion follows two patterns: (*a*) small amounts of basal insulin are secreted continuously during the fasting state, and (*b*) postprandial boluses of insulin are secreted in response to a meal. Patients with IDDM and some patients with more than 18 to 20 years of NIDDM need to have both of these physiological patterns of insulin secretion replaced by exogenous insulin; most patients with NIDDM and women with GIP need to have only the basal insulin replaced.

Replacing basal insulin needs is relatively simple with one (rarely) to two (usually) daily injections of an intermediate to long-acting insulin or of a fixed (70/30 NPH/Regular) mixture insulin preparation. For patients with NIDDM and GIP, replacing basal insulin needs allows the pancreas to "rest" so that it can handle postprandial insulin requirements with endogenous insulin secretion (although simplistic, this model of insulin therapy is logical and effective). Initial basal insulin therapy might begin at about 0.3 to 0.4 units of insulin/kg of ideal body weight per day divided into two nearly equal doses. Basal insulin requirements are about the same at night as they are during the day; therefore, the dose should be distributed about 60% in the morning and 40% in the evening. Nocturnal hypoglycemia is rarely a problem if one starts with this dosing regimen.

Replacing total insulin needs is necessary in patients with IDDM or in those with long-standing NIDDM who are poorly controlled with basal insulin therapy alone. These patients will require at least two injections a day, often with mixtures of short-acting and long-acting insulin at each injection ("split-mixed" insulin therapy). This regimen provides the best control but is more difficult to administer. In this method, the total daily insulin requirement (0.5 to 0.75 units per kg of ideal body weight per day) is split into a morning (2/3 total dose) and evening (1/3 total dose) dose; each dose is a mixture of NPH (2/3 to 3/4 each dose) and Regular (1/3 to 1/4 each dose) insulin (Table 28.3). These formulas are helpful guides for initiating therapy, but subsequent adjustments should be based upon home blood glucose monitoring and the patient's response to these initial dosages. These patients may require three or four injections a day to achieve acceptable blood glucose control.

Self-monitoring of blood glucose levels, with adjustment of insulin dosages based on glucose results, is required with these more flexible insulin regimens. A typical algorithm instructs the patient to decrease the insulin dose by 2 units if the blood glucose level is less than 60, to make no changes for blood glucose levels between 60 and 120, to increase the dose by 2 and 4 units for blood glucose levels between 120 and 150, and 150 and 200, respectively. This regimen may vary, based on individual sensitivity to insulin. Sliding-scale algorithms are usually based on regular insulin administration.

Monitoring the Regimen

Both the patient and the physician must have some sense of how the patient is doing. Three strategies exist for monitoring blood glucose levels in a NIDDM patient: (*a*) periodic testing of glycated hemoglobin, (*b*) periodic office measurement of fasting blood glucose levels, and (*c*) self blood glucose monitoring at home. The first two should be recommended for all patients, with the third for some patients in particular situations (e.g., patients requiring total insulin therapy). Table 28.4 summarizes these tests and gives the nondiabetic, excellent, acceptable, and poor ranges for each.

Whatever modality of monitoring is employed for the individual patient, it is imperative that each patient leave the office after each office visit with knowledge of their blood glucose levels. A

Table 28.3. Insulin Pharmacokinetics

Insulin	Route/Onset (hr)	Peak (hr)	Duration (hr)
Rapid-acting			
Regular (Neutral)	SQ/0.5	1–2	4–7
	IM/0.1–0.5	0.5–1	2–4
	IV/Immediate		<1
Semilente (insulin zinc suspension prompt)	SQ/1–1.5	4–9	12–16
Intermediate-acting			
NPH (isophane insulin suspension)	SQ/1–1.5	4–14	18–24
Lente (insulin zinc suspension)	SQ/1–2.5	7–15	18–24
Long-acting			
Ultralente (insulin zinc suspension extended)	SQ/4–6	10–30	>36

Table 28.4. Indices of Metabolic Control in Diabetes

Test	Nondiabetic	Acceptable	Poor
Fasting plasma glucose (mg/dl)	115	140	>200
2-hr Postprandial plasma glucose (mg/dl)	140	200	>235
Glycated hemoglobin (%)	6	8	>10
Fasting plasma cholesterol (mg/dl)	200	<240	>240
Fasting plasma triglyceride (mg/dl)	150	200	>250

patient education handout can be used to communicate this important information. In addition, lipid values, blood pressure, weight, and smoking status should also be monitored regularly in these patients.

Glycated Hemoglobin Test. This laboratory assay measures the percentage of hemoglobin molecules that are bound to glucose. The reported value is directly proportional to the average blood glucose concentration over the life span of the patient's circulating red cells (120 days). Thus, a glycated hemoglobin test result provides an average measure of glucose levels over the previous 3 months. To help the patient understand the rationale for this test, the average blood glucose concentration over that period can be calculated by the following equation:

$$[\text{Average BG}] = 33.3\,(\text{Hgb}_A) - 86.$$

The glycated hemoglobin assay does not give any information about the range of blood glucose levels over the same time. A mean glucose level of 200 mg/dl might occur with a range between 150 and 250; the same mean concentration could occur with a range that varied between 50 and 350. These two vastly different situations call for different therapeutic responses, but they both result in the same glycated hemoglobin value. Despite these limitations, the glycated hemoglobin assay is an important feedback tool for physicians and their patients with diabetes. Regular use of this test results in improved glucose concentrations in patients with IDDM.

Fasting Blood Glucose Levels. Periodic measurements of fasting glucose concentrations are particularly useful in patients with NIDDM. Among these patients, the fasting glucose level is relatively stable and a general indication of the severity of disease. This is not the case for patients with IDDM, where fasting glucose concentrations are much more variable.

Home Blood Glucose Monitoring. Another means of monitoring a patient's glucose metabolism is with home blood glucose monitoring, essential for IDDM patients and useful for many patients with NIDDM. These monitors are now very easy to use, and newer models (e.g., One Touch II) require no wiping or timing to produce very acceptable results. Home monitoring is especially useful to the patient who can use the results as a form of biofeedback to learn how various ac-

tivities (e.g., cutting the grass, eating a piece of cheesecake) affect blood glucose.

For this monitoring to be helpful to the physician, the patient must record the results in a logbook (or store the results in the machine's memory) for review by the physician, and the physician must review and summarize the contents of the log in the medical chart. Perhaps the most appropriate way to use these results is to help develop explicit guidelines for the patient (e.g., "If your fasting glucose is less than 140 and if you plan to exercise between breakfast and lunch, take only one-half tablet instead of one whole tablet", or "If your blood glucose reading before supper is greater than 250, take your medication and either eat less for supper or take a 30-minute brisk walk after supper").

PUTTING IT ALL TOGETHER: THE ROUTINE OFFICE VISIT

Diabetic patients should be seen at least every 4 months. Ideally, these visits are preceded by a laboratory visit at least 1 week prior to the office visit, so that the physician has the results of a glycated hemoglobin and other pertinent laboratory tests.

At the beginning of a visit, ask how the patient is doing. Are there any problems? Any medical complaints? Any symptoms of complications? Next, quickly ascertain the pattern of blood glucose concentrations since the last visit. Review the patient's blood glucose monitoring log, if there is one. Get a sense of the average fasting concentration and the average blood glucose reading before dinner. Have there been any hypoglycemic episodes? If so, how severe have they been? Occasional (two to three times a month), mild reactions are nearly unavoidable if one is going to achieve acceptable or excellent ranges of glucose concentration; recurrent, severe reactions should be avoided. Has there been any significant nocturia or polyuria? If results from a recent glycated hemoglobin test or that day's fasting glucose determination are available, discuss that value as well.

There will not be enough time for a complete physical examination at each visit. Try to alternate between the head (eye, retina, and periodontal), the cardiovascular system (heart and major arteries), and the lower extremities (including feet). In this way, each of these three important areas gets documented at least once a year. During the examination, discuss the appropriate care of that area of the body. Patients should also be encouraged to keep regular visits with their ophthalmologist and dentist.

Next, review the patient's previous behavioral goals in a friendly, nonjudgmental way (e.g., "How are you doing with your smoking? I remember last time you said you wanted to cut back to one-half pack a day," or "How is your walking program going? Have you been able to do what you want to with that?"). This part of the visit should be friendly and nonconfrontational. Patients should feel comfortable enough to share with you their failures as well as their successes. When problems are uncovered, move into a collaborative, problem-solving mode. For example, "So it's just not working out for you to walk after you get off work? You are probably too busy getting supper ready for the family. I can understand that. Perhaps you might consider some other time to walk." To be successful with this aspect of patient care, it is essential to work with patients to help solve their problems; do not try to solve their problems for them.

The visit is concluded by summarizing your findings to the patient. Ideally, patients should be given visual, printed feedback about their range of blood glucose concentrations and how their level corresponds to what is desirable. The important behavioral domains that influence glucose concentrations should be reviewed: activity level, eating habits, and stress management techniques.

Goals should be negotiated and summarized. The patient may choose to reaffirm a previous goal that was difficult to meet, or to set a new behavioral goal that moves beyond the current program. The physician's role at this point is to clarify the goal, to make it as specific as possible, and to write the goal down legibly for the patient to review later. Limit the number of goals to three per visit.

CONCLUSIONS

Diabetes is common. All physicians will care for patients with diabetes. Although the diagnosis of diabetes is straightforward, the evaluation of these patients requires a comprehensive, systematic approach. Treatment is complex and requires a continuity relationship with a primary care physician. A friendly, nonthreatening doctor-patient relationship is important to maximize adherence to complex behavioral and medical treatment plans.

As in many areas of primary care, a preventive, self-care approach involving both patient and family members is critical to successful management. By remembering the principles of family medicine, the care of these patients can be a rewarding and enjoyable experience, providing the satisfaction that comes from preventing tragic complications.

REFERENCES

1. *Diabetes Surveillance*, 1980–1987. Division of Diabetes Translation, Center for Chronic Disease Prevention and Health Promotion, Centers for Disease Control, Atlanta, April 1990, pp 17–36.
2. Barrett-Connor EL, Cohn BA, Wingard DL, Edelstein SL: Why is diabetes mellitus a stronger risk factor for fatal ischemic heart disease in women than in men? The Rancho Bernardo Study. *JAMA* 265: 627–631, 1991.
3. Singer D, Nathan D, Fogel H, Schachat A: Screening for diabetic retinopathy. *Ann Intern Med* 116:660–671, 1992.
4. Helmrich SP, Ragland DR, Leung RW, Paffenbarger RS Jr.: Physical activity and reduced occurrence of non-insulin-dependent diabetes mellitus. *N Engl J Med* 325: 147–52, 1991.
5. American Diabetes Association: Nutritional recommendations and principles for individuals with diabetes mellitus: 1986. *Diabetes Care* 10:126–132, 1987.

SUGGESTED READINGS

Jensen NCM, Moore MP (eds): *Learning to Live Well with Diabetes*, Minneapolis, International Diabetes Center, 1985, pp 53–67.

This section provides a complete discussion of exercise for patients with diabetes.

Lebovitz HE (ed): *Therapy for Diabetes Mellitus and Related Disorders*. Alexandria, VA, Amercian Diabetes Association, 1991.

This easy-to-use text provides a comprehensive and practical reference for the general management of, and all of the conditions associated with, diabetes.

Marble A, Krall LP, Bradley RF, Christlieb AR, Soeldner JS (eds): *Joslin's Diabetes Mellitus*, ed. 12. Philadelphia, Lea & Febiger, 1985.

This is perhaps the most comprehensive text covering the range of topics related to diabetes to date. With 1000 pages, 45 chapters, and over 60 contributors, it contains excellent tabular information in a readable text.

Rifkin H (ed): *The Physician's Guide to Type II Diabetes (NIDDM): Diagnosis and Treatment.* New York, American Diabetes Association, 1984.

This spiral-bound, 100-page text, is complete with succinct information and excellent tables and references; excellently indexed. Chapters include Diagnosis and Classification, Pathogenesis, Management, Helping the Patient Cope, Detection and Treatment of Complications, and a Bibliography.

Sims DS (ed): *Diabetes: Reach for Health and Freedom.* American Diabetes Association, St Louis, Mosby, 1984.

This basic text is written for well-educated lay people, as well as health professionals. It espouses well-informed self-care for diabetics and includes understandable physiological and anatomical reasoning underlying the recommendations.

chapter 29

CHRONIC CARDIAC DISEASE

Donald O. Kollisch and Philip D. Sloane

The ongoing management of chronic cardiac disease, the leading cause of disability in the United States today, takes place largely in the offices of primary care physicians. Most heart patients are elderly, which makes sense, since the cause of most cardiac problems is atherosclerosis or degenerative change. One of the implications of this is that cardiac problems tend to occur not as the patient's only problem but in the context of other medical problems as well. Therefore, the diagnosis and management of cardiac ailments always should be focused on the patient, rather than the diagnosis. There is no one right way to treat any heart problem, and—because the heart is such a powerful metaphor for life itself—there is no heart problem that doesn't have a significant effect on the patient's sense of self.

Cardiac disease is the leading cause of death in the United States for people above age 65. The physician can always relieve pain and discomfort and often prolong life. But, although recent advances in technology and pharmacology are impressive, we are not yet able to *beat* death. Most elderly patients understand this, and we hope their physicians do as well.

THREE COMMON SYNDROMES OF HEART DISEASE

In managing patients with heart problems, it is useful to conceptualize three separate (but interrelated) systems: (*a*) a muscular *pump* to push fluid (blood) around the body, (*b*) a *network of electrical wiring*, and (*c*) a series of *vascular conduits* supplying the muscular and electrical systems. Derangements of each system causes distinct syndromes, but as with any complex machine, failure in one system often leads to problems with another.

Pump problems result in too little blood reaching other organs and/or in the blood being backed up trying to get into one of the ventricles. These are the syndromes of *congestive heart failure* (CHF):

- When not enough blood is getting out to the body, such problems as hypotension, renal failure, and fatigue result.
- When blood backs up behind the right ventricle (*right-sided heart failure*), fluid collects in dependent regions such as the ankles or peritoneal cavity. Thus, peripheral edema, ascites, hepatic enlargement, and engorged neck veins develop.
- When the left ventricle fails (*left-sided heart failure*), increased hydrostatic pressure in the pulmonary veins causes fluid to collect in the alveoli and/or the pleural spaces. Clinically, this increased fluid presents as dyspnea on exertion, paroxysmal nocturnal dyspnea, chest rales, and pleural effusion.

Problems with initiation of the electrical impulse or conduction of the impulse through the heart's wiring, result in *arrhythmias* of various types, usually with a fairly good correlation between the anatomical location of the insult and the type of arrythmia produced. Arrhythmias cause clinically important syndromes primarily because they interfere with the normal rhythm of the pump.

Derangements of the coronary artery circulation lead to *angina pectoris* or *myocardial infarction*, which in turn can trigger various CHF syndromes by causing the myocardium to work less efficiently. Simply stated, heart muscle hurts when it doesn't get enough oxygen; so angina pectoris typically occurs when the heart is asked to perform more work than its vascular supply can support.

265

APPROACH TO THE PATIENT

Although family physicians often make a diagnosis of angina, failure, arrhythmia, or valvular disease, many of the cardiac patients we see have already been identified as having a heart problem. Much of what we do, then, is manage a chronic illness rather diagnosis an acute one. Patients with stable cardiac disease are usually seen in the office for follow-up at intervals ranging from 1 to 6 months, depending on their other illnesses, their likelihood to progress to worse disease, the side effects of the medications they are on, and the personalities of both them and the physician.

In managing patients with a chronic cardiac disease, maintenance of the best possible function over the longest possible time is the goal of treatment. When decisions are to be made, the risks and side effects of medical and surgical treatments must be carefully weighed against benefits in function. Patients may need your counsel, encouragement, and assistance in doing things that are important to them, whether it's visiting family in another town or merely being more active at home.

The New York Heart Association (NYHA) has developed criteria for staging the impact of heart disease on a patient's everyday life. These are useful in assessing the severity of illness due to either angina pectoris or congestive heart failure. Table 29.1 presents the NYHA criteria.

Many sophisticated tests are now available to evaluate and monitor these patients. Before ordering any test, ask yourself what you will do with a positive result, with a negative result, and with an equivocal result. Be sure that the test will truly help you make management decisions. If you are uncertain, seek consultative help from a cardiologist whose judgment you trust.

One of the biggest challenges is determining how urgently to proceed when a patient reports a change in symptoms. For example, a telephone call about worsening symptoms in a patient with known CHF could represent an unimportant fluctuation in symptoms (e.g., too much salt the night before) or an entirely new problem (e.g., the onset of atrial fibrillation). One's ability to accurately assess such situations is improved by experience and by the knowledge of the patient that comes from providing care over time. As a general rule, however, one should err on the side of seeing the patient urgently when the problem is cardiac disease.

ANGINA PECTORIS

Diagnosis

The pain of angina pectoris reflects hypoxia of heart muscle. In simplistic terms (which are useful for patient education), one can think of angina as a myocardial "charley horse." Oxygen demand is primarily a function of myocardial work (contractile state and mass) and heart rate; thus, an increase in either of these can result in increased oxygen demand, which may or may not be met by the available delivery system, the coronary circulation.

The most common alteration in this balance occurs when coronary atherosclerosis or coronary spasm diminishes the available blood supply to the myocardium during physical exertion or emotional stress. Angina is triggered (at least initially) when a temporary need for more oxygen in peripheral muscles causes the heart rate to go up. The myocardium has to work harder and in turn puts more demand on the coronary circulation. Myocardial oxygen needs can be increased chronically as well, such as when there is ventricular hypertrophy due to long-standing hypertension or after a myocardial infarction (heart attack) results in scarring of a portion of the ventricle, with resultant compensatory hypertrophy of the remaining muscle.

Table 29.1. New York Heart Association Functional Criteria for Patients with Heart Disease[a]

Class	Functional Limitation	Description
I	No limitation	Ordinary physical activity does not cause undue fatigue, dyspnea, or palpitation. Tolerance to intensive physical activity may be reduced.
II	Slight activity limitation	Comfortable at rest. Moderate physical activity (e.g., climbing stairs) results in fatigue, palpitation, dyspnea, or angina.
III	Marked activity limitation	Comfortable at rest. Very modest physical activity will lead to symptoms.
IV	Inability to carry out any physical activity without discomfort	Dyspnea due to CHF is present at rest. Any physical activity results in increased discomfort.

[a]Adapted from Braunwald E (ed): *Heart Disease*, 3d ed. Philadelphia, WB Saunders, 1988, p 12.

Assessing the Patient

Chapter 21 has described the presenting symptoms of angina pectoris. As you evaluate and manage patients with known ischemic heart disease, it is more important to learn from the patient about the triggers, frequency, and severity of attacks than to get detailed descriptions of the pain. Since changing symptoms may not be dramatic, patients should be encouraged to discuss their lives in many realms, including their response to cold weather, meals, and sexual intimacy, as well as asking specifically about physical exertion. Reported changes in angina symptoms are likely to be frightening to the patient and should always prompt a careful review.

Particularly important is the assessment of risk factors for atherosclerosis. Review patient records to make sure that you know about relevant family and personal history of ischemic heart disease, diabetes, hyperlipidemia, hypertension, and cigarette smoking. Obtain information that is absent or needs updating.

The physical examination is usually normal in patients with angina. Murmurs heard in the aortic region or the left sternal border raise the possibility of aortic stenosis, aortic regurgitation, and hypertrophic cardiomyopathy, all of which can cause angina even in the absence of coronary artery disease. Occasionally, an S_3, an S_4, or a murmur will be audible during an episode of chest pain (e.g., during a treadmill test), indicating that the coronary ischemia is severe enough to cause temporary cardiac dysfunction.

LABORATORY AND ANCILLARY EXAMINATIONS

Blood tests are primarily useful for looking at the risk factors of diabetes and hyperlipidemia, thyroid disease, anemia, and polycythemia. Chest x-rays are occasionally useful for picking up concommitant congestive heart failure.

Resting 12-lead electrocardiograms (ECGs) are useful at the time of diagnosis and during an episode of pain. At the time of diagnosis, the ECG may suggest that ischemic heart disease is present by demonstrating a previous myocardial infarction or a conduction disturbance. About half the time, patients with angina will have a normal resting ECG. The demonstration of ECG abnormalities during the pain is more sensitive and specific. The most specific changes of acute angina are depression of the ST segment more than 1 mm and inversion of the T wave, with reversion to normal when the pain goes away.

Exercise tolerance ("stress") tests can help make a diagnosis if the history and resting ECG are not sufficient. The test's overall sensitivity is at best 85%, but there are two important issues imbedded here. The first is that the test can be negative in 15% of patients with the worst disease (i.e., either significant blockages in three of the major coronary arteries or in the left main coronary). The second is that a negative test result does not rule out less-dramatic coronary lesions. Enhancing the stress test with thallium imaging increases the sensitivity of the test but also quadruples the cost; such tests should only be ordered if the additional information will aid in patient management.

Coronary arteriography ("cardiac catheterization") makes it possible to ascertain with fairly good accuracy the extent and location of coronary occlusion. It is an invasive procedure and should, therefore, be reserved for patients in whom the information will change your management. Specifically, angiography is considered (a) if you or your consultant are seriously considering coronary bypass surgery or percutaneous angioplasty or (b) if other tests are equivocal and it is important to make a definitive diagnosis or to rule out coronary artery disease, either because the patient's symptoms are disabling or because the patient has a high-risk lifestyle (e.g., is an airplane pilot).

Always be aware that equivocal results or false-positive results can trigger a "cascade" of further tests, ordered "just to be sure." It is fairly common, unfortunately, to have such a cascade end in coronary arteriography, with resulting expense and emotional trauma. Fortunately, angiography is no longer very dangerous. In addition, new technologies, such as transluminal ultrasonography, may in the future provide better diagnostic data with reduced risk.

Management

General goals of patient management in angina pectoris include:

- Reducing risk factors for atherosclerosis;
- Maximizing the patient's functional ability;
- Minimizing the frequency and intensity of anginal pain;
- Preventing premature death.

268

SECTION III: COMMON PROBLEMS

Risk-factor reduction limits the progression of coronary artery disease; whether or not it can cause disease regression is controversial. Implementing the above goals involves extensive patient education, the use of medications, treatment of coexisting conditions that exacerbate the illness (most specifically hyperthyroidism and hypertension), and consideration of operative "revascularization."

What we call patient education is the sum of your communications with the patient and is far more than just providing a pamphlet on the disease (see Chapter 17 for a detailed discussion of patient education). Educational efforts should focus on realistic risk reduction strategies that assist your patients who smoke or have hyperlipidemia. They should also help patients comply with lifestyle changes and medications that are prescribed as treatments for hypertension, diabetes, hyperlipidemia, and the angina itself. In addition, you should attempt to remain in close touch with the meaning of the illness for the patient as an individual and a family member, helping your patients modify daily activities in ways that least disrupt their sense of identity.

MEDICATION

Medications can help improve patient comfort and function. The medications most commonly used to treat angina pectoris are presented in Table 29.2. When prescribing these medications and monitoring their effects, you should be alert for possible adverse effects and drug interactions. Among the important issues to keep in mind are the following:

- Tolerance has been described in patients on long-acting nitrates. To prevent this, patients on these medications should have a period of at least 6 to 8 hours a day without the medication.
- β-Adrenergic blocking drugs reduce myocardial oxygen consumption by limiting the heart's rate and contractility. Therefore, they must be used with caution, if at all, in patients who also have congestive heart failure. Propranolol was the first β-blocker marketed; it remains the least expensive, but has the greatest number of side effects. Metoprolol, atenolol, nadolol, and others offer some advantages in dosing and side-effects, but are more expensive.
- Among the calcium channel blockers, diltiazem is often the best choice because it causes less hy-

potension and less reduction in cardiac contractility than other agents.
- In patients who also have congestive heart failure, medications to improve contractility and reduce myocardial demands, such as digitalis, diuretics, and angiotensin converting enzyme inhibitors, may have a salutory effect on angina as well.

PERCUTANEOUS TRANSLUMINAL CORONARY ANGIOPLASTY (PTCA) AND CORONARY ARTERY BYPASS SURGERY

Percutaneous transluminal coronary angioplasty (PTCA) is a technique of inflating a balloon inside a stenotic lesion to restore patency of the coronary artery. It is performed in the catheterization laboratory and is useful for selected patients with one- or two-vessel disease. The most common problem with the procedure is rapid restenosis. Coronary artery bypass grafting (CABG) is useful in patients with three-vessel disease, or those with left main coronary disease. It provides excellent relief for patients with severe angina; its long-term benefits are less clear-cut.

When the family physician is considering angioplasty or surgical treatment for a patient with ischemic heart disease, a good relationship with a consulting cardiologist is invaluable. On occasion the need for coronary angioplasty or coronary bypass grafts is absolute and obvious. More often, symptom relief and possible increase in longevity must be weighed against the patient's surgical risks, including morbidity, mortality, discomfort, and cost. In these circumstances it is extremely helpful to have the advice of a consultant whose philosophic approach is similar to yours and whose judgment you trust.

CONGESTIVE HEART FAILURE
Diagnosis

As a four-chambered pump, the heart's function depends on having strong ventricular contractions, walls with just the right amount of compliance, appropriately proportioned chamber size, and valves that open fully and don't leak. When the pump fails to meet the demands of the body, congestive heart failure (CHF) results. The four most common causes of pump failure are coronary artery disease, cardiomyopathy (usually idiopathic or viral, occasionally alcoholic or toxic), hypertension, and valvular disease (see Table

Table 29.2. Medications Commonly Used to Treat Angina Pectoris and Congestive Heart Failure[a]

Drug	Typical Dosage Range	Usefulness[b] In Angina	CHF	Cost	Common Adverse Effects
Short-acting nitrates					
Nitroglycerin	0.3–0.4 mg sublingual	+++	0	$	Headache, transient hypotension
Long-acting nitrates					
Nitroglycerin paste	7–27 mg/day	+++	+	$	Headache
Isosorbide dinitrate	40–320 mg/day	+++	+	$	Headache
Transdermal nitroglycerin	0.4–0.8 mg/day	+++	+	$	Headache, contact dermatitis
β-Blockers					
Propranolol	30–480 mg/day	+++	– –	$	Bronchospasm, depression, fatigue, nightmares
Metoprolol	100–200 mg/day	+++	– –	$$	Same as propranolol but less intense
Atenolol	25–100 mg/day	+++	– –	$$	Same as metoprolol but less intense
Calcium channel blockers					
Diltiazem	60–320 mg/day	+++	0	$$$$	Hypotension, headache
Nifedipine	30–90 mg/day	++½	–	$$	Same as verapamil
Verapamil	120–250 mg/day	++½	–	$$	Conduction problems, bradycardia
ACE inhibitors					
Captopril	25–150 mg/day	0	++	$$$	Cough, hypotension
Enalapril	2.5–20 mg/day	0	++	$$$	Same as captopril
Fosinopril	10–20 mg/day	0	+	$$$	Same as captopril
Vasodilators					
Hydralazine	50–200 mg/day	0	+½	$	Reflex tachycardia, postural hypotension
Prazosin	1–10 mg/day	0	+	$	Hypotension with first dose
Diuretics					
Furosemide	20–240 mg/day	0	++	$	Polyuria, hypotension, hypokalemia, hyponatremia, hyperuricemia
Hydrochorothiazide[c]	12.5–100 mg/day	0	+	$	Same as furosemide
Metazolone	1.25–10 mg/day	0	++	$	Same as furosemide
Digitalis					
Digoxin	0.0625–0.25 mg/day	0	+	$	Toxicity (confusion, yellow-green vision, GI upset, arrhythmias) is common because of low toxic-to-therapeutic ratio

[a]Table prepared with the assistance of Timothy Ives, Pharm.D., M.P.H.
[b]Key: +, favorable effect; –, unfavorable effect; 0, no effect.
[c]Occasionally used in combination with triamterene (e.g., Maxzide, Dyazide).

29.3). Coronary artery disease is responsible for two-thirds of patients with end-stage failure. It causes CHF (*a*) by a large or multiple myocardial infarctions knocking out significant amounts of myocardium or (*b*) by gradual ischemia causing contractile failure.

Most CHF failure occurs during systole, with the ventricle impaired in its ability to pump forward. Some failure—particularly that caused by hypertension—can be diastolic, with a stiffened and hypertrophic left ventricle that doesn't distend well. More commonly, a patient will have a combination of both systolic and diastolic dysfunction. The degree of failure can be measured as an "ejection fraction," which is usually 50 to 60% but can in severe CHF be less than 25%.

Table 29.3. Common Causes of Congestive Heart Failure

Coronary artery disease
Hypertensive heart disease
Dilated cardiomyopathy
Advanced valvular disease (e.g., mitral stenosis)

SYMPTOMS AND SIGNS OF CHF

Dyspnea and edema are the cardinal signs of CHF. Dyspnea is a sensitive but not specific symptom of increased left atrial pressure and pulmonary congestion. In particular, you should be listening for descriptions of dyspnea on exertion, orthopnea, and paroxysmal nocturnal dyspnea. Peripheral edema is generally the presenting sign of right-sided CHF. Increasing fatigue, a sign of low cardiac output, is often the earliest symptom of CHF. Another early indication of developing or worsening CHF is weight gain, which often precedes frank dyspnea or visible edema.

Unlike with angina, the physical examination in CHF is extremely important. Right-sided failure is marked by jugular venous distention and hepatojugular reflux, which are, unfortunately, difficult to discern. Easy to detect, but less specific, are pedal edema and ascites. Decreased left-sided output is marked by cool extremities, hypotension, and tachycardia. Pulmonary congestion is manifested by rales (usually bibasilar) or the dullness of pleural effusion (which is usually more prominent on the right side). Listen carefully to the heart for an S_3 gallop or the systolic murmur of mitral or tricuspid regurgitation.

MAKING A DIAGNOSIS AND SEARCHING FOR PRECIPITATING FACTORS

Congestive heart failure is a serious diagnosis. Its prognosis approximates that of many malignancies, with a 5-year survival of around 50% (1). It is often relatively easy to identify, but in many cases the causes are multiple and are not readily apparent. For these reasons, the onset of congestive heart failure in a patient with no prior history of CHF should prompt a vigorous and prompt search for both an underlying diagnosis (Table 29.3) and for precipitating factors (Table 29.4). The evaluation should include a careful history and physical, directed at the identification of underlying causes and precipitating factors, and selected laboratory

Table 29.4. Precipitants of Worsening Congestive Heart Failure in Patients with Known Disease

Noncompliance with medication or diet (or both)
Uncontrolled hypertension
Atrial fibrillation/atrial flutter
Infection (especially bronchitis or pneumonia)
Myocardial infarction
Medication with negative inotropic effects (e.g., β-blockers or calcium channel blockers)
Sodium retention secondary to nonsteroidal antiinflammatory drugs (NSAIDs)
Excessive fluid loads (especially in hospitalized patients)
Anemia
Pulmonary embolism
Thyrotoxicosis
Paget's disease

tests. A two-dimensional echocardiogram is particularly useful; it can estimate the left ventricular ejection fraction, discern valvular abnormalities, and observe ventricular wall motion. Occasionally, consultation with a cardiologist aids in establishing a definitive diagnosis and a management plan.

In patients with an established diagnosis and chronic CHF, worsening symptoms should also lead to a search for precipitating factors (Table 29.4). Often, the clinical history will identify an obvious factor, such as medication noncompliance. At other times, the physical examination will identify a new arrhythmia, such as atrial fibrillation.

In searching for precipitating factors, review medication use carefully. Doses and prescriptions can be confusing, and the failure to take medications properly is one of the leading causes of worsening of CHF. Also review salt intake, because dietary indiscretion can easily lead to worsening failure. At the time of initial evaluation, review the past history carefully for distant myocardial infarctions or hypertension. Unrelated medical problems, such as pneumonia, anemia, or hyperthyroidism, can disturb the delicate balance that many patients with failure maintain, so you must be prepared to juggle two or more diagnoses.

Management

The first step in managing congestive heart failure (CHF) is to treat all precipitating factors. This is often enough to overcome a crisis or to provide some clinical improvement. Next, the underlying cardiac diagnosis should be treated. If the patient has hypertensive heart disease and an elevated blood pressure, then blood pressure reduction should be a priority. If the patient's underlying diagnosis is ischemic cardiac disease, antianginal medications (Table 29.2) may be indicated. If the patient has underlying valvular disease, the pros and cons of surgical intervention should be evaluated.

Patient education should be aimed at explaining the disease to the patient and family and at helping the patient make lifestyle adjustments that will maximize comfort and physical function for as long as possible. In talking with patients, be aware of the ominous sound of the term "heart failure." Be sure to explain carefully what is meant by failure or, better yet, to use a less emotionally loaded term, such as "fluid in the lungs."

Next comes the difficult task of aiding your patient in making lifestyle changes. Education should be aimed at reducing salt intake to less than 2 g per day in all cases, and less than 1 g if the CHF is moderate or severe. Achieving these dietary goals can be difficult for many patients, and you may need the help of a dietician to individualize the advice. Since exertion leads to dyspnea, most patients need help adjusting to decreased activity patterns.

Medications are necessary in most people with CHF, but there is a lot of controversy about which agents to use. Table 29.2 presents comparative data on the commonly used agents. Diuretics are probably the most popular first-line agent. The "loop" diuretic furosemide is useful to reduce even mild symptoms of failure; sometimes a thiazide diuretic does just as well. In using diuretics, however, the physician must monitor carefully for hypokalemia, a common side effect. Most patients require potassium supplements.

Another popular class of agents is the angiotensin converting enzyme (ACE) inhibitors. There is some evidence that early use of an ACE inhibitor may retard progression of myocardial decompensation, and these agents are effective in patients with moderate to severe disease as well. ACE inhibitors should be used with caution in patients with renal disease, because they can aggravate renal artery stenosis, occasionally leading to renal failure. In diabetic nephropathy, they appear to have a favorable effect and have been shown to reduce proteinuria. Unfortunately, they are moderately expensive and may cause hypotension and cough.

The most controversial agent is the old standby digoxin, which may help many patients with failure, especially those with atrial fibrillation. Digoxin and diuretics are cheap; so the patient's ability to pay for medications may play a role in your recommendations.

In patients who cannot tolerate or afford ACE inhibitors, a combination of hydralazine (to reduce afterload) and isosorbide (a long-acting nitrate, to reduce preload) may help. In patients with diastolic disfuntion, β-blockers or calcium channel blockers are useful. Otherwise they are to be avoided because of their negative effect on contractility. In some patients with atrial fibrillartion, very low ejection fraction, or history of previous embolization, warfarin (Coumadin) or aspirin might be indicated to prevent thrombosis.

If aortic stenosis is contributing to the congestive heart failure, then referral to a cardiologist may be indicated to help determine if surgical valve replacement might help.

ARRHYTHMIAS

Although there are a few congenital arrhythmias (e.g., the Wolff-Parkinson-White syndrome), this discussion will focus on acquired or degenerative arrhythmias, which are more common. In approaching patients with rhythm disturbances, it is useful to recall the electrical wiring of the heart. The sinoatrial (SA) node houses the dominant pacemaker cells with automaticity, and their signal is transmitted through the atrium to the atrioventricular (AV) node. The bundle of His transmits the signal through the top of the interventricular septum and then splits into the bundle "branches," which go to the left and right ventricles, respectively. Disturbances of the wiring cause arrhythmias that correspond to the region of anatomy involved. Stretching of the atria from congestive heart failure or valvular disease results in atrial arrhythmias, particularly atrial fibrillation. Myocardial infarctions can result in bundle-branch blocks in various combinations. Most commonly, MIs cause ventricular irritability, which permits increased automaticity of ventricular cells and ventricular ectopy. In its more severe forms, ventricular ectopy can become repetitive and sequential, leading to ventricular tachycardia. In turn, this rhythm can degenerate into a lethal ventricular fibrillation.

Ventricular tachycardia and ventricular fibrillation generally precipitate unconsciousness and apparent cardiac arrest. The management of these arrhythmias is a medical emergency and is well covered by standard textbooks of cardiopulmonary resuscitation and of emergency medicine. This chapter addresses the less lethal rhythms, which are the ones commonly seen and managed in the family practice office.

Diagnosis

Arrhythmias present in a variety of ways. Many are asymptomatic and are detected only during a physical examination or on a routine electrocardiogram (ECG). Others present as "palpitations," abnormal sensations the patient perceives, usually described as either a fluttering in the chest (rapid heartbeat), an irregular heartbeat, or a "thump" or "empty feeling" in the chest (skipped beat). Two other presentations, congestive heart failure and worsening angina pectoris, have already been discussed in this chapter. Finally, arrhythmias may present as syncope, dizziness, or sudden death.

The history should pay particular attention to identifying factors that might have precipitated the arrhythmia. Common precipitants include drugs (e.g., caffeine, alcohol, nicotine, digitalis, some psychotropic agents), emotional upset, and lack of sleep. Other clues can come from the past medical history, particularly if it contains a history of cardiac disease.

The physical examination is often helpful in establishing a probable diagnosis. The pulse should be taken both peripherally (at the wrist) and centrally (by auscultating the heart), because in some arrhythmias the amount of blood pumped varies from beat to beat, causing some beats to be difficult to detect in the radial artery. Rate and regularity of the pulse will help narrow your differential diagnosis. The heart examination may provide further clues, such as the presence of cardiomegaly or a murmur suggesting mitral valve prolapse. In patients with tachyarrhythmias, carotid sinus massage may also be a useful part of the physical examination. Atrial flutter, atrial fibrillation, and some atrial tachycardias will reduce their rate markedly with carotid sinus massage.

The electrocardiogram rhythm strip provides the definitive diagnostic test in most cases. For patients with intermittant symptoms, 24-hr ambulatory (Holter) monitoring will often make the diagnosis. For specifics of diagnosing the common arrhythmias by electrocardiography, please refer to the recommended readings at the end of this chapter.

Management

Several general principles apply to the management of most arrhythmias:

- Look for risk factors;
- Identify precipitants;
- Decide how acute the problem is;
- Treat the underlying heart disease;
- Tailor the treatment to the rhythm and the patient;
- Define the goals of therapy.

Toxic, drug, or metabolic factors can often trigger arrhythmias. Coffee, alcohol, and tobacco are probably the most common offenders. Electrolyte disturbances, especially hypokalemia, hypomagnesemia, and hypocalcemia, can also provoke or exacerbate abnormal cardiac rhythms. Hyperthyroidism is another possible cause.

By defining the goal of therapy, you will be able to identify whether or not your treatment is successful. In some cases (e.g., premature ventricular contractions (PVCs)), reassurance will be your treatment goal. In other cases (e.g., frequent attacks of paroxysmal supraventricular tachycardia (PSVT)), prevention of the arrhythmia will be your objective. In still other cases (e.g., new-onset atrial flutter), termination of the abnormal rhythm will be your treatment goal. Finally (e.g., many patients with atrial fibrillation), rate control and the prevention of complications will be your goals.

PREMATURE ATRIAL CONTRACTIONS (PACS)

PACs have no prognostic significance and therefore should generally not be treated. Often, PACs are provoked by caffeine or by emotional stress, and control of these risk factors can markedly reduce the number of PACs, providing symptomatic relief for patients with palpitations.

New-onset PACs can, however, be a marker for underlying cardiac or pulmonary disease. In that setting, they may precede atrial flutter or atrial fibrillation, often by several years. Therefore, patients with new PACs should be reviewed carefully to be sure that a reversible or treatable diagnosis is not being overlooked. Pulmonary embolism (acute or recurrent), mitral stenosis, incipient cardiac failure, and chronic obstructive pulmonary disease are some of the diagnoses that can present as PACs.

PREMATURE VENTRICULAR CONTRACTIONS (PVCS)

The importance of PVCs depends on the clinical setting. In patients with no underlying cardiac disease, PVCs carry no clinical significance. If the patient is having a myocardial infarction, PVCs signify an increased risk for more serious ventricular arrhythmias. In patients with known heart disease who are not immediately post–myocardial infarction, the significance of PVCs is controversial. For years many such patients were treated with antiarrhythmic medication. Currently, the feeling is that treatment does not favorably affect prognosis, and that most patients should not be treated with medications (2).

General measures can reduce the frequency of PVCs in symptomatic patients. Reducing caffeine intake and stopping smoking are two particularly valuable measures. In patients taking digoxin, hypokalemia may cause PVCs (and other ventricular arrhythmias) and should be corrected.

PAROXYSMAL SUPRAVENTRICULAR TACHYCARDIA (PSVT)

These patients typically have episodes characterized by a very rapid ventricular rate (150 to 250 beats per minute) lasting minutes to hours, accompanied by palpitations. If the patient has underlying cardiac disease or the arrhythmia persists for hours, chest pain and dyspnea often develop, reflecting the myocardial stress imposed by the rapid heart rate. Most PSVT is benign and self-limited, and treatment should be aimed at improving patient comfort and helping the rhythm spontaneously resolve. Vagal maneuvers, such as carotid sinus massage, Valsalva maneuver, or immersing the face in cold water, will usually terminate the arrhythmia and should be taught to the patient. For recalcitrant cases, intravenous verapamil or adenosine is generally used.

When a patient first presents with PSVT, look for evidence of the Wolff-Parkinson-White (WPW) syndrome, especially if the patient is young. In most cases, the patient will not have WPW syndrome, and your management will consist of education and reassurance.

ATRIAL FLUTTER AND ATRIAL FIBRILLATION

Atrial flutter and atrial fibrillation are related, because both tend to arise in patients whose atria are dilated. Atrial flutter is relatively unstable because it is often associated with varying degrees of atrioventricular block. The goal of treatment is typically to terminate the arrhythmia; it should be managed in consultation with a cardiologist. Atrial fibrillation is more stable and persists in many patients with chronic cardiac disease.

New-onset atrial fibrillation should be investigated carefully. It may represent a previously unrecognized cardiac disease, such as mitral stenosis, or an underlying medical problem, such as pulmonary embolism or thyrotoxicosis. If a treatable cause can be identified, then therapy should be directed toward that cause.

When atrial fibrillation first develops, it is generally worth trying to restore normal sinus rhythm. This is especially true if the patient's atria are not markedly dilated and a treatable cause can be found. The urgency and method of cardioversion depends on how well the patient is tolerating the fibrillation. In general, patients can be digital-

ized; this slows the rate and sometimes converts the patient to sinus rhythm. If the patient has been digitalized and remains in atrial fibrillation, either other antiarrhythmic drugs or electrical cardioversion can be the next step.

The most common situation in the family practice office is the patient who has chronic atrial fibrillation. These patients typically have one of the four common causes of congestive heart failure (Table 29.3), with a chronically dilated left atrium. Their rhythm is stable; if they are cardioverted, they will go back into atrial fibrillation. The goal of management of these patients is to keep the heart rate in a range that optimizes left ventricular function, i.e., between about 60 and 90 beats per minute. Digoxin and propranolol are the agents that are most commonly used for rate control in chronic atrial fibrillation.

A special concern in the management of patients with atrial fibrillation is thromboembolic disease. The fibrillating atria provide a fertile site for thrombus formation, with potential embolism to the brain, the mesenteric circulation, or other critical areas of the body. Patients who have intermittant atrial fibrillation are especially at risk, because when they revert to sinus rhythm the ensuing atrial contractions can dislodge thrombi that formed during fibrillation. This explains why anticoagulation is considered before elective cardioversion in patients who have persistent atrial fibrillation. Patients with chronic atrial fibrillation are also at risk for thromboembolism; over 10 years, approximately one-third of patients in chronic atrial fibrillation will suffer an embolic stroke. Thus, the pros and cons of anticoagulation must be considered in the management of patients with chronic atrial fibrillation.

SICK SINUS SYNDROME

This is the most common reason why patients receive pacemakers. Sick sinus syndrome (also called tachycardia-bradycardia syndrome) is characterized by (a) episodes of sinus bradycardia not caused by medication, (b) conduction disturbances, (c) episodes of sinus arrest, and (d) alternating periods of slow heart rate (bradycardia) and rapid atrial arrhythmias. The syndrome has a number of potential causes, but in most patients it arises from degenerative disease (fibrosis) within the conduction system.

Clinically, such patients present with dizziness, syncope, and palpitations. They generally are elderly and often have coexisting ischemic cardiac disease, as well as other medical problems. Medications generally are not helpful; in fact, they generally aggravate one or another of the rhythm disturbances. Thus, the therapeutic choice rests between treating the patient supportively (i.e., by preventing metabolic disturbances and iatrogenic problems) and referring the patient for a pacemaker. These patients should be managed in consultation with a cardiologist; management decisions should be tailored to the patient's symptoms, risks, and desires.

REFERENCES

1. Arai AE, Greenberg BH: Medical management of congestive heart failure. *West J Med* 153:406–414, 1990.
2. Anderson JL: Reassessment of benefit-risk ratio and treatment algorithms for antiarrhythmic drug therapy after the cardiac arrhythmia suppression trial. *J Clin Pharmacol* 30:981–989, 1990.

SUGGESTED READINGS

Dubin D: *Rapid Interpretation of EKGs*, 4th ed. Tampa, Cover Publishing, 1989.

Excellent introductory book for medical students who want to learn the basics of electrocardiography.

Marriott HJL: *Practical Electrocardiography*, 8th ed. Baltimore, Williams & Wilkins, 1988.

Best reference text on electrocardiography. Has separate chapters devoted to each of the major arrhythmias.

Braunwald E (ed): *Heart Disease: A Textbook of Cardiovascular Medicine*. 3d ed. Philadelphia; WB Saunders, 1988.

Hurst JW, Schlant RC, Rackley CE, et al. (eds): *The Heart: Arteries and Veins*. 7th ed. New York, McGraw-Hill, 1990.

The above two books are excellent comprehensive references on cardiac disease. The chapter on arrhythmias in the text by Hurst et al. is outstanding.

chapter 30

DYSURIA

Jeffrey W. Furman

Dysuria—pain with urination—accounts for over three million office visits per year in the United States. One-quarter of all adult women experience an episode of acute dysuria each year, and over 50% will experience one or more episodes at some time in their lives. Dysuria is second only to respiratory illness as a cause of visits to physicians by sexually active women. Men also experience acute dysuria, though much less frequently than women. Since premenopausal women most often present with dysuria, this chapter focuses mainly on the approach to dysuria in that population. Other groups of patients and special situations are briefly considered at the end of the chapter.

ETIOLOGY

There are several causes of acute dysuria (Table 30.1). Although urinary tract infections account for the majority of cases of dysuria, physicians must approach this common symptom in an orderly fashion to make the correct diagnosis and treat accordingly. What are the causes of dysuria?

Vaginitis

Vaginitis can be due to *Monilia*, *Gardnerella*, *Trichomonas*, or nonspecific causes. Vaginitis has been cited as the cause of dysuria in 10 to 15% of cases of dysuria in the primary care setting. It is the most common cause of dysuria in the adolescent age group.

Urethritis

This can be due to *Chlamydia*, *Neisseria gonorrhoeae*, herpes simplex, *Trichomonas*, or *Candida*. Chlamydial urethritis has been reported in up to 20% of women with acute dysuria and negative urine cultures.

Lower Urinary Tract Bacterial Infection (LUTI; Cystitis)

Escherichia coli is the most common (80 to 90%) cause of uncomplicated LUTI. *Staphylococcus saprophyticus* is the second most common cause of LUTI in sexually active females. Other Gram-negative bacteria causing LUTI include *Proteus mirabilis* (especially associated with calculi), *Enterobacter* spp, *Klebsiella pneumoniae*, and *Pseudomonas aeruginosa*.

Subclinical Pyelonephritis

Subclinical pyelonephritis is caused by the same organisms as LUTI. This entity was reported by Komaroff to be the cause of dysuria in up to 30% of patients in a primary care setting and up to 80% of patients in emergency rooms serving indigent populations among those patients who have only dysuria and no symptoms of acute pyelonephritis (1). This was demonstrated in studies using ureteral catheterization, bladder washout tests, and antibody-coated-bacteria assays. This infection actually involves renal tissue and is harder to eradicate than LUTI.

Subclinical pyelonephritis may smolder for long periods of time and may explain why some studies show initial treatment failure rates as high as 10 to 15%, with high recurrence. Fifteen percent of these patients will relapse 1 to 2 weeks after standard treatment regimens, and 30 to 70% will relapse after single-dose therapy.

Noninfectious

These causes should be considered once the above causes have been ruled out or if treatment failures occur. Noninfectious causes of dysuria are outlined in Table 30.2.

Table 30.1. Causes of Acute Dysuria in Premenopausal Women

Suspected Cause	Clinical Aspects	Laboratory Findings
Acute pyelonephritis	Ill-appearing, fever, flank pain, costovertebral angle tenderness, +GI symptoms	UA[a]: pyuria, bacteriuria, WBC casts UC[b]: $>10^5$/ml
Subclinical pyelonephritis	Suspect if: underlying urinary tract disease, diabetes, immunocompromised, urinary infections as child, symptions 7–10 days before seeking care, relapse infection with same organism, more than three UTI in 1 year, history of acute pyelo within 1 year	UA: pyuria, bacteriuria UC[b]: $>10^5$/ml
Chlamydial urethritis	New sexual partner, sexual partner with recent urethritis, slow onset of symptoms (>7 days), no hematuria, cervical mucopurulent discharge	UA: pyuria UC: negative
Gonococcal urethritis	Sex partner with recent urethritis, recent history of gonorrhea in patient or sex partner	UA: pyuria UC: negative, Gram's stain of cervical or urethral discharge: Gram-negative intracellular diplococci, culture positive for *N. gonorrhoeae* on Thayer-Martin
Vaginitis	Discharge, pruritus, irritation	UA: usually negative except for WBCs and trichomonads, saline and KOH preparations diagnostic
Lower urinary tract bacterial infection ("cystitis")	None of above. May have urgency, frequency, hematuria, suprapubic discomfort, back pain	UA: pyuria, bacteriuria UC: $>10^2$/ml
Noninfectious	Consider irritants, trauma, estrogen deficiency, etc.	UA: negative UC: negative

[a]Urinalysis.
[b]Urine culture.

Table 30.2. Noninfectious Causes of Acute Dysuria

Poor perineal hygiene
Allergic reactions
Chemicals and irritants
    Soap, bubble bath
    Contraceptive foams, jellies, sponges, etc.
    Vaginal lubricants
    Deodorant sanitary pads and tampons
    Feminine hygiene products
Trauma
Sexual abuse
Foreign bodies
Postmenopausal estrogen deficiency

APPROACH TO DIAGNOSIS

Now that we know the various causes of acute dysuria, we can design an approach to make the appropriate diagnosis. As always, this begins with a careful history. The history is most valuable in making your physical examination and laboratory evaluation efficient and cost-effective. You will notice that we do not assume that cystitis is the cause of dysuria. The following approach to diagnosis of dysuria is recommended.

Step 1. Consider Vaginitis

It is important to ask about vaginal discharge or irritation and dyspareunia, since these symptoms are often not volunteered. The dysuria associated with vaginitis is often described as "on the outside" (external dysuria), with the pain felt on the inflamed labia, usually at the initiation or end of micturition. Frequency and urgency of urination are usually absent. If the history suggests vaginitis, a pelvic examination should be performed to inspect the genitalia and obtain a sample of discharge.

A growing number of physicians have suggested that a pelvic examination can be eliminated by having the patient obtain a swab of her own vaginal secretions. This approach can save time and cost, but more studies are needed to compare the quality of swabs obtained by patients with those obtained by physicians. Others argue that cervicitis may be missed if the cervix is not visually inspected by the physician.

Step 2. Consider Subclinical Pyelonephritis

Once you have explored vaginal symptoms, more details of the urinary symptoms should be obtained. Infection of the urinary tract is suggested if vaginal symptoms are absent and the dysuria is felt "on the inside" of the body (internal dysuria). Symptoms such as fever, chills, and flank pain suggest acute pyelonephritis. Some infections, however, involve renal tissue (upper tract) but do not have the clinical symptoms of acute pyelonephritis. These infections are called subclinical pyelonephritis and are treated differently than lower urinary tract bacterial infections.

The following history suggests a high likelihood of upper tract infection: known underlying urinary tract disease, history of diabetes mellitus, immunocompromised patient, history of urinary tract infections as a child, documented relapse of urinary tract infection, symptoms 7 to 10 days before seeking care (also suggests *Chlamydia*), history of acute pyelonephritis within 1 year, or history of three or more LUTIs in a year. The physical examination in subclinical pyelonephritis may be unremarkable. Costovertebral angle tenderness and flank pain are absent.

Step 3. Consider *Chlamydia* or Gonococcal Urethritis

Historical factors that raise the suspicion of chlamydial infection include new sexual partner, sexual partner with recent urethritis, and gradual onset of symptoms. A clear vaginal discharge with dysuria could signify a concomitant cervicitis. Urinalysis that shows pyuria without bacteriuria or hematuria in a female complaining of dysuria strongly suggests chlamydial infection. If there is a history of gonorrhea or of a sexual partner with a recent discharge, swabs from the urethra, cervix, and perianal area should cultured on Thayer-Martin medium to diagnose gonococcal infection. In- and-out catheterization may help to distinguish urethritis from LUTI, since urine from the bladder will have no WBCs in urethritis.

Step 4. Consider Lower Tract Bacterial Infection (LUTI)

This is the entity commonly called cystitis. Most healthy sexually active women with acute dysuria will fall into this category. Dysuria is internal and is often felt throughout micturition. Other historical features suggesting this diagnosis include urinary frequency (can be up to every 15 minutes with small volumes), urgency, incontinence, hematuria, and nocturia. Patients may also experience malaise, low-grade fever, and a flu-like feeling. Back pain and suprapubic discomfort may be present, but high fever, flank pain, and toxic appearance suggest acute pyelonephritis.

Physical examination in LUTI reveals a normal abdominal examination, the absence of costovertebral angle tenderness, and, usually, some mild suprapubic tenderness. If symptoms of vaginitis are also present, perform a pelvic examination. In cases of recurrent LUTI, pelvic examination may reveal a cystocele, urethrocele, or urethral diverticulum.

LABORATORY EVALUATION

Not every patient with dysuria needs a urinalysis or urine culture; guidelines for performing these tests are offered here. If the history suggests vaginitis, a wet preparation should be performed.

If the history suggests urinary tract involvement, urinalysis should be performed. This is best done on a clean-voided midstream urine sample and requires careful and explicit instructions to the patient to be obtained properly. The patient should spread the labia and clean the area with three gauze sponges soaked with soap, the washing accomplished by making a single front-to-back motion with each sponge. One is used to clean the area on one side of the meatus, the next used for the other side, and the third directly across the meatus. One dry sponge is then used with a single front-to-back motion to remove the soap and dry the area. While the labia are still held apart, a small amount of urine is voided into the toilet. Then a midstream specimen is collected in a sterile container.

The urine should be examined under the microscope initially for vaginal epithelial cells (Figure 30.1). If these cells are present, vaginal contamination is suggested and another clean voided urine specimen should be obtained or a catheterization considered.

The most sensitive indicator of infection is pyuria (more than five WBCs/high powered field in the urine). Pyuria can be detected by microscopic examination or by dipstick (leukocyte esterase assay). The leukocyte esterase assay has a specificity of 94 to 98% (2 to 6% false positives) and a sensitivity of 74 to 96% (4 to 26% false negatives). Microscopic examination is more sensitive than dipstick for hematuria and bacteriuria and is the only way to detect casts (Figure 30.2.). While a sensitive indicator of infection, the presence of pyuria cannot distinguish the site or type of infection.

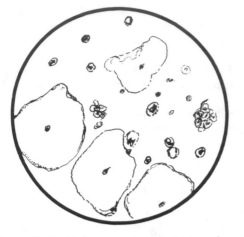

Figure 30.1. High-power microscopic view of a urinalysis with vaginal contamination. Note the large number of vaginal epithelial cells. The presence of a large number of squamous cells indicates a vaginally contaminated sample., In such cases, it is impossible from the sediment to ascertain if WBCs are vaginal or urinary in origin.

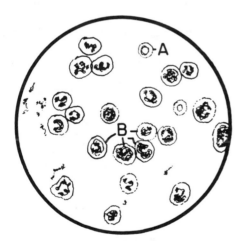

Figure 30.2. High-power microscopic view of a urinalysis suspicious for bacterial urinary tract infection. Note an occasional red blood cell (*A*), large numbers of WBCs (*B*), and no vaginal epithelial cells. Usually few, if any, free-floating bacteria are seen. Pyuria and not bacteria is the major microscopic sediment marker of active urinary tract infection in symptomatic women.

Urine culture with more than 10^5 colonies/ml bacteria is no longer the gold standard for determining the presence of a LUTI. Recent evidence has shown that as many as 50% of women with proven coliform LUTI had cultures with 10^2 to 10^4 colonies/ml. For best culture results, the clean-voided midstream urine should be planted on the culture medium within 20 minutes. This avoids falsely elevated colony counts caused by bacterial overgrowth. If more than 20 minutes will pass before the specimen will be plated, it should be refrigerated.

Current evidence suggests that urine culture is not needed in most episodic LUTIs; the presence of pyuria in women with acute dysuria can predict at less cost which patients will benefit from antimicrobial therapy. In 1983, Stamm reported finding pyuria in 90 to 95% of patients with more than 10^5 colonies/ml, over 70% with 10^2 to 10^4 colonies/ml, and only 1% in asymptomatic patients with negative cultures (2). Urine cultures and sensitivities should be obtained in the following situations: recurrent infections with the same organism, signs of upper tract infection, urinary tract infection contracted during or posthospitalization, infections associated with catheterization or instrumentation, history of urinary stone, history of diabetes or other medical complications, and during pregnancy. If gonorrhea is suspected as a cause of cervicitis or urethritis, the discharge should be cultured on Thayer-Martin medium. Gram's staining for the presence of Gram-negative intracellular diplococci is not a reliable predictor of *N. gonorrhoeae* infection. If the history suggests *Chlamydia* infection and the urinalysis shows pyuria without bacteriuria, the patient should be treated for *Chlamydia*. *Chlamydia* cultures are available but are relatively expensive. Antibody tests for *Chlamydia* are available at less cost than cultures.

APPROACH TO MANAGEMENT

The approach to management of acute dysuria is summarized in Figure 30.3. Several important points should be stressed. Be sure to ask about vaginal symptoms as well as urinary symptoms, since some patients will have two infections. If urinary infection is suspected and acute pyelonephritis is ruled out, decide if the patient is at high risk for subclinical pyelonephritis (see criteria presented earlier in the Etiology section). If the patient is at high risk for subclinical pyelonephritis, perform a urinalysis and urine culture. If pyuria or casts are seen or if the culture grows more than 10^5 colonies/ml, the patient should be treated with a conventional regimen for 10 to 14 days (e.g., a trimethoprim-sulfamethoxazole (TMP-SMZ) double-strength tablet twice a day or amoxicillin 500 mg three times a day). Follow-

DYSURIA

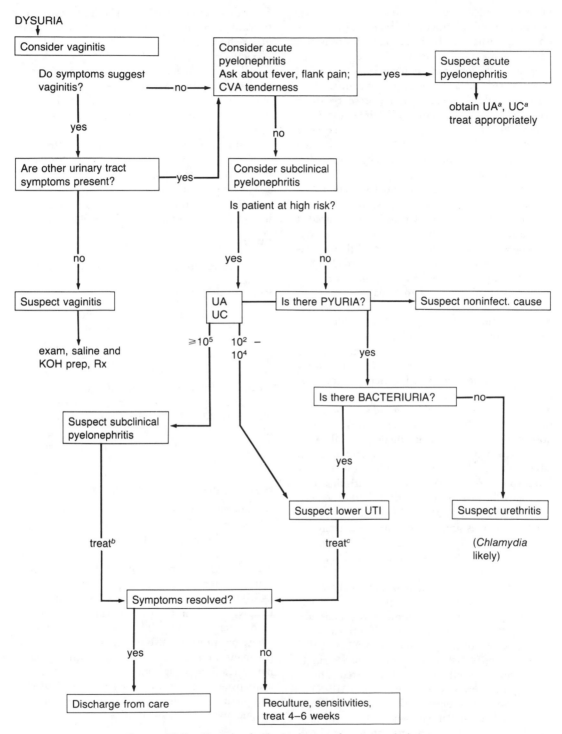

Figure 30.3. Algorithm for the evaluation of women with dysuria.

up urine culture is recommended 2 to 4 days after completion of treatment if subclinical pyelonephritis is suspected. If the second culture is also positive, obtain sensitivities and treat with an appropriate antibiotic for 4 to 6 weeks. If the patient is not at risk for subclinical pyelonephritis, perform a urinalysis only. If pyuria is present without bacteriuria, treat for chlamydial infection (e.g., doxycycline 100 mg twice a day or tetracycline 500 mg four times a day for 14 days). Suspected gonorrhea should be treated as appropriate and documented with a culture.

The presence of pyuria and bacteriuria in a low-risk patient suggests cystitis (lower urinary tract bacterial infection). Urine culture is needed only if the patient has had three or more episodes of cystitis within a year. Conventional therapy has used appropriate antibiotics (e.g., amoxicillin 500 mg three times a day or trimethoprim-sulfamethoxazole twice a day) for 10 to 14 days.

There is much information about alternatives to the traditional 10- to 14-day treatment regimen for uncomplicated cystitis. Some clinicians still advocate single-dose therapy. The advantages of this approach compared with traditional 7- to 10-day regimens include improved patient compliance, decreased cost, and fewer side effects (including a marked decrease in vaginal moniliasis caused by the treatment). The most commonly used single-dose regimen for treating uncomplicated lower urinary tract infections is three double-strength tables of trimethoprim-sulfamethoxazole (TMP-SMZ 160 mg/800 mg). Cure rates with this regimen have been reported at 65%. Other agents, such as amoxicillin (3 g) or sulfisoxazole (2 g), have also been used as single doses but are generally felt to be less effective. The quinolone class of antibiotics may have an 80% cure rate when used as single-dose therapy (4).

In general, however, early optimism about single-dose treatment has been replaced by evidence suggesting that 3-day treatment regimens are probably the best alternative to conventional treatments. Review of the published data suggests that a 3-day regimen is more effective than a single dose regimen for all antimicrobials tested. Three-day regimens (most commonly with TMP-SMZ or the newer quinolones) will cure simple LUTI in virtually all cases. Patients who fail this regimen usually have occult upper tract infection and will need to be treated longer.

The newer quinolone class of antibiotics is highly effective against most bacteria responsible for urinary tract infections. The high concentrations in urine after an oral dose of these agents make short-term (i.e., 3-day) therapy of LUTI very effective (4, 5).

All patients need careful follow-up. If symptoms recur or do not resolve after any of these regimens, a urine culture should be obtained and the patient should be treated for 4 to 6 weeks, since an upper tract infection is likely.

Remember that monilial vaginitis is a frequent complication of antibiotic therapy. Patients with a history of yeast infections associated with antibiotics should be given miconazole (Monistat) or clotrimazole (Gyne-Lotrimin) to use concomitantly with the antibiotic or at the onset of vaginal itching.

SPECIAL SITUATIONS

A few special situations require brief comments.

Recurrent Dysuria

Most cases are reinfection with a new organism. Relapse with the same organism within 14 days of completing treatment signifies an uneradicated upper tract infection. After sexual intercourse, the concentration of bladder bacteria transiently increases 10-fold. Some suggest that urination soon after intercourse may decrease this concentration more rapidly and, therefore, make infection less likely. Other advice for patients with recurrent dysuria includes voiding frequently and drinking lots of fluids.

Asymptomatic Bacteriuria

Asymptomatic women with pyuria and more than 10^5 colonies/ml on urine culture have a high frequency of urinary tract abnormalities, such as renal scars, on intravenous pyelogram. There is no evidence that treatment of this bacteriuria prevents further scarring. Asymptomatic bacteriuria (ASB) is associated with increased mortality in the elderly, but again, there is no evidence that treatment alters mortality. The one group of patients where treatment of ASB is extremely important is pregnant women. Left untreated, ASB in pregnancy leads to a high incidence (up to 40%) of acute pyelonephritis, which in pregnancy is associated with low birth weight babies, premature labor, neonatal sepsis, and death.

Dysuria in Men

This is most frequently caused by urethritis. The most common organisms causing infectious urethritis in men include *Neisseria gonorrhoeae*, *Chlamydia trachomatis*, and *Ureaplasma urealyticum*. *Chlamydia* is responsible for 50 to 60% of cases of nongonococcal urethritis, and *Ureaplasma* for most of the others. Severe dysuria and yellowish discharge are usually present with gonorrhea; nongonococcal urethritis discharge is usually clear or white, and dysuria is milder.

Herpes simplex virus may also produce severe dysuria, but the diagnosis usually becomes obvious as penile herpetic lesions appear. Dysuria in men can also have noninfectious causes such as local trauma, chemicals and irritants (e.g., soaps and contraceptive foams), and allergic reactions.

Prostatitis is another cause of dysuria in men. Patients with prostatitis may also complain of malaise, fatigue, lower abdominal pain, low back pain, or rectal pressure. The prostate may be enlarged, tender, and soft. Since the treatment of prostatitis and urethritis differs, it is important to localize the site of the inflammation.

In men, one way to localize the source of inflammatory cells or bacteria is the three-glass procedure described by Stamey (3). Three separate samples of urine are obtained and examined microscopically for pyuria and bacteriuria. The first 5 to 10 ml voided represent the urethra, the midstream aliquot represents the bladder, and a postprostatic massage specimen represents the prostate.

Treatment regimens for urinary tract infections discussed earlier for women also apply to men. If a urethral discharge is present and Gram's stain and culture for *Gonococcus* are negative, the patient should be treated for *Chlamydia* (doxycycline 100 mg twice a day or tetracycline 500 mg four times a day for 14 days). Since uncomplicated urinary tract infections are much less common in men than women, some authors suggest that men with documented infections of the urinary tract (lower or upper) be evaluated for medical complications (e.g., diabetes mellitus) and anatomical or structural anomalies (e.g., obtain an intravenous pyelogram and consider cystoscopy).

Elderly Patients

Elderly patients with urinary tract infections should be evaluated carefully because of the many physiological changes that occur with aging and concomitant pathologies that may be present. Two common urologic syndromes that can cause UTI in the elderly are obstructive uropathy and urinary incontinence. Effective treatment in these situations depends on resolving the underlying problem, in addition to appropriate antimicrobial therapy.

REFERENCES

1. Komaroff AL: Acute dysuria in women. *N Engl J Med* 310:368–375, 1984.
2. Stamm WE: Measurement of pyuria and its relation to bacteriuria. *Am J Med* 75(1B):53-58, 1983.
3. Stamey TA: *Urinary Infections*. Baltimore, Williams & Wilkins, 1972.
4. Powers RD: New directions in the diagnosis and therapy of urinary tract infections. *Am J Obstet Gynecol* 164(5, pt.2):1387-1389, 1991.
5. Andriole VT: Use of quinolones in treatment of prostatitis and lower urinary tract infections. *Eur J Clin Microbiol Infect Dis* 10(4):342-350, 1991.

SUGGESTED READINGS

Greenberg RN, Reilly PM, Luppen KL, Weinandt WJ, Ellington LL, Bollinger MR: Randomized study of single-dose, three-day and seven-day treatment of cystitis in women. *J Infect Dis* 153:277-282, 1986.

This review article covers the treatment of uncomplicated UTI, including several treatment regimens; 62 references.

Hooton TM, Stamm WE: Management of acute uncomplicated urinary tract infection in adults. *Med Clin North Am* 75(2):339–357, 1991.

This review article covers the treatment of uncomplicated UTI, including several treatment regimens; 62 references.

Komaroff A: Urinalysis and urine culture in women with dysuria. *Ann Intern Med* 104:212-218, 1986.

The value of urinalysis and urine culture in distinguishing the various clinical entities causing acute dysuria in women is examined.

Mulholland SG: Female urinary tract infection. *Prim Care* 12:661-673, 1985.

This useful summary of female urinary tract infections covers epidemiology, pathogenesis, diagnosis, organisms, and treatment.

chapter 31

VAGINITIS

Melanie Mintzer

The annoying and often uncomfortable symptoms of vulvovaginitis are the most common reason why young women visit family physicians and gynecologists. This problem represents several different diagnoses, which require quite different treatments. Some infections can be diagnosed by examination of a wet preparation slide alone; however, pelvic examination is often necessary to determine the type of infection and to rule out concurrent sexually transmitted diseases (STDs) and other gynecologic conditions that may contribute to the increased vaginal discharge. Many cases of vaginal discharge herald the diagnosis of upper genital tract disease.

Vaginal discharges can reflect a wide spectrum of disease, from simple candidiasis to cervical dysplasia. Vaginal infections are a frequent cause of dysuria (see Chapter 30) and can be mistaken for cystitis or urethritis. Many patients are self-diagnosing vaginal conditions now that treatment for candidiasis is sold over the counter. However, in many cases, the diagnosis is complicated. Thus, there is no substitute for an office visit with a thorough evaluation of the patient's symptoms and a definitive laboratory diagnosis, if possible.

Patient education and involvement in the treatment plan can prevent reinfection. Patients can reduce the incidence of vaginal infections by keeping the perineal area dry and clean, wearing cotton underwear, avoiding tight clothing such as slacks or panty hose, and wiping from front to back after a bowel movement (many vaginal infections are caused by rectal contaminants).

NORMAL VAGINAL SECRETIONS

Every woman normally secretes a watery mucous discharge. This normal discharge contains secretions from the mucous membranes of the vagina and cervix, and desquamated vaginal and cervical epithelial cells. It reflects the hormonal changes of her menstrual cycle, and other physiological changes such as pregnancy, stress, sexual excitement, or illness. The normal vagina also contains many bacterial organisms and yeasts that are in a dynamic state of flux and respond to environmental changes such as pH and glucose concentration. When changes occur, overgrowth of the normal bacteria can result. The dominant organism in normal vaginal discharge is a commensal that helps maintain homeostasis and prevent infection.

The normal secretion is usually transparent or milky colored and often filmy and nonhomogenous. When dried on clothing, it can appear yellow. It generally has little odor and causes no symptoms of vulvar irritation, vaginal burning, or irritation on urination. The amount of vaginal discharge and its consistency varies from woman to woman, but most women experience changes in relationship to their menstrual cycle. The amount is usually smallest right after menses ends and gradually increases throughout the cycle, becoming thicker and more alkaline (its pH is normally mildly acidic) as ovulation approaches. When discharge drains onto the vulva or perineum or pools in the introitus, this often indicates that infection is present.

APPROACH TO THE PATIENT WITH VAGINAL DISCHARGE

Vaginitis and Vaginosis

Certain infections, usually due to *Trichomonas vaginalis* or *Candida albicans*, induce an inflammatory response in the vaginal mucosa. This inflammatory response, termed *vaginitis*, is characterized by an increased number of leukocytes in the vaginal fluid. In other conditions, a polymycrobial infection is caused by an increase in anaerobic organisms, but there is no evidence of inflammation (i.e., no leukocytosis in the vaginal fluid). This situation is termed *vaginosis*.

Different mechanisms are thought to explain the changes in vaginal flora observed in vaginitis and vaginosis. In vaginosis, disturbed vaginal antibiosis is postulated. It was once believed that lactobacilli produced acidic compounds that decrease the vaginal pH, making the milieu unfavorable to certain microbes. It is now thought that the antibiosis exhibited by vaginal lactobacilli is mediated by an endopeptidase that inhibits a variety of bacterial species. This antibacterial effect may also be related to changes in the receptors of organisms that colonize the vagina. Another influence on the vaginal ecology is differences in estrogen states (i.e., secretory changes that accompany puberty, pregnancy, menopause, and the use of oral contraceptives).

The long-term effects of vaginitis and vaginosis are currently under study. Organisms occurring in the vagina of women with bacterial vaginosis may spread to the upper genital tract and be associated with pelvic inflammatory disease and resultant infertility. Lower genital tract infections such as human papilloma virus (HPV) are currently associated with cervical neoplasia. Studies are underway to investigate the possibility that vaginitis and/or vaginosis may increase the patient's susceptibility to the human immunodeficiency (HIV) virus. Such an increased risk has been demonstrated for genital lesions caused by *Haemophilus ducreyi* and *Chlamydia trachomatis* (1).

Patient Evaluation

Increased vaginal discharge is common and does not always represent vaginitis or cervicitis. Noninfectious causes include congenital cervical erosion, cervical polyps, foreign bodies in the vagina (including tampons or contraceptive sponges), chemical irritation by douches or contraceptive gels or creams, and early pelvic cancers, as well as bacterial and viral infections of the vagina and cervix (Table 31.1).

Taking a good history with special attention to certain features, performing an adequate physical examination, examining both saline and KOH preparations (vaginalysis), and testing for sexually transmitted diseases will help you make the appropriate diagnosis with little difficulty. Important points to clarify when taking a history include specific symptoms of burning and itching, and the relationship of the discharge to the menstrual cycle.

Table 31.1. Common Causes of Vaginal Discharge*

- Physiological variations in normal secretion and epithelial desquamation with no associated symptoms of vaginitis
- Congenital cervical erosion, usually with no associated symptoms
- Chronic cervicitis and/or cervical polyps
- Trichomonal vaginitis
- Monilial vaginitis
- Bacterial vaginosis
- Atrophic vaginitis
- Foreign bodies (variety of objects in children, usually tampons or contraceptive sponges in adult women)
- Gonorrheal cervicitis, urethritis, skenitis, bartholinitis
- Chlamydial cervicitis
- Irritating douches, contraceptive creams or gels, or other chemical irritants
- Early cervical, endometrial, or vaginal cancers
- Condyloma acuminata or herpes simplex infections of the lower genital tract

*Adapted from: Green T: *Gynecology: The Essentials of Clinical Practice.* Boston, Little, Brown & Co., 1977, p 229.

Temporal events, such as sexual intercourse, pregnancy, use of antibiotics, or concurrent illnesses such as diabetes or cancer, and menopause, may help determine your diagnosis.

Increased vaginal discharge is normal at midcycle, just before menses, during pregnancy, and in cases of cervical erosion (a normal variant where some of the outer surface of the cervix is covered with columnar epithelium, like the endocervix).

Monilial or *Trichomonas* vaginitis primarily presents with burning and itching. At menopause, women often complain of a burning vaginal discharge without the itching. This is often due to the decreased number of epithelial cells and secretions, caused by diminished circulating estrogen. This presentation is often misdiagnosed by physicians as *Monilia* and then is exacerbated by use of antifungal preparations.

Monilial vaginitis is often more symptomatic right before a period, improving after the period. It often occurs after antibiotic therapy (especially broad-spectrum agents such as ampicillin, sulfamethoxasole-trimethoprim, and tetracycline) and is more common in diabetes and in pregnancy. It can coexist with other vaginal infections and prevent their diagnosis. Trichomoniasis symptoms are worse after a period and often present with spotting or frank vaginal bleeding.

The physical examination in a patient with problematic vaginal discharge is straightforward and very helpful. Carefully examine the vulvar, vaginal, and cervical areas for evidence of inflammation, cervical erosion, leukoplakia, herpes, and frank malignancy. Using a speculum and being careful to avoid patient discomfort, look for foreign bodies, such as a retained tampon, and evaluate the vaginal mucosa for estrogen exposure. In a sexually active woman, culture for gonorrhea and *Chlamydia* if the history suggests these are possible. If you suspect a cervical or vaginal malignancy, a Pap smear is helpful. In cases of inflammation and infection, Pap smear readings are often distorted by the presence of inflammatory cells; in such cases, postpone the Pap smear until the infection has been cleared.

A *wet preparation* should be performed in all presentations of vaginal discharge. This examination is performed by swabbing the vaginal mucosa along the walls and the vaginal vault with two cotton-tipped sterile 6-inch swabs. If there are pooled secretions in other parts of the vagina, these areas should also be swabbed. Often, residual discharge on the speculum can be retrieved when the speculum is removed. The swabs are then placed in a clean centrifuge tube containing 1 ml of sterile normal saline, and the swabs are mixed in and out of the saline. A large drop of this mixture is placed on each of two clean microscope slides. One slide is covered with a coverslip. A drop of 10% KOH is added to the second slide, and a coverslip is placed. The two specimens are then ready to be evaluated for the various types of vaginitis. Table 31.2 provides a summary of the visual and microscopic appearance of the vaginal discharge in the common causes of vaginitis.

Making the correct diagnosis involves weighing the evidence, particularly in cases where the patient has received previous treatment or where the wet preparation is nondiagnostic. In such situations, the pH of the vaginal fluid and the presence or absence of WBCs (see Table 31.2) may aid diagnosis.

Before instituting treatment, review the history for frequency of recurrences, douching agents and frequency, symptoms present in partners, and whether the sexual partner is circumcised or not. This information will help you decide on the appropriate length and type of therapy.

DIAGNOSIS AND TREATMENT OF SPECIFIC TYPES OF VAGINITIS
Monial or *Candida* Vulvovaginitis

Monilial vaginitis (a yeast infection) is the most common cause of vaginal complaints. *Candida albicans* is usually the pathogen if the vagina is cultured, but other *Candida* species such as *C. tropicalis*, *C. pseudotropicalis*, *C. stellatoidea*, *C. glabrata*, and *C. krusei* have been implicated as causative agents. On microscopic examination of a wet preparation or KOH preparation, *Candida albicans* appears in two forms; (*a*) as a yeast, a small round organism, often with budding, or (*b*) as filaments called pseudohyphae (see Fig. 31.1). Its identification is more difficult in the yeast phase. Yeasts are normal constituents of the vagina and can be cultured from asymptomatic women. Vaginitis from an overgrowth of these organisms cannot be considered to be a true STD like herpes or gonorrhea. However, these organisms can be spread from one person to another through sexual intercourse, as the organism has been cultured from partners of women with recurrent candidiasis. Moniliasis is most often seen in premenopausal women. It commonly occurs in women who have been treated with antibiotics, in diabetics, and in individuals under stress. Pregnancy, oral contraceptives, and exogenous estrogens also predispose to candidiasis because they lower the vaginal pH, and *Candida* thrives in an acidic environment.

Itching and an increased, often thick, vaginal discharge, are the classical symptoms of vaginal candidiasis. Affected women have irritated, red vulvar and vaginal tissue, which is often excoriated because of intense itching. Dysuria, burning on urination, and dyspareunia during intromission or following intercourse are frequent accompanying complaints. The vaginal discharge varies from scant to copious, and can be liquid or thick. The classic description is a "cottage-cheese-like" discharge, which results from clumping of yeast plaques in the vagina. The organism can be visualized in the saline preparation but is more easily identified in the KOH preparation, because the potassium hydroxide lyses confusing cellular debris, leaving *Candida* (with its sturdy cell wall) intact.

Treatment for monilial vaginitis consists of topical imidazole antifungal agents such as nystatin, miconazole, or clotrimazole. In recurrent or recalcitrant cases, a topical agent can be combined with oral nystatin or ketoconazole. A 7-day dosage schedule of a topical agent is recommended, although shorter treatment schedules often suffice. Patients who are asymptomatic may also benefit from treatment; many will realize after treatment that they have less irritation, discomfort, and discharge. Recurrent monilial

Table 31.2. Vaginal Discharge in Common Diagnoses[a]

	Normal Vagina	Atrophic Vaginitis	Bacterial Vaginosis	Trichomonas vaginitis	Chlamydia trachomatis	Candida albicans	Doderlein's cytolysis
Color	Slate grey	Grey-yellow, purulent, serosanguinous	Grey	Green, thin white, or grey	May have purulent discharge	Thick white	Thick white
pH	<4.5	7.0	>4.7	>5.5	<4.5	4.0–4.5	3.5–5.0
Odor	None	None	Foul, fishlike	Foul	None	None	None
Consistency	Liquid, thin, homogenous	Liquid, thin, homogenous	Liquid, thin, frothy, homogenous	Liquid, frothy, homogenous	Thick	Thick, with plaques	Thick white curds or watery
Physical findings	No abnormal findings	Pale, pink, smooth vaginal and cervical epithelium	No significant changes	Erythema, petechial hemorrhages	Erythematous columnar epithelium	Erythema of vulva and vagina	Erythema of vulva and vagina
Microscopic findings	A few WBCs with very few bacteria; many squamous epithelial cells	Many parabasal epithelial cells; moderate WBCs	Squamous epithelial cells laden with bacteria (clue cells); bacteria in clumps; rare lactobacilli; rare WBCs	Motile trichomonads on wet prep; many WBCs, many basal epithelial cells, and many bacteria	Many squamous epithelial cells; many WBCs; many bacteria	Pseudohyphae; budding yeast; many WBCs; few lactobacilli; squamous epithelial cells	Many lactobacilli and lysed epithelial cells; massive desquamation of epithelial cells
Treatment	None	Estrogen	Metronidazole, clindamycin	Metronidazole	Tetracycline, erythromycin	Nystatin, miconazole, clotrimazole, gentian violet	Baking soda douche, Aminocerv cream

[a]Adapted from: Faro S (ed): *Diagnosis and Management of Female Pelvic Infections in Primary Care Medicine.* Baltimore, Williams & Wilkins, 1985, p 107.

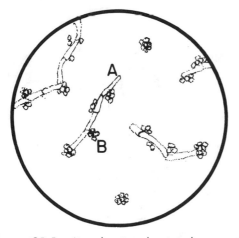

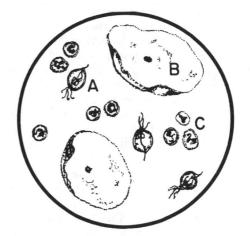

Figure 31.1. Line drawing showing the appearance of *Candida* species under the microscope. (A) Pseudohyphae. (B) Yeast phase, with budding.

Figure 31.2. Line drawing of A, *T. vaginalis*; B, squamous epithelial cells; and C, white blood cells. Approximates magnification with high dry objective.

vaginitis is a frequent problem in office practice, and medical treatments are often unsatisfactory. Stress, warmth, and moisture appear to be contributing factors. Other risk factors include the sexual partner as carrier and the use of oral antibiotics or estrogens. The first step in treatment is to minimize these risks. Avoiding tight clothing and nylon underwear helps. Frequent douching disturbs the normal vaginal flow, but douching once or twice weekly with a mild baking soda solution or with sweet acidophilus milk (which contains lactobacilli) may help. Oral lactobacillus tablets are sometimes helpful. Treating both the patient and the sexual partner with antifungal creams *and* with oral nystatin or ketoconazole, and using condoms during treatment, also decreases the incidence of recurrent infection. It is important to note that persistent candidal infections can be a marker for HIV disease.

Trichomoniasis

Trichomonas vaginalis is a pleomorphic protozoan with four undulating flagella, which is commonly a little larger than a white blood cell (Fig. 31.2). Found in vaginal secretions and urine of humans, its only known reservoir, it grows very well in high glucose and acidic environments. It causes approximately 20% of cases of vulvovaginitis. It is usually acquired through sexual intercourse, though it is possible to pass the organism on washcloths, towels, and intimate clothing such as underwear and bathing suits. Its incidence is highest among prosti-

tutes, and it is found coincidentally in 10% of gonorrhea cases. It is also found in 12 to 15% of men with urethritis. Infected women complain of a copious yellow-green-gray vaginal discharge that is watery and has a foul odor. When the cervix is inflamed, small amounts of bleeding can result. The patient may also complain of dysuria and dyspareunia, but less commonly than in monilial infections.

Metronidazole is the drug of choice in treatment of trichomoniasis. A carcinogen in laboratory animals, metronidazole is now considered safe for humans and can be used in the second and third trimesters of pregnancy without worry. All sexual partners need to be treated. One dose (2 g) and 3- to 10-day dosage (250-500 mg three times a day) regimens of metronidazole are effective. Treatment failures are common and are attributed to reinfection or failure to complete the entire course of medication. Metronidazole often causes gastrointestinal upset and leaves a metallic taste. When taken in conjunction with alcohol, an antabuse-type reaction (nausea and vomiting) occasionally occurs. Topical metronidazole has been approved for use in a 7-day treatment regimen.

Bacterial Vaginosis

Formerly known as nonspecific vaginitis, *Haemophilus vaginalis* vaginitis, *Corynebacterium vaginalis* vaginitis, and *Gardnerella* vaginalis, bacterial vaginosis is now believed to be a polymicrobial infection caused by an increase in anaerobic organisms and a decrease in lactobacilli (the predominent flora in the normal vagina). The pathogenic organisms include *Bacteroides*, *Peptostreptococcus*, *Mobiluncus*, *Eubacterium*, and *Fusobacterium*. The result is a bothersome, malodorous, burning, itching, vaginal discharge. In its most severe form, it is a profuse gray-green discharge with a fishy odor, accompanied by external dysuria and lower abdominal pain. It can be transmitted sexually; pathogenic organisms have been recovered from the urethras of male partners of infected women.

Diagnosis is made by examining a wet preparation for characteristic clue cells, which are vaginal squamous epithelial cells that are studded with coccobacilli (Fig. 31.3). White blood cells are usually absent on wet preparation, and clumps of small coccobacilli replace the normal rod-shaped vaginal bacteria. Addition of KOH to the discharge usually produces a fishy odor. If a Gram's stain is done, clumps of Gram-negative coccobacilli (*Mobiluncus*) can be seen adhering to the clue cells.

No antibiotic is completely effective. The most effective treatment is metronidazole, 500 mg twice a day for 7 to 10 days for both patient and partners, but it causes nausea in many patients and is contraindicated in pregnancy. Ampicillin has been used in the past and is effective in about half of the patients. Clindamycin is an effective alternative; it can be used both orally (300 mg twice a day for 7 days) and topically (intravaginally at bedtime for 7 days) and can be used during pregnancy. Like other STDs, both sexual partners should be treated simultaneously in cases of recalcitrant vaginosis to prevent reinfection; intercourse should be avoided or condoms used until the treatment has been completed.

Chlamydia trachomatis Infections

Chlamydia trachomatis is an obligate intracellular parasite that cannot be seen under the bright-field microscope or on Gram's stain, and which is difficult to culture. It causes many sexually transmitted diseases including lymphogranuloma venereum, trachoma, inclusion conjunctivitis, nongonococcal salpingitis, urethritis, and cervicitis. Cervical infections with *Chlamydia trachomatis* cause a mucopurulent cervical exudate that can present as yellow vaginal discharge without other symptoms. Vaginal burning is usually absent, but dysuria or urinary frequency is often present. Because *Chlamydia* is a frequent cause of salpingitis, pelvic pain

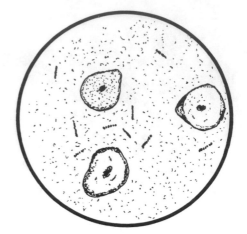

Figure 31.3. Line drawing of clue cells. Note the paucity of normal rods. Approximates magnification with high dry objective.

and cervical motion tenderness on examination often accompany the discharge and help confirm the diagnosis.

Chlamydia cervicitis is often asymptomatic, and diagnosis in this subclinical phase is often one of exclusion. Even symptomatic infection has been difficult to diagnosis, because the organism cannot be seen and is very difficult to culture. The presence of more than five white blood cells on a wet preparation in the absence of other organisms, a sexual history of multiple partners or a new partner, or a friable, eroded cervix should make you suspect infection with this organism. Definitive diagnosis can be made by culture or by immunologic assays, but treatment of this infection is often prescribed on clinical grounds.

In recent years, direct specimen testing for *Chlamydia* using immunologic methods (e.g., Microtrak or Chlamydiazyme) has become available. Figures for sensitivity and specificity vary, but the overall predictive value of a positive test result appears good (i.e., over 90%). Collection requires use of multiple cotton swabs to remove mucus from the cervical os, but lack of transport problems and reduced cost make this test highly appropriate for the primary care office.

Treatment of *Chlamydia* infection requires tetracycline or erythromycin (500 mg four times a day); doxycycline (100 mg twice a day) for 7 to 10 days; Azithromycin (1000 mg single dose) to the patient and her sexual partner(s). If symptoms persist or recur, longer treatment may be required.

Atrophic Vaginitis

Decreased production of estrogen by the ovaries results in thinning and wasting of the vaginal epithelium, causing the vagina to become inflamed, dry, and rough. The tissue shrinks and is shiny and friable, often resulting in vaginal bleeding or spotting. A thin, grey-white, occasionally blood-tinged vaginal discharge is often produced, causing vulvar burning, dysuria, frequency, and urgency. For many women, pruritus is the most troublesome complaint. It is often so severe that it prevents sleep and causes women to scratch intensely, causing secondary skin infections. Among menopausal women, this is the most common type of vaginitis. On microscopic examination, you will see bacteria, white blood cells, and many parabasal epithelial cells in the vaginal discharge.

Topical or oral estrogen replacement can ameliorate the symptoms of atrophic vaginitis. Use concomitant progesterone to cycle the patient if she has a uterus, and exclude endometrial cancer if she presented with vaginal bleeding. When estrogen replacement does not improve these symptoms and other infective agents are ruled out, referral to a gynecologist for biopsy is necessary.

Other Causes of a Vaginal Discharge

Infections with the condyloma acuminata and herpes viruses can cause a clear watery vaginal discharge. Condyloma accuminata often presents as foul-smelling vaginal discharge because anaerobic bacteria secondarily infect the condyloma lesions. If no clear vaginal organism causing the discharge can be distinguished on wet preparation, treatment with triple-sulfa or clindamycin cream usually ameliorates the discharge and may aid in the treatment of the condyloma lesions.

Doderlein's cytolysis is a frequently misdiagnosed or underdiagnosed condition which is often confused with other types of vaginitis. The clinical history is that of a patient who has had numerous visits to the doctor for vaginal discharge and has often been treated with antifungals, antibiotics, or hormone replacement therapy for its symptoms. Doderlein's cytolysis is often confused with *Candida* vaginitis, as their symptoms are similar: vaginal itching, white discharge, which can be watery or curdlike, and burning sensations in the vagina and on the labia after urination. On physical examination, one often sees erythema of the vulva or vulvar excoriations, as well as a whitish discharge that is not malodorous. On wet prep, epithelial cells are seen that have a "moth-eaten" appearance, and many long slender rods of varying length are present, which reflect an overgrowth of lactobacilli. Treatment options include a sodium bicarbonate douche (1 tablespoon of baking soda in 1 quart of warm water, nightly for 1 week) or use of Aminocerv cream (1 applicator applied vaginally BID for 1 week) to sustain an alkaline pH (5.5) in the vagina and to normalize the vaginal ecosystem.

Cervical infection with the herpes simplex virus can present as a clear vaginal discharge. Pain at the site of the lesions is common, however, particularly if there are vulvar, vaginal, or urethral lesions as well. Treatment with acylovir may reduce the duration of viral shedding and the intensity of the symptoms, but it does not eradicate the virus. Long-term suppression with oral acyclovir (400 mg three times a day) decreases the frequency and intensity of outbreaks. Symptomatic treatment of the vulva and vagina with Betadine douches or sitz baths can promote good perineal hygiene and prevent bacterial secondary infection.

In postmenopausal women, Gram-negative bacteria are the most common pathogens causing vaginitis. This bacterial vaginitis often causes a purulent discharge and virtually always accompanies atrophic vaginitis. Treatment is with topical antibiotics (triple-sulfa cream or Betadine douches) for a week and with estrogen preparations.

REFERENCES

1. Greenblatt RM, Lukehart SA, Plummer FA, et al.: Genital ulceration as a risk factor of human immunodeficiency virus infection. *AIDS* 2:47–50, 1988.

SUGGESTED READINGS

Addison LA, Fischer P: *The Office Laboratory*, 2nd ed. East Norwalk, CT, Appleton-Century-Crofts, 1990.

> A definitive text on office laboratory procedure, techniques and interpretation. It is a practical book, well written and comprehensive.

Boston Women's Health Book Collective: *The New Our Bodies, Ourselves: A Book By and For Women*. New York, Simon & Schuster, 1984.

> The first major book on self-help women's health care written by women for women. It contains both factual information about health and individual women's reflections on being a woman. Available in paperback.

Droegmuller W, Herbst AJ, Mishell DR, Stenchever MA: *Comprehensive Gynecology*, 2nd ed. CV Mosby, 1992.

A good general gynecology textbook, which includes sections on lower and upper genital tract diseases.

Faro S (ed): *Diagnosis and Management of Female Pelvic Infections in Primary Care Medicine*. Baltimore, Williams & Wilkins, 1985.

An excellent review of infectious diseases in gynecology, which is well written and up to date. It is well referenced and a book a family doctor would want to have handy.

Spiegel C: Bacterial vaginosis. *Clin Microbiol Rev* 4:485–502, 1991.

This reference discusses recent developments in the understanding of bacterial vaginosis.

chapter 32

CONTRACEPTION

Melanie Mintzer

The office visit for contraception is a critical one for most women. This visit often represents the entry of a young woman into the health care system and provides a forum for addressing the important health concerns of women—menses regulation, sexual activity, pregnancy prevention, planned parenthood, infertility, and sexually transmitted disease prevention. A family physician who is concerned, trusted, and comfortable as a health care educator is in an excellent position to provide the necessary counseling about contraceptive methods for both individuals and couples. By explaining the advantages and disadvantages of the various methods, the family physician can facilitate the best choice by the patient and help ensure compliance. By also educating the patient about sexually transmitted diseases, the physician can prevent many causes of infertility. Once a sense of trust and confidentiality between physician and patient has been established, concerns about sexuality and sexual function can be addressed comfortably. The ability of the family physician to discuss these basic women's health care issues contributes to a family's health and psychological well-being. As you will see women of various ages with different contraceptive needs through the course of their lives, it is especially important for you to become facile with contraceptive techniques. The single female college student may choose a different contraceptive method than a woman who has completed her childbearing. In some instances, a man will choose to be the active contraceptor by using condoms or having a vasectomy. Most single women choose their own contraceptive methods, but couples often discuss the choice with their physician.

In addressing contraception with patients, remember to individualize the method to the patient. Consider her age, sexual activity, exposure to sexually transmitted diseases, lifestyle, and moral beliefs. Expect patient choices to change with time. For example, after the birth of a child, a contraceptive method change will often be requested, and the intent of the contraceptive counseling session will likely shift to address the issues of child spacing and breast-feeding.

The past decade has been marked by an increased concern over sexually transmitted diseases (STDs), including acquired immunodeficiency syndrome disease (AIDS). Certain contraceptive devices can foster or inhibit transmission of STDs; so patients with multiple sexual partners should be counseled about the risks. In high-risk patients, many physicians now recommend using a condom in addition to other contraceptive methods.

This chapter includes brief discussions about the contraceptive counseling session, history taking, and physical examination of the patient. In addition, it reviews the choice and prescription of a contraceptive method, and briefly discusses methods for the future.

CONTRACEPTIVE COUNSELING

A contraceptive counseling session has three purposes: (*a*) to provide the patient with information in a nonjudgmental way; (*b*) to explain the risks, benefits, and side effects of available methods; and (*c*) most importantly, to answer your patient's questions. Evaluate each contraceptive method in relation to the patient's age, marital status, childbearing potential, lifestyle, income, religion, and medical history.

A good counseling session is best done either before or after the physical examination is performed, when the patient is dressed, sitting up, face to face with the physician. Separating the

291

counseling and prescribing from the actual physical examination allows the patient to come to her own decision. Choose terms the patient understands. Begin with a brief review of the basics of reproductive anatomy and physiology, using visual aids that show the menstrual cycle and male and female anatomy. Even well-educated patients will have questions about the reproductive cycle.

Next, describe each contraceptive method, using a pictorial chart. Explain the side effects and minor complications that may arise from each method. Just handing out reading material is not sufficient to assure understanding. Materials should be written at the literacy level of the patient; an 8th grade literacy level is recommended by many health educators for most patient education materials.

In counseling and treating teenagers, confidentiality is of utmost importance. Be aware of your personal feelings about prescribing contraceptives for minors and inform the teenage patient about your own ability to maintain a confidential relationship. If you cannot maintain confidentiality, refer the teen to a family planning clinic where confidentiality can be maintained. A discussion of the teen's needs and desires helps build trust between this younger patient and the physician. By assessing the frequency of intercourse and estimating the number of partners, compliance with the chosen method can be significantly improved. For instance, if your patient feels that taking a pill every night will be difficult, the combined use of an injectable progestin or a barrier method and condoms may prove a wiser choice. Regardless of what other method is used, routine use of a condom by the male partner is recommended to prevent possible transmission of human immunodeficiency virus (HIV) disease (for more details on HIV disease, see Chapter 33).

Expert counseling skills facilitate better compliance. A good explanation of a difficult method, including the risks, benefits, side effects, and specifics of use, can enhance successful contraception. Ask about the patient's fear of pregnancy and whether or not she understands its medical side effects. Also inquire about the patient's need for uninterrupted spontaneity in sex, the frequency of intercourse, prior episodes of sexually transmitted diseases, comfort with touching one's own or a partner's genitals, and the quality of communication between partners. Responses to these questions will help you decide which contraceptive methods are most appropriate for your patient.

MEDICAL HISTORY AND PHYSICAL EXAMINATION

Before prescribing a method of contraception, all women need a physical examination. Although examining teenagers is somewhat awkward, it is important to take a complete medical history and to examine the thyroid, breasts, abdomen, and pelvic organs as well as height, weight, and blood pressure. This focused examination will rule out medical conditions that would preclude oral contraceptive pills. Taking the history and performing the physical examination also provides a natural arena to discuss issues of sexuality, and allows the patient to bring up other medical problems or share anxieties about personal or family medical problems.

Subsequent yearly return visits should update the history and physical assessment and repeat the Pap smear. At each contraception-related return visit, the choice of the contraceptive method should be reviewed. A new symptom or condition that precludes using a certain method also may be discovered, e.g., hypertension in an oral contraceptive pill user, or pelvic inflammatory disease in an intrauterine device (IUD) user. Also, your patient may request discontinuing contraception in order to initiate pregnancy.

Since many women use the family planning visit as their yearly health care maintenance examination, many family doctors choose to do a routine urinalysis to rule out renal disease and diabetes, a lipid screen if not obtained beforehand, a Pap smear, a hematocrit, and STD screening tests. Many family physicians do routine *Chlamydia* cultures or *Chlamydia* immunofluorescence tests on their nonmonogamous sexually active patients. HIV antibody screening tests should be a regular part of yearly family planning examinations for high-risk women.

CHOOSING A CONTRACEPTIVE METHOD

More than half of all pregnancies in the United States are unintended. Most occur because of "nonuse" of contraception, "failure" of a specific method, or "discontinuation" of contraception. These reasons are often related to the patient's age and lifestyle, which explains why the choice of contraceptive method must be tailored to the individual patient. For women who are not in a monogamous relationship, a choice of contraceptive methods should be offered that protects against both pregnancy and sexually transmitted diseases.

To be an effective counselor, you should know the safety and effectiveness rates of each contraceptive method. You can avoid much confusion by quoting "actual" rather than "theoretical" failure rates. Table 32.1 outlines the different contraceptive methods and their relative failure rates with typical users.

All contraceptive methods involve risk to the user. Some are safer than others (diaphragms versus oral contraceptives), some have significant untoward complications (such as IUDs), and use of some result in minor but uncomfortable side effects (sponges causing chemical vaginitis). Childbearing potential must also be considered when counseling patients about various methods. For example, the diaphragm or condom provides relative protection against infection and possible infertility compared to the IUD, but they also carry a higher failure rate, which can result in unwanted pregnancy. Finally, when choosing a specific method, one should consider the relative risk of pregnancy compared to the risk of death from daily living. For nonsmoking teenagers, the risk of death from driving a car is one in 6000, while the risk with oral contraceptive use is one in 63,000.

The costs of the various contraceptive methods are not often considered by physicians but should be, as cost is an important factor in patient compliance. Referring your patient to a local Health Department family planning clinic that provides contraceptive services and examinations on a sliding scale or without charge, can reduce cost. If the patient qualifies for the federally funded Title XX family planning funds for indigent clients, she can often receive 1 year's supply of birth control pills, contraceptive jelly, or condoms free. In most states, Medicaid will pay for Norplant insertion and removal. Table 32.2 provides a summary of available contraceptive methods.

Oral Contraceptives

MECHANISM OF ACTION

Used by more than 50 million women in the world, oral contraceptive pills (OCPs) provide women with a reliable, nonsurgical, reversible method of contraception that has an extremely low failure rate (0.1 to 3 failures per 100 woman-years). Oral contraceptives contain estrogen and progesterone components that in combination are very effective in preventing pregnancy.

The mechanism of action of oral contraceptives is complex. Their estrogen and progestin components cause multiple physiological changes. The estrogens inhibit ovulation by suppressing follicle-

Table 32.1. Failure Rates of Birth Control Methods[a]

Method	One-Year Pregnancy Rate with Perfect Patient Compliance (%)	One-Year Pregnancy Rate in the Average User (%)
Tubal sterilization	0.2	0.4
Vasectomy	0.1	0.15
Injectable progestin	0.3	0.3
Implants (Norplant)	0.04	0.04
Combined birth control pills	0.1	3.0
Progestin-only pill	0.5	3
IUD (Progestasert & Copper T)	0.8–2	2
Condom	2	12
Diaphragm (with spermicide)	6	18
Sponge (with spermicide)		
Nulliparous	6	18
Multiparous	9	28
Cervical cap	6	18
Foams, creams, jellies, vaginal suppositories	3	21
Coitus interruptus	4	18
Fertility awareness techniques (basal body temperature, mucus, calendar, and "rhythm")	1–9	10
Chance (no method of birth control)	85	85

[a]Adapted from Hatcher RA, Stewart F, Trussell J, Kowal K, Guest F, Stewart GK, Cates W: *Contraceptive Technology 1990–1992,* ed 15. New York, Irvington Publishers, 1990, p 134.

Table 32.2. Reversible Contraceptives: A Summary

Method	Benefits	Risks/Problems
Fertility awareness with abstinence (rhythm method)	Can be use by any healthy woman with regular menses; little equipment needed; no adverse side effects	Unreliability, especially in women with irregular menses
Condom	Easy to use; protects against sexually transmitted diseases (STDs); reliable and handy	Breakage; care needed during withdrawal; interruption of lovemaking
Diaphragm	Easy to use; may protect against STDs	Possible bladder infection; must be properly fitted; has to be used with cream or jelly; has to remain inserted for 6–8 hours after intercourse
Vaginal sponge	Easy to insert; may protect against STDs	Allergy; increased risk of toxic shock syndrome; can be difficult to remove intact; cannot use while menstruating or immediately after delivery or abortion
Vaginal chemical contraceptives (foams, creams, jellies, suppositories)	Easy to purchase; may protect against STDs	Contact allergy; inconvenience; messiness
Intrauterine device (IUD)	Convenient and effective	Cramping; midcycle bleeding; ectopic pregnancy; heavy periods; expulsion; perforation of uterine wall; infertility; Copper-7 no longer marketed in U.S.
Oral contraceptives	Effective; convenient; some protection against PID	Increased risk of cardiovascular disease in smokers and with increased age; hypertension; nausea; weight gain; mood changes; amenorrhea
Progesterone implant (Norplant), injectable progestins	Extremely effective; convenient; no estrogenic side effects	Spotting; irregular or absent menses; weight gain

stimulating hormone (FSH) and luteinizing hormone (LH) production by the pituitary gland. They also increase the transit time of the egg through the fallopian tubes, thus reducing the available time for fertilization. The progestins change the cervical mucus, making it thicker, more viscous, and decreased in amount. They also inhibit endometrial proliferation, making it less hospitable to a fertilized ovum.

ABSOLUTE AND RELATIVE CONTRAINDICATIONS

There are both absolute and relative contraindications to prescribing oral contraceptive pills, which are outlined in Table 32.3. The absolute contraindications include thromboembolic disorders, coronary artery disease, carcinoma of the breast or other estrogen-dependent neoplasm, pregnancy, benign or malignant liver tumor, or impaired liver function. In women who have strong relative contraindications to pill use, it is important to consider the risks and benefits of pill use before prescribing it. Cost, effectiveness, compliance, number of sexual partners, risk of acquiring sexually transmitted diseases, and risk of pregnancy

must all be considered. There may be cases where the pill as a method of contraception presents the least risk to the patient.

Absolute contraindications to OCPs are rare, and OCPs have few side effects or complications when used by women under 35 years of age who have none of the significant contraindications. In the late 1960s, the discovery linking serious cardiovascular complications to estrogen dose levels promoted confusion and fear among pill takers. Now, after three major prospective studies demonstrated the safety of low-dose oral contraceptive pills, the "pill" is widely accepted as a safe method of contraception for most young women.

Noncontraceptive benefits include reduction of menstrual cramps, decreased menstrual flow, and regulation of menstrual cycles. Other beneficial side effects of OCPs include protection against ovarian and endometrial cancer and a decrease in the incidence of pelvic inflammatory disease.

A number of supposed risks of OCP use have been disproven. Recent studies show no correlation between monilial infections, uterine myomas, or varicose veins and oral contraceptive use. Significant postpill amenorrhea is rare; fewer than 1% of women have amenorrhea lasting more than 12

Table 32.3. Major Contraindications to Birth Control Pills[a]

Absolute contraindications
- Thromboembolic disorder (or history thereof)
- Cerebrovascular accident (or history thereof)
- Coronary artery disease (or history thereof)
- Known or suspected carcinoma of the breast (or history thereof)
- Known or suspected estrogen-dependent neoplasia (or history thereof)
- Pregnancy
- Benign or malignant liver tumor (or history thereof)
- Previous cholestasis during pregnancy

Strong relative contraindications
- Severe headaches, particularly vascular or migraine
- Hypertension with resting diastolic BP of 90 or greater, or a resting systolic BP of 140 or greater on three or more separate visits, or an accurate measurement of 110 diastolic or more on a single visit
- Diabetes
- Active gallbladder disease
- Impaired liver function
- Mononucleosis, acute phase
- Sickle cell disease (SS) or sickle C disease (SC)
- Elective major surgery planned in next 4 weeks or major surgery requiring immobilization
- Long-leg cast or major injury to lower leg
- 40 years of age or older, accompanied by a second risk factor for the development of cardiovascular disease
- 35 years of age or older and currently a heavy smoker (15 or more cigarettes a day)
- Unexplained (abnormal) vaginal bleeding

[a]Adapted from Hatcher RA, Stewart F, Trussell J, Kowal K, Guest F, Stewart GK, Cates W: *Contraceptive Technology 1990–1992*, ed 15. New York, Irvington Publishers, 1990, p 247.

months after discontinuing the oral contraceptives. Neither spontaneous abortion nor congenital anomalies occur more frequently in pregnancies after discontinuance of the pill.

The preponderance of data suggests that OCPs do not influence overall risk of breast cancer. In 1989, the FDA concluded that no overall risk of breast cancer results from OCP use, and there has been no change in OCP labeling. The Cancer and Steroid Hormone Study (CASH), the largest population-based study to address the breast cancer question, suggested a possible association between the use of *older*, high-dose OCPs and breast cancer in certain subgroups of patients (1, 2). However, results across studies are not consistent, and the conflicting evidence has stimulated more specific epidemiologic studies.

Studies exploring the side effects of contraceptives show that women over 35 who are smokers and those who have other risk factors for cardio-

vascular disease such as elevated triglycerides or cholesterol, diabetes, hypertension, or obesity are at highest risk of having the "pill" precipitate serious cardiovascular complications such as stroke, heart attack, or thrombosis. The more of these characteristics a woman has, the more likely she is to have a major complication with oral contraceptive pill use. Table 32.4 lists the relative contributions of OCP and various factors to mortality rates from circulatory causes. If a woman is young and healthy and a nonsmoker, the risk of a major complication is quite low (3, 4).

From the current studies, it can be concluded that women over 35 who smoke should not be prescribed the pill (5). Healthy nonsmoking women who have no other cardiovascular risk factors can continue using low-dose OCPs (30 to 35 μg of estrogen) into their 40s.

Another risk is that of increased low-density lipoproteins (LDL) and decreased high-density lipoproteins (HDL) cholesterol levels, possibly due to progestins. Therefore, women with significant hyperlipoproteinemia should not take oral contraceptives, and women with a family history of hypercholesterolemia should use a low-progestin, low-estrogen pill. Oral contraceptives can also induce hypertension; the Royal College of General Practitioners Oral Contraceptive Drug Study (1974) found hypertension to be 2.6 times higher among OCP users than among controls (4). Lower-dose agents may have reduced this effect.

Other problems are the possibility of the formation of benign liver tumors (1.2 per 100,000 pill users) and an increased incidence of gallstones. There are also many minor side effects, which are summarized in Table 32.5.

PHARMACOLOGY OF ORAL CONTRACEPTIVE PILLS AND ITS RELATIONSHIP TO PILL SIDE EFFECTS

Combined estrogen and progesterone oral contraceptives contain one of two estrogens, either mestranol or ethinyl estradiol, and one of seven progestins: norethindrone, ethynodiol diacetate, norethynodrel, norethindrone acetate, norgestrel, norgestimate, or desogestrel. Combinations of these two hormones account for the types of oral contraceptives on the market, each of which has predictable, specific side effects. As these hormones have different strengths or potencies, it is helpful to think about the available pills in terms of estrogen or progestin potency strength rather

Table 32.4. Relative Contribution of Oral Contraceptives, Smoking, and Age to Mortality Rates from Circulatory Causes[a]

Age	Smoking Status	Ever Used Pill	Never Used Pill
		Deaths/100,000 Woman-Years	
15–24	Nonsmokers	0	0
	Smokers	10.5	0
25–34	Nonsmokers	4.4	2.7
	Smokers	14.2	4.2
35–44	Nonsmokers	21.5	6.4
	Smokers	63.4	15.2
45–49	Nonsmokers	52.4	11.4
	Smokers	206.7	27.9

[a]Adapted from Royal College of General Practitioners' Oral Contraceptive Study. *Oral Contraceptives and Health: An Interim Report from the Oral Contraceptive Study of the Royal College of General Practitioners.* New York, Pitman, 1974.

than actual microgram or milligram amounts of the drug. Table 32.6 illustrates the relative potencies of estrogens and progestins in currently available oral contraceptive pills; it provides a valuable reference for OCP selection.

When examining the differences between various pills, keep these points in mind:

1. Estrogens are responsible for most major pill-associated complications, such as cerebrovascular accidents and thrombosis, as well as for many minor side effects.
2. Progestins are responsible for some minor side effects and contribute to some major estrogen-induced complications, such as increased HDL levels from norethindrone and norgestrel.
3. The potency of estrogens in OCPs cannot be compared on a microgram per microgram basis.
4. The potency of progestins in OCPs cannot be compared on a milligram per milligram basis.
5. Mestranol is broken down in the body to ethinyl estradiol; ethinyl estradiol is the estrogen used most widely in OCPs.
6. Progestins have both estrogenic and androgenic effects. Some progestins are quite estrogenic (ethynodiol diacetate), and some are very androgenic (norgestrel).
7. Progestins also have antiestrogenic effects.
8. Total estrogenic effect reflects both endogenous production in the ovaries and adipose tissue and exogenous intake. Because of individual variation, pills will cause less suppression of endogenous estrogen production in some women than in others.
9. Estrogens produce different side effects in different women.

CHOOSING AN ORAL CONTRACEPTIVE PILL

There are three types of oral contraceptive pills, monophasic, biphasic, and triphasic. The monophasic pills (e.g., Ortho-Novum 1+35) deliver the same amount of estrogen and progesterone for 21 days. Biphasic pills (e.g., Ortho-Novum 7/7/7, Tri-Norinyl) vary the amount of progesterone through the menstrual cycle, raising the concentration around the time ovulation would occur. The triphasic pills (e.g., Triphasil) alter the levels of both the estrogen and progestin throughout the menstrual cycle, theoretically simulating more closely what happens to normal hormone levels throughout the cycle. There are advantages to prescribing triphasic pills: (*a*) lower total dosages of both estrogen and progestin are used, while still suppressing ovulation and preventing pregnancy; and (*b*) fewer metabolic effects on lipids, blood pressure, and carbohydrate metabolism result. The main disadvantages of triphasic OCPs are (*a*) confusion when a patient misses a pill and then does not know which pill to make up, since they are different colors and potencies; and (*b*) more breakthrough bleeding, thus increasing potential pill discontinuation by an anxious pill user.

When starting a patient on an oral contraceptive pill, you should generally use a low-dose estrogen/progestin combination and observe the patient over the first three to four menstrual cycles for side effects. Many common side effects, such as nausea and breakthrough bleeding (spotting), often resolve within the first three cycles of use. If side effects result, choose an alternative pill that is hormonally structured to treat the side effect(s). If your patient is experiencing no side effects, keep her on the same prescription. It is common to have a woman who has taken Ortho-Novum 1+35 for 15 months present with secondary amenorrhea. Often by switching the patient to a more progestin-dominant pill, such as Nordette or LoOvral, you can produce more adequate withdrawal bleeding. Figure 32.1 is an algorithm that summarizes an approach to selecting and changing oral contraceptives. Some of its major points are discussed below.

1. Generally begin with Ortho 7/7/7, Tri-Norinyl, Ortho-Novum 1/35, or Norinyl 1/35—all low-dose formulations with 35 μg or less of estrogen and a progestin dose of about 1 mg of norethindrone. Advise the woman that breakthrough bleeding is common and usually resolves within three cycles. If a patient has severe acne or is very hirsute, start her on an antiandrogenic pill such as Demulen 1/35 or Orthocyclen.

2. The FDA currently recommends starting the patient on the Sunday closest to the first day of her next period or on the first day of menses. Advise the patient to take the pills at the same time each day. If the pills are prescribed after an abortion, the pill can be started immediately to prevent ovulation. After a pregnancy or surgery, allow 2 weeks before starting, due to the risk of thromboembolism.

3. Any newly menstruating, sexually active adolescent should have three to six regular menstrual cycles before taking the pill.

4. Evaluate the choice of pill after three cycles are taken in adult women, because most minor side effects resolve after three cycles of use. Reevaluate adolescents after one cycle. Some teens will discontinue taking OCPs during the first cycle due to minor side effects. If significant side effects are present after three cycles, change the pill prescription (see Fig. 32.1).

5. If spotting occurs during the 21 days the patient is taking hormones, inquire whether the pill is being taken at the same time each day. If bleeding is heavy, changing the prescription to a pill with a stronger progestin usually stops the spotting. If that fails, change to one with more estrogen.

6. If a missed menses occurs, first take the history to see if any pills have been missed. Perform a pregnancy test to evaluate that possibility. If the pregnancy test result is negative, have the patient take another month of pills. If a second missed menses occurs, change the pill to one with more progestin, and if that fails to produce withdraw bleeding, increase the estrogen dose.

7. If nausea persists, try changing the time of day the pill is taken (e.g., switching to evening) or have the patient take the pill with food. If that fails, decrease the dose of estrogen or prescribe a pill with the same estrogen dose but a more antiestrogenic progesterone.

8. If hyperpigmentation occurs, decrease the estrogen dose and advise the patient to stay out of sunlight and use sun block. Some patients must discontinue the pill to eliminate hyperpigmentation.

9. If depression or premenstrual syndrome symptoms occur, increasing the progestin dose or changing to a progestin dominant pill may help.

10. Oral contraceptives cost about $16.00 to $22.00 per monthly cycle, if purchased in a pharmacy. Most are supplied either in 21-day packages (with instructions to the patient to wait 1 week before beginning the next cycle) or 28-day packages (with 7 days of placebo).

MINIPILL (PROGESTERONE-ONLY PILLS)

Progesterone-only oral contraceptive pills contain a microdose of progestin. They are indicated for women who are lactating or in whom estrogen-containing pills are contraindicated. This pill works by altering the cervical mucus, tubal motility, and endometrial lining, thus making it difficult for the fertilized egg to implant. In some women, the minipill also prevents ovulation.

The actual use failure rate, 2 pregnancies per 100 woman-years of use, is higher than that of other oral contraceptives. The side effect of 10 to 30% breakthrough bleeding is troublesome to its users. Other side effects include an increased risk of ectopic pregnancy, amenorrhea, and fluid retention. This pill must be taken daily, and not in a cyclic fashion to prevent pregnancy, and no regular menstrual cycle is established with its use. Many women find it upsetting to not know whether they are pregnant and prefer to use other methods of contraception, usually barrier methods, while lactating.

Intrauterine Devices

The intrauterine device (IUD), when properly used and carefully inserted into a monogamous, parous

Table 32.5. Side Effects of Oral Contraceptives

| | HORMONAL CAUSE | | | | | TIME COURSE | |
| | Estrogen | | Progestin | | Androgen | Worse Initially, Subsides within 3 Months | Worsens with Time on Pill |
	Excess	Deficiency	Excess	Deficiency	Excess		
General symptoms							
Cyclic edema, weight gain	X					X	
Fatigue, tiredness				X			
Increased appetite, noncyclic weight gain			X	X			
Headaches	X			X			
Vascular	X						
Between pill packages			X				
Noncyclic		X					
Hot flashes		X					
Nausea, dizziness	X				X		
Menstrual/gynecologic							
Amenorrhea, decreased menstrual flow		X	X				X
Cervical eversion	X						
Delayed onset of menses				X			
Dry vaginal mucosa, atrophic vaginitis, and dyspareunia	X						X
Increased leiomyoma size							X
Increased vaginal discharge (without infection)	X						
Monilia vaginitis			X				
Painful menses, cramping, heavy menstrual flow				X		X	
Spotting, breakthrough bleeding: Early/mid-cycle		X				X	
Late cycle				X			
Skin and hair							
Chloasma, hyperpigmentation	X						X
Cutaneous angiomata	X						X
Hairless			X				X
Hirsutism					X		X
Oily skin, acne			X		X		
Pruritus					X		

| | HORMONAL CAUSE | | | | | TIME COURSE | |
| | Estrogen | | Progestin | | Androgen | | |
	Excess	Deficiency	Excess	Deficiency	Excess	Worse initially, subsides within 3 months	Worsens with time on pill
Cardiovascular							
Dilated leg veins			X				
Hypertension	X		X				X
Myocardial infarction	X						X
Pelvic congestion syndrome			X				
Thrombophlebitis	X						X
Mood and affect							
Depression		X	X				
Irritability	X	X					
Libido:							
increased					X		
decreased		X	X				
Breasts							
Cystic changes	X						X
Increased size	X		X				
Lactation suppression	X					X	
Tenderness	X		X			X	
Other							
Cholestatic jaundice			X		X		X
Cyclic abdominal or leg pain	X					X	
Hepatic adenoma	X						
Impaired glucose tolerance			X			X	
Poor contact lens fit	X					X	

aAdapted from Dickey RP: *Managing Contraceptive Pill Patients*, ed 3. Durant, OK, Creative Information, Inc, 1983, pp 104–105.

Table 32.6. Relative Estrogen and Progestin Potency of Currently Available Oral Contraceptives, Reflecting the Debate About the Strength of Progestins[a]

Progestin (mg)			DOSE OF PROGESTIN (mg)	NAME(S) OF PILLS	DOSE OF ESTROGEN (mcg)	Estrogen (mcg) RELATIVE POTENCY	
GREENBLATT (1967) Relative Potency	SWYER (1982) Relative Potency	DORFLINGER (1985) Relative Potency					
0.35	0.35	0.35	Norethindrone 0.35	Micronor Nor-QD			1
2.2	.15-.22	.375-.75	Norgestrel 0.075	Ovrette			2
2.0	0.5	1.0	Norethindrone Acetate 1.0	Loestrin 1/20	Ethinyl Estradiol 20	0.7-0.8	3
1.0	1.0	1.0	Norethindrone 1.0	Norinyl 1/50 Ortho 1/50 Genora 1/50	Mestranol 50	1.0	4
3.0-7.5	.10-.375	.5-2.5	L-Norgestrel 0.05/0.075/0.125	Triphasil Tri-Levlen	Ethinyl Estradiol 30/40 30	1.0-1.2	5
9.0	.3-.45	1.5-3.0	L-Norgestrel 0.15	Nordette Levlen	Ethinyl Estradiol 30	1.0-1.2	6
9.0	.6-.9	1.5-3.0	Norgestrel 0.3	Lo/Ovral	Ethinyl Estradiol 30	1.0-1.2	7
3.0	0.75	1.5	Norethindrone Acetate 1.5	Loestrin 1.5/30	Ethinyl Estradiol 30	1.0-1.2	8
0.4	0.4	0.4	Norethindrone 0.4	Ovcon 35	Ethinyl Estradiol 35	1.2-1.4	9
0.5	0.5	0.5	Norethindrone 0.5	Brevicon Modicon	Ethinyl Estradiol 35	1.2-1.4	10
0.5-1.0	0.5-1.0	0.5-1.0	Norethindrone 0.5/1.0/0.5	Ortho 10/11	Ethinyl Estradiol 35	1.2-1.4	11
0.5-1.0	0.5-1.0	0.5-1.0	Norethindrone 0.5/0.75/1.0	Tri-Norinyl	Ethinyl Estradiol 35	1.2-1.4	12
0.5-1.0	0.5-1.0	0.5-1.0	Norethindrone 0.5/0.75/1.0	Ortho 7/7/7	Ethinyl Estradiol 35	1.2-1.4	13
1.0	1.0	1.0	Norethindrone 1.0	Norinyl 1/35 Ortho 1/35 Genora 1/35 N.E.E. 1/35	Ethinyl Estradiol 35	1.2-1.4	14
15	0.5	1.0	Ethynodiol Diacetate 1.0	Demulen 1/35	Ethinyl Estradiol 35	1.2-1.4	15
1.0	1.0	1.0	Norethindrone 1.0	Norinyl 1/80 Ortho 1/80	Mestranol 80	1.6	16
1.0	1.0	1.0	Norethindrone 1.0	Ovcon 50	Ethinyl Estradiol 50	1.7-2.0	17
2.0	0.5	1.0	Norethindrone Acetate 1.0	Norlestrin 1/50	Ethinyl Estradiol 50	1.7-2.0	18
2.0	2.0	2.0	Norethindrone 2.0	Norinyl 2 Ortho 2	Mestranol 100	2.0	19
2.7	2.5		Norethindrone 2.5	Enovid-E	Mestranol 100	2.0	20
5.0	1.25	2.5	Norethindrone Acetate 2.5	Norlestrin 2.5/50	Ethinyl Estradiol 50	1.7-2.0	21
15	1.5	2.5 -5	Norgestrel 0.5	Ovral	Ethinyl Estradiol 50	1.7-2.0	22
15	0.5	1.0	Ethynodiol Diacetate 1.0	Demulen 1/50	Ethinyl Estradiol 50	1.7-2.0	23
15	0.5	1.0	Ethynodiol Diacetate 1.0	Ovulen	Mestranol 100	2.0	24

15 10 5 0   2.0 1.5 1.0 0.5 0   5 4 3 2 1   0   1.0 2.0
Potency Units   Potency Units

[a]Reprinted with permission from Hatcher RA, Stewart F, Trussell J, Kowal K, Guest F, Stewart GK, Cates W: *Contraceptive Technology 1990–1992*, ed 15. New York, Irvington Publishers, 1990, p 261.

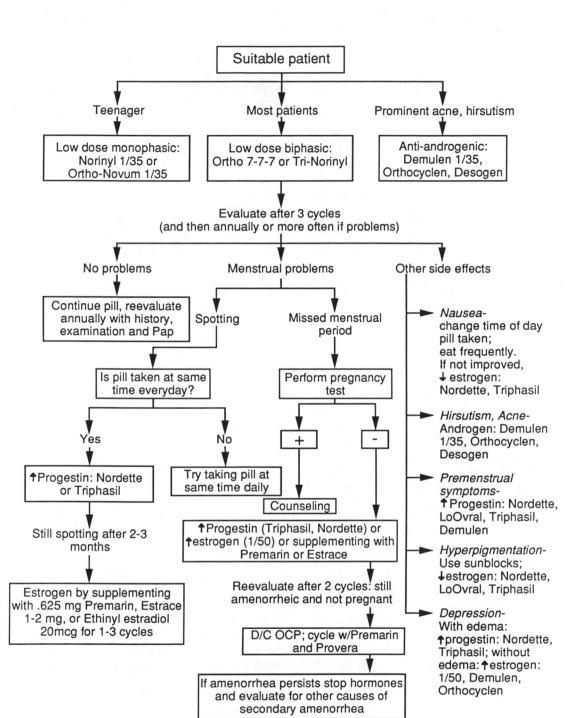

Figure 32.1. Algorithm for selecting an oral contraceptive pill.

woman is one of the most effective forms of contraception available to women. In the past decade, this form of contraception has received considerable negative publicity. A. H. Robins, who produced the Dalkon shield, now off the market, declared bankruptcy after multiple malpractice suits were filed by users and their families. This intrauterine device had a multifilament tail that facilitated entry of bacteria into the uterus, resulting in infection, abscess, sepsis, and death in some women who had the Dalkon shields. Several other intrauterine devices have also been removed from the market because of legal suits, even though many women are at low risk for these complications.

The IUD's theoretical failure rate and the actual failure rate are quite similar (3 pregnancies in 100 women), since the patient has little to do with its use except check that the IUD string is present. IUDs are made of flexible plastic, some with copper wrapped around the device (Copper-7, Copper T380, and ParaGard). Others contain progesterone (Progestasert), which is slowly released into the woman's system. Both copper- and hormone-containing devices lose their effectiveness and must be replaced. Plastic IUDs (Lippes Loops) were designed to be left inside the uterus indefinitely, although the manufacturers suggest replacing them every 5 years to prevent actinomycoses. Most types of IUDs are essentially unavailable in the United States. The Progestasert remains available. In 1988, the ParaGard, a T-shaped copper-coated device designed by Howard Tatum, became available, recommended for monogomous multiparous women with no contraindication.

Non-hormone-containing devices prevent pregnancy by setting up a local inflammatory response that lyses the blastocyst and sperm, and prevents implantation by increasing local production of prostaglandins. In addition to this inflammatory response, copper-containing devices alter carbonic anhydrase and alkaline phosphatase activity and probably interfere with estrogen effects on the endometrium, and progesterone devices provide a microdose of the hormone that prevents implantation. Copper-containing devices are the most common method of contraception in many third world countries.

The Progestasert is particularly suited for women who have dysmenorrhea and heavy periods, as the progesterone in the IUD decreases these two troublesome occurrences. It also seems to help women with significant premenstrual symptoms. It requires yearly reinsertions and often causes breakthrough bleeding.

The IUD is inserted into the patient's uterus during menses, when slight cervical dilation makes insertion easier. The IUD string, which is connected to the end of the device, is cut to leave 2 to 4 cm protruding from the external cervical os. Most women tolerate the insertion procedure well; a preinsertion dose of naproxen 500 mg or ibuprofen 800 mg relieves cramps caused by insertion. A few women have several days of bleeding, cramping, or backache after insertion; time and prostaglandin-inhibiting drugs lessen these symptoms. During the first few months, spotting between periods can occur, and the period itself may become heavier. The position of the device is checked at a 1-month follow-up visit. At this time most major side effects will have subsided.

IUDs are not without problems. Careful patient selection will minimize complications. IUD recipients should have no evidence of genital infection, no evidence or history of unexplained genital bleeding, and no evidence of genital cancer. She should have no condition that precludes the insertion of a foreign body into her body, such as subacute bacterial endocarditis, glomerulonephritis, renal failure, mitral valve prolapse, or immunosuppression. Ideally, IUD patients should not have any of the following risk factors: multiple sexual partners, previous history of pelvic inflammatory disease, risk of gonorrhea or *Chlamydia* exposure, nulliparity, history of infertility, heavy menstrual cramps, or heavy menstrual periods. They should be mentally capable of noting and reporting any IUD-associated infection, the expulsion of the IUD, the possibility of pregnancy, or the occurrence of unusually heavy menstrual periods. Women who have large uteri or who have had children, and who have one sexual partner are ideal IUD candidates, as the IUD can be inserted with little or no difficulty, the expulsion rate is low, and pelvic infections are unlikely.

The most common problems of IUD use are spotting (10 to 15% of users), heavy menstrual bleeding, and bleeding between cycles, which may eventually result in iron deficiency anemia. Other problems include expulsion of the device (5 to 20% of users in the first year, rarely after), shifting location in the uterus, becoming imbedded in the endometrium, and uterine perforation.

The most serious complication is that the IUD seems to promote pelvic infections. Many fine studies have identified an increased risk of pelvic inflammatory disease (PID), which begins slowly and may progress to endometritis, myometritis, and occasionally tubo-ovarian abscess. This illness can present as premenstrual syndrome (bloating, backache, or spotting), as a foul-smelling vaginal discharge, as fever, chills, anorexia, and severe lower abdominal pain, or as infertility. PID can be treated in its early stages as an outpatient illness with ceftriaxone, doxycycline, azithromycin and metronidazole, or with an intravenous cephalosporin and doxycycline in more serious cases. If PID is suspected in an IUD user, the device must be removed immediately.

As with other methods of contraception, the risks and benefits of this method need to be carefully reviewed with the patient before insertion. Careful follow-up of all problems can usually prevent a pelvic infection and its complications.

The cost of the IUD insertion and device vary between $125 and $300. The Progestasert device itself is good for 1 year and costs about $125; the ParaGard costs about $200 and can remain in place for up to 8 years.

Barrier Methods

Barrier contraceptives, (male and female condoms, spermicides, diaphragms, cervical caps, and contraceptive sponges) all function to kill sperm or block their entry into the cervical os. They are readily available to both adolescents and adults, and rarely produce side effects. The theoretical and actual use effectiveness rates vary, because effectiveness depends on proper use by the patient. Diaphragms and cervical caps must be fitted to the individual patient, but the other barrier methods can be used by anyone. All barrier methods are reversible. When used in combination, they are almost 100% effective.

Condoms are the oldest reliable method of contraception for men. Once thought to decrease sexual pleasure, they are now becoming popular because rubber condoms inhibit spread of the HIV virus. Condoms are made of rubber or processed collagenous animal tissue fit over the erect penis. They are easy to apply and are portable. The differences among brands involve slight modifications in shape, the presence or absence of lubricant, and the presence or absence of spermicide on the inside or outside of the condom. They come in different colors and textures, and some have reservoirs for semen collection at the tips.

The more expensive condoms are more comfortable and more flexible.

Female condoms, the newest barrier method to be introduced, will be available in late 1993. One type is a double-rimmed polyurethane tube with a blunt end that covers the cervix. It is inserted like a tampon and, when opened up in the vaginal vault, creates a plastic canal into which the penis is placed. An outer ring lies outside the vagina, covering the labia and protecting them from contact with possible skin lesions, and the internal ring holds the plastic around the cervix to create a fitted cover. The other type is a latex condom pouch worn as a panty. The pouch is pushed up into the vagina when the penis first enters the vaginal vault. This type of condom also provides protection of the labia and perineum from contact with possible skin lesions that can transmit STDs. Thus, both devices provide contraceptive protection and STD protection for the female.

The actual use effectiveness rate is about 10 pregnancies per woman-year, while the theoretical rate is about three pregnancies per 100 woman-years. Three large British studies found the failure rate to be one pregnancy in 10,000 uses. Condoms are contraindicated in men that cannot maintain an erection, as the condom can slip off. Allergy to the rubber or spermicide used in condoms can occur; natural lambskin condoms can be used by these men but provide *no* protection against HIV.

There are many noncontraceptive benefits of condoms, the most important being the prevention of many sexually transmitted bacterial or parasitic infections and inhibition of HIV virus transmission. Male condoms enhance sexual pleasure in men with premature ejaculation, as they reduce glans sensitivity. Although the use of condoms requires the interruption of lovemaking, applying the condom can be incorporated into the lovemaking. The cost ranges from 35 cents to about $5 each. Anyone of any age and either sex can purchase condoms in drugstores.

Spermicides require neither a prescription nor a pelvic examination and rarely cause side effects. Some come in a single-application form, such as preloaded vaginal applicators of jelly or foam, or vaginal suppositories. The convenience and ease of application make them popular with adolescents. Used in combination with condoms, spermicides provide excellent protection from pregnancy. All spermicides act to prevent conception by immobilizing or killing sperm. They are made up of an inert base that holds the spermicide, usually nonoxynol-9. The base helps block the entry of the sperm into the cervical os.

Foam spermicides are more effective than jellies or suppositories, because foam disperses in the vagina more readily. All spermicides must be applied 30 minutes or less before intercourse. In addition to its contraceptive benefit, nonoxynol-9 provides some protection against gonorrhea and chlamydial disease and may provide some protection against viral disease. The only known contraindication is allergy to the spermicidal chemical. A foam kit costs approximately $10 to $12 for 20 applications. A tube of contraceptive jelly (15 applications) costs about $7. They can be purchased in the feminine hygiene section of most major supermarkets or drugstores.

Diaphragms and cervical caps are somewhat more difficult to use than other barrier methods because their efficacy depends on both correct placement over the cervix and an effective spermicide. The appliance must be left in place for at least 6 hours. The rubber cup or cap serves as a reservoir to hold the spermicide against the cervix, preventing conception by acting as both a physical and a chemical barrier to sperm from the cervical os.

A diaphragm must be fitted by a clinician so that it covers the cervix and wedges snugly behind the pelvic bone. Then, the patient must be taught to properly insert and remove the device. Its actual effectiveness rate varies between 6 and 18%, with the more experienced users having greater success than the younger users. Contraceptive failures result from lack of use with every intercourse, improper insertion, improper fit of the appliance, displacement during coitus (most common in the female superior position), a hole in the diaphragm, and failure to use additional spermicide with each additional intercourse. Both the diaphragm and the cervical cap can be used during menses to hold back menstrual flow during intercourse. The major disadvantage of the diaphragm is that it increases the incidence of urinary tract infections in some women.

The cervical cap, which fits over the cervix like a cap, is smaller than the diaphragm and somewhat more difficult to insert. Its failure rates may be slightly higher than those of the diaphragm. Its major advantages are that it can be kept in for 24 hours and that it appears less likely to cause urinary tract infections that the diaphragm.

A diaphragm costs about $15, and the contraceptive jelly or cream used with it costs about $7 for a tube with 15 applications. The cervical cap costs about $70 and does not require the user to place extra spermicide in the vagina with additional intercourse.

The contraceptive sponge is a round, flexible synthetic material that is imbedded with the nonoxynol-9 spermicide. There is a slight dimple in the circle, which fits over the cervix. A polyester loop on the bottom of the sponge is used to remove it from the vagina after 24 hours. As with all other barrier methods, there is no need to wait after insertion before having intercourse. The sponge kills sperm and prevents their entry into the cervical os. Its effectiveness rate is similar to that of foam alone. It is less messy to use than foam or jelly and is a more spontaneous method because no additional spermicide is necessary with repeated intercourse. Its most frequent disadvantage is that the sponge can become lodged at the top of the vaginal vault, making it difficult to remove. It is quite possible to forget about the sponge and leave it in place, which usually results in a vaginal infection. Other side effects, as with all spermicides, are allergy or local irritation of the vaginal mucosa. The sponge costs approximately $1 and can be purchased in most drug stores.

Postcoital Contraception

The use of postcoital contraceptives is controversial. Some people view postcoital contraception as abortifacient, while others view it as a way to reduce the number of abortions performed. As the risk of pregnancy with intercourse is highest (up to 17%) at midcycle, many European nations have developed postcoital contraceptives and are currently testing them for efficacy. In the United States, the FDA has not officially approved the use of oral contraceptives as postcoital contraceptives, but many physicians use them, especially for rape or sexual abuse victims.

A common and effective postcoital contraceptive is two Ovral tablets taken within 72 hours (preferably 12 to 24 hours) after intercourse. Twelve hours later, two additional tablets are taken. The total dose is 200 mg of norgestrel and 200 μg of estrogen. The mechanism of action is to induce a menstrual period within 21 days of administration. It is thought that the failure rate is approximately 2% with this method. Most women feel quite nauseated after taking the tablets; one can counter these symptoms with promethazine (Phenergan) suppositories or pills.

Morning-after insertion of an intrauterine device is also an effective postcoital method, but it has been essentially eliminated as a method because of loss of the availability of Copper-7 and Tatum T devices. Postcoital insertion of the IUD prevents implantation of a fertilized ovum, and it must be done within 4 to 6 days after intercourse.

Injectable Progestins

The use of depo medroxyprogesterone acetate (DMPA or Depo-Provera) and Norethindrone enanthate began after oral hormonal contraception became available. These methods have been used in the third world for the last 20 years and are both effective and safe. The major barrier to their more widespread use is controversy over potential adverse effects of teratogenicity, carcinogenicity, and interference with the return of normal fertility after discontinuation. They have been approved with some reservations by England, Sweden, Canada, and over 100 developing nations. This method acts by inhibiting ovulation, most probably at the level of the hypothalamus, resulting in a reduction of follicle-stimulating hormone (FSH) and luteinizing hormone (LH). There are also effects on peripheral organs, making cervical mucus thick, making the endometrium unsuitable for implantation, and possibly inhibiting ovum transport through the fallopian tubes.

DMPA has the highest efficacy rate of a reversible contraceptive, 0.5 pregnancies in 100 woman-years, and one injection provides protection for 3 months. Both DMPA and Norethindrone enanthate interfere with the normal menstrual cycle, and their effects are unpredictable. Typically, serum levels take a week to peak, and effectiveness lasts for 2 to 4 months. Many women experience intermittent spotting, but by the end of 1 year of use, approximately 50% of users will become amenorrheic. A small percentage of users will have episodes of heavy vaginal bleeding, though treatment of this is not usually required.

Troublesome side effects include bloating, fluid retention, mood changes, headache, dizziness, and weight gain. Carpal tunnel syndrome and alopecia have also been noted. Most studies do not reveal serious changes in blood pressure or liver function.

Injectable progestins were approved by the FDA for use as a contraceptive in early 1993. This method is recommended for women who are very fertile, who have failed other contraceptive methods, who have poor success with barrier methods, who are not good IUD candidates, or who want short term contracepion who have risk factors (such as hypertension or migraine headaches) that preclude using combined oral contraceptive pills. A 150-mg injection costs approximately $25.

Subdermal Progestin Implants (Norplant)

Norplant, a nonbiodegradable subdermal implant, is now marketed in the United States. It consists of six 2.4-mm wide, 34-mm long flexible capsules that release 36 mg of levonorgestrel over 5 years. These capsules can be removed at any time, with rapid return of fertility. Approved for use in the U.S. in 1991, this method is extremely effective, with failure rates averaging 0.04 per 100 users per year. Failure rates increase over the next 4 years, with the average failure rate being 1.1 during the fifth year of use (6).

Advantages include its reliability, reversibility, continuous effect for up to 5 years, and the fact that the user does not need to worry about remembering to use the method. It contains no estrogen, which is an advantage for women in whom estrogen therapy is contraindicated. It is an excellent method for adolescents.

The major disadvantage of Norplant is the production of unpredictable menses. Altered bleeding patterns, including prolonged bleeding and spotting, and absent or scanty menses, are common. Other side effects parallel those of injectable progestins. Insertion and removal of the device requires minor surgery, and the implants are slightly visible.

Contraindications to Norplant use include acute liver disease, jaundice, unexplained vaginal bleeding, pregnancy, and a history of thrombophlebitis, pulmonary embolism, stroke, or myocardial infarction. The device costs approximately $350, plus up to $200 for insertion and removal. If the cost is averaged over 5 years, however, it is lower than that of oral contraceptive pills purchased at a pharmacy.

Fertility Awareness or Natural Family Planning

Fertility awareness methods include the "rhythm" or calendar method in combination with the basal body temperature (BBT) method and the mucus method (Billings) of predicting ovulation. Fertility awareness is now very popular, being used both to predict fertility and to prevent pregnancy. This method requires significant motivation by the couple. It is the only method sanctioned by the Catholic church. Success with this method depends on the couple's ability to pinpoint the days when another method of contraception (or abstinence) needs to be used as a backup, i.e., when the woman is most fertile and conception is most likely.

Couples who choose this method must become facile with all the signs of fertility, such as temperature rise, change in cervical mucus, and pain of ovulation. Family planning experts feel that this method is generally ineffective, with fertility awareness advocates identifying actual failure rates around 25 pregnancies per 100 woman-years (see Table 32.1). Courses to learn fertility awareness, taught by various family planning and state agencies and by planned parenthood clinics, usually cost between $30 and $75 per couple.

Sterilization

For men and women requesting a permanent method, sterilization is often the best option. It is the most common method of contraception for married women in the United States today. The most important issue is informed consent. The patient should fully understand that sterilization must be considered irreversible. Although a slight possibility of pregnancy exists, sterilization is nearly 100% effective.

Vasectomy is a surgical operation that permanently blocks sperm passage by cutting out, ligating, and cauterizing the vas deferens. The sperm are then absorbed in testes and epididymis, leaving the semen sterile. Vasectomy can safely be performed under local anesthesia as an outpatient procedure costing $300 to $500. It is often performed by family physicians. Tubal ligation is a similar procedure on the fallopian tubes. It too can be performed on an outpatient, but spinal, epidermal, or general anesthesia is required. It can be done via a laparoscope through the umbilicus or by making small incisions above the pubic symphysis. The cost of these procedures varies, depending on whether they are performed in an outpatient facility or in the hospital. The average cost is $600; many states provide funding for eligible women over 21 years of age.

REFERENCES

1. The Cancer and Steroid Hormone Study of the Centers for Disease Control and the National Institute of Child Health and Human Development. Oral-

contraceptive use and the risk of breast cancer. *N Engl J Med* 315:405–411, 1986.
2. The Centers for Disease Control Cancer and Steroid Hormone Study: Long-term oral contraceptive use and the risk of breast cancer. *JAMA* 249:1591–1595, 1983.
3. Ramcharan S, Pellegrin FA, Ray R, Hsu JF: *The Walnut Creek Contraceptive Drug Study: A Prospective Study of the Side Effects of Oral Contraceptives*, Vol 3. Bethesda, M.D: US Dept. of Health Education and Welfare, Public Health Service, National Institutes of Health, National Institute for Child and Maternal Health and Human Development, Center for Population Research, 1981.
4. Royal College of General Practitioners: *Oral Contraceptives and Health: An Interim Report from the Oral Contraception Study of the Royal College of General Practitioners*. London, Pitman, 1974.
5. Vessey MP, McPherson K, Johnson B: Mortality among women participating in the Oxford Family Association Contraceptive Study. *Lancet* 2:731–733, 1977.
6. Affandi B, Santoso SSI, Djajadilaga W, et al.: Five year experience with Norplant. *Contraception* 36:417–428, 1987.

SUGGESTED READINGS

Corson SL, Derman RJ, Tyrer LB (eds): *Fertility Control*. Boston, Little, Brown & Co., 1985.

Dickey RP: *Managing Contraceptive Pill Patients*. ed 5. Durant, OK: Creative Informatics, 1992.

Both of the above references are excellent, practical resource books on contraception.

Hatcher RA, Stewart F, Trussell J, Kowal K, Guest F, Stewart GK, Cates W: *Contraceptive Technology 1990–1992*, ed 15. New York, Irvington Publishers, 1990.

This book is the family planning "bible" used by all types of family planning professionals from health educators to physicians. Written in an easy-to-read format, its material is ready to be cited and integrated into standing orders, nursing orders, or clinical protocols.

Lee NC, Rubin GL, Borucki R: The intrauterine device and pelvic inflammatory disease revisited: New results from the Women's Health Study. *Obstet Gynecol* 72:1–6, 1988.

A comprehensive study about IUD risks and benefits.

Neinstein LS: *Adolescent Health Care: a Practical Guide*, ed 2. Baltimore, Urban & Schwarzenberg, 1991.

This book is a must for all adolescent-health practitioners. It is written in an easy-to-use format with a complete index.

chapter 33

PRIMARY CARE OF HIV DISEASE

Cora D. Spaulding and Warren P. Newton

In 10 years, HIV disease has grown from a few cases into a major pandemic. HIV disease is caused by infection with a retrovirus, the human immunodeficiency virus (HIV), which invades and destroys helper lymphocytes (also called T4 or CD4 helper lymphocytes). These CD4 helper cells regulate antibody-producing cells and killer cells. As a consequence of the destruction of CD4 cells, HIV-infected patients experience a progressive and predictable deterioration of their immune systems. They become susceptible to the opportunistic infections and malignancies that characterize the adult immunodeficiency syndrome (AIDS), the most severe manifestation of HIV disease.

In the United States, it is estimated that 1.5 million Americans are HIV-infected. Most are between the ages of 20 and 49 and will die prematurely of AIDS. Already, over 300,000 Americans have died of AIDS (1). The early death of young productive human beings represents a loss to individual families and to society. Medical care for people with AIDS is expensive because of the chronicity and severity of illness.

Over the past 10 years, considerable effort has been devoted to describing the epidemiology and natural history of the infection and to searching for curative or palliative therapies. Despite these efforts, HIV infection has continued to spread. While the care of infected patients continues to be important, more attention needs to be focused on prevention. In fact, prevention of the spread of HIV disease is one of the major challenges of the 1990s. Physicians can aid this effort by recognizing and working with individuals in their practices who are infected or at risk of infection.

This chapter offers a practice-based approach to HIV disease, which highlights prevention. It presents a method for assessing HIV risk and suggests guidelines for counseling patients. A brief overview of the clinical spectrum of disease is provided, and the psychosocial and ethical issues relevant to HIV infection are examined. For a more detailed treatment of the clinical aspects of HIV infection, interested readers can explore the referenced materials.

WHO IS INFECTED OR AT RISK OF INFECTION?

The initial appearance of HIV disease among gay white males led to the misperception that gays were exclusively at risk. When infection was subsequently seen among hemophiliacs, blood transfusion recipients, intravenous (IV) drug users, and their sexual partners, members of these groups were considered to be at high risk. More recently, heterosexual transmission among individuals with multiple partners has been on the rise. With the discovery of the human immunodeficiency virus (HIV) and the availability of a serologic diagnostic test, it became apparent that the common theme among all risk groups was exposure to the virus via contact with an infected bodily fluid.

We now know that exposure can occur as a result of sexual contact or transfer of blood via IV drug use or transfusion, during birth, or in utero. Cases of postnatal transmission subsequent to breast-feeding have been reported. Recognized behaviors that increase the likelihood of infection include unprotected anal intercourse among homosexual or bisexual men, unprotected vaginal or anal intercourse in women, and the use of shared unsterilized IV drug paraphernalia. Risk of infection is raised to a lesser degree by a history of heterosexual intercourse with multiple partners, blood transfusion between 1978 and 1985, or needlestick exposure to blood from a person known to be infected or with a history of high-risk behaviors.

Unfortunately, because the idea of *risk groups* preceded the concept of *risk behavior*, some people continue to operate under the illusion that they are immune to HIV infection as long as they don't belong to a high-risk group. In reality, it is individual behavior, not group membership, that determines risk of infection. This message must be communicated to all of our patients to forestall the epidemic.

SCREENING PATIENTS FOR HIV DISEASE

Risk Assessment

Patients at risk for HIV disease look normal. They have no visible signs that indicate high risk. Only a careful history can identify risk status, and a history of high-risk behaviors takes skill to obtain. Those who are at high risk of infection because of their behavior often minimize that risk or, because high-risk behaviors are stigmatized, don't initiate discussions of sexual and drug use with their physicians.

To determine who is infected or at high risk of infection, physicians must initiate discussions of risk behavior with their patients. Any patient who could potentially be sexually active or engaged in drug use deserves a risk assessment. Particular attention should be given to young people, since they constitute the most sexually active population and are at highest risk for intravenous drug use. Moreover, since adolescence is a time marked by experimentation and infrequent physician visits, risk assessments are appropriate almost any time a teenager is seen.

A risk assessment should include questions on current and past drug use and sexual behavior. Unfortunately, a sexual history is often not done because physicians and patients are uncomfortable talking about sex. To become more proficient at assessing HIV risk, physicians should first assess their level of comfort with sexual history taking and then develop an approach to asking the necessary questions that puts the patient at ease.

Figure 33.1 illustrates one approach to the patient interview. Information that should be elicited includes the number and gender of sexual partners, specific sexual practices (vaginal and anal intercourse, oral sex), use of barrier methods and spermicides, drug use history, and risk behavior of their partners. Discussing these issues requires sensitivity on the part of the physician and a nonjudgmental manner. Reassurance should be pro-

vided that the questions are a routine part of a thorough medical examination and help the physician to tailor preventive care. Along with affirming the sensitive nature of the questions, the physician needs to remind the patient that the information provided will be treated confidentially.

The questions in Figure 33.1 have been organized to streamline the risk assessment and facilitate an efficient yet compassionate discussion of the relevant issues. When the patient has engaged in few high-risk behaviors, the interview will be very abbreviated. When high-risk behavior is acknowledged, more specific inquiries to better define risk are triggered. Additionally, the questions have been formulated with a variety of lifestyles in mind so as not to be exclusive or presumptive.

By combining the information derived from the patient interview, the medical history, and the physical examination, a risk estimate can be generated for each patient. Based on the knowledge from the clinical assessment and the community prevalence, an approximation of the probability of infection between 0 and 100% should be made to guide future actions. In patients at any risk level, safe behaviors can be reinforced and education about unsafe practices can be provided. In patients at higher risk, HIV testing may be indicated.

Case 1. Risk Assessment

Joan M., a 30-year-old accountant who is married and the mother of two children, presents for a well-woman examination. She has no complaints.

Should she be assessed for HIV disease?

Case Discussion

It would be easy to assume that because the patient is married, has a profession and a family, she is not at risk of HIV infection. But it must be remembered that the risk of HIV infection is largely related to behaviors that may not be readily discernible. Risk determination should be based, not on assumptions made about the patient's behavior, but rather on factual information that the patient provides.

An assessment of this patient in fact revealed that she was at risk for HIV infection because of her past history. Joan's first husband was an IV drug abuser who occasionally shared needles and had sexual encounters with prostitutes. Joan divorced him 4 years ago and a year later married her current husband. He is the father of her children and has no known risk factors for HIV disease. Joan's relationship is monogamous, and she denies any drug use. However, based on her ex-husband's risk behavior, Joan is at high risk of HIV infection. She decides to be tested.

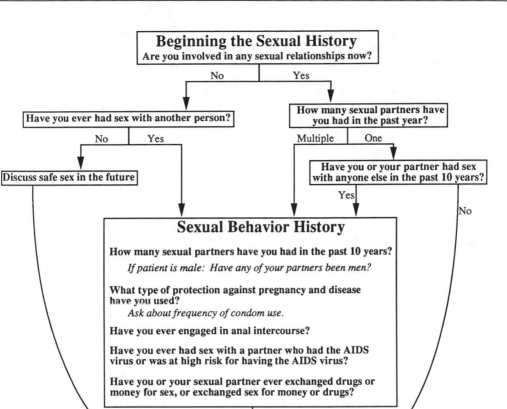

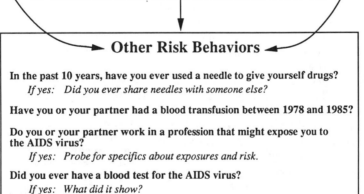

Figure 33.1. Interview guide for HIV risk assessment.

Testing for HIV Infection

HIV testing is a matter of great controversy. At issue are whom to test and under what circumstances and conditions. For example, some people have called for widespread population screening for HIV disease, a practice used by the armed forces and by some insurance companies. Others have called for selective testing of specific populations, such as hospitalized patients or medical workers. Still others support only voluntary testing. For the individual patient and physician, however, we recommend that testing decisions be guided by the estimated probability of infection and consideration of the implications and consequences of testing.

The benefits of identifying HIV patients early are (*a*) the ability to modify behavior to reduce viral transmission risk, (*b*) early antiviral and prophylactic treatment of HIV-positive patients, and

(c) the ability to institute public health measures to identify others at risk. Potential hazards are (a) adverse psychological responses to an HIV diagnosis, (b) loss of insurability, and (c) discrimination in housing or employment. Prior to testing, these considerations should be discussed. The expectations and consequences of testing should be reviewed as part of establishing informed consent. Additionally, patients should understand the rationale for testing, the basic principles that underlie testing, how tests are interpreted, and their options for testing.

Initial infection with HIV results in the production of antibodies directed against the virus. These are usually detectable within 8 to 12 weeks, although the extent and timing of the antibody response varies considerably. Antibodies to specific viral core proteins can be detected by the ELISA (enzyme-linked immunosorbent assay), which is used to screen for prior HIV exposure. The sensitivity of the ELISA is 99%. This level of sensitivity is desirable in the case of HIV infection, because few cases will be missed. The specificity of the ELISA is between 97 and 99%, depending on the test kit. Because false-positive results (people without disease are mislabeled as diseased) occur, a more specific test, the Western blot, should be performed to confirm the results of the ELISA. The Western blot test detects proteins unique to HIV and is 99.8% specific, so fewer false positives result (2).

While sensitivity and specificity are important, clinicians are most interested in the predictive value of a test, that is, knowing what the chances are that the patient has the disease if the result is positive. This varies depending on disease prevalence. Thus, in a population with a low prevalence of the HIV virus, the positive predictive value decreases, and the probability that a positive result truly predicts disease is low. In fact, because the prevalence of HIV disease in the general population is low, many have advised against mass and indiscriminant HIV-testing. This practice would lead to an increase in the number of Western blot tests performed, great anxiety for the patients whose tests are borderline or falsely positive, and extra work for the clinician. A risk assessment can estimate the risk of infection in each patient, and testing can be recommended only if the probability of infection is sufficiently high.

Pretest Counseling

Once the decision to test is made, patients must choose between anonymous and confidential test-

ing, because this will dictate where they are tested. *Anonymous testing* ensures that test results cannot be linked to the patient. It is often available at local health departments or public health clinics. Anonymity protects patients from discrimination based on risk factors (sexual preference, sexual practices, or IV drug use) or the disease itself. However, anonymous testing precludes contact tracing of seropositive patients as is done for other sexually transmitted diseases. Because of the desirability of identifying and treating infected contacts, some clinics offer only confidential testing. With *confidential testing* the test results become a part of the patient's medical record, although efforts are made to protect the privacy of the patient. Critics of confidential testing oppose it because of the potential for violation of anonymity of tested individuals.

Ultimately, each patient must decide her or his own preference in testing, but physicians can assist by being familiar with the relevant issues, local testing practices, and testing sites.

Case 2. HIV Testing

Donald V. is a 35 year-old bisexual hospital nutritionist. A former lover of his recently died of AIDS. He is currently sexually active with two partners and uses condoms.

He tells you that he wants to be tested but is afraid. What do you tell him?

Case Discussion

The first step in dealing with this patient is to identify his fears. Some patients fear the prospect of a positive test result and the implications that it has for their health. Other patients fear the potential for discrimination or alienation should their risk behavior or test results be disclosed. In this case, Donald was concerned that his family would somehow learn of his bisexuality. It is important to explain the differences between confidential and anonymous testing. Donald should understand that if he is tested confidentially, only authorized personnel should have access to his medical record, and the information can be released only on his approval. Any unauthorized release would carry penalties for the offender. However, if Donald is concerned about being tested at the hospital where he works, he could elect to be tested at another site. If Donald remains uncomfortable with any form of confidential testing, anonymous testing is appropriate. As the primary physician, it would be important to emphasize to Donald the importance of notifying his contacts if he is positive, particularly if he is tested anonymously, since contact tracing cannot be done.

Posttest Counseling

After the patient has been tested, the results should be discussed on a return appointment only. If the result is negative, the patient should be reminded that an antibody response may be delayed up to a year in some individuals. If there is a concern about recent infection, repeat testing in 3 months is advised. Each returning patient should be reminded of the risk behaviors that predispose to HIV infection. If the patient requires assistance with modification of high-risk behavior, such as IV drug use, the proper referrals should be made. Future clinical encounters represent an opportunity to follow up on patients previously considered at risk.

If the patient tests positive by ELISA, most laboratories routinely perform a Western blot for confirmation. If the Western blot results are negative or indeterminate, repeat testing in 2 to 3 months is indicated.

Patients who are HIV-positive should be told only in a personal interview. Prior to the office visit, you may wish to advise your patient to bring along a support person. The diagnosis should be stated clearly and simply. Support and encouragement should be offered. Since most patients won't retain many details beyond the diagnosis, multiple visits should be planned to discuss the future implications. Your patient should be given an opportunity to discuss feelings, vent emotions, and ask questions. A follow-up visit should be scheduled soon after to monitor the patient's adjustment to the illness and to stage the infection.

MANAGEMENT OF THE HIV-POSITIVE PATIENT

Who Will Care for Patients with HIV Disease?

Many primary care physicians are already caring for people with HIV infection either knowingly or unknowingly. Given the increasing numbers of people infected with HIV, all of us are likely to encounter HIV-seropositive patients in our practices, irrespective of the medical discipline. At the very least, then, every physician should be familiar with screening practices for HIV and have a basic understanding of the principles of testing.

During the 1990s, primary care physicians will assume a prominent role in caring for HIV-positive patients. Now that most known HIV-positive patients are in early, often asymptomatic, stages of the illness, HIV disease has become more of a primary care problem and less the province of specialists in infectious disease. In addition, the growth of the epidemic has overwhelmed the capacity of infectious disease specialists. As a result of these two trends, the role of infectious disease specialists in HIV disease is being redefined as that of consultants to primary care physicians, who will in the future manage the majority of patients.

Family physicians are well-equipped to provide care for people with HIV disease. Family practice emphasizes the delivery of continuous care, something that HIV-positive patients need. Frequently challenged with complicated medical, psychosocial, and economic problems, HIV-positive patients benefit from the multidisciplinary and comprehensive approach to patient care in which family doctors are trained.

Case 3

Barbara L. is a 26-year-old who comes to your office complaining of swollen glands in her neck. Her history is remarkable for a husband with HIV disease as the result of a blood transfusion. They have used condoms intermittently. The patient denies other risk factors for HIV disease. Her review of systems is negative. The physical examination is notable only for generalized lymphadenopathy. The patient's ELISA and Western blot results are both positive.

What other studies would you order? How should she be monitored? What prophylactic measures should she receive?

Staging

A first step in the optimal medical management of HIV-infected patients is determining the extent of infection (staging). Defining the status of disease as precisely as possible enhances clinical decision making. Staging helps the physician choose between conventional treatment options, determine eligibility for experimental protocols, and identify appropriate prophylactic therapies. It also provides a basis for making a prognosis and alerts the physician to impending complications.

To stage a patient, a thorough medical evaluation should be conducted, including a detailed history, a directed physical, and selected laboratory testing. The medical history should include questions about symptoms that may be HIV-related. During the physical, a careful neurological assessment and examination of the mouth and skin should be performed, although in early infection, abnormalities may not be detected. Most helpful are those findings unique to HIV infection, including hairy leukoplakia and Kaposi's sarcoma. Oral candidiasis is highly suggestive of HIV infection when other immunodeficiency states have been excluded. Other findings on physical examination are related to the stage of infection.

Laboratory studies are also useful in the staging process. Table 33.1 presents the initial tests that should be performed for a patient who is HIV-positive. The most helpful and relatively specific laboratory evidence of HIV infection is the CD4 helper cell count. A depressed CD4 count in the appropriate setting supports a diag-

nosis of HIV infection. The CD4 count is normally above 800 mm³.

After the history, examination, and laboratory studies are completed, the physician has only to decide which classification scheme to use. Several classification schemes for HIV infection exist, using different criteria and having different purposes. A clinically useful classification scheme divides HIV infection into acute, early asymptomatic, late asymptomatic, early symptomatic, and late symptomatic infection. Table 33.2 provides the clinical and laboratory criteria for staging patients with this system.

When first infected with HIV, patients often develop a flu-like illness. These symptoms usually appear within 2 to 6 weeks of infection and last between a few days and a few weeks. The disease then enters the asymptomatic phase, where it may remain for over a decade. With progression to late asymptomatic infection, patients generally become anergic, as evidenced by lack of a measurable skin test response to common antigens such as mumps, *Candida*, and tetanus toxoid. During the early symptomatic phase, constitutional symptoms develop and overt mucocutaneous manifestations are common. In the late symptomatic phase, patients have full-blown adult immunodeficiency syndrome (AIDS), which is characterized by opportunistic infections with organisms such as *Pneumocystis carinii*, *Cryptococcus neoformans*, *Toxoplasma gondii*, and cytomegalovirus. These infections usually signal that the patient is preterminal.

Estimates concerning the average incubation time for AIDS (defined as the time between ac-

Table 33.1. Initial Laboratory Evaluation of the HIV-positive Patient

Complete blood count (CBC) with white cell differential and platelets
Chemistry profile: electrolytes, glucose, blood urea nitrogen, creatinine, serum protein, albumin, aspartate transferase, alanine transferase
Hepatitis B surface antigen (HbSAg)
Hepatitis B surface antibody (HbSAb)
Urinalysis
Glucose-6-phosphodehydrogenase
VDRL
Tuberculin skin test (PPD)
Toxoplasma gondii antibody titer
Cytomegalovirus titer
T lymphocyte profile:
  total T lymphocyte count
  CD4 lymphocyte count
  CD8 lymphocyte count
  CD4/CD8 ratio
Chest x-ray

Table 33.2. Clinical Staging of HIV Infection

Stage	Clinical Manifestations	Laboratory Studies
Acute infection	Fever, malaise, lymphadenopathy, headache, and maculopapular rash lasting 1–2 weeks	Nonspecific hematologic studies typical of any viral syndrome; CD4 count may be normal (≥800)
Early asymptomatic infection	Persistent generalized lymphadenopathy	CD4 count is usually above 400, and typically is between 500 and 750
Late asymptomatic infection	Cutaneous anergy, oral hairy leukoplakia, Kaposi's sarcoma	Anemia, leukopenia, lymphopenia, thrombocytopenia are common; CD4 count is usually decreased (400–600)
Early symptomatic infection	Night sweats, fever, weight loss, profound fatigue, vomiting, diarrhea, seborrheic dermatitis, oral candidiasis	CD4 count 100–500
Late symptomatic infection	Opportunistic infections (*Pneumocystis carinii* pneumonia, cytomegalovirus retinitis and gastroenteritis, *Cryptococcus neoformans* meningitis, CNS infection with *Toxoplasma gondii*); CNS lymphoma; memory problems, ataxia, paresthesias	CD4 count 50–200

quisition of HIV infection and onset of AIDS) have varied widely, depending on the route of infection in the cohort studied. For example, in a group of gay men in San Francisco, 2% developed AIDS within 2 years of infection, 5% within 3 years, 10% within 4 years, 23% within 6 years and 48% within 10 years. Taken together, the evidence suggests an incubation period of 8 to 11 years for adults (3). In general, studies show that the risk of AIDS for HIV-infected persons increases over time. Available data and current trends suggest that most HIV-infected persons will eventually develop signs or symptoms of AIDS.

Therapy for HIV infection is not curative. Antivirals such as zidovudine (AZT) are used to delay progression to AIDS in patients with CD4 counts below 500 and to prolong survival in AIDS patients. Additionally, medications are available to prevent or control opportunistic infections. Careful follow-up of the patient is required to institute medications at the appropriate time. Table 33.3 gives a timetable for laboratory tests and prophylactic medications to optimize health maintenance.

A few laboratory studies predict progression to AIDS. Of these, the CD4 count is currently the best single indicator of disease progression. Thirty percent of patients with a cell count below 200/mm³ develop AIDS-defining illness within a year. Approximately 50% of patients with a cell count between 200/mm³ and 400/mm³ develop AIDS within 3 years. It is estimated that 15% of patients with cell counts above 400/mm³ develop AIDS within 3 years (4).

Psychosocial Issues in the Care of HIV-infected Patients

While treatment of medical problems is a major priority in the care of HIV-infected patients, it is not the only priority. As with other chronic diseases, psychosocial issues in patients with HIV infection are significant determinants of patient comfort and quality of life. Assessment of psychosocial needs involves learning about the fears, stressors, coping mechanisms, feelings, and values of a patient.

There are a number of psychological stressors to which HIV-positive patients are subjected:

- Patients often react to the diagnosis as they would to any major personal loss—with anger, confusion, and feelings of depression.

Table 33.3. Routine Health Maintenance of HIV-positive Patient

Immunizations
Pneumococcal vaccination
Influenza vaccination annually
Haemophilus (HiB), measles-mumps-rubella (MMR), inactivated polio, and Hepatitis B vaccines should be given if there is no evidence of immunity
Diphtheria-tetanus (dT) every 10 years

Monitoring the CD4 lymphocyte count
If the previous count was >500 cells/mm³, repeat in 6 months
200–500 cells/mm³, repeat in 3 months (sooner if the value is falling rapidly)
≤200 cells/mm³, routine CD4 monitoring is not indicated

Other laboratory tests
CBC with platelets:
  if CD4 >500, every 6 months
  if CD4 <500 or the patient is on zidovudine, every 3 months
Chemistry profile: every 2–6 months
PPD: every 12 months until anergic twice
Toxoplasma titer: every 12 months if seronegative at baseline

Prophylactic medication
Zidovudine (AZT): an antiviral agent used to slow disease progression
  if CD4 is below 500, administer 100 mg five times a day
  if CD4 is below 200, increase to 600 mg per day
Trimethoprim/sulfamethoxazole: prophylaxis against *Pneumocystis* pneumonia
  if CD4 is below 200, administer one 160/800 mg daily
Aerosolized pentamidine: prophylaxis against *Pneumocystis* pneumonia; considered a second-line alternative to trimethoprim/sulfamethoxazole
  if CD4 count is below 200, administer 300 mg every 4 weeks

- Because HIV transmission is often tied to willful behavior, patients tend to blame themselves for contracting or spreading HIV infection. They often feel guilty about their past behavior and are anxious about future behavior.
- Many patients are reluctant to share their diagnosis for fear of condemnation and discrimination and, as a result, often feel isolated and alone.
- When the diagnosis does becomes known, patients sometimes experience distancing in their relationships. Misperceptions about transmis-

sion, prejudice, and the fear of AIDS contribute to this problem.

As their disease progresses, patients become increasingly debilitated and require assistance with activities of daily living. Fears of abandonment, dependency, and loss of control become particularly prominent. During this time, it is very important to help the patient maintain as much independence as possible, but steps should be taken to ensure that the patient has access to needed resource persons. Home health agencies and social services organizations can be particularly helpful in this regard.

As the disease progresses, patients must realistically confront fears about death and dying. In fact, all patients should be given the opportunity to talk about their mortality early in the course of illness. Eventually patients will need to make decisions about terminal care (home, hospital, or hospice) and options for life-sustaining interventions. Physicians should encourage patients to think about and to formulate advanced directives for care.

Depression is particularly common among HIV-positive patients. The physician should be very aggressive about monitoring the patient for this condition and instituting treatment when necessary. Suicide risk may be particularly high when the patient develops AIDS, due to the psychologically devastating effect of this diagnosis. Later in the course of the illness, there may be another period of high suicide risk as a result of delirium or dementia, central nervous system complications of AIDS. In one New York study, AIDS patients had 66 times the relative risk of the general population of committing suicide (5).

In general, physicians should seek to develop an honest and open partnership with patients. Patients should be encouraged to make informed choices about their care, based on information provided by the physician and others.

Perhaps the most important contribution to ongoing care for these patients is education and reassurance. Many infected individuals will have profound psychological effects and develop a variety of somatic complaints. Patients and their families must know which symptoms warrant prompt medical attention and which don't.

Additionally, patients need to be counseled about prevention of HIV disease. Physicians should inquire occasionally about risk behaviors

and follow-up. Patients should be counseled about safe sex. Partners of HIV-positive patients should be involved in these discussions. In many places, physicians are mandated to ensure that HIV-positive patients inform their sexual partners of their infection or solicit the help of public health authorities in informing the partner.

Caring for patients with HIV disease has implications for the physician. At the death of the patient, the physician may experience feelings of loss. When this occurs frequently, it can lead to feelings of depression, anger, and frustration. Participation in support groups for caretakers often gives doctors an opportunity to process these feelings. When this is done, care of HIV-positive patients can be very rewarding and intellectually challenging.

CONCLUSIONS

Given that HIV disease is spread largely by engaging in risky behaviors, the potential to influence the course of this epidemic is great. Already, we know that sexual behavior can change. A number of studies conducted during the 1980s in San Francisco demonstrated a change in the sexual practices of gay men in the wake of a safe sex campaign to prevent the spread of AIDS (6). Beyond caring for patients who are already infected, there is an opportunity for family physicians to lead the way in emphasizing risk assessment, risk reduction counseling, and promotion of healthy behaviors.

REFERENCES

1. Centers for Disease Control: HIV prevalence estimates and AIDS case projections for the United States: report based on a workshop. *MMWR* 39 RR-16, 1990.
2. Centers for Disease Control: Update: serologic testing for antibody to HIV. *MMWR* 36 (52):833–845, 1987.
3. DeVita VT: *AIDS: Etiology, Diagnosis, Treatment and Prevention*, ed 3. Philadelphia, JB Lippincott, 1992, p 429.
4. Lifson AR, Rutherford GW, Jaffe HW: The natural history of human immunodeficiency virus infection. *J Infect Dis* 158:1360-1367, 1988.
5. Marzuk P, Tierney H, Tardiff K, et al.: Increased risk of suicide in persons with AIDS. *JAMA* 259:1333–1337, 1988.
6. Becker MH, Joseph JG: AIDS and behavioral changes to reduce risk: a review. *Am J Public Health* 78:394-410, 1988.

SUGGESTED READINGS

DeVita VT: *AIDS: Etiology, Diagnosis, Treatment and Prevention*, Philadelphia, JB Lippincott, 1992.

The text contains an excellent section on the clinical aspects of HIV infection, including disease manifestations, complications, and treatment. It would serve as an excellent reference text for physicians involved in the care of HIV-positive patients.

Rapoza N: *HIV Infection and Disease Monographs for Physicians and Other Health Care Workers*. Chicago, American Medical Association, 1989. Copies can be ordered from Book and Pamphlet Fulfillment: OP014690; PO Box 10946; Chicago, IL 60610-0946.

This monograph provides a more detailed, but readable overview of HIV infection. Chapters on the pathogenesis and the epidemiology of infection are well written. There is also a chapter addressing HIV infection in children.

chapter 34

COMMON SKIN PROBLEMS

John M. Little, Jr. and Darlyne Menscer

Skin diseases are common problems that the primary care physician will be asked to evaluate and treat. One-third of the United States population has some skin pathology that should be evaluated by a physician at least once (1). In one large study, dermatologic complaints accounted for 5.5% of all office visits to family physicians (2). The purposes of this chapter are (*a*) to acquaint the student with an approach to the diagnosis of a patient with a skin problem, (*b*) to introduce a dermatologic vocabulary, (*c*) to explain several common office procedures used in dermatology, and (*d*) to discuss briefly several common dermatologic principles.

APPROACH TO THE PATIENT WITH A SKIN COMPLAINT

Skin diseases are approached in exactly the same manner as all medical problems: history, physical examination, and laboratory tests. The major difference is that dermatology is almost exclusively a visual branch of medicine. Often physicians are adept at analyzing laboratory data and physical abnormalities but find it difficult to evaluate what is immediately before them. A simple approach to the patient with a skin complaint involves three steps.

1. Initial history. What is the problem? When did the original lesion occur? What did the rash look like? Where did it start? Did it spread? If so, in what pattern? What did the rash look like when it was at its worst? Were there any symptoms—itching, pain, etc.? What has the patient used for treatment?
2. Physical examination. Often a large portion of the physical examination can be performed while obtaining the patient's history. Dermatologic examination requires examining the en-

tire skin, including mucous membranes and nails. It is preferable to develop a set pattern for skin examinations; a commonly suggested pattern is nonhairy skin followed, in order, by examination of the hairy areas, intertriginous skin, nails, hair, and mucous membranes. The examination should be performed in a well-lighted room—preferably with natural light.

Initially, examine the patient from a distance. This is analogous to scanning a slide at low power. Notice the distribution, arrangement, and morphology of the skin lesions. Skin diseases may have varied and unusual presentations, but most have typical appearances and locations. Several examples of the areas involved by common skin problems are given in Figure 34.1. Remembering these patterns can greatly assist the examiner in reducing the diagnostic possibilities.

After the initial "scanning view", ask the patient which lesion is typical of the primary (initial) lesion. Examine the primary lesions at a closer level. Try to classify these lesions into a diagnostic category as listed in Table 34.1 and in Figure 34.2. Classification will direct the physician toward distinct diagnostic categories. A listing of diagnostic groups and examples of representative diseases is given in Table 34.2.

Often, by the time a patient seeks medical care, the initial appearance of the skin lesion has been modified by scratching, self-treatment, or the underlying pathological process. The process then evolves into one with secondary lesions. A simple listing of secondary lesions and their definitions is in Table 34.3.

3. After a preliminary history and physical examination, the clinical evaluation is completed by obtaining other pertinent historical data. This

317

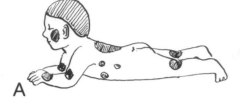

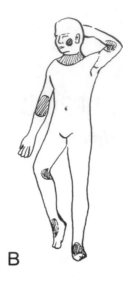

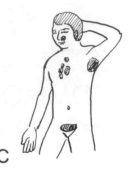

A

B

C

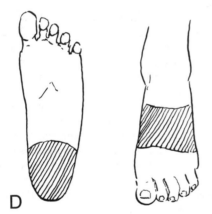

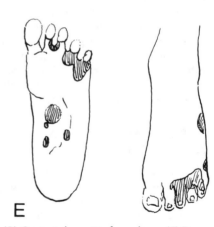

D

E

Figure 34.1. Examples of common rashes with characteristic patterns of distribution (*A*) Atopic eczema (infants). (*B*) Atopic eczema (adults). (*C*) Seborrheic dermatitis. (*D*) Contact dermatitis from shoes. (*E*) Tinea pedis. (Adapted from Sauer GC: *Manual of Skin Diseases,* ed 4. Philadelphia, JB Lippincott, 1980, p 20).

involves obtaining past medical history, family history, social history, and a review of systems. The patient's past medical history includes pertinent hospitalizations, chronic illnesses, and medications. The patient should also be questioned about past dermatologic history; for example, previous skin sensitivity, infantile eczema, and reaction to sunlight. Family history is important because certain diseases such as psoriasis, eczema, and allergies tend to occur in families. Occupational exposures, as obtained in the social history, can often be of etiologic importance in the evaluation of skin diseases. A review of systems will often lead the

physician to consider systemic diseases that can have dermatologic manifestations. A few examples are collagen vascular diseases, sarcoidosis, inflammatory bowel disease, and chronic liver disease. All these facts must be put into context when attempting to narrow the diagnostic possibilities.

Most of the time, after the completion of these three steps, the physician will have a tentative working diagnosis. Usually a treatment plan can be instituted based on this diagnosis. Occasionally, the physician will use laboratory tests to confirm or further define the diagnosis. Simple laboratory measures in the dermatologist's armamentarium include Wood's light examination and KOH preparation to evaluate fungal disease, diascopy (flattening a lesion with a glass slide to distinguish between petechiae and telangiectasia), and punch skin biopsy with examination of the specimen by a pathologist. Blood tests are often useful in the evaluation of systemic diseases.

Often an experienced physician can arrive at a diagnosis almost at a glance, without formally applying the method noted above. This can be particularly frustrating to the inexperienced examiner who is told "this rash must be eczema because that is how eczema looks." While gaining this experience, the student must remember to follow the stepwise approach—including describing the rash in terms of location and primary and secondary lesions.

This brief approach to the patient with a skin problem is obviously not all-inclusive. Many medical students are not familiar with dermatologic examination and vocabulary. It takes practice and experience to become proficient "observers" of the skin.

Table 34.1. Primary Dermatologic Lesions

<1 cm	>1 cm	Varying Size
Macule, papule, nodule, vesicle, petechia	Patch, tumor, plaque, bulla, pupura	Pustule, wheel, telangiectasia

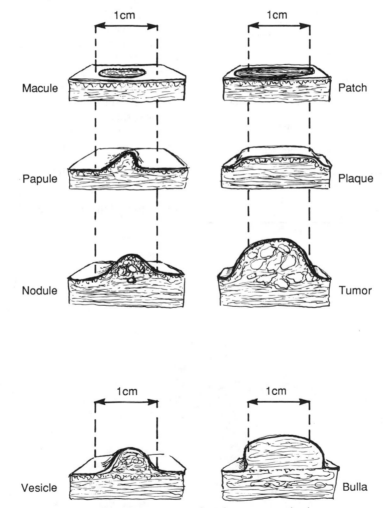

Figure 34.2. Terms to use in describing primary skin lesions.

DIAGNOSTIC PROCEDURES

As mentioned earlier, diagnostic procedures are sometimes necessary to assist or confirm a diagnosis. A few diagnostic procedures are discussed below.

KOH Preparation. This is useful predominantly in the diagnosis of fungal infections. The involved skin is lightly scraped with a scalpel

Table 34.2. Diagnostic Groups and Examples

Diagnostic Category	Example
Dermatitis—scaly	Atopic dermatitis
Maculopapular	Drug eruption, viral exanthum
Papulosquamous	Tinea infection, pityriasis rosea
Vesiculobullous	Varicella
Vacular	Hemangioma
Papulopustular	Acne
Ulcerative	Stasis ulcer
Atrophic lesions	Steroid atrophy

Table 34.3. Secondary Skin Lesions

Crusts—Dried exudates of varying colors

Excoriations—Traumatic skin abrasions, usually secondary to scratching

Scales—Dead epidermal cells shed from the upper layers of skin

Scars—Connective tissue formation representing healing of a skin injury

Lichenification—Thickening of an area of skin secondary to chronic low-grade trauma such as scratching or rubbing

Ulcers—Irregular erosion of the skin

blade, and the resulting material is deposited on a slide. Potassium hydroxide (20% solution) is added, a cover slip applied, and the slide gently heated for 15 to 20 seconds. The slide is then examined for fungal elements.

Diascopy. Diascopy is useful for differentiating erythema from purpura. The glass slide is pressed against the lesion. If the redness is due to capillary dilatation, the lesion will blanch. If the lesion is petechial the redness will persist.

Wood's Light Examination. A Wood's light is an ultraviolet light. Primarily used to detect certain fungi (which cause fluorescence), this type of "black light" also helps in the detection of hypopigmentation.

Biopsy. A pathological examination is sometimes necessary to assist in diagnosis. A *punch biopsy* is performed using a tubular instrument that removes a small (3 to 4 mm diameter) circular core of skin down to the subcutaneous tissue. Either a portion of the lesion or the edge of the lesion and a segment of uninvolved skin can be included. An *excisional biopsy* removes an entire lesion with clear margins. A *shave biopsy* removes only the portion of the lesion projecting above the plane of the skin. The size, shape, location, and type of lesion determines the type of biopsy chosen. Figure 34.3 illustrates these three common types of skin biopsy.

THERAPEUTIC PRINCIPLES

Management of skin problems includes systemic as well as topical therapy. Generally, the treatment of

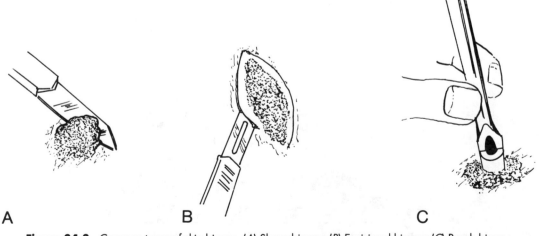

A   B   C

Figure 34.3. Common types of skin biopsy. (*A*) Shave biopsy; (*B*) Excisional biopsy; (*C*) Punch biopsy.

mild and localized skin diseases depends predominantly on topical therapy. Systemic therapy is used only for more severe or extensive disease or if topical therapy fails to give a satisfactory response. Certain conditions, such as fungal infections of the scalp, will not respond to topical therapy and require systemic medications as the initial therapy of choice.

Choosing a topical medication appropriately requires knowledge of (*a*) the pharmacology of the active ingredients, (*b*) the best mode of physical delivery of the drug (e.g., cream, ointment, or lotion), and (*c*) a correct diagnosis. It is important to remember that systemic absorption can occur from topical preparations—especially in already damaged skin and the thinner skin of children. Also, the larger the area being treated, the greater the chance for significant absorption.

Many different drugs are available for dermatologic therapy. Systemic therapy includes the use of antibiotics such as tetracycline and erythromycin for acne and impetigo. Griseofulvin is used for fungal infections of the scalp and nails. Oral or parenteral steroids are sometimes used for extensive or severe skin problems such as contact dermatitis, allergic reactions, and eczema. Topical steroids should be used when local therapy will suffice. For chronic disease requiring long-term therapy, systemic steroids should be used sparingly because of the numerous side effects (e.g., interference with growth and glucose metabolism).

A number of topical agents are commonly used in family practice. Antiparasitic agents such as γ-benzene hexachloride and 5% permethrin are used for treatment of scabies. Miconazole and clotrimazole are two commonly used antifungal agents. Antibiotics such as clindamycin or erythromycin are also available in topical form for acne.

Corticosteroids are widely used in the treatment of skin diseases. Their main pharmacological effects are reducing inflammation and decreasing epidermal cell proliferation. The effect of these drugs depends on absorption of the active drug into the layers of the skin. Absorption can be affected by factors such as drug concentration, skin integrity, and anatomical location. Occlusive dressings increase absorption, thereby enhancing clinical efficacy. Numerous steroids are available for use, so it is important to become familiar with a limited number of these drugs. A sample listing, according to potency, is given in Table 34.4.

The major side effects of local steroid use are skin atrophy and stria formation. Systemic ab-

Table 34.4. Increasing Potency of Steroids

Hydrocortisone	1%
Desonide	0.05%
Triamcinolone acetonide	0.1%
Triamcinolone acetonide	0.5%
Clobetasol proprionate	0.05%

sorption due to topical steroid treatment for longer than 2 weeks can lead to the typical findings of cortisol excess, such as moon facies, edema, and weight gain. These side effects are more likely to occur with the use of the fluorinated (more potent) steroids and with their use in areas where the skin is thinner, such as the face, genitalia, and intertriginous areas. Be particularly aware of the need to use low-potency steroids (e.g., 1% hydrocortisone) in these areas and, at least initially, in most skin conditions requiring steroids in children.

The optimal mode of delivery for a drug varies with the area to be treated and the diagnosis. Many forms of delivery are available, but two of the most frequent methods of topical therapy are creams and ointments. *Creams* are emulsions of oil in water. The active ingredient, such as a steroid, is then mixed with the cream carrier base. Creams are easy to apply and are nongreasy—resulting in a greater cosmetic acceptability for most patients. They do, however, tend to be drying. *Ointments* are of several types, but all tend to be more adherent. They are more difficult to apply and often leave a "greasy" feeling to the skin, which some patients find less acceptable. Their major advantages are greater penetration into the skin than creams and a tendency to reduce dryness.

Numerous other dermatologic agents are available over the counter without a physician's prescription. Shampoos containing selenium sulfide or tar are available for treatment of seborrhea (dandruff). Emollients containing urea, mineral oil, or white petrolatum are also useful for moisturizing and softening the skin. The family physician must be familiar with a limited number of agents from each therapeutic category to use in patients with skin diseases.

Case 1. Rash Diagnosed by Its Appearance and Distribution

An 18-year-old white man comes to your office complaining of a rash on his back, shoulders, and upper arms. It has been present for about 2 weeks now (June), but he had a similar rash only on his shoulders last summer. It itches a little, but mostly it bothers him because it makes his skin look "splotchy." On physical examination you note a slightly pink, scaling rash only in the areas he described. It is macular and in patches.

Case Discussion

The differential diagnosis of a scaling macular rash confined to the torso of an adolescent, which recurs mostly in the summer, is quite brief. *Tinea versicolor* is far more likely than any other possibility (see Fig.

34.4). This can be confirmed by doing a KOH preparation of the scale and identifying the typical "spaghetti and meat balls" configuration of hyphae and spores under the microscope. If this is not identified, an atypical eczema might be suspected, although atypical eczema would be expected to be more pruritic (itchy). There is very little inflammation with this rash, and the surrounding skin may be darker than the affected areas. Therefore, these areas may be mistaken for vitiligo. Pigment is not entirely absent from areas of tinea versicolor, as in true vitiligo, but only reduced.

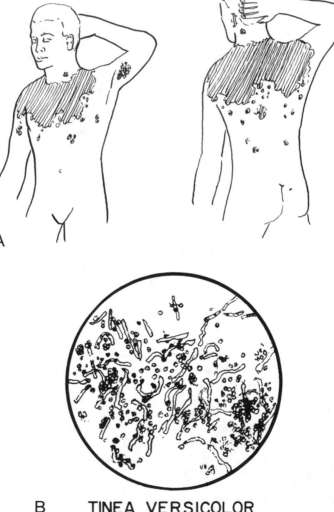

A

B   TINEA VERSICOLOR

Figure 34.4. Typical distribution of tinea versicolor and "spaghetti and meatballs" appearance of KOH preparation. (A) Tinea versicolor. (B) "Spaghetti and meatballs." (Adapted from Sauer GC: *Manual of Skin Diseases*, ed 4. Philadelphia, JB Lippincott, 1980, p 18).

Tinea versicolor can be treated in any one of several ways. If a small amount of skin is involved, topical therapy with miconazole nitrate (Monistat-Derm) or some similar antifungal medication twice daily for 2 weeks is effective. This is an expensive choice if much body area must be treated. Selenium sulfide lotion can also be used and is much cheaper. It is applied and left on overnight, washed off in the morning, and repeated in about 1 week. Regardless of which topical treatment is chosen, the patient should be instructed to treat the area only until the scale is gone, not until the pigment in the skin is the same as in unaffected areas. There will often be postinflammatory hypopigmentation (or, less commonly, hyperpigmentation), especially in darker-skinned individuals, which will take months to resolve. Exposing these areas to sunlight will speed repigmentation.

An alternative to topical therapy is ketoconazole in one 200-mg oral dose daily for 5 days. This is excellent, effective treatment in patients who do not have liver disease. Tinea versicolor is caused by a ubiquitous fungus, *Pityrosporum orbiculare*, which tends to reinfect susceptible individuals. Therefore, a treatment that is safe for the patient to initiate early for recurrences is desirable.

Case 2. Use of Skin Biopsy

A 66-year-old white man comes to your office because he is concerned about three spots on his face. They have been there for at least a few months and each seems to be getting larger slowly. One is on his right cheek and is about 1/2 cm by 1 cm. It is a brown, waxy-appearing plaque, almost seeming to be "stuck on" his face. The second is on his left cheek and is about 1 cm in size. It is somewhat raised and rough, reddish with a grayish irregular surface. The third lesion is on the left side of his nose and is round, about 0.5 cm in diameter. Its center is raised and has a pearly border, giving it a distinct margin. It is slightly red and has a couple of small, nonblanching blood vessels notable in it, called telangiectasias.

The man's hair is white now, but he reports it was a sandy blond in his youth. He is a farmer who frequently worked outside without a hat. He reports no previous skin problems but in surveying his skin you note multiple smaller lesions on his back similar to the one on his right cheek. He has lesions similar to the one on his left cheek on the backs of his hands. He is really only concerned about the ones on his face because they get in his way when he shaves and his wife worries that they may be cancer.

Case Discussion

All of these lesions are abnormal, well-circumscribed new growths—*skin tumors*. All could be removed surgically, but this would leave scars. Biopsy may be used to clarify which if any are worthy of complete surgical removal. The first lesion is typical of a *seborrheic keratosis*, an entirely benign lesion that is sometimes mistaken for a mole. If the lesion is darkly pigmented, it may cause concern regarding whether it is a melanoma. Since this lesion is not very dark and the pigment is even, it would be reasonable to eliminate it by freezing it with liquid nitrogen or electrodesiccating it after local anesthesia. Pathological review of the tissue removed by these methods is not possible but, if malignancy is not suspected, review is not really necessary. The lesions on the patient's back could be similarly treated if he desires.

The lesion on the left cheek is an *actinic keratosis*. These are caused by damage to the skin by sun exposure over many years. They are more common in fair-complected individuals. While they are not often mistaken for anything else, they may progress to squamous cell carcinomas. This process is usually slow and even when malignant transformation occurs, metastases are rarely seen early unless mucous membranes are affected.

If no area of an actinic keratosis is particularly thick or irregular, suggesting malignant transformation, it can be treated with liquid nitrogen in the same manner as seborrheic keratoses and not biopsied. If multiple actinic keratoses are present, 5-fluorouracil may be applied topically for several weeks. Initially this causes the area to become red, inflamed, and tender, but if the patient can tolerate it, the lesions will generally peel off and resolve within several weeks.

Because of its relatively large size and thickness, the lesion on this man's cheek was shave biopsied, allowing full removal of the lesion for pathological evaluation with minimal scarring. Because actinic keratoses are caused by chronic sun exposure, it is helpful to tell affected individuals to reduce their sun exposure in the future by wearing a hat and long sleeves in the sun and protecting their hands or any exposed part of their skin with sunscreen. Sunscreens with a high-numbered rating, such as number 15, are best at filtering out ultraviolet rays.

The lesion on the patient's nose is a *basal cell carcinoma*. It may also be confused with a mole or minor overgrowth of the skin around pores. Basal cell carcinomas are slowly growing cancers that rarely metastasize but may be locally invasive. They should be completely removed, often a difficult task in the cosmetically important areas of the face where they frequently occur.

To prove the diagnosis, a punch biopsy should be done on this patient. It may be possible to curette the lesion deeply enough after local anesthesia to remove it, following up at 3-monthly intervals for several visits and regularly thereafter to check for recurrence. Surgical removal by a plastic surgeon or dermatologist is another alternative. If surgical removal of the basal cell would be particularly difficult, radiation therapy can be an alternative.

Basal cell carcinomas are also induced by sun exposure. It is appropriate to counsel patients to avoid increasing their risk by appropriate use of sunscreens and clothing barriers.

Case 3. Therapeutic Trial

A 21-year-old black woman presents to you complaining of a rash on her hands. She works as a cashier at McDonald's, and her supervisor is concerned that the rash is offensive to the public she serves. The rash bothers her because it itches and occasionally burns. She has noted the rash off and on for several months. She believes it was caused by the soap she must use to clean her work area. She began doing this about 6 months ago but cannot remember if the rash was present before then or not. She asks if she is allergic to the soap. She has not had a rash on her hands before this present condition. When she was a young child, however, she had very dry skin that was treated with moisturizers and cortisone creams. As she grew older, the rash was mostly on her popliteal fossae and antecubital areas. She had not had any rash for about 5 years before the present rash began. She has had allergic rhinitis for several years. The rash is mostly on the dorsum of her hands, irregularly distributed in scaly, maculopapular, erythematous patches. Her palms are dry but have no distinct rash. The nails are not involved. The rash extends for several inches onto her forearms but is not present anywhere else.

Case Discussion

Rashes on the hands are very common, making the differential diagnosis very long. This patient clearly had atopic dermatitis as a child; hand eczema is common in such individuals when they become adults, often as the only residual manifestation. Atopic individuals are more susceptible to the drying effects of irritants than people with normal skin. Fungus infections can affect the hands. Most commonly, however, the palms are more involved than the dorsum, and if the infection has gone on very long, the nails are likely to be involved. Psoriasis occurs on the hands, too, but rarely is present only there. When psoriasis affects the hands, the palms and nails are usually involved. Contact or allergic dermatitis is also in the differential diagnosis. Most people who believe they have developed a rash in response to touching something believe they are allergic to that substance. The hands are often sites of contact dermatitis because many environmental substances come into contact with them.

It is important to understand the difference between an irritant and an allergen. An irritant is a substance that damages anyone's skin if applied in sufficiently strong concentration. Examples include hydrochloric acid and lye. An allergen is a substance to which only some people are sensitive. A susceptible person responds to this substance even when it is present in low concentrations, a response mediated through the immune system. Allergens vary widely in how many people are sensitive to them. About 70% of people are allergic to poison ivy; only a few percent are sensitive to nickel.

Soaps, particularly those used commercially, often contain irritants. As this patient's skin already tends to be dry, it is possible she is more sensitive to the drying effects of soap than some others would be. If there is any doubt, a dilute drop of soap could be placed on her uninvolved skin (often the back), occluded, and allowed to remain for 24 to 72 hours (patch test). If she is allergic to the soap, she should develop an itchy erythematous spot under the patch.

In planning treatment for this patient, distinguishing between contact, irritant, and atopic dermatitis—or a combination of these—is not essential. For each of these, avoiding the soap and applying steroids and moisturizers will be the recommended treatment. The skin of the hands is thick, especially the palms, drastically reducing penetration of steroids; so a strong steroid cream will probably be necessary. Moisturizing the skin is also very important and can be difficult in a person who must put her hands in water intermittently all day. *Ointments* are more moisturizing than creams, but the greasy feel is unacceptable to some patients or in some job settings. Ointments can generally be used at night, however, with cotton gloves over the ointment to increase penetration, if needed. Several applications of steroid cream and hand cream during the day will also be needed. Rubber gloves protect the hands from moisture, irritants, or allergens; however, these need to be used with white cotton linings to absorb moisture. Failure to do this will lead to sweating of the hands inside the gloves, increased itching, and, therefore, scratching. As you monitor the patient during follow-up visits, your further treatment will be based on her response, which will help clarify the underlying diagnosis. A persistent rash will suggest hand eczema or noncompliance, and treatment will need to be modified or prolonged. If her rash remains resistant to treatment, changing her job to avoid repeated exposure to water and irritants may be necessary.

REFERENCES

1. Johnson MT, Roberts J: Skin conditions and related need for medical care among persons 1–74 years, 1971–1974. Data from the National Health Survey. *Vital Health Stat [2]* No. 212. Hyattsville, MD, DHEW publication, 1978.

2. Marsland DW, Wood M, Mayo F: Content of family practice: Part I—Rank order of diagnoses by frequency. Part II—Diagnosis by disease category and age/sex distribution. *J Fam Pract* 3:37–68, 1976.

SUGGESTED READINGS

Arndt KA: *Manual of Dermatologic Therapeutics*, ed 4. Boston, Little, Brown & Co., 1989 (spiral illustration).

Concise, specific recommendations for therapy of the common skin diseases. This manual contains a very good presentation of therapeutic principles in dermatology.

Fitzpatrick TB, Eisen AZ, Wolff K, Freedberg IM, Austen KF: *Dermatology in General Medicine: Textbook and Atlas*, ed 3. New York, McGraw-Hill, 1987.

An excellent reference text for the primary care physician. More detailed than necessary for everyday use but provides in-depth discussion of specific dermatology diseases.

Habif TP: *Clinical Dermatology: A Color Guide to Diagnosis and Therapy*, ed 2. St. Louis, CV Mosby, 1990.

Useful, readable text for the student needing a broad initial exposure to dermatology. Gives a practical approach to the differential diagnosis and therapy of common skin problems.

chapter 35

WEIGHT MANAGEMENT AND OBESITY

Paul F. Dunn and Michele Marshall Tuttle

Obesity affects over 34 million Americans, often leading to harmful medical and psychological effects. It is not difficult to recognize. Its treatment is largely behavioral and is best dealt with in the context of the patient's family and environment. This chapter presents the basic knowledge and skills needed to develop an effective approach to obese patients seen in a family practice setting.

EPIDEMIOLOGY

The National Health and Nutrition Examination Survey of 1976 to 1980 (NHANES II) defined men as overweight if the body mass index (see Figure 35.1) equaled 27.8, and severely overweight if the index score equaled or exceeded 31.1. For women, these cutoff points were 27.3 and 32.3, respectively. The overweight categories correspond to approximately 20% and 40% above the midpoint height/weight scales on the Metropolitan Life Insurance 1983 tables. According to the NHANES II, 34 million adult Americans were more than 20% overweight. Of this group, 12.4 million were more than 40% overweight.

Major risks to health, both in terms of morbidity and mortality, correlate well with increases in body mass index. According to a National Institutes of Health consensus panel, body weight 20% or more above desirable constitutes an established health hazard. The most important risks of obesity include:

- Increased mean blood pressure, with an increased prevalence of hypertension;
- Increased serum cholesterol;
- Increased prevalence of diabetes;
- Increased risk of heart disease independent of the added risk due to elevation of other risk factors;

- Increased rates of colon, rectum, and prostate cancer in men;
- Increased rates of gallbladder, breast, uterus, and ovarian cancer in women;
- Increased mortality rates, particularly in extremely obese individuals (1).

Table 35.1 summarizes known data on many of the above health consequences of obesity. Numerous other risks, which may contribute to morbidity during adult life, are presented in Table 35.2.

The psychological consequences of obesity are immense. In this slimness-oriented society, obese individuals are constantly confronted with their "failure" to conform to accepted standards of health and beauty. Studies have shown that "fat" people are denied jobs, promotions, and educational opportunities. They are more frequently challenged in their right to adopt children. Negative feelings are prevalent from the general public, social workers, employers, graduate school admissions officers, nurses, and physicians. As a consequence, the obese frequently feel ineffective, unsuccessful, and unhappy.

ETIOLOGY OF OBESITY

The cause of obesity is multifactorial, and incompletely understood. Current theories are based on physiological observations about obesity and may help you appreciate some of the barriers patients must overcome in losing weight and staying thin. Some points of interest from current theories (2) are:

- Obesity can result from having more fat cells (hyperplastic adiposity) or from having unusually large fat cells (hypertrophic adiposity).

327

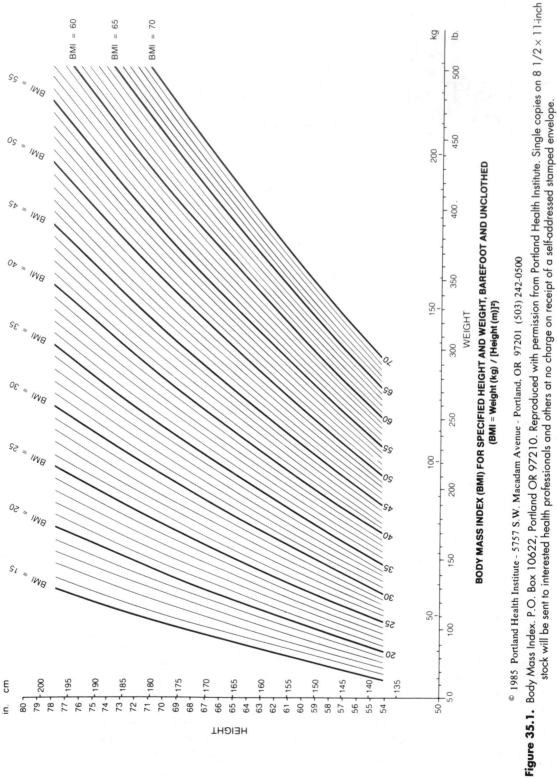

BODY MASS INDEX (BMI) FOR SPECIFIED HEIGHT AND WEIGHT, BAREFOOT AND UNCLOTHED

(BMI = **Weight (kg) / [Height (m)]²**)

© 1985 Portland Health Institute - 5757 S.W. Macadam Avenue - Portland, OR 97201 (503) 242-0500. Reproduced with permission from Portland Health Institute. Single copies on 8 1/2 × 11-inch stock will be sent to interested health professionals and others at no charge on receipt of a self-addressed stamped envelope.

Figure 35.1. Body Mass Index. P.O. Box 10622, Portland OR 97210.

Table 35.1. Quantified Risks from the NHANES II (1976–1980) and American Cancer Society 12-Year (1959–1972) Studies[a]

Study	Disease	Ages	Risk of Obese vs. Nonobese	Relative Risk
NHANES II	Hypertension (160/95)	20–44	BMI >27.8 men 27.3 women	5.6X
		45–74	BMI >27.8 men 27.3 women	11.2X
NHANES II	Hypercholesterolemia (>250 mg/dl)	20–29	BMI >27.8 men 27.3 women	2.1X
ACS	Diabetes	Unspecified	BMI >31.1 men 32.3 women	5.19X men 7.90X women
ACS	Coronary disease		BMI >31.1 men 32.3 women	1.95X men 2.07X women
ACS	Digestive diseases		BMI >31.1 men 32.3 women	3.99X men 2.29X women
LaVecchia et al.	Endometrial cancer		+ 10 lb overweight + 20 lb overweight	6.69X 7.20X
Friedman et al.	Gallbladder disease	20–30	BMI >27.3 women	2.0X

[a]Compiled from Barrett-Connor EL: Obesity, atherosclerosis and coronary artery disease. *Ann Intern Med.* 103:1010–1019, 1985. Bray GA: Complications of obesity. *Ann Int Med.* 103:1052–1062, 1985. Lew EA, Garfinkel L: Variations in mortality by weight among 750,000 men and women. *J Chron Dis* 32:563–576, 1979. Friedman GD, Kannel WB, Dawber TR: The epidemiology of gallbladder disease: observations in the Framingham study. *J Chron Dis* 19:273–292, 1966. LaVecchia C, Franceschi S, Gallus G, Decarli A, Colombo E, Liberati A, Tognoni G: Prognostic features of endrometrial cancer in estrogen users and obese women. *Am J Obstet Gynecol* 144:387–390, 1982.

Table 35.2. Nonquantified, Study-supported Morbidity Correlated with Excess Body Mass[a]

Women	Men	Both
• Heavy menstrual flow	• Decreased serum testosterone	• Increased osteoarthritis of weight bearing joints
• Menstrual irregularity	• Increased estrone and estradiol	• More gouty arthritis
• Excess facial hair		• Cutaneous disease
• Excessive length of periods (>36 days)		• Proteinuria
• Polycystic ovary syndrome		• Increased hemoglobin
• Oligoamenorrhea		• Hepatic steatosis
• Longer labor during childbirth		• Decreased FEV 1
• More cesarean sections		

[a]Adapted from: Bray GA, Complications of obesity. *Ann Intern Med* 103:1052–1062, 1985.

Obesity in infancy tends to be hyperplastic, and these extra fat cells may make it more difficult to stay thin in later years.

• Body weight may have a physiological "set point," to which individuals will return if eating is not restrained. Obese individuals who successfully lose weight may retain an abnormally high set point. Thus, they must continuously restrain their eating to stay thin.

• Metabolic rates vary from person to person. Thin people typically have higher metabolic rates, dissipating more calories through heat loss, than do the obese. This explains why obese people often eat no more than do thinner individuals.

• Dieting can cause the body's metabolism to slow down. This slower metabolic rate persists even after a diet is stopped. For this reason, repeated dieting followed by refeeding often leads to weight gain.

• Patterns of food intake are important. Many obese people eat only one or two meals a day, a situation that encourages the body to store fat. In contrast, lean individuals tend to eat smaller meals more frequently, which both facilitates exercise and reduces fat deposition.

Socioeconomic status is clearly related to obesity. The lower the status the more prevalent the obesity. In the United States, blacks, Hispanics, and Indians are statistically of lower socioeconomic status than whites. Family and cultural factors are also extremely important and may underlie many of the epidemiologic data about obesity. Obesity clearly has a familial preponderance, some of which is genetic but much of which is environmental. Families with obese children tend to use food as a reward more often than do other families, and parents who react to emotional problems by eating model such behavior for their children. When 55 husbands were asked whether they would like their obese wives to lose weight, 91% responded yes. Only 49% said they were willing to assist, however, and many husbands anticipated detrimental marital effects. Fifty-three percent of the husbands feared eating together would no longer be a shared activity; 49% feared they would lose power in marital conflicts if their wives lost weight; and 31% feared their wives would lose marital commitment or would not remain sexually loyal. Recorded mealtime conversations revealed that husbands of obese women were 7 times more likely to talk about food, 4 times as likely to offer food to their wives, and 12 times more likely to criticize rather than praise their wives for their efforts (3).

If culture can be defined as the passage of learned values and behaviors from one generation or group to another, then attitudes and behaviors associated with obesity are a reflection of culture. Thus, although the dominant cultural value in America is that slimness is good and obesity is bad, some obese individuals may fit a subculture where largeness is good. The idea that obesity is the result of poor nourishment is a western conception. Largeness is viewed by some as having plenty of food. Grandmothers who are large may be seen as "grandmotherly." Such individuals may have strong cultural disincentives to weight loss.

Thus, the etiology of obesity is often complex. It is true that general obesity develops because caloric intake exceeds caloric expenditure. On the other hand, individuals who attempt to treat obese patients must recognize the underlying physiological mechanisms and the family and cultural factors that contribute to the development of obesity.

DETERMINING WHEN A PATIENT IS OBESE

The most common reference used by practitioners in defining obesity is the Metropolitan Life Insur-

ance mortality tables. These tables are somewhat controversial, having been derived from insured individuals (and thus being of questionable generalizability) and failing to account for age. A second standard, the body mass index that was used in the NHANES studies, is the most commonly used epidemiologic reference table.

In office practice, however, two other methods have proven especially useful. One is to estimate ideal body weight using the following simple formulas:

Males: 106 lb/5 ft + 6 lb/inch above 5 ft ± 10%.
Females: 100 lb/5 ft + 5 lb/inch above 5 ft ± 10%.

The other, and perhaps most accurate, measure of adiposity (without sophisticated laboratory measurement) is skinfold thickness. These measurements are taken with the use of calipers specifically designed to measure body fat. By testing the skinfold thickness at predetermined anatomical points, the examiner can estimate the ratio of adipose tissue to lean body mass (i.e., the percentage of the body that is fat). Skinfold thickness can be very helpful in long-term counseling on weight reduction, since it directly measures adipose tissue.

While overall body fat content is important, new evidence indicates that the distribution of body fat is more predictive of health risks. Obesity in the abdominal areas carries the greatest risk. Distribution of fat in the hips and periphery, most prevalent in women, is not associated with increased mortality. In men, the waist/hip ratio (waist circumference divided by hip circumference) is a risk factor for ischemic heart disease, diabetes, stroke, and death. This is independent of total body fat mass. In men, the risk of the above diseases rose significantly when the waist/hip ratio rose above 1:1, and in women when it rose above 0.8:1. There was actually a higher associated risk in men with low general obesity (by body mass index) and high waist/hip ratio (4).

APPROACH TO MANAGEMENT

Whether we define it as an illness or not, obesity does lead to medical complications, and reducing weight results in favorable, clinically significant findings. As a family physician treating obese patients, you should realize that several steps must be taken to help patients lose weight. First, patients must be interested in losing weight. Second, health education about the medical consequences of obesity and specific nutritional information is important. Third, the family physician needs to work with the individual in setting realistic goals and subgoals. When possible, family members should be included in the treatment plan, as they can be a good source of positive reinforcement.

Finally, the family physician needs to offer support and continuous positive reinforcement throughout the weight loss process. Family physicians need to be aware of the various approaches to management. Many approaches can and should be used in combination, and long-term lifestyle change should be the ultimate goal of management. Your goal should be to build a program the patient can do and believes in. Generally, such a program will build on positive experiences the patient has had with prior weight loss efforts. Developing such a program involves getting to know the patient's past history of weight loss, family and occupational status, and eating patterns.

Self-Efficacy Theory

Albert Bandura's theory of self-efficacy is a working model particularly appropriate to managing obese patients. In brief, self-efficacy theory states that people are motivated to engage in a new behavior (walking, diet modification, etc.) if:

- They believe that they can do what they are being asked to do;
- They believe that what they are being asked to do will actually make a desirable difference.

If you systematically design a plan for your patient that involves exercise, diet change, and ongoing discussion about stresses, ask the patient the two questions above. If the answer to the first question is no, then your proposed program is unrealistically complex. If the patient can follow the program, but doesn't believe it will really change weight, then you need to investigate and overcome those beliefs. If you do not ask these questions first, your efforts will often be wasted. Make sure you and the patient are in concert with both program content and belief in the end product.

Initial Visit: Contracting and Setting Initial Goals

The initial visit is very important for both the patient and the provider. Most patients who wish to lose weight have been through one or many programs before. Most have stories about why they started, whether they got to a desired weight, how frustrating or embarrassing their experience was, and why they quit. Eighty percent will have regained their original weight or more. Many are depressed and have feelings of worthlessness. The fact that they are now in your office is an opportunity to boost their self-worth by stating the obvious. Part of your job is to get the patient interested by spelling out the program and allowing the patient to chose to start or not. *Always* give support when you can, no matter how small it might seem to you.

A checklist of important first visit questions is presented in Figure 35.2. These questions will help you learn about the patient's beliefs, interests, dietary habits, and previous weight-loss history. Often, patients know where the problems lie and need your help with those problems. At other times, the patients have important misconceptions (e.g., patients often say that carbohydrates are making them fat, when fat intake is the problem). As you ask these and similar questions, try to understand to what extent the patient is motivated to lose weight, and why. In addition, try to encourage favorable attitudes toward a weight-loss program.

GOAL SETTING AND CONTRACTING

An important first step is for you and the patient to establish a contract. The contract usually stipulates the following:

> I, (patient's name), agree to enter this contract with the understanding that Dr. (doctor's name) will provide (*a*) information to assist with changing diet, exercise, and whatever else is required to deal with the issues surrounding this problem, and (*b*) ongoing support without judgment for any effort I make. This comes with the realization that losing weight is an emotionally tough and complicated job that requires support. I also agree to make every attempt to follow the advice given to me and to let the doctor know when something doesn't seem to be working or when additional information or support is needed.

It has been our experience that what people ask for is weight loss. They must be convinced that what they really want is to feel better, move more easily, and gain an improved feeling of well-being. Thus, their goals should be feeling-based and rein-

Views about dieting

1. Who suggested diet counseling? Do you really want to lose weight?
2. What do you think is "wrong" with your current diet or lifestyle?
3. What foods do you think contribute the most to your weight problem?
4. If you try to lose weight, what do you think will happen?

Eating habits

5. How many pounds have you gained in the last 6 months? Why?
6. How much "fast food" do you eat?
7. How much television do you watch? Do you eat while watching?
8. (If the patient cooks for the family): Does your family expect you to cook in a manner that is poor for dieting?
9. Do you ever eat to calm a "nervous stomach"? Does the food help? (this could represent peptic disease or fulfillment of a psychological need.)

Previous attempts to diet

10. How long (in months or years) have you been "overweight"?
11. How many times have you dieted?
12. Were previous weight-control attempts intitated alone or through a public program (e.g., Weight Watchers, TOPS, Nutri-System)?
13. Did previous diet attempts produce weight loss? How many pounds? Was a desired weight reached?
14. Did you exercise during the diet program?
15. Did tension in the family increase during the weight control program? Why?
16. What was the worst part about dieting?
17. What made you stop the program?

Factors that might help or hinder a weight-loss program

18. With whom do you live? To whom are you the closest? Do you think that these people will support you in a weight-loss program?
19. What hobbies do you have? (How sedentary is the patient?)
20. Some people say their spouses really don't want them to lose weight. Could this be true for you?

Figure 35.2. Questions to ask during the initial visit for weight-loss counseling.

forced (e.g., "I want you to have more energy at 7 PM, get behind the wheel of your car more easily, become less irritable, look in the mirror and be able to tell yourself you're working to look and feel better," etc.).

Have the patient identify one *specific* goal during the first visit. If the stated goal is not realistic, then help the patient reframe it into a realistic goal. For example, "I will walk for 15 minutes 3 times a week after supper on Monday, Wednesday, and Saturday" is more realistic than "I'll jog 2 miles a day," if the patient has not been exercising regularly. Similarly, "I will switch to diet Coke and only drink it with meals" may be more realistic than "I won't drink any more soft drinks." Be specific, and tie the goal to daily events such as meals. At the end of your visit, ask the patient to return in 1 week with three additional written goals.

THREE-DAY PROSPECTIVE FOOD DIARY

A food intake history, in which all food and drink (even small items like cough drops) are noted, is important in planning management. At this stage, many physicians introduce a registered dietitian or other practitioner with specific expertise in dietary counseling. This is highly desirable, but not always absolutely necessary. Analysis of the 3-day food diary (on visit 2) can be accomplished by the physician with some background knowledge of food groups, caloric load, and exchange lists. Subsequent visits are usually with this other team member. Figure 35.3 provides a sample 3-day food diary form.

Second Visit: Developing a Weight-Loss Plan

On the second visit, three key issues are discussed or assessed, knowledge recall (which may be an

Food Diary		
Name: _____		
Date: _____ Day of the week: _____		

Exact time eaten	Amount	Item	Comments

Figure 35.3. Sample food diary form.

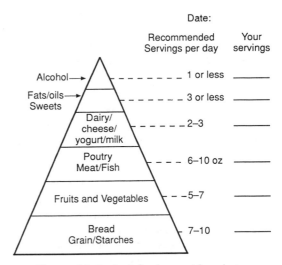

Figure 35.4. Daily food pyramid analysis.

Eat from the bottom of the pyramid. Fifty to 60% of calories should come from starches. Put a mark (indicating one serving) next to each category as you analyze your food diary.
Starch = 4 cal; Veg = 4 cal; Protein = 4 cal; fat = 9 cal.
Are you changing over time? Look at your older pyramids!

indication of literacy), motivational enthusiasm, and the 3-day food history. Potential barriers are discussed by finding the answers to the following questions:

1. What are you able to remember from the last meeting? Did you find the last session useful? What wasn't useful?
2. Did you discuss the last session with anyone at home? Did you find someone to help support your efforts?
3. Did you bring your three additional goals? (Review these.)
4. Did you bring a 3-day food diary today?

The analysis of the food diary is a simple task if you use the "Food Pyramid Analysis" sheet (Fig. 35.4). The purpose of the pyramid is to categorize foods and graphically demonstrate to the patient how to eat. It also assists them in being able to follow changes over time when done repetively. The process takes 5 minutes and gets quicker as you get used to it.

How to Use the Pyramid. Put a mark beside the food group that the patient has written down (e.g., a slice of bread is one mark next to starch (bread). A slice of cheese pizza might be represented by one starch (bread), one meat or diary (cheese), one or two fats (also for the cheese), and 1/2 vegetable (for the tomato sauce). Keep in mind that the pyramid is only an approximation, and that it will not give you the number of calories. It

will give you balance and sources of calories. As the chart says at the bottom, the highest calories are in fats and alcohol. If the total number of marks on the page are high on the pyramid, then most of their calories are from inappropriate sources.

At the end of the pyramid analysis simply direct the patient to eat more from the bottom of the pyramid. Starches, fruits, and vegetables (contrary to popular belief) do not have high calories and will not contribute to a person's weight as much as a few items from the top of the pyramid.

Make a copy for the patient and put one in the chart. Have him/her repeat the diary every month and see if the balance of calories is shifting to the bottom of the pyramid. Constant encouragement and assistance with substitutions (e.g., eat low-fat popcorn for a snack instead of Nabs or potato chips) are always essential to promote behavior change.

If the patient remains committed, the options for sensible weight loss and conditioning/food intake are discussed and an individualized program negotiated. A target weight should be set, with a goal of reaching it in an amount of time that is both feasible and physiologically realistic. Generally, losing 1 to 2 pounds per week during the first month is a sensible goal. Later, with conditioned exercise and fine-tuning of the diet, this can be increased to 2 to 3 pounds/week.

Dieting

A basic premise of dieting is that by reducing caloric intake and increasing energy expenditure, adipose body mass is lost. Few would argue with this.

There is no ideal diet that works for all patients. Consultation with a registered dietitian is very helpful in arriving at a diet plan that fits the individual preferences of your patient. Some diets are based only on caloric intake, and others on the number of exchanges from each food group. What is important to understand is that any short-lived "diet" is unlikely to be successful. Patients should be encouraged to adopt eating patterns that they will feel comfortable with for a long time, rather than short-term crash diets. While the guidelines change frequently, a few important recommendations are included in Figure 35.5.

At the end of the visit and during subsequent visits, always ask the patient to complete another 3-day food diary and bring the list back for discussion at the next visit. Always review the patient's problem list, helping problem solve. Connect the patient with a counselor if needed, but maintain close contact. Patients often need your support more than specific skills. They should get both from you.

Fad Diets and Fasting

Fad diets should be discouraged, as many are imbalanced and unsafe. While fad diets can result in rapid weight loss, the weight is rapidly regained when the person discontinues the diet. In general, dietary advice is more effective if it includes all aspects of eating, including habitual eating, eating to fill an emotional need, poor food choices, and sedentary lifestyle.

Fasting is controversial. It is used by some obese people and generally results in a significant rapid weight loss. As with other rapid weight loss strategies, however, this weight is also quickly regained. The risks of fasting for more than a few days include cardiac arrhythmias and sudden death. Long-term fasts should, therefore, be discouraged.

Because of the risks associated with fasting, protein-sparing modified fasts have become more popular. These are generally safe if used properly by individuals who are carefully screened and monitored. Patients should take supplements, which include animal protein of high biological value, potassium, sodium chloride, magnesium, calcium, phosphorous, and the recommended daily allowance of vitamins and minerals. Patients are encouraged to drink 1.5 liters of liquid per day and consume 400 to 800 calories per day. Close physiological and psychological monitoring is essential. Individuals undertaking this type of fasting must be under medical supervision, with the fast being used only in conjunction with longer-term

---

1. Concentrate on starches, vegetables, and fruits (not fats or sweets) to fill you up.
2. Modify before you eliminate foods. Cutting back from 2 tablespoons to 1 tablespoon of margarine is easier than expecting total abstinence.
3. Eat three meals a day. Skipping meals to cut calories only results in overeating later in the day (often of foods high in fat and simple sugars).
4. If you eat simple sweets or fats, always eat less than normal and always eat them as part of a larger meal, not between meals.
5. Always try to eat soluble fibers (e.g., green peas, lentils, kidney beans, pinto beans, navy beans) during meals, especially if there are sugars and fat in the meal. These fibers slow the absorption of fat and sugar and prevent the roller-coaster effect of lots of sweets on your emotions.
6. Always walk after meals. This is the worst time to watch TV or go to bed, because the food will go into storage rather than be used for energy.
7. Make one change at a time and stick with it until it's under control before changing something else.
8. Look at yourself in the mirror each morning and tell yourself you're stronger and feeling better than yesterday and that you're proud of yourself for making the effort.
9. Always speak frankly with your doctor and dietitian. There's no sense in wasting your time or theirs.
10. When you encounter problems, write them down to bring to the next meeting for discussion. This is how progress takes place. Your doctor has already signed a contract with you that commits his/her support. Expect it.

Figure 35.5. Ten rules for successful dieting.

treatment. For example, this fasting diet could be combined with a behavioral program and/or a community program. A person should not be encouraged to fast without planning to change overall eating habits.

One type of fast that is often helpful involves changing the patient's diet to one food source, such as "only fruit," for 1 day a week. This provides a break in the monotony of a weight-loss regimen and can help trim off additional weight. Complete fasting, even for a day, should be avoided.

Exercise

Much has been written about the benefits of exercise as an adjunct to diet, but the benefits of exercise alone in weight loss are far from clear. The problem is that considerable exercise is needed to burn enough calories to lose measurable weight. For example, one must walk at least 35 miles to lose a pound of fat; so short-term weight loss cannot be built upon exercise alone. Exercise is very important in dealing with long-term weight control and overall improvement in health, however. Some studies also suggest that exercise is an important factor in the prevention of obesity.

Many forms of exercise are not advisable for moderately to severely obese patients; so obese patients should be medically evaluated prior to starting an exercise program. Strenuous weight-bearing exercises on compromised or stressed joints (e.g., jogging) often should be avoided. Maintaining muscle mass through walking or water aerobics is helpful.

Patients will find the greatest results if they exercise in conjunction with decreasing their food intake. While patients on very low calorie diets (400 to 800 calories) may find it difficult to exercise, those on more moderate diets should be able to keep up a modest exercise program. Many obese people have led very sedentary lives and should (*a*) choose an activity they enjoy and (*b*) set realistic, achievable goals. Setting intermediate goals should be encouraged; it helps set the patient up for rapid success. For example, a patient who has not exercised in the past could choose walking (it is easy, inexpensive, and convenient for most) as the form of exercise and choose to walk around the block once each day for 2 weeks. If the patient makes these choices, continuation with the regimen is more likely.

Most research shows that it takes 6 to 8 weeks to develop a habit. Encouragement and praise are important in developing a habit. Therefore, plan on regularly scheduled return visits for your patients to reinforce this new behavior and to assist in setting new goals. You will also want to consider whether your patient is more likely to be successful exercising alone or in a group. Many find it useful to exercise in a structured program.

Group Treatment Programs

While it is difficult to define and measure "success," group treatment programs such as Weight Watchers clearly provide an effective approach for many people. A number of such groups exist, which vary both in philosophy and dietary approach. Each of them seems particularly suited for some individuals.

Weight Watchers, perhaps the most widespread group, encourages participants to set a realistic goal and then assists in achieving it. The low-fat, high-protein diet allows participants a great deal of variety. It focuses less on calories consumed and more on assuring that a specific number of portions of each food group are consumed. Participants are encouraged to attend weekly meetings and weigh in at each meeting. Strategies for cooking, dealing with family, and eating at restaurants are discussed. Members pay an initiation fee and a fee at each meeting.

TOPS (Take Off Pounds Sensibly) is another internationally known group. It requires a membership fee and recommends that all its members seek the assistance of their doctors. Both Weight Watchers and TOPS recommend foods that can be expensive.

Overeaters Anonymous (OA) is also a well-established group. OA has no membership fees; baskets are passed at the end of the meeting for voluntary donation. The only requirement for membership is a sincere desire to stop eating compulsively. OA is not associated with, but is based on the same principles as, Alcoholics Anonymous. The goal of OA is more to assist individuals in changing their addictive eating behaviors than to monitor weight loss.

Psychological and Behavioral Therapy

It is widely accepted that long-term substantial weight loss will only result from lifestyle changes that incorporate both eating and exercise habits. Since the goal is to change lifelong habits, psychological and/or behavioral therapy is often helpful. Psychological therapy is most useful for patients who are compulsive eaters, who have been obese for more than 6 months, or who are having a difficult time dealing with changes in body size and body image. Examples of behavioral strategies that are helpful in this type of counseling include:

- Eliminating the compulsion to eat everything served (the "clean plate syndrome");
- Eating more slowly;
- Pausing in the middle of each meal;
- Eating only at the dinner table, whether it's a meal or a snack;
- Not doing other things while eating (e.g., reading or watching television);
- Doing grocery shopping after meals, not when hungry;
- Weighing oneself only once a week;
- Continued self-monitoring.

As noted earlier in this chapter, initiating weight loss is relatively simple, maintaining the weight loss is more difficult. Behavioral therapy clearly enhances other weight-loss strategies, particularly dieting and exercise. It can effectively curb the problem of dropouts from treatment and should be considered an excellent adjunct to other weight-loss strategies.

Research has borne out that weight loss is most successful when the spouse is actively involved in treatment. This is mostly true, of course, when the existing relationship is stable and supportive. Good wishes are not enough, however. The obese person will be involved in eating habits, activities, and body-image changes that could threaten the marital relationship, so attention to feelings and relationships is important. Involvement of family members in providing support and behavioral reinforcement for a patient in a weight-loss program is crucial for its success. Assessment and on-going interaction with the spouse and children are vital.

Obesity in Children

More often than not, childhood obesity reflects an underlying family systems problem. Therefore, meeting with the family members is essential to the management of obese children and adolescents. Find out whether family members perceive the child's obesity as a problem and whether they are interested in, and capable of, doing something about it. Then, assess the family's eating patterns: who is responsible for meals, whether eating between meals is structured, how the child's time is

spent, and where the sources of inappropriate eating appear to be. Use your knowledge of family dynamics (see Chapter 3) to help plan behavioral management strategies, and involve a professional counselor.

At a community level, a family physician can assist the schools in setting up programs to prevent and treat childhood obesity. Children eat between 1/3 and 2/3 of their meals at school; so the schools should have special programs for children who need weight reduction. Where such programs do exist, you can encourage obese patients to enroll and receive guidance and planned meals.

Drug Therapy

Antiobesity drugs play little or no role in treating obese patients. While research shows that these drugs do result in rapid weight loss, it has also shown that this weight is rapidly regained once the drug is discontinued. Amphetamine derivatives, which were formerly used as antiobesity drugs and are no longer approved for this purpose, had significant side effects and a large abuse potential. More recently, prolonged medication use has been shown to maintain modest weight reduction (5). In general, however, the risks of antiobesity drugs outweigh the benefits. Very rarely, a drug can be given as part of an overall management plan that includes an attempt to modify eating habits.

When patients inquire about weight reduction pills, you should emphasize that these drugs are both dangerous and ineffective (in the long run). Point out physiological principles, such as set point and food intake patterns, that underlie obesity and that must be altered through behavioral change. Know the options available to build a management and support program for any motivated patient.

Surgical Intervention

For massively obese patients, surgery can lead to significant weight loss when other measures have failed. Surgery should only be used when more conservative measures have failed and the benefits outweigh the risks. Patients should be carefully screened and monitored. Jejunoileal bypass surgery results in weight loss partly because of the reduction in food intake and partly because of malabsorption. Morbidly obese patients often lose significant weight postoperatively, but after 2 years there is a tendency for regaining weight as bowel adaption takes place. Immediate complications include a 1 to 2% mortality (usually from thromboembolism, aspiration pneumonia, wound adhesions, and sepsis), profuse diarrhea for months to years, fluid and electrolyte loss, stone formation, and nutritional deficiencies. For these reasons, careful patient selection is important. Patients over 50, those unlikely to follow up, and those with severe psychiatric difficulties should not undergo jejunoileal bypass surgery.

Gastric bypass, another common surgery, has fewer long-term complications than jejunoileal bypass. By surgically reducing the size of the functioning gastric reservoir, most of the stomach is bypassed, and a feeling of satiety occurs after a small meal, resulting in a lower caloric intake and subsequent weight loss. This operation is technically difficult in the morbidly obese and may have side effects that decrease quality of life, such as eating-induced diarrhea (dumping syndrome).

A similar technique, which is easier to perform, is gastroplasty or gastric partition, in which an autosuture stapling machine is used. As with other surgical treatments of obesity, most weight loss occurs in the first 2 to 6 weeks. Both the gastric bypass and gastroplasty can result in severe and persistent nausea and vomiting, renal stones, and hair loss. With all these techniques, the goal of treatment is to create a temporary condition that will compel the patient to break a compulsive eating habit. During the first 3 months after surgery, it is important for the patient to develop a new concept of eating. Pre- and postoperative counseling is therefore essential.

Recently, endoscopically placed gastric balloons have been developed. By partially filling the stomach, these balloons have the same rationale as the above gastric surgical procedures. This technique is currently experimental, with balloon failure and pyloric obstruction being the most frequent complications.

CONCLUSIONS

Effective management of obesity by the family physician illustrates many of the basic principles of family medicine. A broad base of knowledge is required, embracing physiology, family dynamics, psychology, and the use of community resources. An individual assessment and treatment plan is needed, which uses other health team members as consultants and therapists. Effective treatment requires regular follow-up, with the doctor-patient relationship often playing an important role in a patient's success.

REFERENCES

1. National Institutes of Health Consensus Development Conference Statement: Health implications of obesity. *Ann Intern Med* 103:1073–1077, 1985.
2. Nash JD: Eating behavior and body weight: physiological influences. *Am J Health Promotion* 2:5–13, 1987.
3. Stuart RB, Davis B: *Slim Chance in a Fat World; Behavioral Control of Obesity.* Champaign, IL, Research Press, 1972.
4. Björntorp P: Regional patterns of fat distribution. *Ann Intern Med* 103:994–995, 1985.
5. Weintraub M, et al.: Long-term weight control: The National Heart, Lung and Blood Institute funded multimodal intervention study. *Clin Pharmacol Ther* 51(5):581–646, 1992.

SUGGESTED READINGS

Barrett-Connor EL: Obesity, atherosclerosis, and coronary artery disease. *Ann Intern Med* 103:1010–1019, 1985.

This review article presents data from the Metropolitan Insurance mortality studies, the Framingham Heart Study (26-year follow-up), and the NHANES I and II. Methodologic questions, cross-cultural perspectives, and population effects are discussed.

Munro JF, Douglas JG: The management of obesity. *Hum Nutr Clin Nutr* 370:1–19, 1983.

This excellent article discusses the treatment and causes of obesity. Much of the research is based in the UK.

Pacy PJ, Webster J, Garrow JS: Exercise and obesity. *Sports Med* 3:89–113, 1986.

This article provides an in-depth overview of the relationships between exercise and obesity. Some topics covered include mortality and obesity, the impact of physical activity on obesity, and the effect of physical activity on energy intake.

chapter 36

ANXIETY AND DEPRESSION

Matthew Alexander

Anxiety and depression are among the most frequently encountered psychosocial problems that present to family physicians, a circumstance explained by both the high prevalence of these disorders in our society and the relative frequency with which they are associated with medical disorders. Anxiety disorders occur in 30 to 40% of the adult population at some time in their lives, and 27% of patients who present to family physicians with psychiatric symptoms do so with symptoms of anxiety. In addition, approximately 10% of all males and 20% of all females will experience a significant depression during their lifetimes. Many researchers have suggested that depression is the most common psychiatric problem encountered by family physicians.

Both anxiety and depression are, however, underrecognized by family physicians because they often present with somatic symptoms such as pain, palpitations, and constipation. Depression is associated with numerous medications and medical conditions. Medical illness is the most common precipitant of depression among the elderly.

Anxiety and depression result in high costs to society in terms of medical expenses, lost work days, and psychic suffering. Thus, it is important for physicians to be skilled in recognizing and treating both of these common medical problems.

ANXIETY

Definitions of Anxiety

Each of us experiences moments and possibly extended periods of anxiety. In a family medicine practice, you will see patients with a variety of symptoms related to anxiety. Often, anxious patients present with physical complaints such as fatigue, headaches, lower back pain, and insomnia. These symptoms reflect mild to severe reactions to

anxiety, and your goals in dealing with the patients are to identify where they fall along this continuum (Fig. 36.1) and provide appropriate treatment.

Situational or secondary anxiety is a condition you will see frequently. It occurs in response to many of the everyday demands of life, be they job-related, relational, or normal life transitions such as pregnancy, midlife, or old age. Situational anxiety usually remits on its own. People experiencing situational anxiety respond well by talking to others about their feelings and receiving their support. Psychological diagnoses should only be considered when anxiety becomes chronic and/or interferes with on-going adaptation to life events.

Adjustment disorder with anxious mood is the diagnostic category for individuals whose response to stress is severe enough to interfere with daily functioning. Like people with situational anxiety, people with adjustment disorder with anxious mood respond well to support and talking about emotions, and improve with the passage of time.

In contrast to the above diagnoses, anxiety disorders are on-going conditions that are relatively unresponsive to talking therapies, support, and the passage of time. Patients with **anxiety disorders** usually present to their physician with the following symptoms:

- Vague complaints such as stomach upset, pain syndromes, headache, general fatigue, or malaise.
- General feelings of uneasiness, excessive worrying, difficulty concentrating and sleeping, or heightened attentiveness and vigilance. Some patients may simply refer to these feelings as "nerves."
- Panic attacks, which are intense and circumscribed periods of spontaneous fear characterized by any of the following symptoms:

339

Increasing
Severity
	Situational anxiety
	Adjustment disorder with anxious mood
	Anxiety disorder
	   Phobias (ex. disabling fear of heights)
	   Anxiety states (ex. generalized anxiety disorder)

Figure 36.1. Types of anxiety.

faintness, feeling of impending doom, smothering sensations, dizziness, sweating, paresthesias, trembling, and fear of dying or going crazy.

The third edition of *The Diagnostic and Statistical Manual* (DSM-III) classifies anxiety disorders under two broad categories: phobic disorders and anxiety states. Individuals suffering from **phobias** experience persistent irrational fear of specific objects (e.g., spiders, dogs, mice), activities (e.g., riding an elevator, going into a dark basement) or situations (e.g., being alone in a crowd, driving a car, being on a mountaintop). Such fear results in a strong desire to avoid the dreaded object, activity, or situation. To merit diagnosis as a phobic disorder, the individual's fear must be a real source of distress and interfere with social function.

Case 1. Agoraphobia

Ms. L. has a 7-year history of hypertension, hypokalemia, and vague shoulder discomfort. She presents with attacks of nerves, characterized by a feeling of smothering and tightness in her chest and shoulders, rapid heart beat, and sense of impending doom. These attacks occur either in large crowds or at church. Ms. L.'s fear of having these attacks in public has made her increasingly housebound. Social history reveals recent deaths of her alcoholic husband, sister, and son-in-law.

Case Discussion

Ms. L.'s case is an example of agoraphobia, which literally means fear of the marketplace. Agoraphobics are afraid of being alone in public places from which escape may be difficult in the case of sudden incapacitation. Agoraphobics experience recurrent panic (or anxiety) attacks, which lead to anticipatory anxiety (fear of having a panic attack). In turn, this anticipatory anxiety causes them to avoid any situations associated with the attacks. As Ms. L.'s case demonstrates, agoraphobics in the chronic state often become housebound, insisting that a friend or family member accompany them whenever they leave home. Approximately 5% of the population has had agoraphobia at some time in their lives. The disorder is more frequently diagnosed in women, and it may wax and wane

in severity. Drug abuse and depression are two common secondary reactions to the disorder, the most common phobic disorder seen in medical practice.

The second broad category of *anxiety disorders*, anxiety states, refers to feelings of marked fear that arise spontaneously without clear-cut precipitants. *Generalized anxiety disorder* is the most common anxiety state seen in medical practice. The criteria for this diagnosis include persistent, generalized anxiety for at least 1 month and symptoms from at least three of the following four categories:

1. Motor tension: jumpiness, inability to relax, and restlessness;
2. Autonomic hyperactivity: sweating, heart pounding or racing, hot or cold spells, diarrhea;
3. Apprehensive expectation: worry, fear, rumination;
4. Vigilance and scanning: difficulty concentrating, insomnia, feeling on edge.

Differential diagnoses include major depression, hyperthyroidism, and alcohol/drug abuse and dependency.

Case 2. Generalized Anxiety

Mr. P. has borderline diabetes, mild obesity, hypertension, and a long history of anxiety. He speaks in a halting, stuttering voice and appears overly apologetic and unassertive. Ten years ago, a nervous breakdown precipitated by an anxiety attack caused Mr. P. to move his family to another city and switch jobs. He has never felt right since. He complains chronically of worrying, jitteriness, difficulty concentrating, an overactive mind with thoughts running away from him, a racing heart, and difficulty sleeping. He also reports marked feelings of inadequacy, decline in sexual functioning (feeling too tense to have sex), and decreased appetite. He works presently as a janitor and feels others look down on him.

Case Discussion

Mr. P.'s symptoms include all four categories for generalized anxiety listed in DSM-III. Biological or "vegetative" changes in his appetite, sexual functioning, and sleep patterns also suggest depression, a common coexisting condition in many anxiety cases.

Diagnostic Interview for Anxiety

When the patient complains directly about anxiety or "nerves," or when the physician suspects anxiety may be a significant component of the prevailing complaint, the following questions should be asked:

1. Everyone experiences anxiety differently—exactly what is your anxiety like?
2. Is it steady or intermittent?
3. Are there specific situations that lead to your having anxiety?
4. How long have you had this problem with your nerves? days, months or years?
5. Have you ever experienced rapid heart beats? trembling? rapid breathing or shortness of breath? chest discomfort? tingling in your extremities? a sense of impending doom?
6. What changes in your lifestyle have occurred as a result of your anxiety?
7. How have you and others in your family dealt with your anxiety?
8. What is your greatest concern about your anxiety?
9. What do you think is causing your anxiety?
10. What are your thoughts about what would help?

Patients can also be asked to keep an anxiety diary where they can note time, place, feelings, thoughts, and behaviors, both theirs and others, before, during, and after the anxious episode. Involving the patient in collecting personal data reinforces the collaborative nature of medical care. Self-administered questionnaires, such as the Sheehan anxiety scale, can also be helpful (1). Gathering data through the diagnostic interview and the diary will reveal important information regarding the patient's anxiety, will enhance rapport between the patient and physician, and will likely provide therapeutic value itself.

The differences between a stress reaction, adjustment reaction with anxious features, and anxiety disorder are qualitative. Stress reactions and adjustment reactions both remit once the stress ceases, changes, or is met with a more relaxed attitude. Anxiety disorders are, however, more deeply rooted in the individual personality. Panic attacks

indicate a likely anxiety state rather than stress or adjustment reaction.

Anxiety is difficult to distinguish from the somatoform disorders (see Chapter 38, "Somatizing Patients"), and they so often coexist. The critical features of somatoform disorders are physical symptoms, such as back pain, dizziness, abdominal pain, painful menstruation, or pain during intercourse, for which there are no demonstrable organic findings and which are closely linked to psychological factors or conflict.

Treatment for Anxiety
MEDICATIONS

Once a diagnosis of anxiety is established, the physician needs to decide whether or not to medicate. Although antianxiety agents can provide important temporary relief for some anxiety patients, these drugs have the potential for abuse and should be prescribed cautiously.

Medications can be useful in providing sufficient control of both panic attacks and anticipatory anxiety to enable phobic patients to approach and master avoided situations. The tricyclic Imipramine is frequently used to suppress panic attacks. A relatively low dosage, 10 to 75 mg per day, may be sufficient, although higher doses of 100 to 200 mg per day may be necessary. In certain cases, management of anticipatory anxiety can be achieved with a benzodiazepine such as alprazolam (Xanax—0.25 to 0.5 mg three times a day), which may also effectively treat the panic attacks. Due to rapid tolerance and the addictive potential of the benzodiazepines, treatment with Xanax should be episodic and short-term (i.e., less than a month). Tricyclic antidepressants have been found to be an effective pharmacological treatment for some individuals suffering from generalized anxiety as has the nonbenzodiazepine anxiolytic agent, buspirone (Buspar). Propranolol, clonidine, and alprazolam are other medications that have been tried with limited success with this group of patients.

In using pharmaceutics to treat individuals with anxiety disorders, physicians should inform these patients that anxiety itself is part of life and that anxiety problems will resolve. Reassurance should be given that panic attacks themselves are not associated with imminent death, heart attacks, loss of consciousness, or insanity.

Anxious people can often be demanding and needy patients. Many of these patients will request specific medications provided by other physicians.

Clarify your own attitudes regarding use of antianxiety medication prior to working with patients having anxiety symptoms. You should accept patients' feelings and requests for help even if you choose not to support some aspect of the requested assistance, such as medication.

SUPPORTIVE COUNSELING

Patients suffering from stress-related anxiety or adjustment disorder with anxious mood often benefit from a few sessions of supportive counseling with the physician. These patients are often hard-driving and motivated, so they frequently take suggestions well and work hard to get better. The physician's role in such situations is to listen actively, facilitate open exchange, and encourage the patients to develop their own problem-solving skills. The use of open-ended questions is particularly valuable in this regard. The physician should educate the patients regarding the ubiquitous nature of anxiety and seek to help them gain insight into the relationship between their symptoms and life situation. The Holmes and Rahe life change inventory (2) helps clarify for the patients the degree of change in their lives. Since life change is associated with stress, using the inventory improves awareness of how one's life situation is affecting one emotionally.

Some training in progressive relaxation, a technique developed 50 years ago by Dr. Edmund Jacobson (3), is also helpful. This technique teaches people to distinguish between muscle tension and relaxation. The patient then focuses on inducing a state of deep muscle relaxation as a way of relieving stress. Patients can learn this technique with the assistance of commercially available relaxation tapes. Check your local bookstore or library for current tapes or books. Massage, exercise, meditation, listening to music, and other relaxation techniques can help.

WHEN TO REFER

If patients with stress-related anxiety do not improve after a few sessions of supportive counseling, a referral to a qualified mental health professional should be considered. You can receive a list of qualified professionals in your local area by contacting national associations such as the American Psychological Association (APA), American Association for Marriage and Family Therapists (AAMFT), or the National Register for Health Care Providers in Psychology. A more useful approach is to ask fellow health professionals to recommend therapists in your area with whom they have had success in the past.

Referral should especially be considered for individuals suffering from agoraphobia. Therapists typically use a behavioral approach that includes programmed practice with the feared situation. The patient develops a hierarchical list of situations from least- to most-feared. The patient, with the help of the therapist, slowly proceeds through the list, first in imagination and then real life, until the situations no longer evoke unmanageable anxiety. Since one cannot simultaneously experience anxiety and relaxation, progressive muscle relaxation training is used in conjunction with programmed practice.

Patients suffering from panic attacks benefit from the same approaches used with phobics. The physician should be careful to gather a thorough social history. Clinical experience has suggested that spontaneous panic attacks sometimes are associated with extramarital love affairs or persistent grief reactions.

Patients with chronic generalized anxiety may also need therapy from mental health professionals. Patients who are emotionally and financially prepared to address underlying psychological conflicts may benefit from intensive psychotherapy. Some family physicians will choose to provide short-term psychotherapy utilizing a therapeutic supportive relationship. The physician should educate the patient regarding the predictable course of the symptoms and provide reassurance that the patient will not "go crazy." Relaxation techniques and biofeedback are additional nonpharmacological interventions for generalized anxiety.

DEPRESSION

Definition of Depression

All individuals experience sadness at certain times in their lives. Normal sadness or the "blues" occurs in response to loss, either physical loss of loved ones through death/divorce or loss of one's own health, self-esteem, or security. During such times, individuals may experience crying spells, lethargy, and discouragement. Such sadness usually remits with support and time or when the external situation changes. Normal sadness responds to reassurance, involves mild physical changes, and does not interfere with the ability to function.

The DSM-III classifies depression under *affective disorders*, a term that applies to a disturbance of mood not due to any other physical or mental disorder. Mood refers to a prolonged emotion that colors the whole inner life of the individual and generally involves either sadness or happiness. Only when a sad mood interferes with daily functioning or becomes a chronic way of relating to the world does it merit consideration of a DSM-III diagnosis. The DSM-III no longer distinguishes between endogenous (biological) and exogenous (reactive) depression, since all depressions may involve biochemical changes and since it is hard to determine causality.

A more useful distinction involves primary and secondary (or situational) depression. *Primary depression* occurs in the absence of any other medical, psychiatric, or surgical disorder. *Secondary depression* occurs in the context of a serious medical, psychiatric, or surgical problem. For example, secondary depression may occur in response to extended hospital stays; to medical conditions such as cancer, heart disease, or AIDS; and to psychiatric conditions such as dementia or obsessive-compulsive disorder. Patients with a family history of depression may be more likely to suffer from primary depression.

The DSM-III classifies depression, whether primary or secondary, under three general categories as illustrated in Figure 36.2: (*a*) adjustment disorder with depressed mood; (*b*) dysthymic disorder; and (*c*) major depression. The differences between these classifications relate to increasing intensity and duration. Adjustment reaction, however, always occurs with a psychosocial stress or loss.

The following case examples illustrate the different clinical pictures of patients with depression.

Case 3. Adjustment Disorder with Depressed Mood

Mr. P. is a 27-year-old man who presents to his physician with multiple complaints including a sharp pain in his right side, fatigue, and general malaise. Six months ago, he was divorced from his wife of 7 years. Since his wife left him, he has just not "felt well," has been anxious with a poor appetite, and has had diffi-

culty sleeping. The patient wants to know what he can do to "feel better."

Case Discussion

The predominant feature of adjustment disorder with depressed mood is a dysfunctional reaction to an identifiable psychosocial stress. It occurs within 3 months of the onset of that stress and is characterized by such symptoms as sadness, tearfulness, and hopelessness. The maladaptive nature of the adjustment reaction is indicated by either impairment in social or occupational functioning or symptoms that are in excess of normal and expected reactions to the stressor. The depression will eventually end once the stress stops or, if the stress persists, when a new level of adaptation is achieved. This disorder is common.

Case 4. Dysthymic Disorder

Ms. S., a 28-year-old woman, presents to her physician for a birth control prescription. During the course of the interview, she reports feeling depressed, inferior, and pessimistic, feelings that she claims to have had since she was 16 or 17 years old. She has recently started dating a man but expresses doubts about the relationship. She also voices criticism about her boss and her past experiences with the medical profession.

Case Discussion

Dysthymic disorder involves the same symptom picture as major depression (described below), but the symptoms are less severe and more chronic, lasting at least 2 years. The dysthymic person has developed a chronically depressed view of both self and the world, and is usually considered a "depressed personality."

Case 5. Major Depression

Ms. C. is a 48-year-old woman with a long history of migraine headaches. She initially presented to the physician 3 years earlier with premenopausal hot flashes that have been controlled with estrogen. She reports feeling "blue" and fatigued and has had difficulty sleeping in the past few months. More recently, she has lost the desire to communicate with others and seriously wonders if life is worth living. She feels worthless and blames herself for the breakup of her marriage years ago. Now, she has gone for days with-

Increasing Severity	Normal sadness
	Adjustment disorder with depressed mood
	Dysthymic disorder
	Major depression
	Depressive psychosis

Figure 36.2. Types of depression.

out getting out of bed. She works at a stressful job, lives with two grown sons at home, and has no close friends.

Major Depression

The diagnostic criteria for a major depressive episode are:

1. Loss of pleasure in all or almost all usual activities and pastimes (i.e., anhedonia);
2. Vegetative or physical changes such as poor appetite, significant weight loss or weight gain, insomnia or hypersomnia, loss of energy, fatigue, psychomotor agitation or retardation, and decreased interest in sexuality;
3. Cognitive changes such as feelings of worthlessness, low self-esteem, excessive guilt, difficulty concentrating, recurrent thoughts of suicide or wishing to be dead, hopelessness, and helplessness.

These symptoms must have been consistently present for at least 2 weeks. The onset of a major depressive episode may be sudden, and estimates are that half of those individuals experiencing an episode of major depression will eventually have another one.

Diagnostic Interview for Depression

Patients rarely present to their family physician having diagnosed themselves as depressed. More often patients do not know they are depressed and present with complaints such as chronic pain, headache, fatigue, low back pain, chest and abdominal pain, or memory loss. This is often referred to as masked depression. Because patients may not interpret their complaints as depression, the physician must make an accurate diagnosis and interpret this diagnosis in a compassionate and positive manner.

When you suspect depression, begin by assessing symptoms from the "depressed triad": (*a*) disturbance in mood, (*b*) vegetative signs, and (*c*) lowered self-esteem.

Questions to ask include:

1. Have you been feeling "blue" or "down in the dumps" lately? Can you describe those feelings?
2. Have you had changes in your appetite? sleep patterns, particularly early morning awakening? sexual interest? activity or energy level?
3. Do you have difficulty concentrating?

4. How do you feel about yourself? How do you feel about the future?
5. On a scale of 1 to 10, with 1 being not bad at all and 10 being the worst possible emotional pain you could experience, how bad have you been feeling?
6. How long have you been feeling this way?
7. Have there been any recent losses in your life (e.g. person, health, income, self-esteem)?
8. Have you ever felt like this before?
9. Is there a history of depression or antisocial behavior in your family?

A number of standardized questionnaires exist to aid in diagnosis of depression. Among the more popular patient-administered instruments are the Zung depression scale (4) and, for older patients, the geriatric depression scale (5).

Since alcoholism and drug abuse can cause depression, ask specifically about their use. (For information on screening and diagnosis of alcoholism see Chapter 37.) A briefer assessment of depression would target the following: the inability to experience pleasure; physical vegetative signs, particularly sleep disturbance; and cognitive changes (e.g., guilt, loss of self-esteem, and suicidal thoughts).

Asking patients the following three questions will help clarify, in a brief interview, the presence or lack of depression: What do you do for a good time? How is your sleep? How do you feel about yourself?

Assessing Suicide Potential

Comprising the seventh leading cause of death in the United States, an estimated 80% of suicides are associated with severe depression. Since the mortality rate from suicidal depression is estimated to be between 5 and 15%, the physician must routinely ask depressed patients about suicide.

Questions to elicit suicidal intent should be asked at an appropriate time during the interview and can include:

1. Have you been feeling bad enough to have had thoughts about harming yourself?
2. If yes, have you actually had thoughts about killing yourself?
3. If yes, how would you kill yourself?
4. If yes, what is the plan? At this point the physician needs to evaluate the lethality and immediate danger of the plan being carried out.

Additional risk factors to consider in assessing suicide potential are a clear intention regarding the impact of the suicide on others, family history of suicide, past history of a suicide attempt, social isolation, recent separation from a loved one, alcoholism/drug abuse, psychosis, or terminal illness. If the physician, on the basis of the information gathered and a "gut reaction," feels that the patient is suicidal, immediate psychiatric consultation should be sought.

Many drugs and medications can produce or aggravate depression. These include oral contraceptives, steroids, propranolol, antianxiety drugs, cocaine, alcohol, marijuana, amphetamines, and antihypertensives, particularly α-methyldopa and reserpine.

Treatment for Depression

Once you have diagnosed depression, your next step is to develop a treatment plan. In doing so, the key questions to consider are:

1. Should this patient be primarily counseled, and if so, how?
2. Are antidepressant medications indicated?
3. Should the patient be referred to a mental health professional?

SUPPORTIVE COUNSELING

Supportive primary-care counseling (helping the patient understand solutions to problems) without medication or referral should be provided to patients who have a good outside support system and are suffering from a situational depressive reaction related to a recent loss of a person, a job, health, or self-esteem. Your role will be particularly relevant if the depression is related to a recent illness or death in the family. Intervention should include informing the patient of your diagnosis of mild depression and linking this diagnosis with recent changes in the patient's life. Set aside weekly, regular, brief (20 minutes) appointments for supportive counseling. Six sessions are usually sufficient.

Successful counseling approaches include developing a supportive relationship, focusing on the patient's feelings, maintaining a hopeful attitude, clarifying thoughts and feelings for the patient, and allowing the patient to express emotion. It is very helpful to validate the patient's feelings as normal, given the circumstances. Specific criteria for improvement include reduced subjective feelings of sadness, more pleasure in life, later wakening in the mornings, increased sexual frequency, improved appetite, and increased social activity. If several of these criteria are not met after the six visits, outside referral should be considered.

MEDICATIONS

Many patients with depressive symptoms will improve over time with supportive therapy, a change in their environment, or when the natural healing response to loss has taken its course. Some will, however, respond much more quickly to antidepressant medications. Indications for antidepressant medications include (a) vegetative signs (e.g., weight loss, early morning awakening, loss of sexual interest); (b) past history of response to medication; (c) positive family history of depression and good response to somatic treatment of depression; (d) lack of response to counseling; and (e) severe symptoms incapacitating the individual. Tricyclic antidepressants or trazadone are the medications of choice for patients having the above-mentioned positive indicators. Lithium carbonate is useful for patients who experience manic-depression, i.e., strong and powerful mood swings alternating between elation and depression. Because the therapeutic window of lithium carbonate is narrow, initial management of this drug should be handled by a psychiatrist. Urgent consultation and use of electroconvulsive therapy (ECT) may be indicated for patients suffering from acute suicidal depression. Monoamine oxidase inhibitors (MAOIs) should be reserved for second-line treatment, since these drugs have harmful side effects and require strict dietary precautions. Commonly prescribed medications are listed in Table 36.1.

Considerable publicity has been generated regarding the relatively new antidepressant Prozac (fluoxetine). In fact, in 1990 Prozac was the most frequently prescribed of all antidepressants. It is as effective as other antidepressants but has neither the suicide potential nor the adverse cardiovascular and anticholinergic effects associated with tricyclic or MAOI antidepressant medication. Because of its activating effect on the nervous system, it may be particularly well suited to the depressed patient with lethargy and fatigue. To avoid possible drug-related insomnia, however, dosing should occur in the morning or midday. Links with drug-induced violent and/or suicidal behavior have, as yet, not been conclusively established.

Table 36.1. Commonly Prescribed Medications for Depression

Symptom Indicator	Medication	Dosage
Sleeplessness	Amitriptyline	125–200 mg/day
Hypersomnia	Imipramine	150–300 mg/day
Agitation	Alprazolam (short-term use only; i.e., no longer than 3 weeks)	0.5 mg t.i.d.
Lethargy	Fluoxetine	20–80 mg/day
?Suicide risk	Trazodone	200–350 mg/day
?Cardiac problems	Nortriptyline	50–150 mg/day
Elderly	Desipramine	25–100 mg/day

Patients need to be educated about the side effects of these medications and told that therapeutic effects may not occur for up to 4 weeks (possibly up to 8 weeks for Prozac). Positive effects will only occur if the medications are taken daily. When prescribing antidepressants, begin at a low dose, about one-third the maintenance dose for young adults and one-fifth the maintenance dose for elderly patients. Increase the dose gradually. Prescribe limited doses of these medications and bring the patient back frequently for follow-up, since suicide is always a possibility. Unresponsiveness to a particular tricyclic antidepressant may indicate a trial with a medication from another class of the tricyclic antidepressants. When treatment has been successful, plan on tapering after 6 months or more. Depressed patients who are either suicidal or psychotic need to be referred immediately to a psychiatrist. Referral for outpatient psychotherapy should be considered in cases where patients are insight-oriented and motivated to work on their depression and find better ways to cope, have a dysthymic disorder, or have long-term unresolved grief reactions.

REFERRAL

Physicians should refer depressed patients whenever they themselves feel inadequately trained to deal with the presenting problems or do not have the necessary time to treat the problem psychotherapeutically. Several studies have indicated the effectiveness (with or without medication) of outpatient psychotherapy. Other studies have indicated that the most successful results for treatment of depression come when psychotherapeutic and pharmacological approaches are combined. If you are referring your patient, remember that many psychotherapists prefer to be involved in the decision to medicate and to interview the depressed patient before antidepressants are started. It is also advantageous in terms of increasing motivation for

therapy to hold off on prescribing antidepressants until after patients have begun counseling.

Patients referred to mental health professionals should be reassured that they are not crazy, that their physician will continue to follow their medical care, and that the physician, in the patient's shoes, would also consult a therapist. A patient's resistance to the idea of psychotherapy should be carefully discussed. The physician should schedule a follow-up appointment after the patient has contacted a therapist.

Regardless of the specific treatment approach taken, depressed patients will benefit greatly from a caring approach from the physician. Reassurance, empathy, education about the characteristics of the patient's illness, and unconditional acceptance are of great value in the treatment of depression.

REFERENCES

1. Katon W, Sheehan DV, Uhde TW: Panic disorder: a treatable problem. *Patient Care* March 30, 148–173, 1988.
2. Holmes TH, Rahe RH: The social readjustment rating scale. *J Psychosom Res* 11:213–218, 1967.
3. Davis M, Eshelman ER, McKay M: *The Relaxation and Stress Reduction Workbook*, ed 2. Oakland, New Harbinger Publications, 1982, pp 23-27.
4. Zung WWK: A self-rating of depression scale. *Arch Gen Psychiatry* 12:63–70, 1965.
5. Yesavage JA, Brink TL, Rose TL: Development and validation of a geriatric depression screening scale: a preliminary report. *J Psychiatr Res* 17:37–49, 1983.

SUGGESTED READINGS

Benson H, Stuart E (eds): *The Wellness Book: The Comprehensive Guide to Maintaining Health and Treating Stress-related Illness*. New York, Carol Publishing Group, 1992.

A good textbook covering all aspects of the mind-body connection. It presents current research findings that support many behavioral medicine treatment approaches.

Burns D: *Feeling Good: The New Mood Therapy*. New York, William Morrow, 1981.

This book incorporates the behavioral-cognitive approach of Dr. Aaron Beck in treating depression. Pragmatic and effective "homework assignments" for the patient are included.

Davis M, Eshelman ER, McKay M: *The Relaxation and Stress Reduction Workbook*, ed 2. Oakland, New Harbinger Publications, 1982.

An extremely useful book for the medical practitioner. Reviews over a dozen stress-reduction techniques, presenting rationales for use, drawings, and concise and clear explanations of such approaches as self-hypnosis, autogenics, exercise, and progressive relaxation. An excellent source of patient handouts.

Wilson RR: *Don't Panic: Taking Control of Anxiety Attacks*. New York, Harper & Row, 1986.

A very practical and readable book for patients suffering from anxiety problems. The book successfully "normalizes" anxiety reactions and provides anxiety sufferers with useful, nonpharmacological tools for combating anxiety.

chapter 37

ALCOHOLISM AND DRUG ABUSE

Robert E. Gwyther and Michael J. Tyler

Of all the problems the family physician faces, alcoholism is the disease that presents the widest diversity (varied presentations), affects the greatest percentage of patients (one in eight) and families (one in three), and offers preventive medicine its largest potential for cost reduction ($104 billion annually in the United States). Added to that is an enormous impact on the medical, legal and social institutions of the country, caused by the abuse of both illicit and prescription drugs. Family physicians see these problems daily, some presenting overtly and others as the root cause of chronic problems or hidden in subtle patient complaints.

DEFINITIONS

Use—Purposeful ingestion of a chemical substance orally or through the epithelial lining of the nose, rectum or lungs; injection of a chemical subcutaneously, intramuscularly, or intravenously.

Abuse—Purposeful use of a "therapeutic" drug in excess of amounts prescribed or for indications not intended; continued use of drugs and/or alcohol, in spite of adverse consequences on the user or others.

Dependency—State in which a person must continue to use a chemical to avoid withdrawal symptoms.

Withdrawal—Physical and/or psychological symptoms and signs that develop when the use of a chemical is stopped.

Addiction—Continued use of a chemical in spite of accompanying physical, psychological, social, economic, legal, and/or spiritual deterioration.

Tolerance—State of reduced sensitivity to a chemical, caused by increased metabolism of the chemical or decreased bodily reaction to its presence.

Chemical dependency—Generic term referring to dependency on mood- or mind-altering substances.

Alcoholism—A chronic disease, characterized by the compulsion to consume alcohol and the eventual loss of control over its intake, despite adverse social, emotional, and/or physical consequences that follow its use.

ETIOLOGY

Until 1960, when Jellnek published a now-classic treatise entitled "The Disease Concept of Alcoholism," most physicians viewed substance abuse as a moral weakness. Now, we consider its etiology to be multifactorial. We no longer consider there to be an "alcoholic personality." Some individuals are clearly more susceptible than others. A strong genetic component probably exists, as evidenced by a 5-fold increased risk for alcoholism in adopted twins of alcoholic fathers and a 50% alcoholism rate among first-degree male relatives of alcoholic inpatients. Growing evidence indicates that neurotransmitters and their receptor sites in the brain are the locus of the effects of drugs of abuse; addicts may differ genetically from other people at this central nervous system (CNS) interface. Environmental and social components also play a considerable role, with people of lower socioeconomic status, those living in urban areas, and those in selected professions (e.g., painters, construction workers, bartenders) being at higher risk.

All drugs of abuse have CNS effects that patients seek, including euphoria and anesthesia. They also cause a variety of negative CNS effects including agitation, depression, anesthesia, and respiratory depression. Prolonged chemical dependency is associated with delay in normal psy-

349

chosocial development. Long-time abusers in their twenties frequently have not resolved issues ordinarily conquered by teenagers.

Drugs are frequently categorized by their effects on the brain. Stimulant drugs, such as cocaine and amphetamines, differ generally from depressant drugs, such as barbiturates and alcohol; however, this does not mean that all drugs within one category act the same. Two people may react differently to the same drug. Two drugs in one category, such as depressants, may have different effects on the same organ system. For instance, marijuana and alcohol are both classified as depressants, yet marijuana typically causes users to decrease their motor activity, while many alcohol users become aggressive.

Of the many substances of abuse, some appear to be more addictive than others. Alcohol "captures" about 10% of those exposed to its effects; crack cocaine addiction may eventually claim over 80% of those who use it on multiple occasions. Alcohol and drugs of abuse are closely related. For many, alcohol is a "gateway drug," meaning the first one used by people who later become addicted to other drugs. Most drugs (including alcohol) reduce human judgment and inhibition, permitting people to do things while intoxicated that they might otherwise avoid.

Most users have a "drug of choice," one whose effects they prefer. Some people are less discriminating and take several drugs; others will take virtually any drug offered to them. The term *cross addiction* refers to people addicted to more than one drug at the same time; it is especially common among adolescent chemical abusers. People also take drugs to counter undesirable effects of other drugs they have taken. Family physicians must suspect multiple ingestion and cross addiction; work-up and treatment must proceed accordingly.

EPIDEMIOLOGY

The statistics on alcoholism are impressive:

- Eighteen million Americans have drinking problems; ten million are alcoholic.
- More than a third of high school seniors report drinking five or more drinks in a row during the previous 2 weeks; 5% drink alcohol daily.
- In 1987, Americans consumed 2.54 gallons of alcohol per person per year. This is the equivalent of 56 gallons of beer, 20 gallons of wine or 6 gallons of distilled spirits; 30% of Americans do not drink alcohol, while 10% account for *half* of the above consumption.
- Alcoholism costs the nation over $104 billion yearly in direct health care costs, industrial accidents, and lost work time.
- Alcohol underlies many of the nation's premature deaths. Cirrhosis alone is the ninth leading cause. As a major contributor to accidents, suicide, and homicide, alcohol is the most common underlying cause of death in the 25-to-45 year age group.
- Alcoholism is the primary disease affecting 30% of psychiatric admissions, 15 to 30% of medical admissions, and up to 80% of burn unit admissions.

The statistics on drug abuse are equally impressive:

- As of 1988, 66 million Americans had used marijuana at least once, 21 million had used cocaine, and 1.9 million had used heroin.
- Between 1985 and 1988, the number of current users of illicit drugs (those using in the past month) fell 37%, from 23 million to 14.5 million users. The number of users continues to decline; however the frequency of use and the quantity of drugs consumed per individual user continue to increase.
- Cocaine-related emergency room visits increased from 9,539 in 1985 to 49,206 in 1989.
- Simultaneous intravenous use of heroin and cocaine ("speedballing") doubled between 1985 and 1988.
- Two million teenagers continue to use illicit drugs.
- As many as 19% of pregnant women use illicit drugs.
- In 1985, there were 81 million benzodiazepine prescriptions written (down from 100 million in 1975) totaling 3.7 billion pills.

Substance abuse is a common, and often overlooked, diagnosis in the physician's office. Approximately 15% of patients seen in the family physician's office are addicted to alcohol or drugs. Since most family physicians diagnose far less than 15% of their patients, it follows that most of these diagnoses are missed. Patient factors such as embarrassment and fear of legal reprisal are a major reason. Physician factors are also at work, *including* denial of addiction problems.

PATIENT EVALUATION

Case 1 (Part 1) Bill Donovan

Bill Donovan is a 42-year-old white salesman. He is married to Maureen, who is a nurse. They have two children, Susan (12) and Patrick (9). Bill has come to the office of Dr. John Porter, his family physician of 10 years, for a physical examination. He last saw Dr. Porter 3 years previously. His complaints today are persistent epigastric pain and difficulty sleeping. The CAGE questionnaire, administered as an office routine, yields a score of 2: Bill gets annoyed when his wife complains about him drinking during the week, and he feels guilty because of missing his children's school activities.

On taking a history, Dr. Porter learns that Bill began drinking in college, where he was a "party animal." After receiving a B.A. in marketing, Bill successfully launched a sales career, earning "salesman of the year" honors three times during his first 5 years. Drinking with customers at lunch or dinner was a part of his job that gradually became a daily event. Drinking on weekends continued to be a part of Bill and Maureen's social life early in their marriage. Bill reports that he could always drink more than others, never had hangovers, and occasionally had blackouts. Over the past 2 years, his daily lunchtime intake has increased to three cocktails, and he reports drinking two beers or glasses of wine with supper. He reports trying marijuana on a couple of occasions in college and that he and Maureen tried cocaine at a party 2 years ago; he does not use either drug now. He has a prescription for Halcion that Dr. Porter wrote at his last visit and has renewed a few times since. Bill states that he smokes 1 1/2 to 2 packs of cigarettes per day, and has smoked for 22 years.

Further questioning reveals that Bill has traveled increasingly for the past 5 years and is often absent from home. He received a "DWI" 3 months ago, and his driver's license is now restricted to business travel; Maureen must do all other driving. She is irritated by Bill's constant traveling and by her increased childcare responsibilities. She worries about Bill's health and has begun to complain when he drinks during the week. Bill says that Maureen's father was an alcoholic who could not hold a job and verbally abused her when she was young. He also says that his children complain when he fails to attend their school activities because he is tired or sick. They seem hurt if he disciplines them and have recently begun to "blow up" after minor arguments with him. Bill also reports that he has recently had a change of bosses. The new one is not pleased with his productivity. Twice, he has had to call in sick on short notice, and his most recent product presentation went poorly. He is worried about losing his job.

Past medical history is significant only for knee surgery in high school and gastritis, for which Dr.

Porter has prescribed ranitidine and antacids. Review of systems is significant for a nonproductive morning cough, a 12-pound weight gain over the past 3 years, decreased exercise tolerance, and difficulty sleeping.

Bill's father died at age 55 of an MI, and his mother died at age 71 of breast cancer. His father was a heavy smoker and had chronic lung disease; his mother drank too much in her later life. His two sisters are in good health, and he has a brother with ulcers, hypertension, and a bad liver.

Case 2 (Part 1) James Blackwell

James Blackwell, a 24-year-old surgeon's assistant in the local hospital, presents to Dr. Porter's office 2 days after an emergency room (ER) visit for chest pain. On the night of the ER visit, James and a friend had been smoking marijuana and crack cocaine, when James experienced dramatic substernal chest pain, radiating to his neck and left shoulder, accompanied by nausea and profuse sweating. James left for the ER immediately, arriving about 10 minutes later, and the pain resolved shortly after his arrival. An ECG showed sinus tachycardia but was otherwise normal. A stat CPK was also normal. The ER physician obtained a urine drug screen, which was reported positive for marijuana and cocaine the next day. He called James with the results and suggested that James make an appointment with Dr. Porter, his family doctor.

James begins the interview by stating his concern that his job could be in jeopardy if his employer finds out about his drug use. He is also concerned that a positive urine drug screen could result in being charged with illicit drug use. Dr. Porter states that he cannot control the urinary drug results at the hospital and that all medical records could be subpoenaed by a court of law. However, he agrees to divulge no information unless it is requested by a court and reassures James that the results of the urine screen done in the hospital are probably not admissible in court, since the sample was not handled by the "chain of custody" standards legal evidence requires and the tests did not use forensic techniques.

Reassured about confidentiality, James relates that his drug use began at age 15, when he and some high school friends started smoking marijuana at parties. This was usually accompanied by alcohol consumption. James began to smoke cigarettes at age 12. He started using cocaine about 2 years ago, when he and friends would "snort" it at parties. Then, James felt able to control his use of cocaine, limiting it to the Fridays and Saturdays following paydays.

About 6 months ago, James tried smoking crack cocaine for the first time and particularly enjoyed the intense high it gave him. He soon found himself unable to limit his use to weekends and started using it

3 or 4 nights per week. James prefers to roll crack in joints of marijuana, referred to as "woolies." He has never used IV drugs, because of fears about AIDS. James tries to avoid using drugs on nights before surgery but has found himself increasingly unable to avoid them. He reports that he is often preoccupied with thoughts about using crack and that he sometimes has dreams from which he bolts awake, sweating and craving cocaine. It is becoming increasingly difficult to wake up in the mornings; so he has begun taking Sudafed before work, in addition to drinking several cups of black coffee. James has missed work a few times, calling in sick on short notice, which has twice provoked arguments with his supervisor. He worries that his OR performance could be influenced by his cocaine use and that he could hurt a patient. He has recently begun to have financial problems because he spends so much money on cocaine.

James is a high school graduate with 2 years of surgical assistant training. He is heterosexual, single, and involved in no serious relationships. He lives with another man who also uses cocaine, and the two of them frequently party with other users. Once easily able to support himself, James has recently resorted to selling cocaine to help support his lifestyle. He and his roommate often entertain women who enjoy using cocaine with them, and casual sex has become a common occurrence. He has had gonorrhea twice in the past 18 months. He has smoked 1 pack of cigarettes daily for 12 years. He continues to drink beer "socially."

Past medical history includes a fractured clavicle at age 14, an appendectomy at age 18, and a diagnosis of "allergic rhinitis" made about 2 years ago, which has been treated unsuccessfully with antihistamines, nasal steroids, and decongestants. While Sudafed helps him wake up in the morning, it does not decrease the rhinorrhea.

Taking the Patient's History

To improve their success at diagnosing substance abuse, particularly in the early stages, physicians must have a high index of suspicion and search for it, particularly in high-probability situations *and* during physical examination visits. High probability situations include acute psychological changes; automobile, industrial, or boating accidents; cases of violence or abuse; and key target organ diseases such as hepatitis, pancreatitis, gastritis, ulcers, GI bleeding, refractory hypertension, and impotence. Table 37.1 presents diagnoses that should prompt the physician to consider substance abuse.

Table 37.1. Common Presenting Signs and Symptoms of Substance Abuse

Organ/System	History	Physician Findings
Vital signs	Dyspnea, rapid pulse, dizziness	Bradycardia, tachycardia; rapid, slow, shallow or labored respirations; shock hypertension, hypotension
Abstinence syndrome	Stopped drinking, disoriented, "not him/herself," shakes	Delirium, encephalopathy, obtundation, tremors, seizures
ENT	Dentition problems, nosebleeds	Caries, cheilosis, glossitis, leukoplakia, oropharyngeal carcinoma, trauma, nasal ulcer, perforated septum
Respiratory	Recurrent pneumonia	Aspiration pneumonias, Gram-neg. pneumonias, hyperventilation, respiratory depression, hemoptysis
Cardiovascular	Palpitations, chest pain	Tachycardia, syncope, labile hypertension, early MI, cardiomyopathy, SBE
Gastrointestinal	Heartburn, abdominal pain, hematemesis, jaundice, melena, hemorrhoids	GI bleeds, recurrent PUD, gastritis, pancreatitis, acute abdomen, cirrhosis, ascites
Genitourinary	Impotence, decreased libido	Testicular atrophy, erectile dysfunction
Dermatologic	Chronic dry skin, infections, bruising	Chronic dermatitis, pressure ulcers, multiple ecchymoses and lacerations, needle "tracks," cellulitis, telangiectasia
Endocrine	Nervousness, fatigue, polyuria	Euthyroid thyrotoxic state (tremor, tachycardia, and diaphoresis +/– weight loss in face of normal thyroid functions); poorly controlled diabetes
Neurologic	Blackouts (i.e., amnestic events), syncope, seizures, belligerent	Syncope, seizures, neuropathies, (especially ocular and radial nerve palsies), acute psychosis
Psychiatric	Sleep disorders, anxiety, depression, hallucinations	Agitation, anxiety, depression, character disorder, overdose, panic, psychosis, suicide attempt
Hematologic/ immunologic	Fatigue, fever	Macrocytic anemias, frequent and opportunistic infections, anergy
Other	Unstable relationships, frequent job changes, arrests (DUIs, drunk and disorderly), spouse/child abuse/neglect	Drownings/near-drownings, auto accident victims, traumatic injuries, poisoning, falls, AIDS, sepsis

A "routine" physical examination is an excellent opportunity to identify clues to the diagnosis. During physical examinations, physicians should routinely ask questions about tobacco, alcohol, and drug use. To be efficient, some physicians ask two questions, as a brief screen. These are "Have you had a problem with alcohol or drugs?" and "When was your last drink?" If the patient answers "yes" to the first, or "yesterday" to the second (Mondays excepted), it is considered a positive result. Another quick and useful screening technique for alcohol abuse is to ask the four CAGE questions (Table 37.2). These may be modified for drug abuse. If a patient responds with a "yes" to two or more of these questions, the screen result is considered positive.

When suspicious problems present or screen results are positive, a more extensive drug and alcohol history must be sought. Several different strategies have been proposed to help elicit an accurate history. Some suggest entering the subject obliquely, by taking the family history first to start the discussion in a less threatening way, and to discover a chemically dependent family, which is characteristic for substance abusers. Others presume that alcohol and/or drugs are being used and start with questions such as "How old were you when you began to drink?" or "What is your favorite brand of beer?" or "When you are drinking, how many beers do you consume?" These questions skip the illusion of nonuse and give the patient the impression that the physician knows what is occurring and will not accept denial.

The history related by an alcoholic may include a straightforward account of his drinking or it may be dramatically minimized. The latter is often the case, in part due to denial of the problem or to shame in relating the truth. While alcoholics have a variety of stories, there are common themes. They frequently began drinking, smoking, and using drugs in their early teens. They fre-

quently describe *tolerance*— the alcoholic relates that he could always "drink more than his friends" and simultaneously show less of its effects. Another is that alcoholics frequently have minimal to *no hangover* after drinking substantial quantities of alcohol. Alcoholics frequently describe *blackouts*, which are periods of time they cannot remember after they begin drinking. During blackouts, the alcoholic is *not* "falling down drunk"; others report them to be awake and functioning. The alcoholic may awaken in a strange place and not remember how he/she got there, or friends may relate occurrences that the alcoholic cannot remember. Blackouts may begin very early in the patient's drinking. Finally, many alcoholics relate a *loss of control*; once they begin to drink, they cannot stop until they are very drunk or all the alcohol has been consumed.

Of the standardized questionnaires to diagnose chemical dependency, the short Michigan alcoholism screening test (SMAST) is the most suitable for the primary care office. Table 37.3 presents the SMAST questions and its interpretation. Adaptations of these alcohol screens are available for drug abuse. An example is the drug abuse screening test (DAST), based on the MAST. McLellan's addictions severity index (ASI) is useful to determine the severity of psychoactive drug abuse.

Objective tests should be administered in the following situations: (*a*) whenever there is a question about alcoholism or drug abuse being present, such as two positive responses to CAGE questions (if the diagnosis is obvious, a screen is unnecessary); and (*b*) as a learning tool to help the patient recognize the problem. In these situations, the physician can present the questionnaire by stating concern about the diagnosis, with a lack of certainty. If the patient is open to taking the test, both patient and physician may learn more about the patient.

Table 37.2. CAGE Screening Questions for Alcoholism (with drug-use adaptations in parentheses)

1. Have you ever tried to *C*ut down your use of alcohol (drugs)?
2. Have people ever *A*nnoyed you by criticizing your drinking (use of drugs)?
3. Have you ever felt *G*uilty about your drinking (use of drugs)?
4. Have you ever used a drink (drugs) as an *E*ye opener in the morning to get going?

Physical Examination

Physical examination of the substance abuser can be completely normal. Table 37.1 lists physical findings that go along with diagnoses, by organ system. A few important clues are bizarre behavior, alcohol on the patient's breath, needle tracks or numerous small ecchymoses, hepatomegaly, ascites, testicular atrophy, numerous telangiectasia, and pronounced hemorrhoids. If any of these are found in the absence of an alcohol or drug

Table 37.3. Short Michigan Alcoholism Screening Test (SMAST)[a]

1. Do you feel you are a normal drinker? (By normal we mean you drink less than or as much as most other people.) (No)[b]
2. Does your wife, husband, parent, or other near relative ever worry or complain about your drinking? (Yes)
3. Do you ever feel guilty about your drinking? (Yes)
4. Do friends or relatives think you are a normal drinker? (No)
5. Are you able to stop drinking when you want to? (No)
6. Have you ever attended a meeting of Alcoholics Anonymous? (Yes)
7. Has drinking ever created problems between you and your wife, husband, a parent, or other near relative? (Yes)
8. Have you ever gotten into trouble at work because of drinking? (Yes)
9. Have you ever neglected your obligations, your family, or your work for two or more days in a row because you are drinking? (Yes)
10. Have you ever gone to anyone for help about your drinking? (Yes)
11. Have you ever been in a hospital because of drinking? (Yes)
12. Have you ever been arrested for drunken driving, driving while intoxicated, or driving under the influence of alcoholic beverages? (Yes)
13. Have you ever been arrested, even for a few hours, because of other drunken behavior? (Yes)

[a]From Pokorny AD, Miller BA, Kaplan HB: The brief MAST: a shortened version of the Michigan alcoholism screening test. *Am J Psychiatry* 129:342–349, 1972. Copyright 1972, the American Psychiatric Association. Reprinted by permission.
[b]Positive responses are noted in parentheses. Subjects scoring 0–1 positive responses should be considered nonalcoholics; 2 points indicates possible alcoholics; and those with 3 or more points are labeled alcoholics. Individual positive responses to questions 6, 10, or 11 should be considered highly suggestive of alcoholism.

history, the physician should pursue the subject vigorously.

Laboratory Tests

Certain laboratory abnormalities should place alcoholism in the differential diagnosis. These include elevated liver enzyme levels (with SGOT typically higher than SGPT), an unexplained elevated uric acid, elevated serum triglycerides with a normal or depressed serum cholesterol, an elevated serum amylase, and elevated mean corpuscular volume (MCV). The pattern of an elevated GGT (γ-glutamyl transferase) and elevated MCV is highly suggestive of alcoholism. However, alcoholics may have completely normal laboratory tests.

A blood alcohol concentration (BAC) is often helpful in diagnosing a patient. If an adult has a blood alcohol level in excess of 0.1 mg/dl, it is illegal to operate a motor vehicle in most states; a conviction of driving while intoxicated (DWI) suggests abuse of alcohol by the driver. Levels of 0.2 mg/dl should make nonalcoholics appear very inebriated; levels in excess of 0.3 mg/dl are dangerous to the non-alcohol-dependent patient. If an elevated blood alcohol level is obtained, but the patient does not seem as severely impaired as expected (e.g., tolerant employees may perform jobs with a blood alcohol of 0.18 mg/dl and not seem drunk), it strongly suggests alcoholism. A prudent physician should suspect alcoholism in a

patient with a blood alcohol concentration above 0.20 mg/dl.

The law enforcement system has developed the "breathalyzer" as a quick, portable field test. Many emergency departments and alcohol treatment facilities also use breathalyzers. Salivary alcohol test strips can yield quantitative results in seconds.

The laboratory may also be helpful in diagnosing drug abuse. The most widely used test is the urine drug screen on specimens that have been collected under direct observation. Urine screens detect most of the prescription and illicit drugs that patients have taken recently, even in small quantities. Specific blood levels are also available for many of the drugs of abuse. Elevated creatine phosphokinase (CPK) and lactate dehydrogenase (LDH) levels may suggest cocaine use, which elevates skeletal muscle enzymes secondary to rhabdomyolysis, cardiac enzymes from coronary spasm, and pulmonary enzymes from pulmonic vasospasm.

Case 1 (Part 2) Bill Donovan

Positive findings on physical examination include a blood pressure of 160/100, mild obesity, a ruddy complexion, and bibasilar, end-expiratory wheezes in his lungs. His liver edge is palpable just below the costal margin. Laboratory tests ordered in advance of the physical examination included the following abnormalities: a hematocrit of 54%, an MCV of 101, an SGOT of 70 μg/dl, an SGPT of 40 μg/dl, a total cholesterol level of 210 mg/dl, and triglycerides of 280 mg/dl. Office spirometry reveals an FEV1 of 68%.

Case 2 (Part 2) James Blackwell

Physical examination reveals a generally well appearing young black man. His pulse is 70, respirations 14, temperature 37.1, and blood pressure 120/70. Skin examination reveals mild facial acne; no needle tracks were seen. Slight nasal mucosal erythema with clear discharge is noted. Cardiac rate and rhythm are normal; there are no murmurs. The abdominal and neurological examinations are normal.

MAKING THE DIAGNOSIS

When is a patient an alcoholic or a drug addict? No simple answer to the question exists. In general, the disease is likely when alcohol and/or drug use is associated with deterioration in one or more major areas of a patient's life, such as family, health, and/or occupation. Remember that substance abuse is a *clinical* diagnosis, and while objective evidence may be sought, abnormal test results are not prerequisite. Many times the physician and patient agree that a problem is present.

Sometimes, the diagnosis is obvious, such as cirrhosis in the face of years of drinking alcohol; sometimes the patient is in jail, has AIDS, or has otherwise severely disrupted her or his life. The physician must strive to make the diagnosis before these late-stage problems are present. Early recognition is one of the most important keys to successful outcomes in substance abuse treatment. Keep in mind the axiom that common diseases occur commonly. Alcohol and drug abuse should be included in the differential diagnosis of many medical complaints. Table 37.1 lists presenting symptoms and signs that should prompt the physician to consider substance abuse as a possible diagnosis. Chemical dependency is also a diagnosis made over time. Since it is a chronic disease, the physician (and the patient) can see the illness unfold gradually. Indeed, pointing out adverse consequences over time is a tool that can help patients recognize the problem.

Clinicians often refer to the guidelines in DSM IIIR to make diagnoses, particularly when they are working with third-party payers. These guidelines are broadly inclusive of substance abuse symptoms, signs, and laboratory abnormalities, yet provide specific guidelines for making each diagnosis. They include categories for abuse and dependence of both alcohol and drugs.

Barriers to Diagnosis

There are real obstacles to recognizing and diagnosing alcoholism and drug abuse. If alcoholism alone occurs in one out of three families, it is reasonable to assume that a significant number of physicians have had previous experience in their personal or family lives, which may bias their view of its causes and amenability to treatment. Alcoholism and drug abuse carry stronger social stigmas than other diseases; stigma discourages the patient from seeking help and the physician from confronting and treating the disease.

Medical education seems partially responsible for negative attitudes about alcoholism and drug addiction among health professionals. A progressive decline has been demonstrated in medical student attitudes toward alcoholism as students progress from their preclinical to clinical to internship years. Students who see hospitalized patients in later, more refractory stages of their disease develop negative attitudes toward alcoholics and drug addicts, particularly when poor role modeling by their teachers exists.

Another major obstacle to the recognition of substance abuse is its frequent presentation as a mood disturbance. Alcoholics and addicts often present with symptoms of major psychiatric disorders. At these times, the psychiatric disturbances may be very apparent and may mask the underlying alcohol or drug problem. Up to 80% of patients admitted to alcoholism treatment facilities carry major psychiatric diagnoses in addition to alcoholism. Yet, this same population has only a 3 to 5% incidence of psychiatric disorders following 1 year of sobriety. Thus, a significant number of psychiatric disorders are secondary manifestations of underlying alcoholism and/or drug addiction. In fact, it is so difficult to be certain of a psychiatric diagnosis in the chemically dependent patient that patients should be free of alcohol and other mood-altering substances for 6 to 12 months before a chronic psychiatric diagnosis can be made with absolute confidence.

Patients with a true "dual diagnosis," defined as a substance abuse problem *and* a psychiatric disorder, are therefore difficult to diagnose and treat. They present the dilemma of choosing to recommend abstinence from all mind-altering substances, to see what psychiatric picture emerges over time, versus treating a patient's symptoms and behaviors with psychoactive drugs in an attempt to alleviate psychiatric pain and patient/family discomfort. The former tactic risks withholding medication that could potentially alleviate 12 months of patient distress; the latter eliminates the possibility of determining a patient's true psychiatric state without the influence of psychoactive drugs. The authors prefer the first treatment plan when possible, because the vast majority of patients presenting the diagnostic dilemma do not have an underlying psychiatric disorder.

TREATMENT

Conveying the Diagnosis

A big problem with the diagnosis of substance abuse is denial—on the part of the patient, their families, and the medical profession. Once a problem with substance abuse or dependence is diagnosed, the physician is obliged to inform the patient of the diagnosis and try to negotiate some form of treatment. Failure to inform the patient perpetuates denial of the disease and guarantees a continuation of the patient's and family's physical, psychological, and/or social deterioration. In addition, repetition of the diagnosis seems to have an additive effect on acceptance by the patient; many are not convinced in the beginning and accept the diagnosis and subsequent treatment only after hearing their diagnosis several times.

Research indicates that up to 5% of patients will stop abusive use of alcohol or drugs simply because a physician tells them that they have a problem. Although 5% is not large, this approach costs very little and is a worthwhile, initial intervention.

Approach to Management

To effectively treat alcoholics and drug addicts, physicians should have the perspective they are dealing with a lifelong, chronic disease. As with other chronic diseases (e.g., diabetes), the emphasis should be on maintaining optimal function over time, preventing complications, and encouraging self-responsibility in the patient. Crisis management is inevitable at times, but the real strength of therapy is in helping the patient learn, and adhere to, a lifelong treatment program. If the chronicity of chemical dependency is recognized, the intricacies of its symptoms and manifestations learned, and physicians elect to treat it in an unbiased, supportive manner, they will have rewarding patient experiences and a major impact on the overall disease process.

Denial should be expected from the patient. What is apparent to the physician, and often to the family as well, may be vehemently rejected by the patient. Again, the physician's attitude must be one of facilitating change over time rather than expecting an immediate and permanent cure. Attempt to establish a working relationship with the patient and provide anticipatory and predictive counseling, just as should be made with other chronic conditions. Over time, opportunities for helping the patient will arise. Sometimes a life crisis, like losing a job or an arrest for driving while intoxicated, is the final incentive for a properly prepared patient to accept the disease and enter treatment.

Working with the Families of Substance Abusers

Families of alcoholics and addicts are also victims of the disease. Family systems theory suggests that families seek a functional equilibrium. Sometimes instability caused by drinking or using drugs leads to ejection of the substance abuser by desertion or divorce. More often, other family members capitulate to the disease and adjust their lifestyles to allow the alcoholic to drink yet remain in the family. Such adaptations are called "enabling behavior." Enabling can be very destructive to the self-esteem of spouses and children, who feel they must clean up the house, cover social blunders, lie to employers, or endure verbal and/or physical abuse. However, enablers generally benefit secondarily from their behavior; so it is often difficult for them to change. Commonly, an enabler leaves one alcoholic relationship only to become involved in another one. Many enabling spouses have grown up in alcoholic families, and being married to an alcoholic fulfills their perception of married life.

Enabling behavior sometimes becomes ingrained in family members to the extent that they deny their own basic needs. This is called "codependency" and is usually the result of prolonged exposure to an alcoholic or an addict. The codependent receives such secondary gain from the addict's dependent relationship on them that they are said to be "dependent" on the addict's relational dependency. Codependent family members require their own treatment to gain insight into their problem and learn ways to change. Frequently, marriages fail once an addict gains sobriety. Unfortunately, this is true even when the codependent spouse gets help with his/her codependency.

Frequently, both people in a relationship are substance abusers. In these situations, both people contribute to the dynamics that keep the drug and alcohol use going. Communications are generally flawed, and to resolve things, both members must deal with their codependency issues as well as their own addiction problems.

The impact of a substance-abusing member on his/her family can be enormous. Most cases of violence, sexual abuse, and physical abuse involve one or more substance abusers. Financial difficulties are precipitated by the cost of drugs, loss of employment, and damage to property. Legal problems arise out of illicit use, selling illicit drugs, stealing to obtain funds, driving under the influence of alcohol, and lawsuits for property damage, divorce, child custody, or support payments. Shame is often felt by family members because of their alcoholic/addicted members.

A recently described group of substance-abuse victims is the Adult Children of Addiction (ACOAs), who share some similar characteristics. These individuals have been raised with one or both parents being addicted. They frequently describe their childhood experience as one of chaos, having little predictability, feeling a lack of personal safety, an absence of important nurturing figures, and shame at perceived social ostracism of their family. They often report parents as being extremely critical, giving inconsistent messages, and providing no reliable structure to family life. Sometimes the opposite occurs; parents cling, and families become extremely enmeshed. ACOAs frequently have low self-esteem, anhedonia, difficulty accepting positive feedback from others, and feelings of guilt and responsibility for everything that goes wrong. They seem drawn to conflict, and many go into the helping careers. Many ACOAs report themselves to be very critical of themselves and others, controlling of others, to find difficulty with intimacy, and having an inordinate fear of failure.

The syndrome known as fetal alcohol syndrome (FAS) has been described for over a decade. Once called "funny-looking kids," these children manifest craniofacial and cognitive changes that are the result of intrauterine exposure to alcohol. A new chapter in maternal use of drugs and fetal effects is being written in the 90s by the abuse of crack cocaine among pregnant women. Cocaine causes premature uterine contractions and placental separation and may be one of the leading causes of premature birth in certain segments of the pop-

ulation. It also has effects on intrauterine development of the CNS that are just beginning to be understood.

In cases of substance abuse in pregnancy, physicians must bear in mind that they are dealing not just with the abuser, but also with her unprotected child. Programs are available that work aggressively with substance-abusing mothers; these are often in addition to programs for nonpregnant patients. While state laws vary, physicians many times have legal options, such as commitment of the mother to a hospital or inpatient drug rehabilitation center for the duration of her pregnancy. Community agencies are frequently able to help find resources and programs to which these patients may be admitted.

Case 1 (Part 3) Bill Donovan

After the history and physical examination, Mr. Donovan's problem list includes (a) alcohol abuse with possible dependence; (b) hepatitis, probably secondary to alcohol abuse, r/o infectious; (c) hypertension, possibly secondary to alcohol abuse; (d) chronic epigastric pain, probably secondary to alcohol abuse; (e) chronic obstructive pulmonary disease (COPD); (f) possible hyperlipoproteinemia, type IV; (g) family problems secondary to alcohol abuse; and (h) anxiety about job. Dr. Porter informs Bill that he is concerned about his drinking and explains that several of the diagnosed problems are probably secondary to his excessive use of alcohol. He suggests that Bill be admitted to the hospital for detoxification and subsequent referral to an intensive outpatient chemical-dependency treatment program.

Bill confides that he had been worried that his drinking was out of hand, but feels he can quit on his own. Dr. Porter asks that both Bill and Maureen return the next day for a joint counseling session, during which he solicits Maureen's view of the problem. They contracted that Bill will drink only two beers per day and that Maureen will keep a drinking calendar. Over the next 3 weeks, Bill is unable to drink less than 6 drinks per day, experiences severe restlessness, and agrees to enter the hospital for detoxification. There, with continued support from Dr. Porter, Bill is successfully detoxified in 4 days and agrees to enroll in an intensive outpatient substance-abuse treatment program.

Case 2 (Part 3) James Blackwell

Mr. Blackwell's problem list includes (a) cocaine abuse with possible dependency; (b) coronary artery spasm, secondary to cocaine abuse; (c) rhinitis, probably secondary to cocaine abuse; (d) high risk sexual behavior, with recurrent gonorrhea; and (e) nicotine abuse. Dr. Porter informs James that his chest pain was probably secondary to coronary artery spasm from smoking crack cocaine and that continued use of cocaine could lead to a heart attack. While noting the remote possibility that James could have early onset coronary artery disease, Dr. Porter emphasizes that he is far more concerned about the use of cocaine. He points out that cocaine is highly addictive and that it has already been accompanied by negative life consequences: legal risk, poor performance on the job, and financial and STD problems. Dr. Porter suggests that James seek treatment for his cocaine addiction, starting with the Employee Assistance Program (EAP) at the hospital. He also suggests an exercise tolerance test (ETT) to rule out coronary artery disease and an HIV test to screen for the AIDs virus, and he discusses "safe sex" practices.

James agrees to the ETT and HIV testing, says that he will practice safer sex, and promises to "think about" treatment for his drug problem. Two days later, the EAP contacts him directly because of the positive drug screen result from the ER, and James agrees to stop using cocaine. The EAP runs an unannounced urine drug screen 2 weeks later, which is positive again for both cocaine and marijuana. James is told that he will be fired unless he agrees to inpatient treatment for chemical dependency and a follow-up program of random urine testing. James agrees to enter an inpatient treatment program.

Choosing a Treatment Modality

In the United States, options for treatment of substance abuse depend on the drugs used and on the patient's pattern, quantity and frequency of use, social situation, and ability to pay. Inpatient programs that begin with detoxification and progress to educational sessions about chemical dependency; group, family, and individual counseling; and assistance with beginning an outpatient program boast a 50 to 70% success rate, defined as consistent sobriety for 1 year after discharge. Intensive outpatient programs demonstrate similar rates of success.

Intensive involvement in Alcoholics Anonymous (AA), if maintained, will achieve a similar success rate. Narcotics Anonymous (NA) has not been as successful as AA, possibly because it is more difficult to motivate people to stay involved. In choosing a treatment plan for a patient, the family physician may seek help from a social worker or a mental health professional with knowledge of community resources.

Prior to beginning the treatment process, any acute medical or psychiatric problems must be treated. Chronic medical and psychiatric sequelae of chemical use must be noted, and plans made for their eventual care. The overall goal is generally to deal first with the addiction problems, observe what psychological state emerges when the chemical effects wear off, and work hard to maintain sobriety.

Social support is important for successful recovery. Patients are unlikely to recover if they live, work, and/or socialize in settings that revolve around drinking or drug use. Often, some change must be made to increase the likelihood of success. Returning a teenager to the streets or to a social circle of drug-using companions is not likely to result in successful recovery. Similarly, a married couple with a long history of alcoholism will need strong group support; without it, there is a high probability of recidivism.

Some patients, especially if they are in the early phases of addiction, are unconvinced that their substance use is problematic. For these patients, a "brief intervention" may be a helpful second step. This involves contracting with the patient to cut down or discontinue use of alcohol and drugs (to see if it can be done with ease), keeping a calendar and recording the circumstances surrounding any consumption of the substance they are trying to discontinue. With the patient's consent, it is best to solicit help from a family member with this approach. In many cases, patients are surprised to find that they cannot control their use and develop unpleasant withdrawal effects, adding further credence to the diagnosis of dependency.

Occasionally, discontinuation is done with ease, and dependency is not the diagnosis; however, even these patients many times find that they function better with reduced intake or abstinence.

Once a patient accepts that she or he has a problem with alcohol and/or drugs and is willing to undergo treatment, a plan must be developed. Patients with mild disease (short duration of use, absence of physical sequelae), a stable home environment, supportive family and friends, financial means, and a desire to stop may be referred directly to outpatient treatment. Available resources for such a program may include counselors or therapists who deal with addictions; community recovery groups, usually run by substance-abuse therapists, which meet to help members quit drinking and/or using drugs; and lay support organizations such as Alcoholics Anonymous (AA) and Narcotics Anonymous (NA). Many patients are unlikely to successfully overcome their substance abuse without very intensive treatment, either as inpatients or outpatients. Figure 37.1 provides an

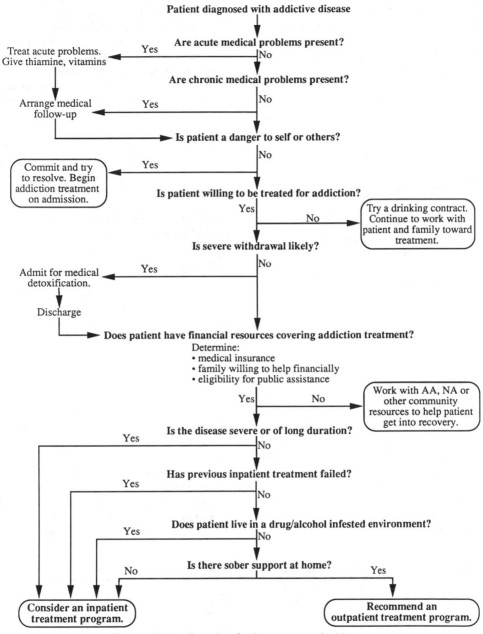

Figure 37.1. Flow chart for the treatment of addiction.

algorithm that can help make initial therapeutic decisions about a patient.

Detoxification and Medical Stabilization

If the quantity of drug being consumed or the duration of its use is such that its discontinuation puts the patient at risk of seizures, delirium tremens, or other serious withdrawal symptoms, the patient should be admitted to a facility for a standard regimen of medical detoxification. For alcohol, there are many "detox" protocols utilizing sedative drugs such as phenobarbital or benzodiazepines. For narcotics, most physicians use methadone and/or clonidine. Detoxification medications are tapered over sufficient time to avoid unpleasant withdrawal symptoms and serious medical sequelae caused by discontinuation of the drugs.

Many patients have altered metabolism or do not eat sufficient nutrients while they are on a drug binge. Consequently, they are at risk for development of vitamin and mineral deficiency syndromes like Wernicke's encephalopathy. For this reason, initial management of severe drug dependency must include the early administration of sufficient vitamins and nutrients, including thiamine and magnesium, to replenish patient stores and avoid these syndromes.

Treatment of the Chemical Dependency

After detoxification and treatment of medical problems, treatment of chemical dependency begins. Change in attitudes and behaviors is the goal of such treatment. Patients must learn what triggers their substance use and develop alternative ways to cope with these stimuli. They need insight into living and working situations, patterns of interpersonal relationships and lifestyles, which may need to be altered to reduce the propensity to use chemicals. Family involvement is crucial; all programs teach family members about addiction, seeking to heal past wounds and involve them in learning techniques for "relapse prevention." Role playing, for example, can help teach relapse prevention (e.g., a patient can rehearse going out to dinner without ordering a drink). These concepts may be learned in either an inpatient or an outpatient setting.

For many years, most addiction treatment in the United States has been based upon the precepts established in the 1930s by Alcoholics Anonymous (AA). The "12-step program," named for the steps to recovery developed by AA (Table 37.4), has been adapted for patients chemically dependent on any substance (e.g., opioids, cocaine, prescription drugs). While several 12-step organizations exist, AA and Narcotics Anonymous (NA) are the largest and are available in most locations in the United States. AA tends to deal with alcohol addiction; NA deals with addiction to all other drugs, whether they are prescription or illicit. However, there is a big overlap between the membership of these organizations because many addicts abuse multiple chemicals and because some people who are addicted to one substance find the meetings of another group more to their liking. On average, NA members are younger than AA members; so many younger alcoholics attend NA meetings because the membership is more contemporary.

Al-Anon and Nar-Anon are 12-step programs for the families of alcoholics and drug abusers. Their focus is on educating members about chemical dependency and living with dependent people. Coping strategies, suggestions for changing enabling behaviors, and general support are available in these groups.

Economic Issues

Payment for addiction treatment in the United States is a perplexing problem. The 1980s saw the evolution of many inpatient treatment programs that were initially supported by the public and private health insurance. However, since about 1988, third-party payers have been less willing to pay for inpatient treatment. They claim that the hotel costs (food, housing, etc.) are too expensive. This change in reimbursement has led to the develop-

Table 37.4. Original Twelve Steps of Alcoholics Anonymous

1. We admitted we are powerless over alcohol—that our lives had become unmanageable.
2. We came to believe that a Power greater than ourselves could restore us to sanity.
3. We made a decision to turn our will and our lives over to the care of God.
4. We made a searching and fearless moral inventory of ourselves.
5. We admitted to God, to ourselves, and to another human being the exact nature of our wrongs.
6. We were entirely ready to have God remove all these defects of character.
7. We humbly asked Him to remove our shortcomings.
8. We made a list of all persons we had harmed, and became willing to make amends to them all.
9. We made direct amends to such people wherever possible, except when to do so would injure them or others.
10. We continued to take personal inventory and when we were wrong, promptly admitted it.
11. We sought through prayer and meditation to improve our conscious contact with God, praying only for knowledge of His will for us and the power to carry that out.
12. Having had a spiritual awakening as the result of these steps, we tried to carry this message to alcoholics, and to practice these principles in all our affairs.

ment of "intensive outpatient" programs, most of which continue to encourage 12-step participation. Many outpatient programs work closely with employee assistance programs (EAPs) to keep people working during the day and use the evening hours for treatment activities.

Another economic problem is treatment of substance abuse among uninsured and underinsured populations. Because substance abuse often leads to a decline in the socioeconomic status of an addict, many of its victims have lost the ability to pay as a direct result of the disease. This pushes the cost of treating these patients into the public sector. Finding funds to treat a patient is frequently a red-tape nightmare.

Medications as Adjuncts to Treatment

The use of medications for the treatment of chemical dependency is controversial. A key dynamic that most recovering addicts must *unlearn* is their tendency to respond to problems with alcohol or drugs. Nevertheless, some medications have been used for the treatment of addictions. Disulfiram (Antabuse) is a drug that causes protracted nausea and vomiting if patients consume alcohol when they have Antabuse in their system. Antabuse may deter impulsive drinking in patients who can manage to take the medication before the temptation to drink overcomes their resolve. However, this treatment is easily defeated by discontinuing Antabuse, and patients can blunt its effect by taking large doses of vitamin C and diphenhydramine (Benadryl). More importantly, patients may concentrate on their pills instead of their underlying chemical dependency; so Antabuse may actually retard the development of self-reliance in abstaining from alcohol.

Many alcoholic patients manifest clinical signs of depression when they get into treatment. These signs are often related to guilt or remorse because of the negative life events that motivated their getting into treatment and not manifestations of chronic endogenous depression. Antidepressants may lift the mood of patients and help with initial treatment. However, "mood-altering" drugs are the very ones that predispose to relapse, and the controversy over whether to prescribe them continues to rage. AA generally advises members against taking *any* mood-altering substances. However, many physicians feel antidepressants are a successful adjunct to treatment.

Methadone hydrochloride is a synthetic narcotic that does not cause the euphoria of heroin, morphine, and other opiates. Many patients who cannot withdraw themselves from opiates enter treatment programs that dispense methadone daily. Incentives to stay in such a program can include (*a*) functioning at a job, (*b*) avoiding withdrawal symptoms, and (*c*) avoiding the expense, criminal behavior, and danger inherent in the street life of drug users. Most programs dispense a daily dose of methadone that is sufficient to extinguish a patient's craving for narcotics. They then maintain that dose, or less commonly, attempt to gradually withdraw the drug. Programs require abstinence from other drugs of abuse to participate and periodically test patient urine samples for drugs.

AFTERCARE

Successful long-term treatment requires constant reminders of chronicity and vigilance against relapse. Although some patients are successful on their own at discontinuing drugs and alcohol, most need support. This may come from close spousal relationships, one-on-one counseling, therapy groups, church groups, or friends. No potentially successful source of patient support should be overlooked. Alcoholics Anonymous, Narcotics Anonymous, Al-Anon, and Nar-Anon are widely available for the patient and family trying to maintain long-term sobriety. "Ideal" 12-step program recommendations generally include 90 AA meetings in 90 days and three to four Al-Anon meetings per week for the alcoholic and the family, respectively. A program of random urine or saliva testing for drugs and/or alcohol can help some patients, especially if failure to stay drug-free leads to loss of a professional license (e.g., recovering physicians or nurses).

There is a need for close, regular physician follow-up, regardless of the support system(s) chosen. Weekly office visits (at a minimum) should be scheduled initially, to monitor progress in physical and emotional recovery. Physicians treating alcoholic patients should avoid prescribing medications that are known to have central nervous system effects and that may precipitate the resumption of drug and/or alcohol use by recovering patients. These medications include narcotic analgesics, tranquilizers, sedative hypnotics, elixirs containing alcohol, antihistamines, cough suppressants and antidiarrheal agents. It is important to know alternative methods or preparations for treating common problems (e.g., ibuprofen or in-domethacin for pain, terfenadine or astemazole for allergy) and to be certain to properly withdraw patients if a potentially addicting drug cannot be avoided (e.g., narcotic use followed by clonidine taper for severe postoperative pain).

Relapses are common among substance abusers. If a patient has relapsed, the physician should recognize this as the natural history of the disease, realize that the family is probably severely stressed, and offer support. Family physicians can proceed by discussing the precipitants of relapse with the patient, offering any necessary detoxification, and encouraging resumption of support activities like AA meetings. If the patient is not motivated to discontinue use of substances, the physician should seek to provide support for the family.

SUGGESTED READINGS

Fleming MF, Barry KL (eds): *Addictive Disorders*. St. Louis, Mosby–Year Book, 1992.

An excellent, quick reference text on all aspects of alcohol and drug abuse.

Johnson VE: *I'll Quit Tomorrow*, New York, Harper & Row, 1980.

An excellent review of the alcoholism disease process with practical approaches to specific problems. It is "must" reading for anyone seeking more information about alcoholism intervention.

Mooney AJ: Alcohol abuse and dependence. In Taylor RB (ed): *Family Medicine: Principles and Practice*, ed 2. New York, Springer-Verlag, 1983, pp 1632–1650.

A good resource for the basic disease process, effects on the family, approach to alcoholism, etc.

chapter 38

SOMATIZING PATIENTS

William A. Hensel and William R. Marshall

Patients with emotional problems frequently come to a family physician with physical symptoms rather than emotional complaints. In our current culture, physical symptoms are perceived as less demeaning than complaints of an admittedly emotional nature. For somatizing patients, physical symptoms are often the "ticket for admission" to the medical care system. Because family physicians are usually the physicians of first contact, they often provide most of the treatment, whether counseling or psychotropic medication, for people with emotional problems who seek medical attention. To provide proper care, the physician must look beyond the presenting physical symptoms and search for the patient's actual reason for coming (ARC) to the office. Often, patients are unaware that emotions are at the basis of their symptoms; they only know that they do not feel well and express this feeling in terms they understand. Only when the underlying problems are identified and appreciated, can the physician begin to help the patient feel better.

Many physicians have difficulty getting beyond the patient's presenting symptom(s). No laboratory test proves conclusively that physical disease is absent or that somatization exists. As a consequence, physician anxiety about potentially hidden organic pathology often fuels a futile search for an underlying physical ailment while the patient's ARC remains undiscovered. In fact, the stronger the physician's focus on the somatic complaints, the more convinced the patient may be that an undiagnosed ominous illness is the cause. A vicious cycle is established in which the patient complains bitterly of a variety of unrelieved symptoms while the physician futilely explores more improbable obscure diagnoses to explain the nonspecific symptoms. This scenario leads to both the patient's discontent, distrust, and disbelief in the medical profession and the physician's frustration and efforts to discharge or minimize contacts with the patient.

An alternative exists to this unfortunate sequence of events. The correct diagnostic approach to a somatizing patient is not only ruling out organic disease. Rather, the physician must bring up and begin to address emotional issues early in the evaluation. Only by understanding the patient's psychosocial stressors and unmet emotional needs will the physician know the patient well enough to make an accurate diagnosis based on these underlying factors. Thus, the puzzle of the patient's multiple complaints can be solved, and appropriate intervention strategies implemented.

In this way, somatizing patients can be cared for successfully, with both the patient and physician being satisfied with the relationship.

ASSESSING THE SOMATIZING PATIENT

You will often first suspect somatization when someone presents with multiple complaints but no significant changes in functional level. For example, the patient with horrible, intractable abdominal pain, nausea, and/or diarrhea who loses no weight over time. At other times, a single complaint that seems appropriate and reasonable on the first visit will be replaced by others on subsequent visits, and only after many visits does the pattern of multiple shifting complaints become obvious. Other clues that suggest somatizing are a depressed feeling when you enter the examination room (particularly if you have known the patient for a while), feelings of frustration at being unable to make the patient better, and (often) the patient's willingness to continue multiple diagnostic and therapeutic trials without questioning their cost or value. Other clues that should raise a suspicion of a somatizing disorder are listed in Table 38.1.

The approach to patients with multiple complaints is complicated by the broad range of symptoms that can suggest both organic and somatized problems. The physician should carry out whatever workup is necessary to be convinced that the patient's complaints do not indicate serious organic disease. Tests should be ordered only as required by ordinary reasonable standards of medical practice. Such appropriate tests will reassure the physician and may even reassure the patient. Ordering multiple tests or procedures only to "prove" to the patient that organic disease is absent is discouraged, since extensive testing usually does not reassure the patient and contributes to the vicious cycle described above. A simple screening test or consultation is helpful in reassuring the patient about a specific fear such as "anemia," "mono," or "arthritis." The presence of organic disease does not, of course, rule out somatized disorders and vice versa. Chronic health problems become more bothersome during times of stress, isolation, or depression. A patient's physical and emotional health are inextricably intertwined. Physicians must care for the whole patient in order to give optimum treatment.

Table 38.1. Clues to Suspecting Somatizing Patients[a]

Multiple vague complaints involving several different organ systems
Shifting complaints, usually GI or musculoskeletal
Incongruities between symptom severity and lack of indicators of chronic ill health
Demands for tests and drugs
Unrelieved anxiety when the diagnosis and treatment plan are suggested
History of numerous workups with insignificant findings
Polypharmacy/polyphysicians
Stubborn conviction that there are external sources for problems, e.g., diseases, toxic substances
Unwillingness to discuss life aside from medical complaints
Poor interpersonal relationships
Demanding yet disparaging of physician
Hostile/provocative or dependent/clinging attitude
Dwells on or seems proud of suffering
Mood disturbances
Multiple drug allergies

[a]Modified from Marshall WR: Chronic somatizers. In Rogers CS, McCue JD, Gal P (eds): *Managing Chronic Disease.* Oradell, NJ, Medical Economic Books, 1987, p 366.

Patients who present with multiple somatic complaints actually represent a divergent group of disorders. Differentiating between these disorders is based on the wide variety of psychosocial stressors and emotional needs that patients express through somatic complaints. Key questions to ask yourself that will help in understanding and specifically diagnosing these patients are:

1. Is this an acute problem in a previously healthy patient or do the expressed problems fit into a long-standing pattern of somatic concerns?
2. Is there any recent reason for unusual bodily preoccupation such as recent illness in a family member or friend?
3. What psychological stress factors exist? Are those factors acute or chronic?
4. What benefits (secondary gains) does a patient get from being sick? These benefits may vary widely from increased attention from loved ones to disability payments and the excuse to quit working.
5. Are there reasons to suspect deeper psychological problems? Is the patient's affect depressed? Is the patient's thought process appropriate?

Once these questions are answered, the diagnosis and treatment of these patients can be approached with some intellectual precision. The disorders will generally fit into one of the categories listed in Table 38.2.

Syndromes Representing Minimal Psychopathology

Any person is subject to transient somatic concerns. These may be appropriate age-related concerns or exaggerated concerns triggered by an external stressor. For example, a change in bowel habits would not concern a 20-year-old but may cause worries about cancer in a 65-year-old. Also, a 45-year-old man may rush to his physician for concerns about heart disease immediately after a business associate suffers a heart attack. These concerns are understandable and not considered to represent psychopathology. The third edition of the *Diagnostic and Statistical Manual* (DSM-III) recognizes a category of diseases labeled "psychological factors affecting physical conditions," which also does not imply significant psychopathology.

Table 38.2. Diagnostic Groupings and Treatment Approaches for Patients with Functional Somatic Complaints[a]

Diagnosis	Treatment
Syndromes of minimal psychopathology Includes psychological factors affecting physical conditions	Appropriate but not excessive evaluation and treatment of the organic pathology; thorough understanding of patient's environmental stress factors; education and reassurance usually effective; lifestyle readjustment strategies occasionally needed.
Somatiform disorders Somatization and hypochondriasis	Caring, steady, long-standing relationship with primary care physician; minimize evaluations and medications; focus attention away from symptoms
Conversion reaction Psychogenic pain	Referral to psychologist or psychiatrist Minimize evaluation and pain medication; referral for psychological evaluation and treatment
Masked psychiatric disorders Depression and schizophrenia	Treatment of the underlying problem using appropriate medication and/or psychotherapy; referral to a psychiatrist or a psychologist may be appropriate
Factitious disorders and malingering	No known treatment; confrontation is appropriate; avoid unnecessary workups, procedures, and medications

[a]Modified from Marshall WR: Chronic somatizers. In Rogers CS, McCue JD, Gal P (eds). *Managing Chronic Disease.* Oradell, NJ, Medical Economic Books, 1987, p 367.

Psychological Factors Affecting Physical Condition

Although psychosocial factors play a role in most organic diseases, these disorders have both strong organic and emotional components: hypertension, muscle contraction and migraine headaches, irritable bowel syndrome, asthma, inflammatory bowel diseases, fibrositis, and peptic ulcer disease. To date, attempts to demonstrate that stress or emotions somehow "cause" these diseases and illnesses have been inconclusive.

These disorders are best considered as parallel medical and psychological problems. Peptic ulcer disease, for example, requires medical attention such as change in diet, H2-blockers, and avoidance of gastric irritants. Optimal treatment also requires an understanding of exacerbating (or perhaps causative) emotional stressors that accompany the illness.

SOMATIFORM DISORDERS

The somatiform disorders represent a distinct diagnostic category in DSM-III classification. Although each disorder in this group can range from mild to severe, these disorders represent an abnormal expression of psychic stress through somatic concerns.

Somatization

Patients with this disorder tend to have a lifelong preoccupation with bodily function and physical illness. The DSM-III criteria for this diagnosis are (*a*) vague physical symptoms beginning prior to age 30 and (*b*) at least 14 symptoms (12 for males) from the following seven groups:

1. Reports being sickly most of their adult life;
2. Pain;
3. Cardiopulmonary symptoms;
4. Gastrointestinal symptoms;
5. Conversion or psychoneurological symptoms, e.g., difficulty swallowing, loss of voice, deafness, memory loss, muscle weakness, urinary retention;
6. Psychosexual symptoms;
7. Female reproductive symptoms—patient judges that her symptoms are more severe than those of the typical woman.

Unfortunately, the relationships of such patients with their physicians often involves interactions that are either hostile and provocative or dependent and clinging. Prominent features of this disorder are the patient's inability to establish satisfying interpersonal relationships and the attempt to gain affection and caring through illness or somatic complaints.

Hypochondriasis

This disorder is narrowly defined to include patients with a preoccupation about "one" symptom, unrealistic interpretation of sensations, or an unalterable belief that a specific disorder is present, (e.g., the interpretation of any abdominal discomfort as a sign of a malignant tumor). The onset of this disorder is not restricted to any particular age, but the elderly may be more prone to hypochondriasis, especially if isolation reduces their outside interests and social contacts. Note that this definition differs significantly from the common usage of the terms hypochondriac and hyponchondrial.

Conversion Reaction

In this disorder, primary and secondary gains must be considered. The sudden occurrence of a symptom (e.g., paralysis or blindness) allows the patient to achieve some secondary benefit or relief and obscures the underlying psychological conflict. The diagnosis is based on recognition that (a) the symptom itself indicates a physical infirmity that the patient can be shown "not" to have, (b) the symptom is precipitated by severe psychological stress, (c) this is a distinct episode and not part of a long-standing somatization or schizophrenic disorder, and (d) the symptom is involuntary (not malingering).

Psychogenic Pain

This disorder is related to conversion reaction in that it serves a similar psychological function. The pain is severe and protracted, disproportionate to any physical disease, and used to avoid a threatening situation or achieve another secondary gain. The pain is a discrete symptom and not part of another mental disorder. The distinction between psychogenic pain and malingering is important because they require different treatments. Unlike malingerers, these patients are not faking pain. Their perceived pain is real but out of proportion to physical findings.

MASKED PSYCHIATRIC ILLNESSES

Unlike the somatiform disorders, somatization is not the primary problem in diseases of this category. Rather, it is important to understand and treat the underlying psychiatric disorders.

Depression

Most depressed patients initially present with somatic complaints, and 20 to 50% of somatizing patients have underlying depressions. Dysphoric mood is the predominant factor differentiating this group of patients from other somatizers. The patient's mood may be either clearly evident or hidden, requiring elicitation by the physician's careful questions. The interview is likely to reveal vegetative signs of depression (e.g., anorexia, weight loss, insomnia, constipation, sexual dysfunction) (See Chapter 36 on Anxiety and Depression). Unlike other somatizers, the depressed patient will report symptoms with intense guilt, sadness, worthlessness, and despair, yet the anger and hostility of many somatizers will be conspicuously absent.

Schizophrenia

Important components of this disorder are the internalized focus and the withdrawal of external interest that accompany exacerbations of the condition. Probing questions are likely to show that the concerns about bodily function are excessive and even bizarre in nature. As the psychosis develops, the symptoms are often replaced by full-blown delusions. For patients who are able to maintain function with only periodic disruption by psychotic episodes, increased somatic complaints may serve as a barometer of the patient's loosening psychic boundaries and movement toward another psychotic episode.

MALINGERING AND FACTITIOUS DISORDERS

In both groups of disorders, the somatic complaints expressed by the patient are under the patient's voluntary control. The patients create symptoms for a specific purpose. It is critical to recognize these patients because their pain (or other symptom) is contrived, not real. These patients represent only a small minority of patients with somatic concerns.

In malingering, the specific purpose is readily identifiable. A high index of suspicion of malingering should be maintained if the patient has (a) a medicolegal context in the presentation, (b) a marked discrepancy between the objective findings and claimed disability (especially if workman's compensation or disability certification is at stake), (c) a lack of cooperation with diagnostic or therapeutic regimens, or (d) a preexisting antisocial personality disorder.

In factitious disorders, the specific goal is not as clear. Apparently, these individuals have the goal of assuming the "patient" role. Often they are willing to subject themselves to potentially harmful diagnostic or surgical procedures in order to assume this role. While the correct DSM-III diagnosis is chronic factitious disorder with physical symptoms, the more familiar clinical diagnosis is Munchausen syndrome.

TREATMENT

Since patients with multiple somatic complaints can have dramatically different underlying disorders, the first and foremost step in treating these patients is establishing an accurate diagnosis. Table 38.2 briefly summarizes the treatment approach for each diagnostic category.

Syndromes Representing Minimal Psychopathology

In this diagnostic group, the physician is dealing with patients whose psychological makeup is basically normal. Therefore, no major intervention is needed. Reassurance and educating patients about the role that emotions and stress play in the illness will usually be sufficient. Occasionally, stress reduction and/or lifestyle adjustment strategies are needed. If the physician is not skilled in these techniques, referral to a psychologist is appropriate. Prognosis for this group of disorders is excellent.

Somatiform Disorders

Understanding these patients is important for family physicians, since they will have primary longitudinal responsibility for patient management. Three of these disorders, somatization, hypochondriasis, and psychogenic pain, are by definition on-going disorders that require longitudinal care. The primary goal of therapy is to establish a healthy, therapeutic doctor-patient relationship. Do not assume the traditional medical goals of diagnosis, treatment, and cure. Since these are chronic disorders, a primary goal of cure, i.e., relief of all symptoms, is doomed to failure. A therapeutic relationship between doctor and patient, based on trust and understanding, can lead to effective treatment.

The usual treatment approach is to schedule frequent, brief, office visits. Appointments should be regularly scheduled so that the patient does not need to develop a symptom to justify a visit to the doctor's office and, also, so that the appropriate relationship can develop more quickly. The sessions should be brief, 10 to 20 minutes, with the doctor and patient focusing on one or two major concerns. Over time, the physician gradually shifts the conversation from primarily somatic concerns to other events in the patient's life. Other treatment suggestions are listed in Table 38.3.

Table 38.3. Treatment Strategies for Patients with Somatization or Hypochondriasis[a]

Appropriate	Inappropriate
Provide a "sustaining" approach	Belittle complaints
Regularly (biweekly or monthly) scheduled, short (10 to 20 min) appointments	Ignore complaints
	Say "there's nothing physically wrong"
Contracting	Call the person a hypochondriac
Allow patient to maintain defense (illness) with minimum of suffering and medical resources utilization	Use psychological explanation for complaints
	Label the complaints as psychosomatic
Consider one symptom at a time	Offer premature reassurance
Order only studies necessary to convince physician that organic pathology is absent	Offer definitive reassurance
	Use placebos
Any diagnosis should imply chronic but benign disease	Use insight or confrontation approaches
Focus your interest on life issues rather than symptoms	Promise cures
Help the patient renew life interests	Directly refer to psychologist or psychiatrist—usually not accepted by patient
When medication is necessary, use the lowest dose of the mildest medication that the patient will accept with the goal of discontinuing use as soon as possible	Treat with potentially addicting medications
Minimize "as necessary" medications, especially those that have psychoactive effects	Continue to test, hospitalize or refer patient in search of obscure organic illness
Encourage more frequent appointments during time of stress	
Reinforce healthy behaviors, e.g., exercise	
Involve significant others in treatment plans	

[a]Modified from Marshall WR: Chronic somatizers. In Rogers CS, McCue JD, Gal P (eds): *Managing Chronic Disease.* Oradell, NJ, Medical Economic Books, 1987, p 370.

For patients with psychogenic pain, specific pain reduction strategies are often necessary. In addition to brief, frequent visits to the family physician's office, referral to a psychologist or pain clinic may be required to implement these strategies.

Patients with conversion reactions are treated differently than patients with other somatiform disorders. Conversion reactions are acute events. With appropriate and timely intervention, usually by a psychologist, these reactions can be dramatically reversed. Once the conversion reaction is eliminated, the therapist and patient can focus attention on the underlying factors that predisposed the patient to such a reaction.

Prognosis for the treatment of patients with conversion reactions is excellent. Prognosis for somatization, hypochondriasis, and chronic pain depends on how success is defined. Prognosis for complete cure is poor. All of these patients can be helped, however, and their prognosis for improvement is excellent if they are properly managed.

Masked Psychiatric Illnesses

For these patients, treatment of the underlying disorder is critical. However, it is beyond the scope of this chapter to discuss the specific treatments of schizophrenia and depression. Depending on the severity of the illness and the level of expertise of the doctor and the particular needs of the patient, the family physician may treat these patients primarily or refer them to a psychologist or psychiatrist for primary management.

Malingering and Factitious Disorders

These patients feign symptoms to trick the physician. The patient's goal may be to abuse drugs, obtain disability status, or, in the case of factitious disorders, be admitted to the hospital and have procedures performed. Regardless of the goal, once this diagnosis is suspected, confrontation is necessary. These disorders thrust the family physician into the uncomfortable role of patient adversary. A firm statement of the physician's unwillingness to meet inappropriate patient demands is usually sufficient confrontation. Hostile, open confrontations should be avoided if possible.

Prognosis is poor for this group of patients. Once the physician clearly states that unreasonable demands will not be met, the patient usually moves on to another physician.

CONCLUSION

Patients with multiple somatic complaints represent a wide variety of underlying issues. Without a good understanding of diagnostic possibilities and the patient's underlying motivations and concerns, the physician will have trouble meeting the patient's needs. With the special understanding and insight gained from a longitudinal relationship, these patients can be among the most grateful, loyal, and rewarding in the office practice.

SUGGESTED READINGS

Adler G: The physician and the hypochondriacal patient. *N Engl J Med* 304:1394–1396, 1981.

> Emphasizes the long-term nature of treatment of chronic complainers and ways to deal with personal reactions to such patients.

Anstett R, Collins M: The psychological significance of somatic complaints. *J Fam Pract* 14:253–259, 1982.

> Reviews clues to the functional nature of somatic complaints and the diagnostic possibilities that such symptoms present.

Barsky AJ: Patients who amplify bodily sensations. *Ann Intern Med* 91:60–70, 1979.

> Describes a rationale and framework for collecting psychological information relevant to the patient's presenting symptoms.

Drossman DA: The problem patient. *Ann Intern Med* 88:366–372, 1978.

> Provides guidelines for evaluating and treating patients with multiple somatic complaints in a comprehensive approach using biological, psychological, and sociological determinants.

Groves JE: Taking care of the hateful patient. *N Engl J Med* 298:883–887, 1978.

> A discussion of dreaded patients whose behaviors lead them to be subdivided into four groups: dependent clingers, entitled demanders, manipulative help reflectors, and self-destructive deniers. A description of the behavior, physicians' negative reactions, and appropriate psychological management for these patients is provided.

Ries RK, Bokan JA, Katon WJ, Kleinman A: The medical care abuser: differential diagnosis and management. *J Fam Pract* 13:257–265, 1981.

> This article considers the somatizing patient from the perspective of protecting both patients and physicians from unnecessary expenses and potentially litiginous medical interventions.

Rittelmeyer LF: Coping with the chronic complainer. *Am Fam Physician* 31:211–214, 1985.

Provides strategies for effectively dealing with patients who produce chronic complaints.

Sapira JD: Reassurance therapy: what to say to patients with benign diseases. *Ann Intern Med* 77:603–604, 1972.

A discussion of the appropriate strategy for providing reassurance to those patients for whom it is appropriate.

chapter 39

ACHES AND PAINS

Peter Curtis

"Doctor, I seem to be all aches and pains lately. Is this something I should expect at my age?" This type of question is asked by patients almost every day in the physician's office, and is yet another example of nonspecific symptoms that the generalist must clarify and manage.

The term "aches and pains" implies mild to moderate discomfort that usually comes from muscle, joints, bones, or inflamed tissues. Symptoms may be localized to one region of the body or move from one area to another in acute, recurrent, or chronic patterns. Causes of aches and pains vary considerably with age and come from a wide range of diseases, syndromes, and psychological problems.

EVALUATION

As with all other nonspecific symptoms, a careful focused history that covers medical, social, and behavioral areas is important to elucidate clues or patterns of significance. Questions should cover the following:

- Description of the sensation by the patient. This should include the onset and duration of symptoms, what parts of the body are affected, aggravating and relieving factors, and any family history of musculoskeletal disease.
- History or presence of any other current systemic disease (for example, psoriasis is often associated with arthropathy) and a list of prescription and over-the-counter medications taken by the patient. Some pharmaceutical products can produce muscle or joint pains.
- Identification of the patient's occupation, stresses, and family dynamics, as well as the patient's mood. Physically exhausting or repetitive jobs can produce symptoms, while life stress and

depression are often associated with nonspecific pain.

Clinical examination should include palpation of muscles, joints, and bones in the areas complained of by the patient, followed by briefly testing range of motion in the hands, shoulders, hips, knees and feet. It is a good idea to ask the patient to reproduce the discomfort and, if no symptoms are apparent at the time of the visit, to have the patient return when the pain is worse. More than one visit may be needed to get the patient's full history and to observe response to discussion, reassurance, and often empiric pain management.

Laboratory tests are directed toward excluding serious or systemic disease that might be presenting with nonspecific aches and pains. It is important to start with low-cost simple tests such as CBC, erythrocyte sedimentation rate (ESR), and urinalysis. Normal results of these tests will usually screen out many rheumatic and collagen vascular disorders. It is easy but costly to order a barrage of hematologic, rheumatologic, and endocrine tests before developing a working diagnosis—the danger being a slide into the cascade of overinvestigation and equivocal and false positive results.

Case 1. "These pains are getting me down"

Ms. Haynes, age 45 years, comes to the office complaining of pains in her shoulders, thighs, and knees over the previous 5 months. There is a family history of osteoarthritis. Clinical examination is completely normal. The physician orders a CBC, ESR, rheumatoid factor, C-reactive protein, antinuclear factor, LE factor, and SMA 6. The CBC shows mild hypochromic anemia, the ESR is equivocal at 30 mm/hr, and the rheumatoid factor is mildly positive. Radiographs of the joints involved are normal.

She is placed on a nonsteroidal antiinflammatory medication (NSAID), but after several monitoring visits, she says that she is no better. As the physician probes further, it becomes apparent that she is a single mother who has lost her job recently. She admits to crying spells, sleep disturbance, and difficulty concentrating. Therapy with an antidepressant, counseling, and referral to a social worker lead to improvement of her aches and pains.

Case Discussion

Mrs. Haynes has *depression*, a condition that frequently produces heightened awareness of body functions (palpitations, breathlessness, and muscle and joint pains). Her anemia was the result of poor nutrition, and the other test results were not significant, given her normal clinical examination. However, the workup (especially the x-rays) cost this woman, who had no insurance, about $200. More attention to *all* aspects of her history would have led to earlier diagnosis at less cost.

ACHES AND PAINS DURING CHILDHOOD

Aches and pains are frequent presenting complaints in all age groups, except perhaps for children below the age of 5 years. It is quite common for parents to bring a child or teenager in to see the family physician with a story of nonspecific aches and pains, and the cause may be difficult to identify. The more frequent causes of these pains in children are shown in Table 39.1.

Case 2. "Growing Pains"

Johnny, aged 8, is brought to the family physician by his mother, who says that he has been complaining of aching in the lower back and legs for 4 months. It can be bad enough to make him cry at times. He has no fever or swelling of the joints and walks and runs quite normally. He can keep up with the other children's activities. He eats well and seems otherwise

happy. The pains usually last about an hour. Johnny's father apparently had the same problem when he was a child. Clinical examination is completely normal.

Case Discussion

"Growing pains" are a common problem, affecting between 10 and 15% of children. Generally they are defined as intermittent limb pain lasting for more than 3 months, with no joint involvement but causing some disruption of normal activities. There is no known cause. Characteristics of this problem include (*a*) pain in the thighs and calves (occasionally in the back and arms), which can range in intensity from mild to quite severe, (*b*) vague localization, and (*c*) in many cases, occurrence of the pain at night. Pathology is rarely found in these children (<5% of cases).

The history and examination of a child with aches and pains should be aimed at ruling out serious causes needing treatment and looking for indicators of benign disease. Thus, your evaluation should include looking for these warning signs:

• Fever during the episodes;
• Localized joint, muscle, or bone pain/tenderness;
• A persistent limp.

You should also rule out joint hypermobility, which can cause similar complaints. Signs that would point to a self-limited problem, such as "growing pains," include a history of episodes of pain, with the child appearing normal in between, a family history of similar problems, and a correlation between pains and stress or activity levels.

Therapy of benign "growing pains" involves home massage, mild analgesics, conservative monitoring over time, and strong reassurance for a good prognosis. Counseling on home stresses and excessive athletic activity is also an important strategy.

Table 39.1. Common Causes of Aches and Pains in Children

Acute	Chronic	Recurrent
Arthralgia	Rheumatoid arthritis	Tenosynovitis
°Rheumatic fever	Headaches	Sickle cell disease
°Rubella	Scoliosis	Growing pains
°Varicella	Osteochondritis	Episodic arthralgia
°Mumps	Postimmunization	
Trauma	Psychosomatic	
Allergy (bee sting)	Lyme disease	
Acute synovitis		
Henoch-Schönlein purpura		

°Infectious etiology.

ACHES AND PAINS IN ADULTS

There are a large number of causes of musculo-skeletal aches and pains in adults. The more common ones are listed in Table 39.2.

In making a diagnosis, the history is of particular importance. Pay attention to detailed descriptions of the pain, such as onset, rapidity, frequency, time of day, associated fatigue, and aggravating and relieving factors. Stiffness, especially if present first thing in the morning and persisting for several hours, is a common symptom suggesting an inflammatory rheumatic disorder. Table 39.3 identifies the disorders in which stiffness is a prominent feature. Unremitting fatigue is another symptom of rheumatic disease, but it is less specific.

When aches and pains are associated with joint swelling, especially of the hands and feet, the differential diagnosis is still broad. In general, *osteoarthritis* is associated with minimal morning stiffness, mild to moderate disability, very little soft tissue swelling, but significant irregular bony swelling around the joints. Joints characteristically affected are the shoulders, knees, hips, and distal interphalangeal joints of the hands and feet. The ESR is normal.

In contrast, *rheumatoid arthritis* and its variants more commonly affect the metacarpal, carpal, and metatarsal joints. The knees, shoulders, and cervical spine are often severely involved. There is marked swelling of the soft tissues around the joints, significant deformity and muscle wasting, and considerable morning stiffness.

Other aspects of the evaluation of adult aches and pains include paying careful attention to nonarticular features of rheumatic disease and the role played by stress in a number of disorders. Table 39.4 identifies some of the nonarticular

signs and symptoms that should raise your suspicions for rheumatic disease in a patient with aches and pains. Table 39.5 identifies the most common conditions in which aches and pains are brought on by, or are aggravated by, emotional stress.

Although the history and physical examination are major diagnostic determinants, a number of tests may be of value in a puzzling case or one that has specific evidence of arthritis. Among the tests that may be considered in such patients are:

- *CBC.* A normocytic, normochromic anemia is seen in rheumatoid arthritis and variants; a hemolytic anemia may be present in systemic lupus erythematosus (SLE); and an elevated platelet count suggests inflammatory disease.
- *Serum creatinine.* This may be elevated in SLE, vasculitis, or drug toxicity.
- *Erythrocyte sedimentation rate (ESR)* and *C-reactive protein.* Both are acute phase reactants and are nonspecific. High levels are typical of rheumatoid arthritis, polymyalgia rheumatica (and temporal arteritis), neoplasms, and infection.
- *Urinalysis.* Proteinuria, red cells, and casts suggest renal disease and may reflect underlying SLE or a vasculitis.
- *Rheumatoid factor.* This is positive (mainly IgG in a titer >1:160) in 80% of patients with rheumatoid arthritis, 33% of patients with scleroderma and SLE, and 90% of patients with Sjögren's syndrome or hepatitis. The test is nonspecific, however; detectable titers are present in 33% of healthy people over 65 years old.
- *Antinuclear antibodies (ANA).* This is a good screening test for connective tissue disorders, particularly SLE (positive in 95%), Sjögren's syndrome (80%), rheumatoid arthritis (40–60%),

Table 39.2. Common Causes of Aches and Pains in Adults

Acute	Chronic	Recurrent
°Systemic infections	Osteoarthritis	Lyme disease
°Viral syndrome	Rheumatoid arthritis	Myofascial syndrome
°Mononucleosis	Gout	Gout
°Rocky Mountain fever	Pseudogout	Premenstrual syndrome
Rheumatoid arthritis	Hyperparathyroidism	
Polymyalgia rhematica	Hyperthyroidism	
Temporal arteritis	Hypothyroidism	
Stevens-Johnson syndrome	Neuromyopathies	
Trauma	Depression	
Gout	Fibromyalgia	

°Infectious etiology.

Table 39.3. Disorders with Stiffness as a Symptom

- Rheumatoid arthritis
- Seronegative arthropathies
- Generalized osteoarthritis
- Polymyalgia rheumatica
- General infections
- Prolonged bed rest
- Ankylosing spondylitis

Table 39.4. Nonarticular Features of Rheumatic Disorders

- Skin and nail changes
- Cutaneous/subcutaneous nodules
- Conjunctivitis/uveitis/dry eyes
- Chest pain, cough, dysnpnea
- Diarrhea and/or abdominal pain
- Dysuria/urethral discharge

Table 39.5. Aches and Pains Related to Stress

- Depression—psychogenic rheumatism
- Fibromyalgia
- Myofascial syndromes
- Osteoarthritis
- Rheumatoid arthritis and variants

and scleroderma (60%). The pattern observed provides a key to the underlying diagnosis.

- *Radiology.* Joint destruction is generally evident on plain films or on a bone scan within 2 to 7 days in septic arthritis, within 4 to 5 months in rheumatoid arthritis, within 3 to 4 years in gout, and within 5 to 6 years in osteoarthritis.

In using laboratory tests in evaluating the patient with aches and pains, remember that the lower your clinical suspicion of a disease before you perform the test, the more likely an abnormal test is to represent a false positive.

A review of the myriad causes of aches and pains is not feasible in this chapter. The following cases, drawn from the author's practice, illustrate some of the more common diagnostic and management problems seen in the primary care office.

Case 3. Pain in the Back

Mr. M., aged 60, presented with a 5-month history of intermittent aching pains in the muscles of both arms and the upper trunk. He also complained of mild fatigue, and a 5-pound weight loss. The pains seemed to move from place to place and were made worse by

activity. He worked as a teacher, had a satisfactory home life, and had no significant stresses. Clinical examination was normal, and routine NSAID therapy did not help his symptoms. Screening CBC and ESR were normal. X-ray films of the shoulders and spine showed only mild osteoarthritic changes compatible with his age.

Because the persistent nature of his complaints remained unexplained, the next step was to exclude metabolic bone disease. Serum calcium, phosphate, and alkaline phosphatase levels were ordered. These were normal, except for minimal elevation of the serum calcium at 10.9 mg/100 ml (the upper limit of normal in this laboratory is 10.5). Two further calcium levels are also slightly elevated; so a parathormone level was obtained, which was normal. Next, Mr. M. was referred to a rheumatologist, who found no evidence of rheumatic disease but repeated the parathormone level and found it to be elevated. Subsequently, the patient was found to have a parathyroid tumor, and his symptoms abated after its surgical removal.

Case Discussion

It is often wise to repeat tests because of diurnal and pathophysiological variation in levels of hormones, minerals, and metabolites in the blood. There has been increasing realization that mild or subclinical hyperthyroidism and hyperparathyroidism are relatively frequent and can present with musculoskeletal symptoms.

Case 4. Riding Accident

Ms. S., aged 35, comes to the office complaining of aching and stiffness of the shoulders, hips, lower back, and knees for 6 months following a riding accident. Her symptoms are made worse by cold wet weather and stress. She is currently considering marriage. She reports lethargy, anxiety, and tension at times during the day and some wakefulness at night. Clinical examination is normal apart from a number of tender areas in the neck, shoulder, and paraspinal muscles. She is also tender over the iliac crests and the medial aspects of the knee joints. A CBC and ESR are normal.

Case Discussion

This patient has *fibromyalgia syndrome*, which has a prevalence of 19% in the adult population. It typically presents with aching pain or stiffness involving at least 3 muscle groups and persisting for at least 3 months. Tender "trigger points" are characteristically found in one or more of the following locations: the medial border of the scapula, the upper trapezius, the buttocks, the anterior costochondral junctions, the lateral elbows, and the medial knees. Mood disturbances and a non-rapid-eye-movement (REM) sleep disorder are also common in fibromyalgia. Treatment consists of explanation, reassurance that this is not a serious problem and will improve, and moderate conditioning activities. The sleep disturbance is treated with antidepressants, since it is thought that muscle deconditioning occurs during sleep in this syndrome. After 4 months of therapy, Ms. S. is symptom free.

In the case of Ms. S., the differential diagnosis could include depression, but the clinical findings of multiple tender trigger points with a preciptating injury pointed toward fibromyalgia.

Case 5. Leg Cramps

Ms. McG., aged 70, comes to the office with 6 months of nocturnal leg pains, involving the calves and feet. Sometimes it is just a mild ache, at other times she gets severe cramps. Clinical examination is completely normal. Laboratory test results, including an ESR and a serum calcium level, are normal.

Case Discussion

This lady has *nocturnal leg cramps*, a common problem with no known cause. It occurs at night and usually in the elderly. Congestive heart failure appears to be a predisposing factor. Treatment includes massage and dorsiflexion of the foot during an acute cramp. Prevention entails using a bedboard or pillow for the feet, sleeping prone, exercising before bedtime by stretching the calf muscles (leaning into a wall with the feet 1 foot away from the wall works well), and wearing properly fitting shoes. Quinine 200 or 300 mg (both dosage strengths are available over the counter) or quinine sulfate 260 mg (available by prescription) often provides marked relief. This condition should not be confused with the *restless leg syndrome*, a neurological disorder that consists of bi-

lateral drawing or creeping sensations associated with an uncontrollable urge to move the legs, and which responds to benzodiazepines (e.g., clonazepam).

MANAGEMENT

Most patients with rheumatic symptoms can be well managed by the generalist. Patients with chronic, disabling rheumatic disorders may be difficult management problems, particularly in the areas of functional remediation, medication regimens, and surgical interventions. These patients and others who are persistent diagnostic puzzles are appropriately referred to rheumatologists for consultation or shared care. Indications for consultation or referral include (*a*) uncertain diagnosis, (*b*) the need for specialized studies (i.e., synovial biopsy), (*c*) severe, persistent symptoms, (*d*) rapid deterioration or disability, (*e*) the need for comprehensive rehabilitation, and (*f*) advice on high-risk therapies such as gold or cyclophosphamide.

SUGGESTED READINGS

Corman LC, Bell CL, Edwards NL, Harmon CE (eds): *Rheumatology for the House Officer*. Baltimore, Williams & Wilkins, 1990.

Highly readable, succinct, easy-to-carry volume that is packed with valuable information, management strategies, and descriptions of pharmaceuticals and physical therapy modalities.

Katz WA (ed): *Diagnosis and Management of Rheumatic Diseases*, ed 2. Philadelphia, JB Lippincott, 1988.

Very comprehensive text on rheumatic problems. Excellent reference for browsing.

chapter 40

LOW BACK PAIN

Peter Curtis

Low back pain is extremely common, so common, in fact, that 70% of the world's population will have at least one disabling episode in their lives; but most of those people, even in developed countries, will manage their problem without seeing a health professional. In the United States, backache is the most frequent cause of limitation of activity under the age of 45, and it is the commonest type of chronic pain seen in office practice. The morbidity of chronic back pain in the working population is significant, since employees with more than 6 months of absence have only a 50% chance of returning to work, and those absent for a year with back pain have only a 25% chance of ever returning to work. Eleven percent of industrial workers are off work for 1 to 6 months, and 4% have permanent disability. The annual national cost of this problem is $20 billion, of which one-third are medical costs. Medical, environmental, or social factors may contribute to low back pain. Table 40.1 lists some of these factors.

Despite these statistics attesting to its frequency and severity, low back pain is poorly understood and often poorly treated. Diagnostic and treatment strategies abound, some diametrically opposed to each other. It is noteworthy that low back pain is the only common medical problem for which the public largely bypasses orthodox medical care in favor of an alternative philosophy and method, i.e., chiropractic.

This chapter explains how to approach the patient with low back pain in a rational, systematic way, so that an effective treatment plan can be developed despite the areas of uncertainty in our current knowledge of this condition.

EPIDEMIOLOGY

Although there is no clear explanation for this, episodes of backache seem to occur in a bimodal distribution, with greatest frequency in the third and in the fifth and sixth decades (Fig. 40.1). In about 80% of first attacks, the specific lesion causing back pain cannot be identified. Only 6 to 8% of cases show a proven disc prolapse. Several studies have shown that over half of all attacks resolve within 2 weeks, but there is a high incidence of recurrence months or years later. Five to 10% of people with acute low back pain develop chronic problems.

In many cases we cannot pinpoint the pathophysiological cause in back pain; so diagnosis and treatment are often nonspecific. Moreover, pain affects the patient's psyche and often causes a feeling of helplessness, especially in a previously fit person. Consequently, both physicians and patients become frustrated. A plethora of treatments has emerged, indicating the medical profession's attempts, often unsuccessful, to deal with this problem. Likewise, the many kinds of healers low back pain sufferers visit indicate the patients' frustration. Family physicians, internists, gynecologists, emergency room physicians, orthopaedists, neurologists, neurosurgeons, osteopaths, chiropractors, faith healers, acupuncturists, and massage and physical therapists all treat low back pain.

Diagnosis and treatment very much depend on which physician or healer the patient visits first. For example, a patient visiting a neurosurgeon first is much more likely to have a myelogram or CT scan. A person visiting a chiropractor is likely to have a series of manipulations performed.

CAUSES OF LOW BACK PAIN

Table 40.2 lists the causes to consider when a patient presents with low back pain. These causes can be divided into structural and nonstructural. Nonstructural causes are those independent of the function of the back itself, such as rheumatoid

Table 40.1. Factors Contributing to Low Back Pain

Medical	Environmental	Family/Individual
Respiratory disease	Work-related	Marital problems
Trauma	Sitting for long hours	Young children
Pregnancy	Subordinates in an organization	Depression
	Poor job satisfaction	Anxiety
	Transient jobs	Excess alcohol intake
	Truck/automobile driving for long periods	Smoking associated with cough

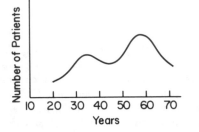

Figure 40.1. Epidemiology of low back pain.

arthritis, carcinomatosis, and aortic aneurysm. Diagnosis of such nonstructural conditions is important and often urgent.

The great majority of patients with low back pain have a structural cause that reflects the local anatomy and physiology of the back. The structural causes of low back pain are the subject of much on-going dispute because a number of local conditions can produce similar symptoms. Moreover, these conditions often coexist because they are mechanically connected. For instance, vertebrae articulate via three separate joints: the two facet joints posteriorly, and the disc anteriorly. This tripartite system is called the motion segment and is illustrated in Figure 40.2. A torsional strain of one such motion segment may cause a tear in the annulus fibrosus of the disc and a capsular sprain of one or both facet joints, together with injury to some of the ligaments and muscles that also connect the two vertebrae. Any of these injuries may cause similar pain, the physical findings may be nonspecific, and radiographs are nondiagnostic.

Once you have excluded nonstructural causes of low back pain, pinpointing the specific structural lesion is often difficult. This uncertainty must be acknowledged in your diagnosis and treatment.

The most common cause of low back pain is soft tissue injury of the muscles and ligaments, which can occur as a result of direct trauma (e.g., falling on the ice) or from twisting or bending. In the latter case, one theory is that an apophyseal (facet) joint between two lumbar vertebrae slips out of alignment, damaging the joint capsule and the surrounding soft tissues. Another theory is that the sacroiliac ligaments may be strained in lifting or pushing. Many soft tissue injuries are associated with local muscle spasm and inflamed tissue. This "myofascial syndrome" is identified by small movable tender lumps in the lower back area.

Common precipitating factors for soft tissue injuries are twisting and stressing the back by lifting. Sitting, however, may be even more significant, for it is in this position that the highest pressure is exerted on the lumbar discs, thereby predisposing them to progressive injury. Clinically, mild disc disease is often indistinguishable from other structural problems. Severe disc disease is likely when pain radiates to one or both legs and is accompanied by sensory and/or motor deficits.

Finally, osteoarthritis of the lumbar spine is a common cause of backache, producing disc damage, mechanical instability, and osteophyte formation. Osteoarthritis is the most common cause of low back pain in the elderly.

EVALUATION OF THE PATIENT WITH BACK PAIN

The most useful diagnostic approach in the office is the "safety net strategy," a series of internal questions you ask yourself while interviewing and examining the patient. They are:

1. What is the likely diagnosis, given the age and history of this patient?
2. What serious disease should *NOT* be missed? (These usually are malignancy, fracture, or bone infection.)
3. What illnesses are often missed? (Think especially about ones that present atypically or subclinically, such as urinary infection or ankylosing spondylitis.)

Table 40.2. Causes of Low Back Pain[a]

Structural	Nonstructural	

Degenerative disease(+ +)[b] (discs, facets)	Neoplasia
	  Primary
	  Metastasis
		Visceral
		  Prostatitis
		  Endometriosis
		  PID(+)

Intervertebral strain(+ +)		Renal disease
Myofascial syndromes(+ +)	Infection	Aortic aneurysm
Kyphoscoliosis	Osteomyelitis	Pancreatitis
Fractures(+)	Paraspinous abscess	Cholecystitis(+)
Osteoporosis(+)	Epidural abscess	Peptic ulcer
Spondylolisthesis	Bacterial endocarditis	Osteonecrosis
Spinal stenosis		

	Inflammatory arthritis
	  Ankylosing spondylitis(+)
	  Rheumatoid arthritis(+)	

	Paget's disease	

[a]Adapted from: Deyo RA: Early diagnostic evaluation of low back pain. *J Gen Intern Med* 1:328–338, 1986.
[b]Key: (+) frequent causes of low back pain
     (+ +) very frequent causes of low back pain

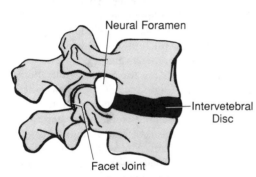

Figure 40.2. The intervertebral motion segment: two vertebrae articulating via a disc and two facet joints.

4. Is the patient depressed? (Psychological disorders, exaggerated illness behavior, and depression may be offered to the physician as back pain.)
5. Does the pain hide the actual reason for coming (ARC)—underlying stress, alcoholism, family dysfunction, malingering, need for compensation, drug dependency?

Taking the History

Keeping in mind the five internal questions, you ask the patient questions in the following areas:

1. General health—appetite, weight, malaise, fever, energy level;
2. Past history of back problem—episodes, tests, therapy, recovery;
3. Current function—sleep, work, dressing, sex, recreation, attitudes, family function, previous violence or abuse;
4. Past illnesses—other illnesses, family history of arthritis, rashes;
5. Medications/drugs—analgesics, steroids, NSAIDs, drugs, ethanol;
6. Pain patterns.

Your history should include the following data: occupation of the patient; time course; details of any trauma; the number of attacks; treatments and medications used; surgery; character of the pain; aggravating factors (coughing, sneezing, sitting, bending forward, walking up or down stairs, lying on back, stomach, or side); alleviating factors (standing or lying down, heat, cold, drugs); detailed neurological symptoms (numbness, radiating pain, paresthesia, weakness); disability; and pending litigation or workman's compensation. The history should include questions about other medical problems such as visceral or systemic symptoms (weight loss, urinary problems, etc.) and family/personal stresses.

The pattern of the pain can help suggest a diagnosis.

- Throbbing suggests inflammation;
- Deep aching, diffuse pain suggests referred pain;
- Steady, superficial pain suggests muscle strain;
- Deep, boring pain suggests malignancy or Paget's disease;

- Sharp, stabbing pain suggests nerve root compression.

Sciatic pain ("sciatica") is back pain that radiates into the buttocks and produces tingling in the posterior thigh and posterolateral calf to the lateral malleolus. It is often attributed to disc prolapse, however disc disease is only one of many causes. Other causes of sciatic pain are spinal stenosis, entrapment neuropathy, lateral stenosis, obturator neuritis, piriformis syndrome, back pocket syndrome, direct trauma, sciatic nerve inflammation, ischiogluteal bursitis, and osteoarthritis.

In asking questions, use standard descriptors (site, type, radiation, episodes, aggravating and relieving factors). Ask about the dynamics of the pain—whether it is getting worse, better, or staying the same. Be sure to ask about the relationship of pain to day/night. Ask also about associated features—fever, malaise, urinary symptoms, cough, and sensory loss.

Find out how the symptoms interfere with functioning. Ask about daily tasks—climbing stairs, dressing, and driving. Find out details of work content and the patient's perceptions of disability.

The patterns of aggravating and relieving factors can also give clues to the underlying diagnosis. Some common patterns are noted in Table 40.3.

The physical examination for low back pain is outlined in Table 40.4.

Further Investigations

In most young patients up to the age of 50 years, no further workup (blood or x-ray) is needed for a first attack of back pain, since the probability of serious disease is very small. Additions to the workup are needed in the following situations:

1. When fever is present, blood count, sedimentation rate, plain x-ray films, and bone scanning

are indicated. Your concern is for inflammatory disease or infection.
2. In males under 40 with slow onset of back pain and morning stiffness, x-ray films, sedimentation rate, and HLA-B27 are indicated. Your concern is ankylosing spondylitis.
3. In females over 40, breast and thyroid examination is indicated to rule out cancer.
4. In males over 60, examination of the prostate gland and prostate-specific antigen (PSA) levels are needed to rule out prostate cancer.
5. For prolonged pain in all age groups (more than 4 to 6 weeks), a general physical examination, x-ray films, serum calcium and phosphorus levels, alkaline phosphatase, blood count, and sedimentation rate may be indicated to rule out systemic or bone disease.

There is much evidence that x-ray films are of little diagnostic value in most patients with backache. The drawbacks are radiation to gonads, a low yield of useful findings, and high cost. One lumbar spine x-ray series gives gonadal doses equal to a daily chest x-ray for 6 years. Indications for early x-ray are: age over 50; fever; weight loss; previous malignancy; serious trauma; motor neurological deficits; long-term corticosteroids; substance abuse; history and findings suggesting rheumatoid arthritis and ankylosing spondylitis; and potential litigation (road traffic accidents, workers' compensation cases).

X-ray Ordering. Anteroposterior and lateral views are adequate and should be specifically requested to avoid other low-yield views being done as a routine by the radiologist. Myelography is used to delineate prolapsed intervertebral discs when intervention is contemplated. It will delineate nerves, nerve roots, and the extradural space. Sensitivity is in the region of 90%, but there is a high false-positive rate, so that clinical correlation is very important. CT scans and

Table 40.3. Patterns of Pain Aggravation and Relief in Selected Diagnoses

Aggravating Factors	Relieving Factors	Suggested Cause
Cough, sneeze, strain	Lying flat	Disc prolapse
Sitting forward	Upright	Spinal tumor (rare)
Standing, walking	Sitting	Spondylolisthesis
Hard walking	Resting	Spinal canal stenosis
		Ischemia
Turning in bed	None	Ankylosing spondylitis, disc prolapse, SI joint strain
Movement, any direction	Stay still	Malignancy, fracture

Table 40.4. Physical Examination

Technique	Reason
1. Inspect the unclothed back	To identify scoliosis, kyphosis
2. Get patient to walk and observe	To identify gait problems
3. Discreetly watch patient undressing, if possible	Gives an idea of patient's mobility and whether he or she may be "putting it on"—it is difficult to simulate limited mobility while undressing
4. Check range of motion	The degree of restriction and its pattern (flexion vs. extension) gives clues to the cause of pain
5. Palpate the back in area of pain	To identify areas of muscle spasm, trigger points, tender bony points
6. Measure lower limb length	To check whether one lower limb is shorter than the other. One to 1.5 inches is significant and can cause back pain

7. Check lower limb reflexes
    Knee-root L3/4
    Ankle-root S1
	To identify neurological deficit

8. Check power in legs
    Quadriceps (straighten leg deficit out from
      knee-bent position) L3/4
    Dorsiflex big toe L5
    Plantar flexion S1
	To identify neurological deficit

9. Check sensation
    Inner thigh L4
    Outer calf and top of foot L5
    Outer edge of foot S1
	To identify neurological deficit

10. Straight leg raising to 90°	Limitation suggests nerve root irritation

magnetic resonance imaging (MRI) are being used increasingly to identify discs and disc rupture and are largely replacing myelograms at many centers.

CLINICAL FINDINGS IN COMMON DISEASE ENTITIES

One or more of the findings in Figure 40.3 may be present at the same time. The common ones are listed below.

Myofascial Syndrome

Tender nodules are similar to the trigger points found in other parts of the body (shoulder, neck). These myofascial trigger points are often felt as mobile, tender, rubbery nodules at the sacroiliac area and iliac crest. Figure 40.4 shows trigger points associated with myofascial syndrome.

Sacroiliac Strain

Often due to the tearing of sacroiliac fibers or possibly due to slippage of the sacroiliac joint, sacroiliac strain causes local tenderness in the dimple area of the back. This pain is made worse by flexing the knee on the hip and pushing the knee medially with the patient lying on his back. Sometimes, sacroiliac pain radiates down the leg.

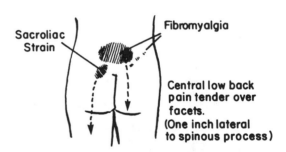

Figure 40.3. Common clinical findings (one or more may be present).

Paraspinous Pain

Diffuse pain on both sides of the spine is called paraspinous. Often, tenderness between the spinous processes or at the facet joint of a vertebra (1 inch lateral to the spinous process) can be noted. Common causes include injury to facet joints, muscular strain, or minor tears of the disc annulus.

Prolapsed Disc

Symptoms are similar to those above but with very limited straight leg raising and often a neurological deficit with referred pain. See Table 40.5 for details of findings at commonly affected disc levels.

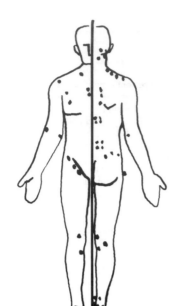

Figure 40.4. Trigger points associated with myofascial syndromes.

Table 40.5. Common Signs of Herniated Disc

L5 root compression (L4-5 interspace)
  Limited straight leg raising
  Sciatic/popliteal nerve tenderness
  No reflex change
  Decreased sensation at outer aspect of calf and top of
    foot
  Weakness of dorsiflexors of ankle and great toe
S1 root compression (L5-S1 interspace)
  Limited straight leg raising
  Sciatic/popliteal nerve tenderness
  Decreased ankle reflex
  Decreased sensation on back of calf and outer side of
    foot
  Weak plantar flexion of foot and great toe
Central disc
  Bilateral leg pain
  Loss of bowel and bladder function

THERAPY

Approach to Management

Back pain is a classic example of the biopsychosocial model of illness, partly because pain is modulated by cortical and thalamic centers (the gate control theory of pain perception). This paradigm has been the basis for the growth of interventions such as biofeedback, hypnosis, transcutaneous nerve stimulation, and acupuncture. Psychological distress and abnormal illness behavior contribute 30%, and severity of pain 40%, to the disability of low back pain. The psychological distress and illness behavior come from previous experiences of stress and pain, family and work contexts, and personal belief systems of the patient. Understanding and addressing these issues is an important path to recovery and is worth the investment of time by the physician. Severe frustration in managing the patient may be avoided in the future by using these principles.

1. Find out what the patients believe is the cause of pain. Do not discount their opinions!
2. Provide a clear, confident explanation of why they have pain.
3. Reassure the patient that this pain will improve—disability is not likely.
4. Have sympathy for the patient's pain and dysfunction.
5. Tell the patient that a variety of scientific and nonscientific therapies can be tried, one of which may work effectively.
6. Use models or diagrams to explain the anatomy.
7. In chronic pain or prolonged episodes, invite the spouse or friend/family to participate in discussions.
8. Many patients with chronic pain have histories of physical or sexual abuse as children. Check on their past.
9. Give clear instructions on exercises, posture, functional activities, and lifestyles or refer to someone who can.

WHAT PATIENTS SAY AND THINK ABOUT LOW BACK PAIN

Patients have explanatory models of the cause of their pain based on their belief systems. These include:

- Misuse of the body—bad habits, wrong movements, bad car seat, exposure to cold, dampness;
- Mind/body effect—stress, personality type;
- Guilt—penalty for bad behavior, deserving to suffer;
- Heredity—all the family are prone to low back pain;
- Aging—expect this as one gets older;
- Work—heavy labor or work positioning are the main cause.

Effects and limitations that seriously concern patients with low back pain include their ability to:

- Be a parent of young children;
- Work and provide for the family;
- Do household duties, such as cooking, cleaning, and yardwork;
- Drive or take public transportation;
- Sleep, have sex, or socialize with friends;
- Undertake physical/leisure activities;
- Pay for their health care.

Patients cope with their pain and situation by "living with it," (i.e., overcoming their pain by will); by "living through it" (i.e., continuously seeking remedies and therapy); or by allowing the pain to dominate their existence. Patients often feel that the medical system/provider has no good explanation of what the problem is, is not really interested in their pain, only their body, does not want to touch them where their pain is, and offers inadequate advice on how to cope with daily living activities.

Physicians can do a much better job of managing low back pain if they find out more about the belief systems and coping styles of their patients, particularly as these affect their daily lives and those of their families.

In planning therapy, you can often be guided by these key questions:

1. Is the cause structural or nonstructural? The answer is often clear from the history. If the pain began with a mechanical strain, and the patient is young and otherwise well or has no predisposition to a nonstructural problem, the diagnosis is likely some kind of structural backache.
2. Should the patient be referred to a specialist? Several factors have to be weighed here. There are a few conditions that mandate urgent referral to an orthopaedist or neurosurgeon (acute leg weakness and disturbance of bladder or bowel function). For most low back pain, even when associated with sciatica, the chance of spontaneous recovery is high enough that a short period of rest and analgesia is appropriate. If referral is not mandatory, your choice will depend on the severity of symptoms, the extent and duration of the patient's disability, history of previous episodes, and on the availability of local specialist services such as physi-

cal therapy. Table 40.6 provides guidelines for specialist referral.

3. Is the problem likely to resolve spontaneously? This depends much more on the history than on the examination findings. If the patient strained the back doing a very strenuous task that will not be repeated (e.g., helping a neighbor move a piano), the patient will probably get better quickly unless daily activities include tasks that mechanically reproduce the initial injury. On the other hand, if the patient hurt the back performing an activity that is repeated many times daily, spontaneous recovery may be less rapid and less complete. If no mechanical stress can be implicated, the symptoms are probably the culmination of repetitive microtrauma from daily activities, and prognosis without treatment is again less assured.
4. If not, what specific treatment is indicated? The answer once again depends more on the history than the examination findings. If the problem is likely to improve spontaneously, treatment should provide pain relief and safety, i.e., avoiding mechanical stress that might delay healing.

A large number of studies have attempted to demonstrate improved outcomes with specific types of treatment such as exercise, traction, bed rest, the use of corsets, analgesics, spinal manipulation, and transcutaneous nerve stimulation. Most have suffered methodology problems—nonrandomization, heavy patient attrition from the study group, poor compliance with the regimen, or inadequate standards of diagnosis. Table 40.7 lists the orthodox therapies available for patients with low back pain.

Table 40.6. Guidelines for Specialist Referral

Urgent referral
    Intractable pain to pain clinic or surgeon[a]
    Progressive neurologic deficit to neurologist or surgeon[a]
    Fractures to orthopaedist
Standard referral to subspecialty internist
    Neoplasia
    Infectious disease
Optional referral to subspecialty internist
    Arthritis
    Renal disease
    Gastrointestinal disease
    Bone disease

[a]Neurosurgeon, orthopaedist.

Some clinical predictors of poor outcome can be helpful to the clinician. These include:

- Pain lasting >1 week before visit to provider predicts the need for a follow-up visit 2 weeks later and moderate disability 4 weeks after the first visit.
- Gradual onset of pain.
- Limited straight leg raise (SLR) of less than 60° predicts disability at 4 weeks after the first visit; <30° is even worse.
- Referred pain below the knee.
- Neurological deficit. This predicts a long absence from work, independent of pain duration. (This may be due to the clinician's anxiety about neurological problems.)

Table 40.7. Available Therapies for Nonspecific Low Back Pain

Oral drugs	Injected drugs
Muscle relaxants	Systemic cortico-
Analgesics	steroids
Antiinflammatory agents	Local corticosteroid
Antidepressants	injections
	Epidural steroid injec-
Physical measures	tions
Bed rest	Epidural anesthetic
Corsets/braces	injections
Traction	
Exercises	*Counterstimulation*
Spinal manipulation/	Transcutaneous elec-
mobilization	trical nerve stimula-
Massage	tion (TENS)
Weight loss	Acupuncture
Local heat (radiant,	Cold massage
short-wave diathermy)	

- Pain on dorsiflexion of the foot in the straight leg raise position predicts a high disability at 4 weeks and work absence for 2 weeks.
- These patient factors: a tendency to somatic complaints, a history of anxiety/depression, or cigarette smoking.
- Workman's compensation case.
- Diagnosis by the clinician of prolapsed disc or a possibility of a prolapsed disc.
- The patient is a manual laborer.

The only therapies that have been established as being somewhat effective by clinical trials (compared with placebo) are isometric flexion exercises, traction in which the patient controls the force applied, nonsteroidal antiinflammatory drugs, muscle relaxants, and spinal manipulation (which produces early improvement but no difference in long-term outcome). Tricyclic antidepressants have been shown to reduce by 40% the need for analgesics in chronic low back pain, without altering physical activity levels.

In light of our ignorance on effective therapeutic measures, practical therapy must take into account other factors for the patient, e.g., cost, length of therapy, and practicality.

THERAPY OF THE ACUTE EPISODE WITHOUT SIGNS OF HERNIATION

Fifty percent of patients are well within 1 week and 80% within 2 weeks of an acute episode, so the approach should be simple, safe, cheap, and quick, in the hope of getting the patient back to full functioning. The guidelines for treatment of the common structural causes of low back pain are listed in Table 40.8.

Table 40.8. Treatment Options for Common Structural Causes of Low Back Pain

Myofascial syndrome and nonspecific diagnosis	
Step 1:	Aspirin, Tylenol or nonsteroidal antiinflammatory drugs
Step 2:	Physical therapy: massage to relieve spasm
Step 3:	Local injection therapy
Step 4:	Preventive measures and exercise program
Sacroiliac strain	
Step 1:	Nonsteroidal antiinflammatory drugs
Step 2:	Specific exercise program
Step 3:	Spinal manipulation to readjust sacroiliac joint surfaces
Step 4:	Local analgesic/steroid injection
Central low back pain	
Step 1:	Nonsteroidal antiinflammatory drugs often combined with muscle relaxants
Step 2:	Decreased activity or bed rest for 2 to 5 days if severe pain
Step 3:	Gentle exercises to reduce stiffness; abdominal strengthening exercises to improve posture; physical therapy program
Step 4:	Spinal manipulation to readjust facet joints

PLAN OF THERAPY SEQUENCE

The physician may often undertake treatment interventions in parallel. In treating the patient, the physician should do two other things. First, it is essential to clarify the problem and educate the patient about the anatomy of the back, about prognosis, and particularly on ways of avoiding further injury (such as switching from a lifting to a less stressful job). Second, an empathic physician with an ability to deal with the frustrations of disappointing or slow clinical progress will make a tremendous difference to the outcome of the patient's illness.

Patients should be instructed to avoid unsupported and forward sitting, bending slightly while vacuuming, washing, lifting, straining, jumping, jogging, prone sleeping (face down), and the use of a soft mattress.

These patients should be encouraged to sit with a backrest, knees and hips flexed, to flex knees when lifting, and to be sure that work areas are at an adequate height. A firm mattress should be used for sleeping, and pillows should be positioned to tilt the body while sleeping. (A pillow between the knees while sleeping on the side prevents sacroiliac strain.) Swimming, walking, and gentle exercises (isometric, abdominal, flexion) should be suggested to the patient. Patients should receive guidance in prevention measures that will help strengthen postural muscles and improve the mechanics of daily living. This is most efficiently done by a physical therapist.

Many physicians are not trained in spinal manipulation, injection techniques, and other therapeutic modalities. Referral to specialist therapists is therefore often necessary.

THERAPY OF CHRONIC BACK PAIN AND/OR DISC DISEASE

A long or relapsing course occurs in 10 to 15% of patients and is characterized by more than three previous episodes of acute back pain, gradual worsening of symptoms, and/or pain referred to the lower limb. Many of these patients have had stresses or psychological problems and if not, may well develop them after prolonged suffering. The physician should obtain psychological evaluation; referral to a multidisciplinary pain clinic will often help clarify these complex issues and lead to recommendations for treatment. In these patients, physical therapy, back corsets and braces, drug

therapy, and exercise programs are commonly used in combination or alone. When acute attacks of pain occur, spinal manipulation, injections, and counterstimulation methods may be used. The history of chronic low back pain may vary over a lifetime, often improving in the later years.

Surgery has been used increasingly for the treatment of low back pain, some would say excessively, since 65 to 90% of patients with chronic sciatic pain are either coping well or improved after 10 years if treated conservatively. Surgery is generally performed for (a) intractable pain unrelieved by conservative measures; (b) progressive neurological symptoms secondary to nerve root compression; (c) cauda equina syndrome (disc rupture affecting bowel or bladder function) urgent referral needed; and (d) prolonged disability. The outcome of surgery is best in patients with severe sciatica and clear radiographic signs of a disc rupture.

Some physicians test the patient's emotional and psychological status before deciding on surgery in those people with chronic pain. Certain patients present with backache as an hysterical conversion syndrome, and surgery in these cases usually does not help and often makes the conversion syndrome worse. Signs that suggest major psychological factors contributing to symptoms are:

1. Ability to straighten leg in the sitting position compared with raising leg while lying flat;
2. Strange neurological deficits unexplained by anatomy/physiology concepts;
3. Overreaction to the examination (facial, verbal, tremor, sweating);
4. Exaggerated reaction to sensory testing or palpation.

Some doctors refer the patient for psychological testing. The Minnesota multiphasic personality inventory (MMPI) is the test most commonly used.

The overall success rate for surgery is 54%, which is not too different from either conservative therapy or chance. As many as 10 to 20% of patients have negative explorations when operated upon, i.e., no obvious cause is found. The most common surgical procedure is vertebral laminectomy with excision of the prolapsed disc.

SUGGESTED READINGS

Deyo RA: Early diagnostic evaluation of low back pain. *J Gen Intern Med.* 1:328-338, 1986.

Excellent review of general approach to low back pain.

Deyo RA: The role of the primary care physician in reducing work absenteeism and costs due to back pain. *Spine* 2:77–30, 1987.

Excellent review article with good references.

Grieve GP: *Common Vertebral Joint Problems*. New York, Churchill Livingstone, 1981.

Marvelously huge and comprehensive book on back problems.

Kirkaldy-Willis WH: *Managing Low Back Pain*. New York, Churchill Livingstone, 1988.

Excellent, readable book with particular tolerance toward manipulative therapy.

Lee JC, Genshwi ME, Fowler WB, (eds): *Principles of Physical Medicine and Rehabilitation in the Musculoskeletal Diseases*. Orlando, FL, Grune & Stratton, 1986.

Broad-ranging, useful description of many physical therapy techniques.

Paterson JK, Burn L: *Back Pain: An International Review*. Boston, Kluwer Academic Publications; 1990.

Succinct, explores many myths about research into back care. Easy to read.

Travell JG, Simons DG: *Myofascial Pain and Dysfunction: The Trigger Point Manual*. Baltimore, Williams & Wilkins, Vol 1, 1982, and Vol 2, 1992.

Volume 1 is the definitive work on myofascial pain and trigger points.

Waddell GA. A new clinical model for the treatment of low-back pain. *Spine* 2:632–644, 1987.

Interesting article suggesting that the epidemic of low back pain is a societal symptom and that orthodox medical approaches need to be rethought.

Weinstein JN, Weisel SW: *The Lumbar Spine*. Philadelphia, WB Saunders, 1990.

Comprehensive, current text on back care that covers the waterfront, even manipulation.

chapter 41

NECK PAIN

Peter Curtis

CAUSES OF NECK PAIN

The two major symptoms associated with neck diseases are pain and limited motion. The pain may be only in the neck or radiate to the shoulder and down the arm. The most common cause, considering all age groups, is myofascial syndrome, a condition of localized muscle spasm. Degenerative arthritis in the cervical vertebrae is the other common cause of neck pain, particularly in the older patient, and is known as cervical spondylosis. Trauma, particularly motor vehicle accidents, can lead to whiplash and other neck injuries. Sedentary occupations (e.g., desk work and driving motor vehicles) are often associated with pain, but the precise anatomical cause of pain is in many cases uncertain.

EVALUATION

Most acute neck pain is caused by structural problems such as myofascial syndrome, muscle spasm, and traumatic ligament sprains. Diagnosis of these common conditions is clinical, relying entirely on the history and physical examination. Subacute and chronic neck pain is also most commonly structural, with osteoarthritis becoming more likely with increased age. Stress and biomechanics (e.g., positioning at work or in bed) are often important contributing factors to both acute and chronic neck pain, so they should be sought. Less common but serious conditions must also be considered in developing a differential diagnosis; the causes of neck pain are listed in Table 41.1.

In taking a history, the following items should be recorded: the patient's occupation, daily postural habits, stresses at work and at home, the onset of pain (sudden or gradual), the main focus (arm, shoulder, back), and the character of the pain (sharp, dull, or aching).

Trauma, whiplash, or persistent unusual activity (such as home remodeling) often produces acute pain with limited neck movement, which improves with rest. Pain over the lower pole of the scapula and posterior aspect of the shoulder, radiating into the neck, is often caused by myofascial syndromes and is associated with stress or poor posture. A persistent aching or piercing pain going into the occipital area or down the arm suggests nerve root compression. Pain that came on gradually and improves with rest is particularly worrisome; it may be caused by infection or malignancy in a vertebra.

As you move to the physical examination, focus your attention on the neck, occiput, and arms. Test the range of neck motion in flexion, extension, rotation, and side-bending, to establish the degree of limitation and the movements that cause pain. Press the top of your patient's head gently down into the shoulders; increased pain down an arm suggests root compression. Then carefully palpate the neck anteriorly and posteriorly, checking for lymphadenitis, muscle spasm, and particularly tender areas of muscle or bone ("trigger points"). Palpate the region of each cervical facet joint, approximately 1 inch lateral to the cervical spinous process. Facet joint tenderness suggests malalignment, a frequent cause of acute neck pain.

Next examine both arms for neurological deficits, which would indicate injury to one or more cervical nerve roots. Check the power of major muscle groups and the sensation in each dermatome. Test the biceps (C-5 and C-6) and triceps (C-7) reflexes. Many patients have subjective pain or paresthesias in root distributions, but relatively few have objective neurological findings. Subjective neurological symptoms with a normal examination reflect referred pain from damaged

387

soft tissue such as ligaments, facet joint capsules, or muscle. True radiculopathy, on the other hand, is confirmed clinically by specific neurological deficits such as muscle weakness, atrophy, diminished tendon reflexes, and sensory loss (as outlined in Table 41.2). Such findings are suggestive of disc disease but can also occur transiently in severe sprains.

Rarely, central spinal cord compression affects descending tracts, causing upper motor neuron findings. In this case, there is spasticity and increased muscle tone instead of flaccidity, and heightened rather than decreased deep tendon reflexes.

Another unusual but important condition is the thoracic outlet syndrome. This involves compression of the neurovascular bundle (brachial plexus, subclavian vessels) as it passes out through a narrowing between the clavicle and first rib. Symptoms consist of pain and numbness down the arm as well as weakness. The syndrome occurs predominantly in women in their 20s and 30s. The symptoms can often be replicated by simple clinical maneuvers:

a. Have the patient sit upright and thrust the shoulders backwards with hands on thighs; or
b. Abduct the arm to 180° and rotate it externally while the patient sits upright.

During both of these maneuvers, monitor the radial pulse and listen with a stethoscope over the supraclavicular area. A positive result is indicated by a reduced or absent pulse and/or a bruit heard in the clavicular area.

Laboratory studies are indicated only when the history suggests systemic or bone disease (e.g., fever or symptoms in other organs). These symptoms, or persistent pain and disability for more than 3 weeks in a patient over 40 years, should prompt the ordering of a sedimentation rate, blood count, x-ray films, and possibly calcium studies.

X-ray findings are often nonspecific. By age 50, half of patients have radiologic evidence of cervical spondylosis, and at 65 years, 85%, but these findings are usually asymptomatic. Thus, finding osteoarthritic changes on x-ray films does not mean that they are responsible for a patient's neck pain. On the other hand, x-ray films are useful in looking for bony metastases, Paget's disease, myeloma, or ankylosing spondylitis. CT scan and MRI have become much more valuable but costly tools in diagnosing nerve root compression, disc disease, and other pathology in the neck. If entrapment neuropathy (e.g., carpal tunnel syndrome) is suspected, an electromyogram (EMG) and nerve condition studies can be abnormal and can also help confirm nerve compression syndromes.

Table 41.1. Causes of Neck Pain

Structural	Nonstructural	Other
Myofascial syndromes (+ +)[a]	Ankylosing spondylitis	Stress (+ +)
Facet joint asymmetry (+)	Rheumatoid arthritis	Occupation (+ +)
Osteoarthritis (+)	Bone infection	
Muscle spasm (+ +)	Neoplasia—primary metastasis	
Fracture	Lymphadenitis	
Disc prolapse		
Outlet compression syndrome		

[a](+) Frequent cause of neck pain; (+ +) very frequent cause of neck pain.

Table 41.2. Neurological Findings Associated with Cervical Root Lesions

Roots	Motor Weakness	Sensory Loss
C4	Shoulder abductors	Shoulder
C5	Elbow flexors	
	Diminished biceps/brachioradialis reflex	Lateral arm
C6	Wrist extensors	Thumb/index fingers
C7	Elbow extensors	Middle ring finger
C8	Intrinsic hand muscles	Little finger
T1	Finger flexors	Medial arm

ISSUES IN MANAGEMENT

Most causes of acute or chronic neck pain can be managed by simple measures such as ice or heat, analgesics, rest, and the more specific therapies listed below. Findings of persistent or progressive neurological deficit, systemic disease, or bony destruction on patient evaluation should lead to a neurological, orthopaedic, or neurosurgical consultation.

A number of therapeutic modalities are used to manage neck pain. Because the most common conditions causing pain are osteoarthritis of the cervical spine, muscle spasm, and minor trauma, the outcome will be good if therapy is directed toward reassuring and supporting the patient, relieving pain, reducing mechanical stresses, and relieving muscle spasm. Clinical studies have not definitively ascribed benefit to one therapeutic modality over another. Therefore, you should try various approaches, based on the severity and chronicity of the pain, patient preferences, and the cost of treatment. Recommendations for the management of common neck problems are outlined in Table 41.3.

Supportive management, such as moist heat, helps promote muscle relaxation. Heat can be applied by taking a warm bath (15 to 20 minutes), with a heating pad, or with a hydrocollator pack. A soft collar, positioned to produce the least pain, allows the cervical muscles to relax by supporting the head. These collars relieve strain on the cervical muscles and restrict flexion/extension movements (see Fig. 41.1). For patients with chronic severe neck pain, a molded plastic collar may be necessary for several months.

For relief of pain and inflammation, a variety of drugs can be used. Aspirin or acetaminophen is usually sufficient for pain relief. For severe pain, particularly at night, a narcotic such as codeine may be necessary. Any of the nonsteroidal antiinflammatory drugs may be tried and, in some cases,

be effective. Muscle relaxants may be of some benefit beyond their sedative effects, especially when acute muscle spasm is present, but they too have side effects. Patients should take extra care when they drive.

In treating a prolonged acute episode or chronic neck pain, intermittent traction is often helpful. This can be done in a physical therapy department or, more economically, using a home traction kit obtainable from the local drug store (Fig. 41.2). The traction force should be at least equivalent to the weight of the head (about 7 pounds) and is usually between 7 and 15 pounds. In a few patients, traction makes the pain worse and should be discontinued after a brief trial. Continuous traction is rarely indicated but is given to some patients suffering from intractable pain. This must be done in the hospital, and then only for a period of 3 to 4 days.

Increasingly, mobilization and spinal manipulation are being used to treat chronic neck pain and prevent recurrence of symptoms. Mobilization involves careful and gentle movement of the neck through its physiological range of motion, often using gentle traction with the hands. Manipulation moves a specific joint to its anatomical limits, with the final movement being a short, high-velocity thrust. It is performed by many different kinds of health providers with osteopaths and chiropractors most commonly trained in the procedure. Although its efficacy is not well supported by controlled studies, patients often report that manipulation relieves pain and spasm. Neurological symptoms following a manipulation are a rare event but can affect older people, particularly as a result of injury to the vertebrobasilar artery.

Stretching and strengthening exercises are also helpful, particularly in the late recovery phase. To prevent recurrence, exercise should be included in most neck rehabilitation programs. Figure 41.3 outlines several neck exercises.

Table 41.3. Management of Common Neck Problems

	Physical Measures	Medication
Osteoarthritis	Heat, exercises	Aspirin, NSAID[a]
Muscle spasm	Relaxation techniques, massage, heat, stress management	Aspirin, acetaminophen, muscle relaxants
Traumatic sprain	Rest, ice, cervical collar	Aspirin, acetaminophen
Myofascial syndromes	Deep massage, injection therapy, relaxation techniques	Muscle relaxants
Facet joint asymmetry	Rest, mild traction, spinal manipulation	Aspirin, acetaminophen, NSAID

[a]A nonsteroidal antiinflammatory drug.

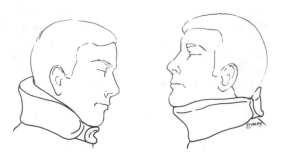

Figure 41.1. Positions for applying soft collar.

Local injections of xylocaine and/or steroids are also commonly used to treat acute neck pain, particularly if a trigger point is identifiable. The procedure is only undertaken below the third cervical disc level to avoid the vertebrobasilar artery as it winds up to the occiput. To perform the procedure, position the patient prone, with the neck flexed. Use 1 to 2 ml of 1% xylocaine with or without an additional milliliter of crystalline steroid suspension (25–40 mg). Insert a long needle (3 cm) 1 inch lateral to the spinous process (midline) and push down through the posterior ligament into the joint area. Then, the mixture is injected at several points around the joint.

A small number of patients with intractable pain or progressing neurological deficits may be considered for surgery. This is usually considered only after medical management has failed.

Whiplash Injuries

Whiplash injuries are flexion-extension injuries of the neck, which usually occur in traffic accidents. Anterior cervical structures (muscles, larynx, esophagus, temporomandibular joint, ligaments) are stretched and sometimes torn. In mild to moderate cases, the victim may be unaware of the injury until several hours later, when muscles become painful or the patient develops "wry" neck. In all such cases, it is important to carry out a detailed neurological examination and to obtain an appropriate x-ray film of the cervical spine to look for a fracture or dislocation. Soft tissue swelling anterior to the cervical vertebrae, increasing the space between the bone and the pharyngeal air space, is a diagnostic sign of whiplash in x-ray films of patients who have intact bony structures.

Therapy includes rest (using a soft cervical collar), analgesics, and local ice/heat treatments. Injection of local anesthetic into trigger points may

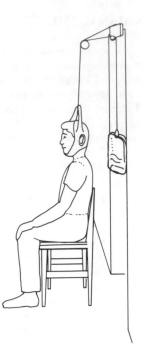

Figure 41.2. Home traction kit.

be helpful. If the symptoms persist for more than 4 weeks, gentle cervical traction (7 to 15 pounds) may help relieve pain. If root signs and symptoms appear, myelography may be indicated to exclude a lacerated cervical disc. At this stage, particularly if litigation is involved, the clinical picture frequently becomes confused by compensation issues. Severe cases of whiplash should be admitted to the hospital for evaluation and referred to a neurologist or neurosurgeon, since there is danger of neurologic damage.

Chronic Neck Pain Syndromes

Some patients develop chronic neck pain syndromes that do not respond to the usual therapeutic modalities. These are often associated with environmental stress, emotional illness, or personality disorders, and are very difficult to manage. They may require alternative methods of pain relief such as transcutaneous nerve stimulation (TENS), biofeedback, hypnosis, or referral to a psychologist, psychiatrist, or pain clinic.

SUGGESTED READINGS

Bland JH: *Disorders of the Cervical Spine and Diagnosis and Medical Management*. Philadelphia, WB Saunders, 1987.

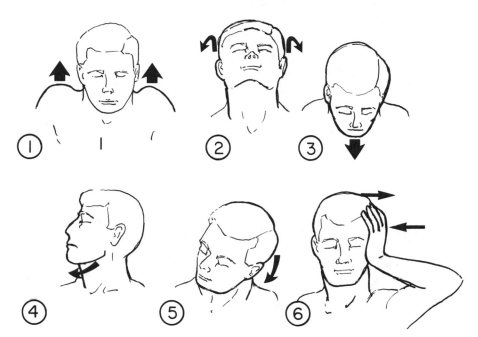

Figure 41.3. Neck exercises. 1. For relaxation, hunch shoulders up high. 2. Bend head backwards as far as you can, so you can see the ceiling directly above your head. 3. Put chin down to your chest. 4. Turn head to the right trying to bring your chin over your right shoulder. 5. Try to bring your left ear down to your left shoulder. 6. Place left hand against left side of head. Push your head against the heel of your palm without allowing it to move. Hold.

Excellent book, deals with disability determinations and a whole spectrum of neck problems.

Bonica JJ, Caillet R, Sola AE: General considerations of pain in the neck and upper limb; neck pain. In Bonica JJ (ed): *Management of Pain*, ed. Philadelphia, Lea & Febiger, 1990, pp 812–847, 848–867.

Review of anatomy, physiology, and mechanisms of neck pain with approaches to management. Part of two huge volumes on pain.

Cloward RB: Acute cervical spine injuries. *Clin Symp Ann* 32:1–32, 1980.

Good illustrated review of the emergency management of acute cervical spine injuries.

Grieve GP: *Common Vertebral Joint Problems*. Edinburgh, Churchill Livingstone, 1981.

An excellent book giving comprehensive guidance on physical examination, mobilization, and manipulation techniques and a critical look at a wide range of therapeutic modalities used in joint disease. Over 1300 references.

Hirsch LF: Cervical degenerative arthritis: possible cause of neck and arm pain. *Postgrad Med* 74:123–130, 1983.

A view of degenerative arthritis with an emphasis on the neurosurgeon's approach.

chapter 42

SHOULDER PAIN

Peter Curtis

The causes of shoulder disorders, like those of many other musculoskeletal problems, are in a spectrum from biomechanical to degenerative. As a broad rule, below the age of 45, biomechanical causes, especially repetitive trauma, predominate; degenerative conditions become increasingly implicated in shoulder problems with advancing age. These two categories are connected: mechanical stress accelerates degenerative processes, and degenerative changes often only become symptomatic because of mechanical stress.

ANATOMY

The shoulder consists of two functioning joints, the glenohumeral and acromioclavicular, and three gliding surfaces, the long head of the biceps, the subacromial bursa, and the musculotendinous cuff (see Fig. 42.1). The musculotendinous or rotator cuff is a group of muscles that strengthen the capsule of the joint. The five rotator cuff muscles are: supraspinatus, infraspinatus, teres minor, subcapsularis, and the long head of the triceps.

In shoulder syndromes, pain frequently arises from inflammation. Among the structures most frequently involved are the capsule of the glenohumeral joint, the supraspinatus tendon, and the subacromial bursa.

CAUSES OF SHOULDER PAIN

Although many specific conditions are described in orthopaedic texts, most shoulder problems are either myofascial syndromes or one of a continuum of interrelated traumatic or degenerative soft tissue processes such as bursitis, tendonitis, rotator cuff syndrome, or adhesive capsulitis.

Myofascial syndromes, the most common causes of shoulder pain, are characterized by "trigger points"—very localized areas of tenderness in and around muscles. On firm pressure with the finger at a trigger point, the patient may wince or withdraw. You should feel for a nodule, an indurated or ropy area in the muscle. Comparison with a noninvolved muscle in the opposite shoulder is helpful. Common sites of trigger points are:

- Superior medial aspect of the scapula;
- Muscles just below the nuchal tuberosity in the neck region;
- Trapezius and sternomastoid muscles;
- Intercostal muscles, pectoral muscles, lateral aspect.

Trigger points result from a variety of factors including genetic propensity, poor muscle conditioning (mechanical trauma), and emotional stress. Once established, these painful sites become self-sustaining despite elimination of the original stimuli, since tension, pain, and fatigue create a feedback cycle that promotes further local muscle spasm.

Bursitis, tendonitis, and the rotator cuff syndrome are a related series of disorders that are parts of a single chronic process and are often clinically indistinguishable. This process often begins in the supraspinatus or bicipital tendon, which has a relatively poor blood supply and can become frayed and inflamed under unusual or repetitive mechanical stress. The inflammatory process can then involve other tendons and bursae and ultimately the entire capsule and acromioclavicular (AC) joint. Patients may present with pain from any of these structures. These conditions are more common in middle-aged "weekend athletes," in patients between 50 and 60 years old, in women, and in the winter months. The disease process is unilateral in 75% of cases. For a summary of clinical features that help distinguish between these overlapping disorders, see Table 42.1 and Figure 42.2.

Bursitis is an inflammation, usually associated with a small effusion of fluid, of one of the several bursae in and around the shoulder joint. Bursae normally provide a lubricating mechanism for easy muscle movement at the shoulder. Bursitis is often precipitated by minor trauma. The onset is often slow, and the condition may persist with exacerbations and remissions for up to 2 years. Improvement is also slow.

Tendonitis is an inflammation (with or without a partial tear) of the tendon insertions of shoulder joint muscles. Rotator cuff syndrome comprises inflammation, strain, or degeneration of the shoulder joint capsule where it is reinforced by muscle tendon sheaths.

By the age of 50, close to 25% of people have some wear and tear of the rotator cuff, thus mak-

ing it susceptible to injury. Partial or full tears of the cuff, therefore, usually present in middle age following trauma, often a fall on the outstretched arm. The pain is acute, and the patient complains of weakness of the arm, reduced range of motion, and pain at the limits of internal and external rotation. Partial tears are often associated with other inflammatory or degenerative disorders of the shoulder.

"Adhesive capsulitis" (frozen shoulder) occurs as a result of the marked reduction in volume of the glenohumeral joint, with tightening and thickening of the joint capsule. The peak incidence occurs between 50 and 70 years of age and is higher in women. The cause may be trauma, but adhesive capsulitis usually arises from immobility. Often, lack of shoulder movement results from a condition such as stroke or an arm fracture. Within as little as 2 to 4 weeks, particularly in elderly in-

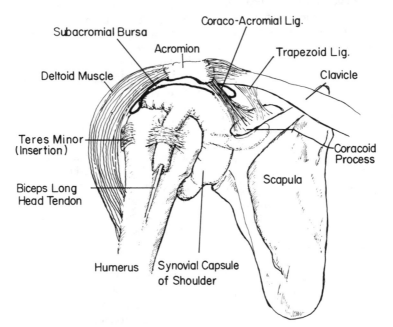

Figure 42.1. Deep anatomy of the shoulder.

Table 42.1. Examination Clues to Common Causes of Shoulder Pain

Problem	Examination Techniques	Findings
Bicipital tendonitis	External rotation of arm or shoulder	Tender in bicipital groove
Supraspinatus tendonitis	External rotation of arm or shoulder, abduction of arm	Pain on movement in this direction: (painful arc 45 to 120°)
Subacromial bursitis	Internal rotation of arm or shoulder, abduction of arm	Pain on movement in this direction: (painful arc 45 to 120°)
Rotator cuff syndrome	Mobility testing in all directions	Pain on movement in all directions

dividuals, immobility produces a tight, painful shoulder joint.

A more insidious type of adhesive capsulitis is associated with clinical conditions such as myocardial infarction, long-term intravenous infusions, thyroid disease, diabetes, and depression. The symptoms include generalized loss of motion and chronic pain. Symptoms develop over several months and last up to 2 years. Examination reveals limitation of active and passive motion in all directions, often with very little tenderness to palpation.

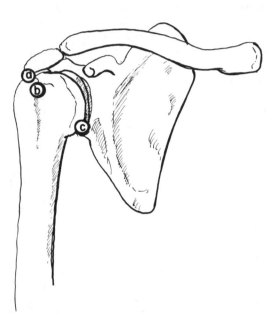

Figure 42.2. Sites of tenderness in the following conditions: *a*, subdeltoid bursitis; *b*, bicipital tendonitis; *c*, adhesive capsulitis.

While shoulder pain is usually caused by musculoskeletal disorders of the shoulder and neck, it may also arise from structures outside the shoulder, such as cervical vertebrae, heart, lungs, or diaphragm. Table 42.2 provides a more complete differential diagnosis of shoulder pain.

CLINICAL EVALUATION

History

Shoulder pain that develops acutely usually results from trauma (e.g., a direct blow, or fall onto an outstretched arm), repeated unusual use (e.g., spring cleaning), or acute cervical nerve root compression (e.g., ruptured disc). More often, both pain and decreased mobility develop over a few weeks. In degenerative diseases, the pain onset is gradual, and it may fluctuate over weeks or months. Usually with degenerative processes, some joint mobility is preserved, and the patient complains more about pain on specific movements than about limitation of motion.

The distribution of pain can provide valuable clues to the specific diagnosis. Pain from any of the structures of the shoulder joint except the acromioclavicular (AC) joint is referred along the same dermatome (C5) that includes the shoulder and the lateral surface of the arm to the hand. In conditions affecting the joint surrounding the capsule and tendons, the earliest and most intense pain is often felt over the deltoid muscle. Later, it may spread to involve the entire shoulder or radiate downward into the lateral or anterior aspect of the arm.

Physical Examination

The shoulder joint should be inspected for swelling and symmetry, palpated for areas of ten-

Table 42.2. Differential Diagnosis of Shoulder Pain

Trauma	Systemic disease
*ᵃAcute or chronic dislocation	Inflammatory diseases: gout and pseudogout, infectious
* Fractures; humerus, clavicle, acromion	arthritis, polymyalgia rheumatica, rheumatoid arthritis
* Rotator cuff tears	Cancer: primary, metastatic
Nerve compression at brachial plexus	
Nerve compression at C4-C6 disc nerve root	
Musculoskeletal syndromes	Neurovascular
* Degenerative arthritis:	Bachial plexus injury
(osteoarthritis)-glenohumeral joint, acromioclavicular joint	Thoracic outlet syndrome
* Tendonitis-biceps	Cervical root compression
* Rotator cuff syndrome	Reflex sympathetic dystrophies/syndromes
* Bursitis-subacromial	
* Myofascial syndromes	

ᵃ*Indicates common problems.

derness, and then put through a range of passive and active movements, while comparing it with the "normal" shoulder. Mobility testing should include abduction, adduction, flexion, extension, circumduction, and internal and external rotation. Passive examination movements are performed by the doctor on the patient. Active movements are performed alone by the patient.

Pain only on active movement implicates muscles and bursae as the main cause of pain rather than the joint itself. Pain with only one movement suggests that the problem is with the muscle or tendon mainly involved in that movement. For instance, pain on initiation of abduction, decreasing later as the angle of abduction increases, incriminates the supraspinatus. Pain on passive movement warrants careful interpretation. It may be due to movement of inflamed tendons or bursae or restricted mobility of the joint capsule itself. The better you know the anatomy of this joint, the better you will be able to establish a precise diagnosis from the clinical examination. A brief examination of the neck and a screening neurological check of the arms (see Chapter 41, "Neck Pain") should be included.

MANAGEMENT OF COMMON PROBLEMS

Myofascial Syndromes

The treatment of myofascial pain begins with identifying precipitating factors such as the wrong chair height or back support for an employee with a desk job; a peculiar body position while working or studying; or an unusual way of doing a repetitive task, such as lifting overhead on an assembly line. This analysis may take time and some imagination to sort out, but it is vital to the success of treatment; the shoulder will stop hurting only when the patient stops doing things in ways that hurt it.

Myofascial syndromes should be treated as use-related musculoskeletal disorders with local heat, massage, active range of motion movements, and stretching exercises; but the most important treatment is coaching the patient in using different movements to execute the tasks that are perpetuating the muscle dysfunction. Muscle relaxants have not proven to be effective. If trigger points are found, anesthesia of the area can usually be obtained by injecting 5 to 10 ml of 1% xylocaine using a 1-½ inch 22-gauge needle. This breaks the pain/spasm/stress/pain cycle and will

often provide long-term relief. If a first injection does not effect complete relief, a second injection may be used. If two injections fail to provide relief, your diagnosis should be reassessed. Several other techniques, most of which involve deep massage, stretching the affected muscles passively and exercising other muscles, can be taught by physical therapists skilled in occupational and other overuse syndromes.

Bursitis, Tendonitis, and Rotator Cuff Syndrome

Bursitis, tendonitis, and rotator cuff syndrome are clinical diagnoses. No diagnostic workup is indicated unless pain and disability persist for more than 4 to 6 weeks, in which case x-ray films of the shoulder joints should be obtained. These may be normal or show degenerative changes in the joint or calcium deposits in the supraspinatus tendon. Patients with symptoms and signs indicating serious, acute rotator cuff injury should have arthrograms, since early surgical repair, usually within 2 weeks, produces the best outcome.

The mainstays of treatment are a brief period of rest followed by physical therapy, which assists restoration of normal motion before secondary weakness and stiffness compound the problem. Indeed, there is evidence that early remobilization actually accelerates healing of injured periarticular tissues. In addition, local steroid injections into periarticular tissue are helpful if specific areas of local inflammation can be identified. When identified, inject 1% xylocaine to determine if your localization is correct. Pain relief should be immediate. If so, inject the equivalent of 40 mg of prednisone in the form of crystalline steroid (Celestone, Aristocort, Depo-Medrol) mixed with 1 to 2 ml of 1% xylocaine. Patients should be warned that pain in the shoulder is likely to increase over the 12 hours following an injection, since the onset of action of steroids is between 12 and 36 hours. This problem often can be avoided by the use of a longer-acting local anesthetic such as Marcaine instead of xylocaine. Repeated injections of steroids into the same site can produce atrophy and tendon rupture; therefore, not more than two or three injections should be given over a 12-month period.

Physical therapy may include analgesic modalities such as local heat, ice, and massage; but it is important to appreciate that these should only be used to increase the ease with which the patient can begin passive and active exercises. The patient

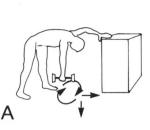
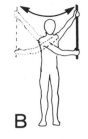
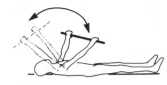
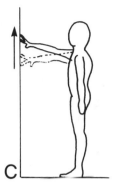
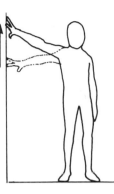
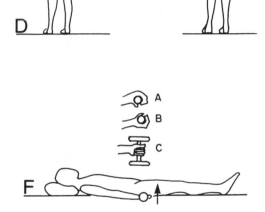
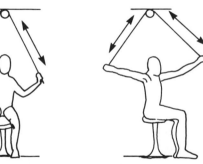
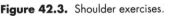

Figure 42.3. Shoulder exercises.
Do 3 repetitions of each at 3 different times a day.

A, Circumduction exercise (pendulum)—hold a 1- to 2-pound weight (such as a sock filled with pebbles) in one hand, arm pointing at floor. To steady yourself, hold onto furniture with the other hand. Make circles in both directions and then straight lines, beside you and then across front.

B, Broomstick stretches—holding a walking cane, yardstick, or broomstick handle. 1) With one hand at each end, take stick out to one side and then the other, using good arm to gently push weaker arm. 2) With hands shoulder-width apart, take arms over head. Do this lying and progress to standing.

C, Finger walking—1) Facing the wall, walk your fingers up as high as possible. Lightly mark with pencil and date. Record your progress weekly. 2) With your weak side to the wall, walk your fingers up with the arm sideways. Again, record your progress weekly.

D, Towel stretch—1) After bath or shower, grasp each end of a towel as if drying your back. With weak arm at waistline pull other arm up and out, causing lower arm to come up back. 2) Reverse positions and pull weak arm from top of shoulder down toward waistline behind.

E, Pulley exercise—construct an overhead pulley (over a doorway works well). Use 10 feet of rope, with loops at each end for handles. 1) Exercise sitting. Take arms up over head, using the stronger one to stretch the weaker or tighter one. 2) Then, sit sideways in the chair and pull the tight arm sideways, elbows straight.

F, Muscle strengthener—lie on back, arms beside body, holding a weight in hand. Keeping elbow straight, lift hand up just enough to clear weight. Do lifts in three positions: (A) palm down, (B) thumb up, and (C) palm up. Gradually increase the weight from 1 to 5 pounds.

can perfectly well apply heat and ice at home; the physical therapist's role is to help restore function, not just to treat the pain. Criteria for referral to a physical therapist are highly individual and depend on several factors such as the availability and convenience of physical therapy and the extent to which the family physician wishes to carry out this part of the treatment plan. Exercises for patients are shown in Figure 42.3.

Medications, if used at all, should be selected carefully, especially if a prolonged course is envisaged. Acetaminophen and propoxyphene derivatives reduce pain but are not antiinflammatory. Nonsteroidal antiinflammatory drugs (NSAIDs) are used extensively for musculoskeletal shoulder syndromes, although there are no well-controlled studies that show significant benefits except in acute inflammatory conditions. The agents produce both an analgesic and an antiinflammatory effect and may be given as a therapeutic trial for 1 to 2 weeks. No one agent is established as better than another. Salicylates (600 to 900 mg every 6 hours) are inexpensive and effective. Other commonly used NSAIDs include ibuprofen (Motrin), sulindac (Clinoril), naproxen (Naprosyn), and indomethacin (Indocin). Patients may respond better to one NSAID than another, so it is worth switching agents if there is no initial improvement. The possible side effects of these drugs (indigestion, gastric erosion, and rash) should be reviewed with patients before prescribing. Table 42.3 summarizes the dosages and side effects of some commonly prescribed NSAIDs.

Adhesive Capsulitis

With a diagnosis of adhesive capsulitis, the age of the patient often raises the possibility of an underlying organic or neoplastic disease. Therefore, a general physical examination and possibly laboratory tests and x-ray films are indicted. Arthrogra-

phy, if performed, will show a marked decrease in joint space and often local osteoporosis. Therapy consists of heat, analgesic medications for pain, and active exercises. A physical therapist should be consulted early, to preserve as much mobility as possible.

Degenerative Osteoarthritis

Degenerative osteoarthritis is often associated with osteoarthritis of other joints such as knees, hips, and fingers. It is common in older patients or in people who have a history of previous shoulder injury (dislocation or fracture). Generally they complain of intermittent, chronic, aching pain, often in both shoulders, which is worse in damp or cold weather. The pain tends to be localized to the joint and not referred down the arm. Movements may be slightly limited but not in any one particular direction. Crepitus (grinding) is commonly felt over the joint when it is in motion.

X-ray films can help to clarify the extent of the osteoarthritic process and exclude other rarer disorders, such as gout, crystalline synovial disease, and rheumatoid arthritis. A blood count and sedimentation rate are also helpful. As a general rule, an acute flare-up of arthritic pain requires a brief period of rest, heat, and antiinflammatory medication. A long-term exercise program may alleviate the chronic, underlying condition.

Other Causes of Shoulder Pain

The shoulder joint may also be affected by infections, inflammatory arthritis, metabolic disease, and cancer. Shoulder pain may be referred from structures outside the shoulder, such as cervical vertebrae, heart, lungs, or the diaphragm. Usually the history and clinical examination will provide strong evidence for these causes and suggest further specific investigations.

Table 42.3. Selected Nonsteroidal Antiinflammatory Drugs—Dosages and Side-Effects

Genetic	Proprietary	Usual Daily Dosage (mg)	Side Effects[a]			
			GI	Blood	Mental	Renal
Ibuprofen	Motrin	1200–2400	+			+
Sulindac	Clinoril	300– 400	+			
Naproxen	Naprosyn	500– 750	+			+
Indomethacin	Indocin	75– 200	+	+	+	+
Acetylsalicylic acid	Aspirin	4000–6000	+			

[a]GI symptoms: indigestion, nausea, gastric erosion; Blood: dyscrasia—leukopenia; Mental: confusion, dizziness, especially in the elderly; headaches; Renal: edema, impaired function, and interstitial nephritis

SUGGESTED READINGS

Cogen L, Anderson LG, Phelps P: Medical management of the painful shoulder. *Bull Rheum Dis* 32:54–58, 1982.

Nice short review of therapeutic measures in shoulder problems.

Escobar PL, Ballesteros J: Myofascial pain syndrome. *Orthop Rev* 16:708–713, 1987.

Review article. Useful, easy to read.

Gray RG, Tenenbaum J, Gottlieb NL: Local corticosteroid injection treatment in rheumatic disorders. *Semin Arthritis Rheum* 10:231–254, 1981.

Excellent discussion of joint injection.

Lee JC, Gershwin ME, Fowler WM (eds): *Principles of Physical Medicine and Rehabilitation in the Musculoskeletal Diseases*. Orlando, FL: Grune & Stratton, 1986.

Useful description of physical therapy modalities.

Section I: The painful shoulder. *Clin Orthop* 173:1–124, 1983.

Major journal issue on shoulder problems with a number of articles on diagnosis and management.

chapter 43

KNEE INJURIES

Peter J. Rizzolo

The knee is the most fragile and vulnerable of our weight-bearing joints. Constructed to allow flexion and extension but very little lateral movement or rotation, the knee is readily injured by lateral stress and by twisting. Such stresses are common in football, basketball, and, to a lesser degree, tennis; so knee injuries are common in these sports. Chronic use is another mechanism of knee injury, which is why long-distance runners frequently have knee problems.

For the family physician, several general approaches should guide your care of knee injuries. First, knee injuries represent a situation in which physical diagnosis is particularly valuable. By knowing knee anatomy, you can evaluate injuries to determine which structure is likely to be injured. Secondly, most knee problems can be managed without specialist referral, however, the physician must learn which require referral. Finally, rehabilitation of the healing knee is extremely important. Good primary care of knee injuries, therefore, requires careful follow-up and guidance regarding knee rehabilitation.

ANATOMY

Although the knee essentially functions as a hinge joint, there is slight external rotation of the tibia during extension of the leg and slight internal rotation of the tibia during flexion of the leg. This is accomplished without the action of the muscle groups that internally and externally rotate the leg, but by the ligamentous attachments in and around the knee joint. In addition there is a forward gliding action of the femur on the tibia during flexion.

The distal femur has two rounded prominences, the medial and lateral condyles, (see Fig. 43.1) which fit into shallow concave areas of the proximal tibia. Between the femoral condyles is a groove in which the patella rides, constituting the anterior portion of the knee joint. The medial and lateral menisci are attached to the margin of the proximal tibia and act as shock absorbers between the femoral condyles and the tibial articular surfaces. The joint is stabilized by the muscles that traverse it and by internal and external ligaments.

Muscles That Help Stabilize the Knee Joint

The quadriceps group consists of four muscles, the rectus femoris, vastus medialis, vastus lateralis, and vastus intermedius (see Fig. 43.2). At their distal end they come together to form the quadriceps tendon that incorporates the patella and inserts on the tibial tuberosity, affording considerable anterior joint stability.

The iliotibial band inserts on the tibia and is a major structure providing lateral stability to the knee.

The hamstring group (see Fig. 43.3) inserts on the posterior aspect of the tibia and assists in preventing hyperextension of the joint.

Major Ligaments of the Knee Joint

The five ligaments of the knee joint are shown in Figure 43.4 and are discussed below.

Lateral Collateral Ligament. The lateral collateral ligament extends from the lateral femoral epicondyle to the fibular head. This ligament crosses the joint line over the lateral posterior aspect. It can be felt deep and anterior to the biceps femoris tendon where it inserts on the fibular head. It is best felt with the knee flexed 90° and in adduction.

Medial Collateral Ligament. This ligament consists of a superficial portion and deep fibers that connect the medial femoral epicondyle and

401

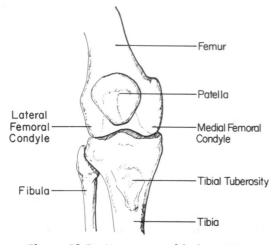

Figure 43.1. Anterior view of the knee joint.

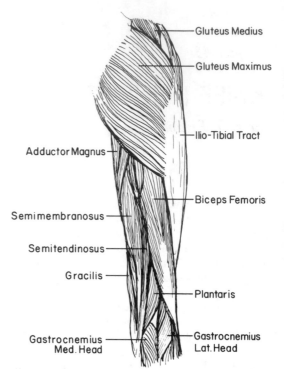

Figure 43.3. Posterior view of the knee: major muscles.

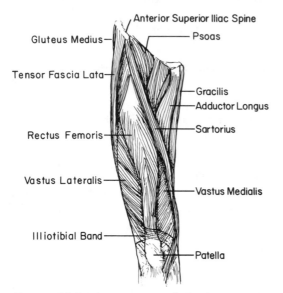

Figure 43.2. Anterior view of the knee: major muscles.

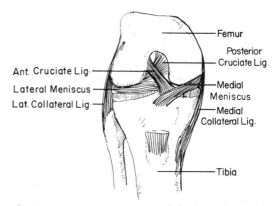

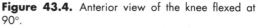

Figure 43.4. Anterior view of the knee flexed at 90°.

the medial aspect of the tibia. It is actually incorporated into the joint capsule. The deep fibers insert along the edge of the tibia, and the superficial portion extends more distally to insert on the tibial flare. The superficial portion provides stability in all degrees of knee flexion. The deep portion of the ligament lends stability mainly with the joint in full extension.

Anterior Cruciate Ligament. This ligament arises in the anterior intercondylar area of the tibia and inserts on the posterior medial aspect of the

lateral femoral epicondyle. It limits the degree of forward motion of the tibia in relation to the femur.

Posterior Cruciate Ligament. This ligament arises from the posterior tibia and traverses the joint space to insert on the medial aspect of the medial femoral epicondyle. This ligament limits the degree of posterior motion of the tibia in relation to the femur.

Medial and Lateral Menisci

These cartilaginous structures help "center" the femoral condyles as they rotate on the tibial plateau. The menisci attach to the medial and lateral margins of the tibia by the coronary ligaments. The lateral meniscus is more mobile than the medial meniscus, which may account for the lower prevalence of lateral meniscal tears. The menisci are best palpated with the knee in flexion, as shown in Figure 43.4.

Patella

The patella is a large, disc-shaped sesamoid bone located in front of the knee. It lies within the common tendon sheath of the extensor muscles of the knee (the quadriceps group, made up of the rectus femoris, vastus intermedius, vastus lateralis, and the vastus medialis). The patella stabilizes the joint and improves the mechanical advantage of the quadriceps muscles as they cross the knee to insert on the tibial tuberosity.

When the knee extends, the patella is normally pulled vertically and slightly medially. Hypermobility of the patella is thought to be present when the quadriceps are inadequately strengthened and toned, at least relative to the hamstrings. In such persons, the patella does not ride correctly in the patellar groove. The resulting *patellar tracking syndrome* (formerly called chondromalacia) presents as knee pain with tenderness around the lower medial aspect of the patella or the adjacent tibial plateau. Characteristically, the pain is worst when walking down stairs and can be reproduced by firm compression of the patella into the medial femoral groove while the knee is in slight flexion. Runners are prone to this condition, known as runner's knee, if they do not exercise to strengthen the quadriceps and stretch the hamstring.

EXAMINATION OF THE KNEE

Inspection

1. Observe the person walking. In an acute injury, shortened stride length and reduced weight-bearing time will be present on the affected side. These combined changes create the appearance of a hobble.
2. Look for evidence of muscle atrophy, especially in the quadriceps group. Muscle atrophy suggests a chronic problem.
3. Look for swelling about the knee joint. It may represent either fluid accumulation within bursae or intra-articular fluid.
4. Standing, the knees are normally fully extended. Persistent flexion may represent knee, hip, or even foot contractures or other pathology causing pain on extension.

Palpation and Range of Motion

With the patient sitting with knees flexed, check for range of motion. Note that extension of the leg is accompanied by external rotation of the tibia. The reverse occurs as the leg is flexed. Generally flexion will be approximately 135° (from the fully extended position) and internal and external rotation approximately 10°. Checking for specific structural integrity involves the following important structures: (*a*) cruciate ligaments, (*b*) collateral ligaments, and (*c*) menisci.

Anterior Cruciate Ligament. This ligament prevents the tibia from riding forward in relation to the femur. With the patient sitting, place one hand behind the upper tibia and the other over the patella. Attempt to force the upper tibia forward to test the integrity of the anterior cruciate ligament. Reversing the force by placing one hand over the anterior part of the upper tibia and the other hand behind the lower femur, test for posterior cruciate stability. If laxity is detected, compare the opposite knee. Abnormal movement on testing the cruciate ligaments is often referred to as the drawer sign, because the tibia moves forward or backward below the femur like a drawer pulls in or out.

Other structures, such as the joint capsule and the medial and lateral ligaments, lend secondary support in preventing anteroposterior instability. However, without cruciate ligament integrity, these secondary supports are not sufficient to maintain joint stability.

Medial Collateral Ligament. This is the knee ligament most commonly injured. With the leg in full extension, secondary structures lend considerable stability to the knee against valgus stress. The secondary support structures are the joint capsule and the cruciate ligaments. You may miss a significant injury to the medial collateral ligament if you test only in full extension. Therefore, test this ligament with the knee flexed 30°, stabilizing the femur by placing one hand over the lower lateral aspect. With the opposite hand placed around the ankle, force the leg laterally (valgus stress).

Lateral Collateral Ligaments. To test these ligaments force the leg medially (varus stress). Look for abnormal displacement or, in a recent injury, pain at the site of the injured ligament. The more acute the injury, the more gentle the force exerted, to minimize patient discomfort. Again, if laxity is noted, compare with the opposite side.

Testing for an Acute Meniscal Injury. This injury typically results in a dramatic inability to flex or extend the joint. The mechanical "locking" is caused by a displaced or edematous meniscus. After the acute phase, locking may become intermittent.

With the patient sitting and the knee flexed, locate the joint line just lateral and medial to the midportion of the patellar tendon. Using the medial femoral condyle as a fulcrum, rotate the tibia internally as you palpate the anterior lateral joint line. A pop or tenderness indicates lateral meniscus injury. Using the lateral femoral condyle as a fulcrum, rotate the tibia externally and forward; tenderness or a pop over the medial joint line indicates injury to the medial meniscus.

Evaluation for Joint Effusion. Large amounts of effusion in the knee cause obvious swelling. Tense effusions cause pain and disability in movement that can be greatly relieved by a therapeutic joint aspiration. Smaller amounts of effusion can be detected by balloting the patella. With the knee in full extension, compress the suprapatellar bursa just above the knee cap with one hand and press firmly on the patella with the other thumb. If the patella is resting on bone, no ballotment will be felt. If some effusion is present, it will lift the patella, and pressing will cause it to travel some distance (ballot) down onto the bones.

DIAGNOSIS AND MANAGEMENT

Classification of Injury

Grade 1. Mild pain and tenderness, minimal swelling, and no instability or significant disability.

Grade 2. More severe pain and tenderness, moderate swelling; difficulty walking, and partial joint instability with moderate disability.

Grade 3. Severe pain, marked swelling, marked instability, and inability to use the knee.

Principles of Management

Treatment of knee injuries depends on the estimated severity of the problem and the suspected diagnosis. If the mechanism of injury is compatible with a fracture and the examination is suggestive or the patient cannot bear weight, obtain x-ray films. If a fracture is present, the knee should be immobilized with a cast or a knee brace (depending on the specific injury). If a cast is applied, extend it from just above the ankle to the upper thigh. Fiberglass casts, being lightweight and waterproof, are preferred. Knee braces come in a variety of sizes and extend from below the calf to approximately midthigh.

Even if the x-ray film fails to confirm a fracture, any patient who has pain on weight bearing should be given crutches and asked to return in 48 hours for a reexamination. During the interim, the patient should ice the knee and should not bear weight.

If the injury is ligamentous, a complete tear (grade 3 injury) generally needs surgery, although not necessarily immediately. An orthopaedic surgeon should be consulted within 7 to 10 days of such an injury. Other ligamentous injuries should be treated with immobilization and a gradual increase in activity. Meniscal injuries do not heal, so they almost always need eventual surgery.

Although grade 2 injuries are commonly casted, removable immobilization splints are usually effective and may prevent excessive muscle loss and avoid the necessity for prolonged rehabilitation. A padded knee brace with rigid stays and Velcro fasteners is a reasonable alternative to a cast. This facilitates examination on return visits, application of ice or heat, gentle range-of-motion exercises, and potentially earlier mobilization.

There is little danger in taking your time making a diagnosis, as long as the patient does not bear weight on a painful knee. Thus, a trial of immobilization and crutches is indicated for most knee injuries.

Since one cannot predict how long an injured ligament will take to regain anatomical and functional normalcy, frequent follow-up visits are essential. Table 43.1 lists the indications for x-ray films and immediate referral.

Immediate Management

Regardless of the severity of the injury, the goals of immediate management are reduction of swelling and pain relief. Compression and ice, when used early, can help reduce swelling. If elastic wrap is used, the 6-inch width is best. Although firm compression is indicated, instruct the

Table 43.1. Indications for X-ray Films and Immediate Referral for Arthroscopy and Possible Surgery

All grade 3 injuries
Tense effusion that comes on quickly
Severe trauma with an inability to bear weight
Severe pain
Obvious bony deformity
Persistent locking of the knee

patient to look for lower leg swelling and to reapply the wrap with less tension if swelling is noted. Ice massage can be used to minimize swelling in the first 48 hours after injury. Gentle massage over the injured area for 15 minutes every 4 hours is recommended.

After 48 hours (some wait for edema to subside), application of heat for 30 minutes three or four times daily may facilitate healing. A heating pad, hot water bottle, or heating lamp are all acceptable.

Pain relief is important for patient comfort. Acetaminophen alone or with codeine may be indicated initially, but if analgesia is required beyond 48 hours, you should suspect more serious injury. A nonsteroidal antiinflammatory drug may be useful after the first week to reduce inflammation and promote compliance with the rehabilitation regimen.

Rehabilitation

The primary goal of rehabilitation is to decrease the inevitable losses associated with forced inactivity. We are concerned about not only the healing of injured structures, but also the condition of other supporting muscles and ligaments and total body fitness. Collagen fibers, ligament strength, and general muscle tone all suffer losses within weeks and even days of inactivity.

Exercises can be divided into two general categories, static (isotonic) and dynamic. Two types of dynamic exercise equipment are widely available, variable resistance (e.g., Nautilus, Universal) and accommodating variable resistance (e.g., Cybex, Orthotron). For the average person, isotonic exercises are adequate, and the equipment is readily accessible or can be improvised. When speed as well as strength is important, e.g., for the athlete, exercise using variable-resistance equipment is helpful. The Canadian Air Force exercises achieve general body conditioning; books describing these and other conditioning exercises

are available in most bookstores. Exercises are graded according to the individual's general level of physical fitness.

Once the symptoms have subsided, resistance exercises can be started. These exercises are aimed at strengthening the quadriceps group as well as the hamstring muscles. With the patient in a sitting position begin with the foot on a low stool and the knee extended about 150°. Then extend the knee as close to 180° as is comfortable. This avoids the area between 130° and 150°, referred to as the crepitant range, which represents the position of maximal patellar stress. Begin without weights, repeating 10 times. Gradually add ankle weights (pennies in a sock will do). Progressively increase both the weight and the number of repetitions, depending on the patient's general strength and comfort. Knee bends are recommended, but flexion must be limited to 40°.

Return athletes to their sports activity as early as can be safely allowed. A simple side-to-side exercise described by Montgomery and Steadman can be used to determine when they can resume competitive activity. With the feet spread slightly beyond shoulder width, the subject hops from one foot to the other for 10 minutes or until discomfort occurs. When this exercise can be completed without pain, full activity can be resumed.

CONCLUSIONS

Knee injuries are the most common cause of disability in sports. The knee is the most vulnerable joint during weight bearing, both on the job and at play. The common injuries described in this chapter are easily diagnosed and managed in family practice. Not many family physicians choose to be team physicians, but all will have to evaluate knees and advise treatment for the common injuries.

SUGGESTED READINGS

Collins HR: Screening of athletic knee injuries. *Clin Sports Med* 4:217–230, 1985.

Especially useful for the team doctor or trainer; discusses on-site evaluation.

Jensen JE, Conn RR, Hazelrigg G, Hewett JE: Systematic evaluation of acute knee injuries. *Clin Sports Med* 4:295–312, 1985.

Comprehensive coverage of acute knee injury examination and evaluation. Presents useful form for objectively documenting degree of injury and function.

Montgomery JB, Steadman JR: Rehabilitation of the injured knee. *Clin Sports Med* 4:333–343, 1985.

Excellent review of rehabilitation following knee injuries. Clearly described with emphasis on readily
available modalities.

Polisson RP: Sports medicine for the internist. *Med Clin
North Am* 70:469–489, 1986.

Outlines how you approach a patient with a painful
knee. Nice differential of overuse syndromes of the
knee.

chapter 44

ANKLE INJURIES

Peter J. Rizzolo

Ankle injuries are among the most common orthopaedic problems seen by family physicians. Their incidence is likely to increase further with the escalating public enthusiasm for fast-paced sports. There are two keys to effective management:

1. A proper appreciation of the functional anatomy of the joint;
2. A planned progression from the initial immobilization phase of treatment to an active rehabilitation program that will return the patient swiftly, but safely, to full and normal activity.

ANATOMICAL CONSIDERATIONS

Three bones form the ankle joint: the fibula and tibia superiorly and the talus inferiorly. The recess formed by the distal tibia and fibula is referred to as the ankle mortise. The articular surface of the talus is wedge-shaped, with the anterior transverse diameter being wider than the posterior diameter as shown in Figure 44.1.

Because of this, when the foot is in dorsiflexion, the widest portion of the talus fits snugly into the joint mortise, increasing joint stability. With the foot in plantar flexion, the narrowest portion of the talus fits into the joint mortise, causing a looser fit and increasing the instability of the joint.

The ankle joint is stabilized by ligaments both lateral and medial to the joint. The lateral ligaments are: the anterior talofibular ligament, the calcaneofibular ligament, and the posterior talofibular ligament. The lateral ligaments are relatively lax and allow for considerable internal rotation of the foot. They are depicted in Figure 44.2.

Over the medial aspect of the ankle are the superficial and deep deltoid ligaments, which connect the tibia to the talus, navicular, and calcaneous bones. The superficial deltoid consists of three ligaments: the tibionavicular, the calcaneotibial, and the superficial talotibial. The deep deltoid ligament consists of the anterior talotibial and the posterior talotibial ligaments. Figures 44.3 and 44.4 show the medial ligaments of the ankle.

Traversing the joint are several tendons involved in flexion and extension of the foot as well as inversion and eversion. These tendons serve as a secondary support system for the ankle joint.

MECHANISMS OF INJURY OF THE ANKLE

Forced inversion of the ankle causes 90% of all ankle injuries. The specific ligament injured will depend on the position of the foot at the time of the injury. With the foot in plantar flexion, the anterior talofibular ligament is placed under tension. This is the ligament most likely to be injured if the foot is now forcibly inverted. With the foot dorsiflexed, the posterior talofibular ligament is under tension, and inversion will now injure this ligament. With the foot in a neutral position, forced inversion will most likely injure the calcaneofibular ligament.

The medial ligaments of the ankle joint (deltoid ligaments) are very tight and allow much less motion than do the lateral ligaments. Consequently, forced eversion accounts for less than 10% of all ankle injuries. Deltoid ligament injuries are caused by forced eversion of the ankle, usually accompanied by internal rotation of the tibia on the foot. Because of this rotational force, the anterior component of the deltoid ligaments is usually injured first.

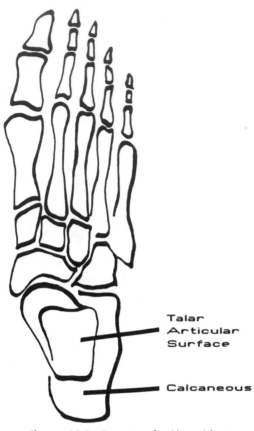

Talar
Articular
Surface

Calcaneous

Figure 44.1. Top view of ankle and foot.

CLASSIFICATION OF ANKLE INJURIES

Ankle injuries are classified in two ways. We can describe the anatomical changes in the ankle ligaments, such as a minor partial tear of the ligament, major partial tear of a ligament, or complete tear of a ligament. A more useful classification for the family physician is one based on the functional status of the ankle. This classification is outlined below.

Grade 1 injury.
A partial ligamentous tearing but of insufficient degree to cause joint instability.
Grade 2 injury.
A partial ligamentous tear, but joint motion is abnormal when the ankle is stressed by manipulation of the joint.
Grade 3 injury.
A complete tear of the ligament causing frank instability of the ankle joint.

EVALUATION OF ANKLE INJURIES

Initiate the history taking with an open-ended question about how the accident happened. A complete description should include answers to the following: Did the foot invert or evert during the course of the injury? Was there a twisting motion of the leg? Was the foot in plantar flexion or dorsiflexion at the time of the injury? Where does it hurt? (Ask the patient to point with one finger.)

Ask what happened immediately after the injury. If the patient was able to get up and walk around or continue activity, a serious ligamentous injury or fracture is less likely. If the ankle became swollen and discolored within minutes after injury, a severe soft tissue injury or even fracture should be suspected.

The physical examination should include inspection and palpation. During inspection, look for swelling in the area of the internal and external malleoli. Compare the landmarks with those of the opposite foot. Any deformity suggests either localized swelling or bleeding and helps to localize the area of injury. Additionally, skin discoloration indicates bleeding into the tissues. A small amount of discoloration suggests partial ligamentous damage, whereas marked discoloration is commonly associated with a fracture or a more extensive ligamentous injury.

Palpate for areas of tenderness, which will help localize the injured structures. Compare the passive range of motion of the injured ankle with the opposite ankle. Crepitus is often associated with a fracture. A useful maneuver is the *anterior drawer sign*. In doing this maneuver, the injured foot is placed in a plantar-flexed position, and with one hand stabilizing the tibia, the opposite hand is placed behind the heel, and the foot is drawn forward. The degree of forward motion is compared with that of the opposite foot; if exaggerated, it suggests disruption of the anterior talofibular ligament.

X-ray films are not necessary for most ankle injuries. Indications for x-ray films include (*a*) a history of not being able to bear weight immediately after the injury; (*b*) an ankle that develops marked swelling and discoloration soon after the injury; (*c*) marked pain on range of motion and manipulation of the ankle and those areas that you would presume to be most stressed in a particular injury; (*d*) crepitation on palpation or movement of the ankle; (*e*) instances in which litigation may be an issue, such as following motor vehicle accidents, injury in a public place, or suspected abuse.

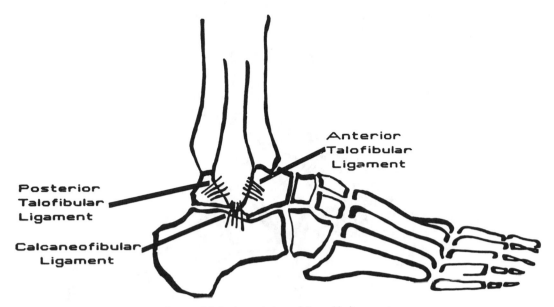

Figure 44.2. Lateral view of the ankle ligaments.

Anterior
Talofibular
Ligament

Posterior
Talofibular
Ligament

Calcaneofibular
Ligament

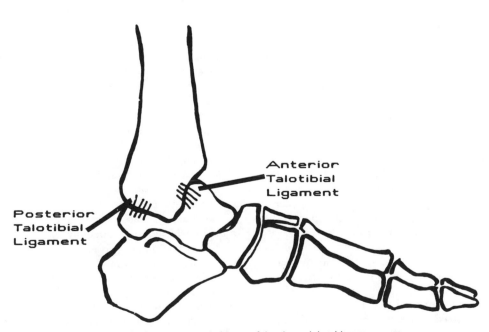

Figure 44.3. Medial view of the deep deltoid ligaments.

Anterior
Talotibial
Ligament

Posterior
Talotibial
Ligament

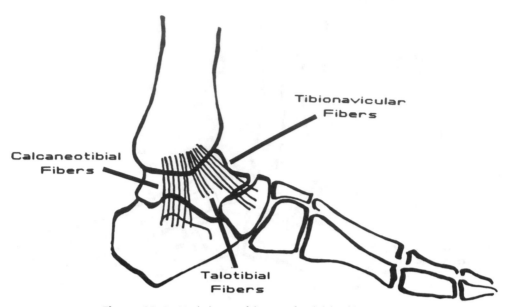

Figure 44.4. Medial view of the superficial deltoid ligament.

TREATMENT OF ANKLE INJURIES

Treatment of ankle injuries involves two phases: (*a*) acute care, which is aimed at relieving pain and reducing swelling, and (*b*) rehabilitation.

Acute Care

Treatment routinely focuses on compression, ice, elevation, pain control, use of braces, casting, and instruction in the proper use of crutches. The grade of injury will dictate variations in the use of each of these potential treatment approaches.

Compression and elevation limit the leakage of blood and extracellular fluid around the injured area. By reducing swelling, these measures help an ankle injury heal faster. Generally, compression is done using elastic bandages such as the Ace wrap. Total pressure on the ankle is related to the degree of stretching and the number of turns around the ankle. If compression is done improperly and too much pressure is applied over the ankle, edema distal to the dressing may occur. Elevation of the injury promotes venous return by decreasing venous pressure in the lower extremity, thereby decreasing edema. When sitting, the patient should be positioned so that the ankle is elevated to hip level.

An effective method that combines cold and pressure is soaking one or more Ace bandages in ice water and applying them immediately after an ankle injury. The cold Ace bandage can be applied to the ankle and after a turn or two some ice incorporated into the wrapping. After the ice is removed from the ankle, a dry bandage can be applied.

Fitting crutches properly and teaching their correct use are crucial to treatment and rehabilitation. Crutches provide the patient with safe mobility during convalescence only if they are used correctly. Crutches that are too short for the patient are ineffective in weight bearing. A pair that is too long and that fits closely to the armpit will strain the axilla and may cause neuromuscular damage. Proper fitting should be done by experienced personnel.

Since early ambulation is the key to more rapid and complete recovery after ankle injury, ankle braces that allow dorsiflexion and plantarflexion, while limiting internal and external rotation, are useful. The *pneumatic compression brace* is especially useful since it is rigid enough to maintain good lateral and medial support while being able to adjust to the individual's ankle anatomy and varying degrees of edema. In persons with grade I and II injuries, ambulation can often be started as soon as the individual can stand without pain. Additionally, since the brace can be removed readily, application of ice or heat is greatly facilitated.

A crucial, but often neglected, aspect of treatment is adequate follow-up care. After the initial assessment, the patient should be seen at 48 hours and again 1 to 2 weeks after the injury. Reevaluation of the injury is imperative to insure that the sprain is healing properly and the patient is complying.

Rehabilitation

The transition from immobilization to rehabilitation is a gradual one. As soon as pain at rest is gone, gentle range-of-motion exercises are begun, often augmented by ice massage or heat. Gradually, the patient progresses to walking and running. While ligaments are healing, keeping the muscles well-toned will add support for the ankle. Thus, rehabilitation tries to keep the muscles toned by using particular exercises.

As with acute treatment, rehabilitation exercises differ, depending on the grade of injury. With grade 1 injuries, the rehabilitation program begins during the first office visit. The patient is placed on crutches and instructed to partially bear weight. This helps maintain the strength of the dorsiflexors and plantiflexors. After 48 hours, the patient is instructed in range-of-motion and isometric exercises.

In children, range-of-motion exercises can be easily done by asking them to write with their affected foot in midair, imagining a pencil between their toes. This activity puts the ankle through a full range of motion, and they can do this four times daily. Adults can be instructed in how to put the foot through the full range of motion: inversion, eversion, dorsiflexion, and plantarflexion. This again can be done four times daily. It should be done gently, without springing or snapping motion.

Isometric exercises can also be started. The ankle itself is not moved during the course of the exercise, but force is applied through the foot as though moving the ankle in that particular direction. For example, to strengthen invertors with isometric exercise, place the foot against a bedpost and force the foot inward while it is snug up against the post. This does not permit the foot to move, but it does strengthen the muscles. Maintain the force for 5 seconds. Likewise, the lateral surface of the foot can be placed against the bedpost and force exerted as though everting the foot. In a similar way, with the person lying supine, the foot can be hooked under the edge of the bed rail and force applied in the dorsiflexion direction. Again, the foot can be placed in front of the bed

rail and plantarflexion force applied. The force is maintained each time for 5 seconds. Advise five repetitions in each of the four directions, four times daily.

By 2 weeks, the patient with a grade 1 injury should have progressed to full weight bearing. Then isotonic exercises can be started. In this instance the foot is moved through a range of motion against a fixed weight or force. A very simple way to do this is have the person start to run figure eights. As people run around the loop in one direction they will be building up the muscles that evert the foot, and as they circle and run around in the other direction, they are building up the muscles that invert the foot. With runners, to avoid reinjuring the ankle, have them run on a flat surface for a few weeks.

With grade 2 injuries, weight bearing is not allowed for 48 hours or until standing is no longer painful. At that point, encourage partial weight bearing with crutches. As with grade 1 injuries, if there is discomfort or swelling, stay with isometric exercises. Once the pain and swelling subside, usually within a few days, isotonic exercises can be started as with grade 1 injuries.

Management of grade 3 ankle injuries should be done in consultation with appropriate orthopaedic specialists.

OTHER MANAGEMENT TECHNIQUES

Using a small block of ice to massage a healing injury has many proponents among sports-oriented physicians. An ice block can be made by partially filling a paper cup with water and placing it in the freezer compartment of the refrigerator. The ice block can be removed from the paper cup when needed. The injured area is gently massaged with the ice block for 10 to 15 minutes three or four times daily or after exercising. Since heat tends to dilate peripheral vessels, warm soaks may actually promote bleeding during the first day or two after an injury. In fact, how soon to start warm soaks is controversial, and many do not advocate the use of heat until all swelling is gone.

After the ankle has healed, taping it prior to strenuous physical activity may provide stabilization and prevent a repeat injury. Taping is particularly recommended for individuals who have repeatedly injured an ankle. The technique of taping an ankle is simple but does require some practice. Figure 44.5 shows one approach to ankle taping.

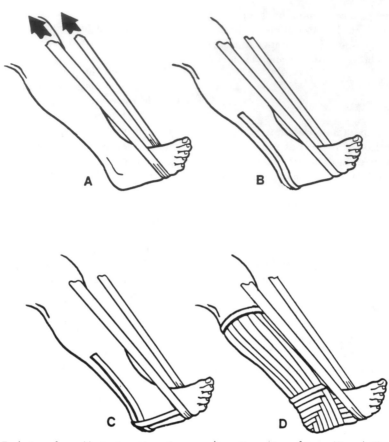

Figure 44.5. Technique for ankle taping. Have the patient use tape or a strap to hold the ankle at 90° dorsiflexion (A). Then, beginning near the heel, apply alternating strips of tape (B and C), which create a tight support by overlapping each other (D).

SPECIFIC TREATMENT RECOMMENDATIONS

Grade 1 Injuries

1. Apply ice as soon as possible and for 20 minutes every 2 to 4 hours for the first 48 hours.
2. Apply an elastic wrap or pneumatic compression brace.
3. Elevate the foot when sitting (hip level).
4. Restrict to partial weight bearing with crutches for first 48 hours or until standing is no longer painful.
5. Use analgesics, acetaminophen, or acetaminophen with codeine for pain.
6. Return visit after 48 hours. At that time advise the patient to (*a*) begin range-of-motion and isometric exercises, (*b*) progress to full weight bearing as tolerated (a cane may help the transition), and (*c*) use intermittent warm soaks (discontinuing ice packs).
7. Reevaluate in 1 week. If symptoms are minimal, allow full weight bearing. Start gastrocnemius-strengthening and heel-cord-stretching exercises. Aim toward full activity by 2 weeks. Taping is often helpful for vigorous sports activity.

Grade 2 Injuries

1. Apply ice immediately and for 20 minutes every 2 to 4 hours.
2. Apply pneumatic compression brace or Ace wrap; casting is controversial.
3. Use crutches and no weight bearing for 48 hours or until standing is no longer painful. Then allow partial weight bearing (with crutches) and progressive ambulation.

4. Begin exercise program described for grade 1 injury.
5. Return visits at 48 hours and approximately weekly thereafter.

Grade 3 Injuries

Consultation with an orthopaedic specialist is indicated for all grade 3 injuries. The choice between nonoperative or operative management depends on many factors. The patient's age, general health, usual physical activities, and avocations all must be taken into consideration. At one time, all grade 3 injuries were thought to require open surgical treatment. However, at the present time, many orthopaedic surgeons are tailoring the treatment of these injuries to the factors already noted.

Fractures

All ligaments connect two bones. Occasionally, the bones themselves rather than the ligaments give way, leading to fracture. This is particularly common in children, where the growing epiphyseal plates are often weaker than the corresponding ligaments. At any age, severe injuries can affect both ligaments and bone, often leading to joint instability, rapid swelling, and pain on weight bearing. Localized tenderness over bone, very rapid swelling after injury, marked pain on standing still, and obvious bony deformity suggest fracture and should prompt x-ray films. All fractures must be immobilized, with the type and duration of immobilization varying according to the severity of the injury and the age of the patient.

Case 1

A 30-year-old mildly overweight woman who recently started an aerobic exercise program visits you because of ankle pain. On her second visit to the aerobic center, she stepped backward, stepping on someone's foot and turning her left ankle. The ankle turned in toward the midline, causing severe pain and a tearing sensation on the outside of her ankle. It became swollen and discolored within a few minutes. A friend drove her home, where she took two aspirin and applied a heating pad to her injured ankle. As her physician, you see her the following morning, 16 hours after the injury.

You obtain a detailed history of the mechanism of injury, onset of symptoms, and course of events following the injury. You determine that she is nonathletic with no previous history of ankle injury and that her ankle turned inward and probably sustained a significant ligamentous tear, based on the severity of symptoms and the early onset of swelling and bruising. Significant findings on your physical examination include tenderness when you palpate over the anterior talofibular and calcaneofibular ligaments of her left ankle. Manipulations that would predictably stress those ligaments cause increased pain. Because of her excess weight, severity of pain, and rapid onset of swelling and bruising, you decide to obtain an x-ray film; it does not reveal any evidence of bony injury.

You diagnose a grade 2 ankle injury and initiate analgesia with acetaminophen, compression with a Ace wrap, elevation to hip level, application of ice for 20 minutes every 4 hours, and non-weight-bearing with crutches for 48 hours, which is when you ask her to return.

Reassessment at 48 hours reveals a trace of edema and slight tenderness to palpation over the lateral ligaments. She is anxious to get back to her exercise program, convinced that she will gain 10 pounds sitting around the house. After demonstrating in the office that she can stand straight on the ankle without increasing pain, you advise her to partially weight bear on her ankle. She is instructed on partial weight bearing with crutches and on using heat when all traces of swelling have disappeared. You advise either a hot water bottle applied for 20 minutes every 4 hours, or a heating pad with the same duration and frequency. She is to continue using a compression bandage and is asked to return in 1 week (approximately 9 days following her injury).

On her return visit her symptoms are much improved, and she can tolerate gentle range of motion. She does not require any analgesia. You instruct her about isometric exercises and ask her to do them for 15 minutes, four times daily. She is also given written instructions on exercises and instructed to switch from crutches to a cane for partial weight bearing. She is instructed in the proper use of the cane.

She will be seen approximately every 2 weeks until you determine full healing has occurred. Whenever the ankle can be placed through a full range of motion without eliciting pain you can begin isotonic exercises to help build muscle strength. Subsequently, her rehabilitation program will include walking, then running on a level surface, and then running figure eights, following each exercise session with a 20-minute ice massage. At that point she can return to full activity, including her exercise program.

SUGGESTED READINGS

Garrick JG: The athlete's ankle and other injuries. *Emerg Med* 14:178–209, 1982.

Very practical approach with common sense rationale for a variety of therapeutic modalities.

Guise ER: Rotational ligamentous injuries to the ankle in football. *Am J Sports Med* 4:1–6, 1976.

Useful for individuals working with athletes. Discussion of rehabilitation limited.

Seligson D, Gassman J, Pope M: Ankle instability: evaluation of the lateral ligaments. *Am J Sports Med* 8:32–42, 1980.

Emphasis on evaluation of lateral ankle instability. Useful, but limited focus.

Smith RW, Reischl SF: Treatment of ankle sprains in young athletes. *Am J Sports Med* 14:465–471, 1986.

Emphasis on treatment complements other articles that stress other aspects of ankle injuries.

Stover CN: Recognition and management of soft tissue injuries of the ankle in the athlete. *Prim Care* 7:183–197, 1980.

Excellent discussion of anatomical considerations that predispose to injuries.

chapter 45

MINOR SKIN WOUNDS: LACERATIONS, CONTUSIONS, AND ABRASIONS

Wayne A. Hale

Injuries to the skin are commonly cared for by the family physician. Although there are many different forms of skin wounds, this discussion is limited to contusions, abrasions, and lacerations. These types of wounds were third most frequent among all diagnoses in a large study of family practices (1). Thus, skill in the management of these traumatic injuries is an important component of family practice training.

Wounds can present dramatically. In all situations, the physician must initially focus on the basics of emergency care. An uncompromised airway, control of bleeding, and adequate circulation must be assured before more specific evaluation of the wound can proceed.

A good history of how the injury happened facilitates evaluation and treatment. An accurate examination is essential. This should be summarized by a note in the medical record that describes the age, size, shape, and extent of the wound and the amount of contamination. Descriptions of lacerations, such as linear, irregular, beveled, or flap, help clarify the approach to their repair. Drawings and photographs may be very useful for later comparison.

The key to evaluating skin wounds is to think carefully about the type of injury that occurred and the nearby structures that might be affected. During your examination, palpate for a foreign body or fracture. Plain x-ray films or xeroradiographs should be used if deeper foreign bodies are suspected. Consider the possibility of injury to vital structures near the wound, such as nerves, tendons, or ducts (e.g., the parotid duct). Deep penetration by the injuring instrument or a high-pressure injection injury may make open exploration necessary. Wounds affected by electrical, thermal, or chemical insult need special evaluation and care, as do bites and puncture wounds. In proximal limb injuries, consider and rule out injury to peripheral motor and sensory nerves.

Once your evaluation is complete, if the problem is indeed a minor skin wound, you can proceed to treatment, following the general principles outlined in this chapter. If the wound is complicated or if an optimum outcome is doubtful, obtain consultation after your preliminary evaluation and treatment.

Any time you treat such patients, remember to inquire about *tetanus immunization* status and to give any indicated immunization. A tetanus booster should be given if the patient has not had one within 5 years for dirty wounds or 10 years for clean wounds. If the patient has not had the primary series of tetanus immunization or if the wound is grossly contaminated, tetanus immune globulin should also be administered. Those patients lacking previous immunization (as is true for many elderly) should then be advised to have a tetanus booster in 1 month and again in 6 to 12 months.

CONTUSIONS

A contusion (also known as a bruise or ecchymosis) results from trauma that injures underlying soft-tissue structures while leaving the epidermis intact. Cellular, vascular, and lymphatic damage causes blood and other fluids to leak into the tissue, producing swelling and discoloration. If enough extravasated blood collects to produce a palpable "knot," a hematoma is said to have formed.

Large bruises can take weeks to resolve, particularly if there is accompanying hematoma forma-

415

tion. The area of ecchymosis will gradually change from a blue or purple color to yellow-brown as the blood is converted to hematin and reabsorbed. These ecchymoses may travel to more dependent areas. Often, hematomas around the knee or calf will also result in ecchymoses in the ankle or foot. Hematomas usually clot and become quite firm, then become red, warm, and tender as the clot liquefies. At this stage they may appear to be infected, although this is seldom the case. Instructing patients about the sequence they can expect will reduce their concerns during the healing process.

Initial treatment of contusions and hematomas is directed at minimizing hemorrhage and edema. This is accomplished by elevating the affected part and by applying pressure and ice. Tissue cooling often provides adequate anesthesia, but acetaminophen and occasionally codeine may be needed. In general, hematomas should not be aspirated or otherwise drained because of the risk of infection and their tendency to recur. If the amount of bleeding seems out of proportion to the injury, consider an underlying hemostatic disorder. However, remember that tissue fragility normally increases as people age. After 72 hours, heat may be applied to these injuries to increase local blood flow and hasten resolution.

ABRASIONS

Abrasions are caused by scraping trauma that removes epidermis. Bicycle or motorcycle accidents, for example, which cause the rider to scrape along the pavement, are frequent causes of severe abrasions. These injuries tend to be quite painful because of the exposure of many nerve endings. Before anesthesia, this pain may raise the question of significant underlying injury. As in a second degree burn, the loss of epidermis causes the skin to lose water through weeping and evaporation. These injuries are most often over joint surfaces, and the scab that forms tends to crack open when the joint moves.

The general management of abrasions is to clean them carefully and then treat them like burns. Like burns, these injuries heal best if they are free from infection and are kept moist until reepithelialized. Adequate cleaning usually requires good anesthesia. Topical anesthetic agents may be sufficient for superficial abrasions, but deep or dirty wounds generally require anesthetic injection. The cleansing itself involves irrigation with sterile saline or a mild antiseptic solution. Using forceps, you should remove ground-in dirt as completely as possible, to prevent tattoo formation.

Once the abrasion is clean, apply an antibiotic ointment and a protective dressing. The antibiotic ointment will keep the healing abrasion soft and pliable while protecting against infection. A number of synthetic semiocclusive transparent wound coverings (such as Op-Site) are available; these retain moisture while allowing oxygen to reach the wound. Nonstick absorbent pads, such as Telfa or gauze coated with petroleum jelly, also work well. If the abraded area is extensive, see the patient every day or two in follow-up until healing is assured.

LACERATIONS

A laceration is a slice or tear in the skin or mucosa. Approximating the wound edges with sutures or adhesive strips minimizes scar formation and healing time. Superficial wounds may simply require cleansing and dressing.

Lacerations whose edges are minimally separated can be closed with sterile adhesive strips; cleaning the skin with ether or applying tincture of benzoin greatly improves their adhesion. Larger lacerations and those located in areas of stretch require suture closure.

The timing of wound closure is important. The risk of infection is lowest if a laceration is repaired within 6 hours, although very clean wounds generally do well if closed within 24 hours. Beyond these limits, the wound should simply be cleaned, inspected, and then dressed, because suturing would promote infection by introducing foreign material and preventing drainage. If there is no sign of infection by the third to fifth day and approximation of wound edges is desirable, then the wound may be sutured.

Bites and puncture wounds are particularly susceptible to infection if closed. Human bites, because of the large number of bacteria in saliva, require particularly careful cleaning and observation and generally should be treated as infected from the onset.

Inspection and Cleansing

Evaluation and treatment of larger lacerations require adequate anesthesia. For patients such as young children or demented adults, premedication with narcotics and/or sedatives may be needed. Reassurance, explanation, and firm restraint usually make local anesthetic sufficient. To lessen the pain of injection, use a small-gauge (25- to 30-gauge) needle inserted through the wound into the dermis. Lidocaine (Xylocaine) in 1 or 2% concentration is the most commonly used anesthetic solution. Before injection, it must be ascertained that the patient is not allergic to the medication. Although it is permissible to give up to 7 mg of lidocaine per kg of body weight (the 1% solution contains 10 mg/ml), use the minimum amount necessary, to avoid toxicity. Preparations that combine lidocaine with epinephrine can be used to decrease bleeding and prolong anesthesia. Epinephrine must not be used in areas where its vasoconstrictive effects might cause gangrene by compromising circulation, such as the fingers, toes, earlobes, or penis. Adequate anesthesia is generally produced in 10 minutes.

In some areas, a nerve block may be more effective than local injection. Circumferential blocks work well for injuries of the ear and nose. Block of the mental nerve produces good anesthesia to the lower lip and chin. Most frequently used is a *digital block* of a finger or toe. This can be performed by anesthetizing the dorsal and ventral nerve branches on each side of the affected digit. Alternatively, anesthetic solution can be placed on each side of the digit's metacarpal head to block the digital nerves before they branch. To perform a digital block, you can insert the needle through either the dorsal or palmar surface, but remember that the nerve is closer to the palm and adjacent to the bone. Often, your patient will report a shooting sensation down the digit when your needle touches the nerve. Aspirate through the needle to be sure you are not in a blood vessel, inject 2 or 3 ml of anesthetic, then reposition the needle and inject the nerve on the opposite side of the digit.

Under adequate anesthesia, the wound can be inspected and cleaned. An antiseptic solution, such as povidone-iodine (Betadine) or chlorhexidine (Hibiclens), can be used for initial cleaning of the surrounding skin, but not in the wound. If significant contamination with bacteria or chemicals is suspected, flush the wound profusely with sterile saline. A 19-gauge needle can be used with a 30- to 50-cc syringe or an IV bag with a compression device to provide a high-pressure stream. Gross dirt and other materials may require removal by forceps or by scrubbing with a brush or sponge. Severely contaminated or nonviable tissue should be debrided. This debridement must be done very

judiciously on areas (such as the face) where significant tissue loss can result in deformity. Cutting hair from around the laceration can make suturing easier. Try to avoid shaving eyebrows, because regrowth may be abnormal.

Preparing for Wound Repair

Having inspected and cleansed the wound and decided that it is appropriate for you to close the wound surgically, make certain that all potentially necessary instruments and supplies are at hand. Table 45.1 lists basic supplies for laceration repair.

A number of suture materials are available, and each has its advantages. Monofilament nylon or polypropylene sutures are initially more difficult to handle than silk and other braided suture materials, but they produce less skin reactivity and fewer infections. On the other hand, braided sutures cause less discomfort on mucosal surfaces (such as the lip or tongue) than the stiffer monofilaments. For subsurface or mucosal repair, absorbable materials are preferred. Traditionally, catgut sutures have been used, but stronger materials such as braided polyglycolic acid or polydioxanone (a monofilament absorbable suture) are now preferred.

Attached to the suture is a curved needle, whose size and shape is generally shown on the package. A reverse cutting needle is appropriate in most circumstances. It should be held with a needle holder not less than one-third of the way from the blunt end. The proper grasp (Fig. 45.1), using the largest needle feasible, will minimize needle bending.

Before beginning the procedure, place the patient in a position that will be comfortable and allow optimal access to the wound. Seat yourself so that the wound and instrument tray can be reached

Table 45.1. Basic Supplies for Laceration Repair

Gauze sponges
Sterile gloves
Sterile drapes
Adequate lighting
Toothed pick-up forceps
Two small hemostats
A smooth pick-up forceps
Needle holder
Suture scissors
Small curved scissors
Scalpel with #15 blade
Suture material
Skin hooks (optional)

easily. Have an assistant present who can obtain additional supplies and give surgical assistance if needed.

After the wound is anesthetized and cleaned, and you have positioned the patient and your instruments, you are ready to put on sterile gloves and drape the wound. When the wound involves the head or neck, take care that the drapes do not obstruct your patient's vision or respiration.

Next, examine the wound carefully and plan your repair. Wound edges should be made parallel if this can be done without removing essential tissue. If you will be making an incision to straighten a wound margin, first mark the incision with the scalpel, then use scissors to cut perpendicular to the skin surface. Excisions in hair-bearing skin should be parallel to the hair shafts, to avoid damage to the follicles. Since crushed tissue will not heal well, crushed areas with sufficient adjacent skin should be judiciously cut out with an elliptical incision whose length is three times its width. In areas like the nose, where there is no excess skin, it may be better to simply approximate the wound, planning later scar revision if necessary. After eval-

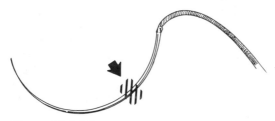

Figure 45.1. Correct position to grasp a suture needle. This provides enough length to rotate the needle through soft tissues; but is far enough forward to minimize bending.

uating the wound, if you do not believe you can perform an optimum repair, consult a surgeon who has the necessary skills.

Suturing Techniques

Appropriate closure technique varies with the depth of the laceration and the body area involved. Single-layer closure is used for superficial wounds and in areas with little subcutaneous tissue, such as the digits and back of the hands. It is also useful in the scalp, where hemostasis can be a problem. Layered repair is preferred for deeper wounds and for lacerations in cosmetically sensitive areas such as the face.

Principles of proper suture placement are shown in Figure 45.2. Insert your needle vertically or angulated away from the wound, with the goal of making the loop wider at the bottom than near the skin surface. This placement is aided by pulling the deeper layers toward the wound. Then, rotate your wrist to bring the needle up through the opposite wound edge, again going wider in the deeper tissue. This is accomplished by scraping the needle point back before puncturing up through the dermis. Ideally, the suture's depth should be greater than its width. This technique produces good results because it approximates the wound edge with some eversion, an optimal situation for healing. Minor differences in elevation of wound edges can often be adjusted by pulling the suture knot from one side to the other.

As a rule, sutures are placed as far apart as they are wide. In areas of skin tension, however, sutures should be closer together and closer to the wound edge. Figure 45.3 demonstrates this principle in the closure of an ellipse. Some surgeons like to

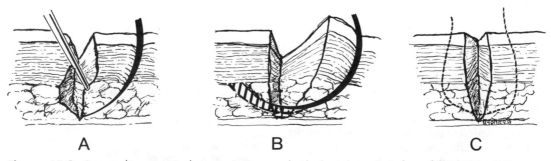

A   B   C

Figure 45.2. Proper skin suture technique. *A*, Perpendicular insertion of the needle is aided by traction at the fat-dermal layer. *B*, The needle point is dragged back along the undersurface of the dermis. *C*, Rotation of the needle while puncturing upward results in a suture wider at its base than at the surface.

close a wound by halving it, but it is probably better to start at one end and work toward the other, thereby reducing the tension on each suture.

Another method useful in lacerations with widely separated edges is the vertical mattress suture (Fig. 45.4). Mattress sutures provide greater strength and better approximation of tissue. They tend to heal leaving visible suture marks, however; so they should be alternated with simple sutures. The mattress sutures can then be removed early, leaving the simple sutures for support. Sterile adhesive strips are preferred by some physicians for surface closure, but they do not evert the wound edges and may not hold well in areas of skin movement.

The best technique for reducing tension on surface sutures is layered closure (Fig. 45.5). Layers that hold sutures are the fat-fascial, the fat-dermal, and the dermal-epithelial interfaces. Placement of deep sutures is aided by undermining the tissue below the layer being closed. In part A of Figure 45.5, undermining has been done in the fatty layer. In this type of tissue it is best to use the curved scissors in a spreading motion to minimize vascular and nerve disruption. Subepithelial sutures should be inverted so that the knots are buried. Most often, it is only necessary to suture the fat-dermal layer before final closure with simple sutures or a running subcuticular stitch. Multiple layer closures have been associated with increased infection, so this risk must be balanced against the benefits of decreased tension on wound edges.

Special techniques are needed in certain situations. V-shaped lacerations are best repaired using the technique shown in Figure 45.6, which minimizes risk of compromise to the blood supply at the tip of the flap.

When closing any wound, it is important to place sutures at equal distances on both sides. Despite efforts to do this, there will sometimes be more skin on one side than the other as the end of the wound is approached. The longer side tends to raise, making it difficult to approximate the edges without bunching on that side. This "dog's ear" can be approached as shown in Figure 45.7. Make the wound edges equal again by extending the wound with an incision at a 45° angle toward the side with excess length. After undermining, the overlapping "dog's ear" is excised, and the incision is sutured. If some excess still remains on that side, the process can be repeated.

AREA-SPECIFIC CONSIDERATIONS

The character of skin and subcutaneous tissue varies greatly over the body. As a result, common

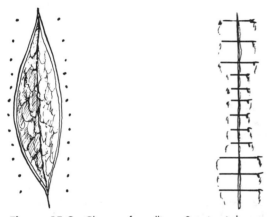

Figure 45.3. Closure of an ellipse. Suturing is begun at one end of the wound. As the middle is approached, sutures are placed closer to each other and closer to the wound edge, to minimize tension on each stitch.

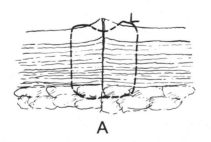

A

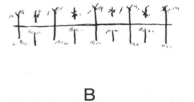

B

Figure 45.4. Repair using vertical mattress sutures. A, Placement of vertical mattress suture. B, Wound closure with simple sutures alternating with vertical mattress sutures.

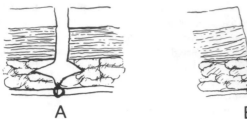 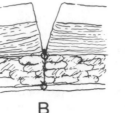 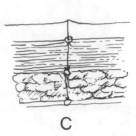

Figure 45.5. Layered closure. *A,* The fat-dermal junction is undermined after closure of the fat-fascial junction. *B,* The fat-dermal junction is sutured. *C,* The dermal-epithelial junction is closed with an inverted suture to bury the knot.

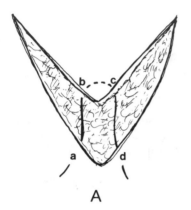 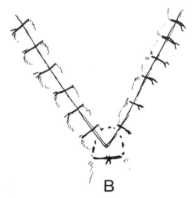

Figure 45.6. Repair of a flap laceration. *A,* The needle is inserted on one side of the wound apex (*a*), passed through the subcuticular tissue of the flap (*b-c*), then brought out on the opposite side of the wound apex (*d*). *B,* Simple sutures are then placed far enough away from the apex to prevent compromise of circulation to the tip.

suturing techniques and materials vary from site to site, as shown in Table 45.2. Lacerations of the scalp are often caused by blows that split the skin to, and sometimes through, the galea. If the galea is lacerated, it should be closed as a layer, after palpating to detect signs of skull fracture. The remaining closure is best performed as a single layer, using a large needle and 3-O or 4-O suture material. This generally provides adequate hemostasis if occasional large bleeders are clipped with a hemostat and coagulated or tied off (exercising care not to injure nerves or other vital structures). After the repair, rinse as much blood as possible out of the patient's hair, because it can be difficult to remove later.

Facial lacerations need particular care to minimize scarring. Revise the wound edges so they are smooth and follow natural skin lines, if this can be done by removing only a small amount of tissue. Use the layered skin closure shown in Figure 45.5, which will minimize tension on the surface. For surface suturing, use thin (6-0 or 7-0) monofilament sutures and remove them early, replacing them with adhesive strips (Steri-strips).

Landmarks such as the vermilion border of the lips should be marked before they are obscured by injection of anesthetic. The first suture can then be placed to assure correct alignment. Lacerations of the tongue do not need to be repaired unless they are very large or bleed persistently despite application of ice and pressure. Similarly, lacerations of the oral mucosa usually heal well without suturing. Lacerations that penetrate from the skin into the oral cavity should have repair of the skin and muscle only. Leaving the mucosal surface open to heal secondarily reduces the chance of infection.

AFTERCARE

An antibiotic ointment promotes wound healing by keeping the epithelium moist and can be ap-

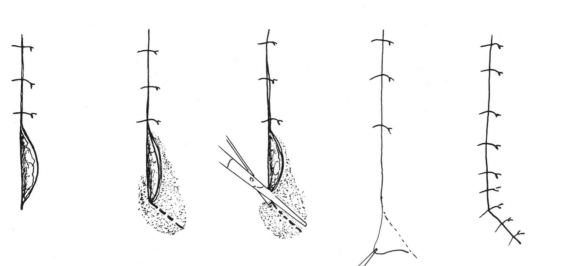

A   B   C   D   E

Figure 45.7. Repair of the "dog ear." *A,* Sometimes, as a wound is being sutured, one side ends up with more remaining tissue than the other, creating an unsightly bulge called a "dog ear." *B,* To begin repair of a "dog ear," a marking incision is made, 45° from the end of the wound toward the longer side. *C,* Scissors are used to cut along the marking, and then used to undermine the shaded area. *D,* The longer skin edge is pulled across the incision line, and the resulting triangle of skin is excised along the line of overlap. *E,* The even skin edges can now be easily sutured.

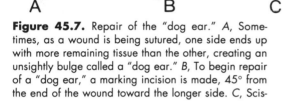

Table 45.2. Guidelines for Suture Selection and Timing of Suture Removal

Location	Recommended Suture Size for Skin Closure	Days to Removal
Face	6–0 or 7–0	3– 5
Scalp	3–0 or 4–0	5– 7
Trunk and extremities	4–0 or 5–0	7–10
Over joint surfaces	3–0 or 4–0	10–14

plied over wound closure tapes. A semiocclusive transparent dressing may be applied if little drainage is expected. For draining wounds, a nonadherent material should usually be applied beneath absorptive and adhesive layers.

Any sutured wound should be kept dry for 24 hours, after which showering is permitted. Lacerations in areas of skin stretch should be supported by splinting the affected part until adequately healed.

Infection is the biggest threat to wound healing. As noted earlier, this is best prevented by aggressive wound cleaning and tetanus prophylaxis. Antibiotic coverage is advisable when a bone, tendon, or joint space has been penetrated and in some contaminated wounds. Whether antibiotics are used or not, the patient should be advised of signs of infection. Wounds likely to become in-fected should be followed closely by the physician. Since infection typically takes 1 to 3 days to become apparent, higher-risk lacerations should be rechecked at 48 hours. Advise your patient of signs of infection: progressive swelling, redness, heat or pain, and increased drainage. Written instructions regarding wound care can be quite helpful, since patients are often distressed and will remember little of the verbal advice they received.

Timing of suture removal varies with the location and type of wound. Table 45.2 lists suture removal times. The goal is to leave sutures in long enough to prevent wound dehiscence, but not so long as to cause suture marks. If infection occurs, some sutures may need to be removed early to allow drainage. To remove a suture, elevate the knot with forceps, cut one side of the loop near the skin, and then put gentle traction on the knot. Do not cut the knot off both sides of a loop, since the free ends may retract into the skin and be difficult to retrieve. To reinforce the wound during the next few days, apply sterile adhesive strips, preparing the wound edges with tincture of benzoin to promote adhesion. These strips come off when soaked; so advise the patient to keep them dry for a few days and then wash them off. Warn the patient that the natural healing process may cause the wound to look red and swollen over the first few months, but that it will have improved by 6 months.

REFERENCES

1. Marsland DW, Wood M, Mayo F: Content of family practice: rank order of diagnoses by frequency. *J Fam Pract* 3:37–47, 1976.

SUGGESTED READINGS

Dushoff IM: A stitch in time. *Emerg Med* 5:21–43, 1973.

A classic review of the important principles of plastic wound closure.

Dushoff IM: About face. *Emerg Med* 6:24–77, 1974.

The principles of wound repair as applied to facial injuries are reviewed in detail.

Ervin ME: Minor surgical procedures. In Schwartz GR, Safar P, Stone JH, Storey PB, Wagner DK (eds): *Principles and Practice of Emergency Medicine*, ed 2. Philadelphia, WB Saunders, 1986, pp 465–475.

A textbook chapter on laceration repair, which includes an excellent description of nerve blocks and other procedures for achieving local and regional anesthesia.

Graber RF: Procedures for your practice: repair of simple lacerations. *Patient Care* 20:149–152, 1986.

This informative and well-illustrated article presents a step-by-step approach to wound repair and reviews several types of suturing techniques.

Graber RF: Procedures for your practice: administering local anesthesia. *Patient Care* 20:137–161, 1986.

This very well illustrated article reviews techniques for injecting anesthetics to obtain local and regional nerve blocks in many areas of the body.

Moy RL, Lee A, Zalka A: Commonly used suturing techniques in skin surgery. *Am Fam Physician* 44:1625–1634, 1991.

A number of techniques for suture closure of lacerations are clearly depicted.

INDEX

Page numbers in *italics* denote figures; those followed by "t" denote tables.